Pediatric Board Recertification

KATIE S. FINE, MD
Private Pediatrician
Charlotte, NC
Co-author of *Blueprints Pediatrics*

Wolters Kluwer | Lippincott Williams & Wilkins
Health
Philadelphia • Baltimore • New York • London
Buenos Aires • Hong Kong • Sydney • Tokyo

Dedicated to Lucy Carpenter Butler, PhD, who gave me life and showed me how to live it.

Acquisitions Editor: Sonya Seigafuse
Managing Editor: Ryan Shaw
Project Manager: Jennifer Harper
Senior Manufacturing Manager: Benjamin Rivera
Marketing Manager: Kimberly Schonberger
Design Coordinator: Steve Druding
Production Services: General Graphic Services

530 Walnut Street
Philadelphia, PA 19106 USA
LWW.com

Printed in the USA

Library of Congress Cataloging-in-Publication Data
Fine, Katie S. (Katie Snead)
Pediatric board recertification / Katie S. Fine.
p. ; cm.
Includes index.
ISBN-13: 978-1-4051-0507-1 (alk. paper)
ISBN-10: 1-4051-0507-0 (alk. paper)
1. Pediatrics–Examinations, questions, etc. 2. Pediatricians—Certification—United States—Examinations, questions, etc. I. Title.
[DNLM: 1. Pediatrics—Examination Questions. 2. Specialty Boards—Examination Questions. WS 18.2 F495p 2008]
RJ48.2.F53 2008
618.9200076—dc22

2007049606

Care has been taken to confirm the accuracy of the information presented and to describe generally accepted practices. However, the authors, editors, and publisher are not responsible for errors or omissions or for any consequences from application of the information in this book and make no warranty, expressed or implied, with respect to the currency, completeness, or accuracy of the contents of the publication. Application of the information in a particular situation remains the professional responsibility of the practitioner.

The authors, editors, and publisher have exerted every effort to ensure that drug selection and dosage set forth in this text are in accordance with current recommendations and practice at the time of publication. However, in view of ongoing research, changes in government regulations, and the constant flow of information relating to drug therapy and drug reactions, the reader is urged to check the package insert for each drug for any change in indications and dosage and for added warnings and precautions. This is particularly important when the recommended agent is a new or infrequently employed drug.

Some drugs and medical devices presented in the publication have Food and Drug Administration (FDA) clearance for limited use in restricted research settings. It is the responsibility of the health care provider to ascertain the FDA status of each drug or device planned for use in their clinical practice.

To purchase additional copies of this book, call our customer service department at (800) 638-3030 or fax orders to (301) 223-2320. International customers should call (301) 223-2300.

Visit Lippincott Williams & Wilkins on the Internet: at LWW.com. Lippincott Williams & Wilkins customer service representatives are available from 8:30 am to 6 pm, EST.

10 9 8 7 6 5 4 3 2 1

Contents

Preface

You need this book.

You're busy. You have patients to see. A business to run. A family to care for. And a life! You don't have time to peruse five years of *Pediatrics in Review*, take a weekend to attend an expensive board seminar, or read through a heavy tome geared to first-time testers. The recertification date is coming up, and the examination isn't cheap. You need one source that gives you everything you need and nothing you don't. You need complete, clear, and concise. This book is for you.

Or maybe you are in academic medicine, research, or a specialty field. You know everything there is to know about sarcoidosis, lung transplantation, or violent injury prevention, but your only recent exposure to general pediatrics is the local weekly Grand Rounds conference, which you attend mainly for the free coffee and blueberry muffins. You'd like to keep your general pediatrics certification current, but it feels like such a hassle to stay abreast of topics you don't really touch on in your day-to-day practice. This book is for you.

Or maybe you are looking for a reliable source for up-to-date information on general pediatrics that also provides required CME credit. Or you are a family practitioner, physician's assistant, or nurse practitioner who evaluates and treats infants and children. Or a pediatrician re-entering active practice after a break to raise children or sail around the world a few times. Or a rural physician with few opportunities for CME beyond internet-based assessment tools. This book is for you.

Pediatric Board Recertification is designed for medical professionals who have a basic foundation of pediatric knowledge, but want to review for the American Board of Pediatrics recertification examination or simply remain current in the field while earning Continuing Medical Education credit. Each chapter in the book encompasses a single subject. Every subject listed in the ABP examination content outline is covered in these pages. The number of pages and questions dedicated to each topic parallels that topic's percentage on the actual test. Tables and figures are complementary to the text, clarifying information rather than bundling ideas together to save space.

It is my sincere hope that, whatever your reason for purchase, you find **Pediatric Board Recertification** to indeed be exactly what you need.

Katie S. Fine, MD

Continuing Medical Education (CME) Overview

Release Date: March 1, 2008

Accreditation: Lippincott CME Institute, Inc. is accredited by the Accreditation Council for Continuing Medical Education to provide continuing medical education for physicians.

Commercial Support: No commercial support has been received for this activity.

Credit Designation: Lippincott CME Institute, Inc. designates this educational activity for a maximum of 30 *AMA PRA Category 1 Credits™*. Physicians should only claim credit commensurate with the extent of their participation in the activity.

Target Audience: This CME activity is intended for pediatricians (both domestic and foreign medical graduates) with an interest in studying for the American Board of Pediatrics recertification examination. It is also appropriate for resident physicians who are studying for their initial certification, as well as for additional practitioners (family practice physicians, nurse practitioners, and physician assistants) interested in the diagnosis, management, and prevention of pediatric disease.

Statement of Need: Each year, approximately 3,000 physicians take the American Board of Pediatrics (ABP) Recertification Examination; another 3,000 take the initial Certification Examination. Recertification is required every 7 years. Board certification is required for participation in most insurance plans and admitting privileges at the majority of US hospitals. In addition, pediatricians must be board-certified in order to obtain the rank of American Academy of Pediatrics Fellow (FAAP).

Although the test is not exceedingly difficult, there is a core body of knowledge that must be mastered and maintained in order to pass the exam. According to the American Board of pediatrics web site (www.abp.org), "pass rates...range from 88% to 100%." Failure to pass the examination can result in loss of certification by the board, which negatively affects the individual's employment opportunities.

The overall goal of this CME activity is to improve the clinical knowledge of participants, which will allow them to be well prepared for the board certification examination or recertification examinations and achieve board recertification as well as help them improve their care of patients. This activity provides the participant with a feel for the formal examination through the use of questions written in the format of those presented on the actual board examination. The topics that are covered by the activity content are those detailed by the American Board of Pediatrics; minimum competency requirements are provided in each general and specialty area. Thus, this content also provides concise, targeted, yet thorough review of all diagnostic, management, primary care, and prevention information deemed essential for the practice of pediatrics by the American Board of Pediatrics.

Participants will be required to complete a CME quiz that helps assess their learning of the activity's content. Participants will also be asked to complete an evaluation assessment questionnaire that gauges: 1) participants' ability to meet of the learning objectives; 2) participants' rating of the activity's overall quality; 3) participants' rating of the activity for its effectiveness in preparing them for the certification or recertification exam; 4) participants' intention to change his/her practice behavior in a manner that would improve patient care and health; 5) participants' perception of commercial bias; and 6) length of time spent in the activity.

In addition, the continuing medical education (CME) credit earned from completion of this review will allow the participant to report 30 hours of dedicated medical review time while preparing for the examination. Individual states generally require an average of 25 hours of CME credit per year to maintain licensure to practice.

Additional Sources: American Academy of Pediatrics, Committee on Pediatric Workforce. Pediatrician workforce statement. *Pediatrics*. 2005;116:263–269.

American Board of Pediatrics PMCP Content Outline 2007 (www.abp.org/ABPWebSite/pmcp/outlines/pmcpoutline.pdf)

American Board of Pediatrics website (www.abp.org)

Freed GL, Uren RL, Hudson EJ, et al. Policies and practices related to the role of board certification and recertification of pediatricians in hospital privileging. *JAMA*. 2006;295:905–912.

PREP® The Curriculum. 2007 Content Specifications and PREP® Study Guide

Faculty Credentials and Disclosure Information: Katie Fine, MD, is in private pediatric practice in Charlotte, N.C.

Dr. Fine has disclosed that she has no financial interests in or relationships with any commercial companies pertaining to this educational activity.

Estimated Time to Complete the Educational Activity: It is estimated that this CME activity should take the average target audience member approximately 30 hours to read the activity's material and answer the CME quiz questions.

Identification and Resolution of Conflict of Interests: Lippincott CME Institute, Inc. has identified and resolved any faculty conflicts of interest regarding this educational activity.

General Learning Objectives: After participating in this CME activity, the physician will be able to:

1. Identify normal and abnormal growth patterns in children and adolescents, and describe the diagnosis and management of conditions associated with disordered growth.
2. Differentiate normal from abnormal development in children and adolescents, and discuss the diagnosis and management of developmental delay and developmental deviancy.
3. Discuss with parents the specialized nutritional requirements of infants, children, and adolescents.
4. Describe the diagnosis and management of caloric and vitamin deficiency and excess.
5. Explain how chronic disease impacts the growth, nutrition, and development of the pediatric patient.
6. Recall the current ACIP recommendations regarding immunization schedules for primary vaccinations, boosters, inoculation against influenza and pneumococcal disease, and catch-up immunizations, including new recommendations regarding vaccinations against human papillomavirus and rotavirus.
7. Outline the age-appropriate anticipatory guidance, preventive care, and appropriate screening at each routine health maintenance visit.
8. Identify the signs and symptoms of accidental and intentional ingestions and environmental exposures.

9. Outline the routine care of the newborn, as well as the disease processes and emergencies in this age group.
10. Recall how prenatal exposures and congenital infections present, and outline their management accordingly, including limitation of long-term sequelae.
11. State the fluid, electrolyte, and acid-base requirements of the healthy pediatric patient; identify systemic disorders which result in imbalance and their management.
12. Define the clinical manifestations of genetic and metabolic disease, including presentations and dysmorphisms, as well as modes of inheritance and methods of pre- and postnatal diagnosis.
13. Recall the pathophysiology of pediatric allergic and immunologic disorders, their typical presentations, and management.
14. Describe the organisms associated with pediatric infectious disease, including bacteria, viruses, fungi, parasites, and atypical organisms; identify their various disease presentations; discuss their appropriate management; and predict complications and long-term sequelae.
15. Point out the presentation of pediatric disorders of the endocrine system and describe appropriate diagnostic studies and management.
16. Identify the presentation of pediatric disorders of the upper and lower respiratory system and describe their diagnostic evaluation and appropriate management.
17. Describe the presentation of pediatric disorders of the gastrointestinal system; summarize the diagnostic evaluation and appropriate management of gastrointestinal symptoms (emesis, abdominal pain, etc).
18. Discuss the presentation of pediatric disorders of the cardiovascular system, including but not limited to congenital heart disease; plan the appropriate diagnostic evaluation.
19. Cite the pathophysiology of pediatric disorders of the blood, including hemoglobinopathies, coagulopathies, membrane defects, anemias, leukocytic disorders, platelet disorders, and neoplasms; describe their diagnostic evaluation and appropriate management.
20. Recall the presentation of pediatric disorders of the kidneys and upper and lower genitourinary system; discuss the diagnostic evaluation and appropriate management of typical symptoms.
21. Define the significance of neurologic signs and symptoms in the pediatric patient and evaluate accordingly; recall the presentation and management of infection, congenital malformations, seizures, strokes, spinal cord disease, peripheral neuropathies, muscular dystrophies, and central nervous system trauma.
22. Recognize the presentation of pediatric musculoskeletal and collagen-vascular disorders; describe the diagnostic evaluation; manage appropriately; and predict complications and long-term sequelae.
23. Describe common pediatric skin lesions, associated findings, and treatment.
24. Discuss the developmentally-appropriate screening, diagnosis and management of congenital and pediatric eye disorders; point out indications for referral.
25. Summarize the presentation of pediatric disorders of the ear, nose, and throat, as well as recommended diagnostic evaluations, therapies, and complications.
26. Describe normal and abnormal physical, psychosocial, and cognitive development in the adolescent.
27. Identify the presentations and managements of gynecologic disorders, substance use and abuse, and psychiatric conditions in adolescent patients.
28. Discuss disorders of cognition, language, learning, attention, and behavior in children and adolescents.
29. Identify the psychological issues and problems that present during specific developmental stages in the child and adolescent, and describe their appropriate management.
30. Plan for emergency and critical care interventions in the pediatric patient, including abuse, burns, wounds, trauma, life support, and cardiopulmonary resuscitation.
31. State the principles of pharmacology relating to pediatric medication, including risks, benefits, adverse effects, conscious sedation, and pain management.

Method of Physician Participation: To earn CME credit, participants must first read the text and complete the CME examination and evaluation assessment questionnaire. Participants can mail a photocopy of the Exam Answer Sheet and Evaluation Assessment Form, along with a check or money order for the $20 processing fee, to Lippincott CME Institute, Inc., 770 Township Line Road, Suite 300, Yardley, PA 19067. Entries must be received by LCMEI by the expiration date of February 28, 2011. Acknowledgment will be sent to participants within 6 to 8 weeks of participation. For more information, call (267) 757-3531.

Normal Growth and Development

GROWTH ASSESSMENT

Growth Parameters

In pediatric medicine, growth is an important indicator of a patient's nutritional status and general health. Routine assessment of growth parameters includes:

- weight in all patients
- length in infants at birth to age 3 years
- head circumference in infants at birth to age 3 years
- height in children ≥2 years
- body mass index (BMI) in children ≥2 years

BMI is calculated by:

- dividing the patient's weight in kilograms by the patient's height in meters squared: (kg/m^2), OR
- dividing the patient's weight in pounds by the patient's height in inches squared, then multiplying the result by 703: (lb/in^2) × 703

Children at risk for abnormal growth patterns include those <5th percentile or >95th percentile, respectively, for weight and/or height. Patients who have BMIs between the 85th and 95th percentiles are considered *at risk of overweight*, and those ≥95th percentile are considered *overweight*. These cutoffs may be modified as BMI gains in standard usage. The real value of growth assessment becomes evident over time; the different parameters form "growth curves" that can reveal sudden and/or unexpected changes in growth velocity, although the patient's actual measurements may still be in the normal range. Children who "fall off" their expected growth curves, especially when measurements cross two percentile lines, warrant further investigation into the cause of their decelerated growth.

Several important rules of thumb regarding growth in children are listed below.

- The average newborn weight in the United States is 3.5 kg (7 lb, 11 oz).
- Newborns lose weight in the first several days after birth; weight loss that exceeds 10% of birthweight is considered abnormal and requires immediate intervention.
- Newborns should regain their birthweight by days of life 10 to 14.
- Breast-fed infants on average lose a greater percentage of their birthweight than formula-fed infants and thus, generally take longer to regain their birthweight.
- Healthy infants double their birthweight at age 4 to 5 months and triple their birthweight by age 12 to 14 months.
- The average newborn length in the United States is 50 cm (almost 20 in).
- Between the ages of 3 and 4 years, a healthy child's stature should reach double that child's birth length.
- The average newborn head circumference in the United States is 36 cm (about 14 in).
- Head circumference is expected to increase by almost 30% during the first year of life (average 47 cm, about 18.5 in).

Abnormalities in Head Circumference

At birth, normal head circumference ranges from about 32.5 to 38 cm (12.8 to 15 in). Head circumference provides an indirect assessment of brain growth.

Microcephaly is defined as a head circumference greater than two standard deviations below the mean. Most cases are due to small brain size. Microcephaly is associated with an increased incidence of mental retardation. Microcephaly may be primary (genetic) or secondary (acquired).

- *Primary microcephaly* is present at birth and is typically familial or associated with specific genetic abnormalities such as Down syndrome.
- *Secondary microcephaly* results from an insult to the brain in utero or during the first 2 years of life. Examples include congenital infections, in utero drug or alcohol exposure, maternal hypertension during pregnancy, meningitis, failure to thrive, and hypoxic encephalopathy. When the cause is a prenatal event, the earlier in development the event occurs, the smaller the head will be. The infant with a normal head circumference at birth and subsequent development of microcephaly has acquired microcephaly by definition. Examination of the head circumference growth chart and a careful history and physical examination usually suggest the diagnosis.

Macrocephaly is defined as a head circumference greater than two standard deviations above the mean (alternatively, >97th percentile). *Familial (inherited) macrocephaly* is typically associated with normal intelligence. These infants are born with large heads, and their head circumference growth curves tract along a consistent percentile. There is no associated cerebral pathology. The development of macrocephaly after birth may result from neurocutaneous disorders, metabolic storage disease, bleeding, or hydrocephalus. *Hydrocephalus* is an abnormal accumulation of cerebrospinal fluid within the ventricles through impaired absorption or increased production. In the infant,

TABLE 1-1
NORMAL DEVELOPMENTAL MILESTONES

Age	Gross Motor	Fine (Visual) Motor	Language	Social/Adaptive
Birth to 1 mo	Raises head slightly in prone position	Follows with eyes to midline only; hands tightly fisted	Alerts/startles to sound	Fixes on face (at birth)
2 mo	Raises chest and head off bed in prone position	Regards object and follows through 180° arc; briefly retains rattle	Coos and vocalizes reciprocally	Social smile; recognizes parent
4 mo	Lifts onto extended elbows in prone position; steady head control with no head lag; rolls over front to back	Reaches for objects with both hands together; bats at objects; grabs and retains objects	Orients to voice; laughs and squeals	Initiates social interaction
6 mo	Sits but may need support; rolls in both directions	Reaches with one hand; transfers objects hand-to-hand	Babbles	Recognizes object or person as unfamiliar
9 mo	Sits without support; crawls; pulls to stand	Uses pincer grasp; finger-feeds	Imitates speech sounds (nonspecific "mama," "dada"); understands "no"	Plays gesture games ("pat-a-cake"); understands own name; object permanence; stranger anxiety
12 mo	Cruises; stands alone; takes a few independent steps	Can voluntarily release items	Discriminative use of "mama," "dada," plus one to four other words; follows command with gesture	Imitates; comes when called; cooperates with dressing
15 mo	Walks well independently	Builds a two-block tower; throws ball underhand	Four to six words in addition to above; uses jargon; responds to one-step verbal command	Begins to use cup; indicates wants or needs
18 mo	Runs; walks up stairs with hand held; stoops and recovers	Builds a three-block tower; uses spoon; spontaneous scribbling	Uses ten to 25 words; points to body parts when asked; uses words to communicate needs or wants	Uses words to communicate wants or needs; plays near (but not with) other children
24 mo	Walks unassisted up and down stairs; kicks ball; throws ball overhand; jumps with two feet off the floor	Builds four- to six-block tower; uses fork and spoon; copies a straight line	Uses 50+ words, two- and three-word phrases; uses "I" and "me;" 50% of speech intelligible to stranger	Removes simple clothing; parallel play
36 mo	Pedals tricycle; broad jumps	Copies a circle	Uses five- to eight-word sentences; 75% of speech intelligible to stranger	Knows age and gender; engages in group play; shares
4 y	Balances on one foot	Copies a cross; catches ball	Tells a story; 100% of speech intelligible to stranger	Dresses self; puts on shoes; washes and dries hands; imaginative play
5 y	Skips with alternating feet	Draws a person with six body parts	Asks what words mean	Names four colors; plays cooperative games; understands "rules" and abides by them
6 y	Rides a bicycle	Writes name	Identifies written letters and numbers	Knows right from left; knows all color names

hydrocephalus may present with rapidly increasing head circumference measurements that form a curve that crosses percentile lines. Other signs include a large, bulging anterior fontanelle and dilated scalp veins. Cranial ultrasonography confirms the diagnosis. Macrocephaly with hydrocephalus is more likely to be associated with subsequent cognitive impairment. Chapter 18 contains a more detailed discussion of hydrocephalus.

NORMAL DEVELOPMENT AND DEVELOPMENTAL DELAY

Although the timetable varies somewhat from child to child, the *sequence* of pediatric neurodevelopment is orderly and predictable. Development generally proceeds:

- in the cephalic-to-caudal direction (head to toe)
- in the proximal-to-distal direction (center to extremities)
- from involuntary reflexes to voluntary, purposeful action
- from dependence on caregivers to relative independence

For organizational purposes, developmental milestones are typically categorized into gross motor, fine (or visual) motor, language, and social/adaptive domains (Table 1-1). Children should be screened for achievement of skills in each of these areas at every health maintenance visit by parental report or through direct assessment. The earlier a delay in development is diagnosed, the sooner intervention and support can be provided to the child and family. Findings suggestive of developmental delay are noted in Table 1-2. Of note, conditions such as prematurity, vision impairment, and hearing loss affect the timing of development in one or more domains; these specific topics are addressed in subsequent chapters. Developmental assessment and disorders of cognition, speech and language, and learning are covered in Chapter 27.

Abnormal development may consist of global delay, isolated delay, or atypical development.

- *Global developmental delay* is diagnosed when a child is functioning at a level at least two standard deviations below the child's expected achievement for age in two or more of the developmental categories listed above. Global delay is associated with mental retardation.
- *Isolated developmental delay* exists when a child is functioning at or below the level described above in only one domain of development. Delay in a single area may adversely affect other developmental streams or may interfere with testing to assess the child's global development.
- *Atypical development* refers to any of the following: (a) divergence from the normal sequence of development such as skipping skills or developing certain skills very early (splinter skills), (b) discrepancies among the areas of development, (c) loss of skills previously achieved, and (d) the presence of atypical behaviors (e.g., echolalia).

TABLE 1-2
FEATURES SUGGESTIVE OF ABNORMAL DEVELOPMENT OR DELAY

General
Skipping skills
Atypical behaviors (e.g., perseveration)
Motor
Abnormally sustained primitive reflex posturing at birth or thereafter
Rolling over at 1 to 2 mo (increased tone)
Tight or persistent fisting at age 3 mo (increased tone)
No visual tracking by 4 mo of age (visual impairment)
Poor head control at 6 mo (hypotonia)
Inability to sit by 9 mo of age (hypotonia or weakness)
Persistence of primitive reflexes beyond 9 mo (neurologic dysfunction)
Hand dominance before 18 mo (contralateral weakness)
Language
No alert to sound at birth or thereafter (hearing impairment)
No babbling with consonants by 9 mo (hearing impairment)
Repetitive, noncommunicative speech (autism)
No use of single words by 24 mo of age (motor dysfunction, speech disorder)
Failure to speak in three-word sentences by 36 mo of age
Unintelligible speech in a child older than 36 mo of age (articulation disorder)
Social/Adaptive
No fixation of visual attention by 2 mo of age
No social smile by 4 mo (visual impairment or attachment issues)
No stranger anxiety 9 to 12 mo (attachment issues)
Inadequate initiation of social interaction (autism)

Language development is the best indicator of future intellectual potential. Delays in language development are more common than delays in other areas. Gross motor development is the least correlative with cognitive potential.

SOURCES

Beker L. Principles of growth assessment. *Pediatr Rev.* 2006;27:196–198.

Dawson P. Normal growth and revised growth charts. *Pediatr Rev.* 2002;23:255–256.

Dixon SD, Stein MT. *Encounters with children: pediatric behavior and development.* St. Louis: Mosby; 2000.

Imseih G, Myers GJ. Question from the clinician: head circumference. *Pediatr Rev.* 2004;25:295.

Johnson CP, Blasco PA. Infant growth and development. *Pediatr Rev.* 1997;18:224–242.

Needlman RD. Growth and development. In: Behrman RE, Kliegman RM, Jenson HB, eds. *Nelson textbook of pediatrics.* 17th ed. Philadelphia: Saunders; 2004:23–66.

Ogden CL, Kuczmarski RJ, Flegal KM, et al. Centers for Disease Control and Prevention growth charts for the United States: improvements to the 1977 National Center for Health Statistics version. *Pediatrics.* 2002;109:45–60.

QUESTIONS

1. Primitive reflexes in the infant should not persist beyond the age of:
A) 1 month
B) 2 months
C) 4 months
D) 6 months
E) 9 months

2. Development in which of the following domains has the best predictive value of future intellectual potential?
A) Gross motor
B) Visuomotor
C) Language
D) Adaptive
E) Social

3. Which of the following statements regarding growth parameters in children is FALSE?
A) All patients should be weighed at each health maintenance visit.
B) Supine length may be used to measure children up to 3 years of age.
C) Stature (height) may be used in children ≥2 years old.
D) Head circumference should be measured at each health maintenance visit from birth until the age of 2 years.
E) BMI should be calculated and recorded for children ≥2 years of age.

4. Patients with BMIs above what percentile for age and gender should be considered "overweight"?
A) 50%
B) 66%
C) 75%
D) 85%
E) 95%

5. You are seeing a 1-month-old female infant for a health maintenance visit. The mother reports that the child watches her face while bottle-feeding and at other times and seems to respond to her voice. The baby raises her head slightly while in the prone position on the examining table. Of the following, she most likely also can:
A) follow objects to the midline
B) track objects horizontally but not vertically
C) briefly retain a rattle placed in her hand
D) smile socially
E) recognize her parent

6. You are seeing a 2-month-old boy for a health maintenance visit. His parent reports that the child is beginning to coo and participate in reciprocal vocalizations. The boy knows his parents and smiles socially. Of the following, he most likely also can:
A) raise his shoulders, chest, and head off the examining table in the prone position
B) reach for objects
C) bat at objects
D) localize sound
E) recognize the examiner as an unfamiliar person

7. You are seeing a 4-month-old boy for a health maintenance visit. The child is squealing and laughing when you enter the room. He looks around for you when he hears you speak. The mother tells you that her baby initiates social interaction with her and his brother. Of the following, he most likely also can:
A) roll over back to front
B) understand that his name refers to him
C) reach for objects with both hands together
D) babble
E) sit with support

8. You are seeing a 6-month-old girl for a health maintenance visit. Her parent reports that the child babbles and sits with support. She can also roll over in both directions. You notice that she can transfer her teething ring from one hand to the other. Of the following, she most likely also can:
A) understand "no"
B) understand her own name
C) imitate speech sounds
D) recognize the examiner as an unfamiliar person
E) sit without supporting herself with her hands

9. You are seeing a 9-month-old boy for a health maintenance visit. When you enter the room, the patient is crawling about the floor. While you are talking with his mother, you notice him pull to standing using a stool. His mother reports that he finger-feeds himself and has started saying "dada," although not in reference to his father. Of the following, he most likely also can:
A) voluntarily release items
B) understand object permanence
C) stand alone for a few seconds
D) follow commands with a gesture
E) come when called

10. You are seeing a 12-month-old girl for a health maintenance visit. Her mother reports that, in some ways, things are getting easier. The child is able to come when called and cooperate with dressing. She can pick up something if the mother asks her to while pointing to it. Of the following, she most likely also can:
A) take a few independent steps
B) scribble with a pen
C) use a cup
D) use a spoon
E) use jargon

11. You are seeing a 15-month-old boy for a health maintenance visit. The child can walk about the room independently. His mother reports that he can say eight words including "mama" and "dada." You would also expect this child to be able to:
A) walk up stairs with his hand held
B) point to three body parts when asked
C) build a tower of three blocks
D) throw a ball underhanded
E) play well with other children

12. You are seeing an 18-month-old girl for a health maintenance visit. You note that she can stoop and recover her cup by herself. Her mother reports that she runs well and can use a spoon. She uses words and gestures to communicate her needs. You would expect her to be able to use at least how many words?
A) 10 to 25
B) 25 to 50
C) 50 to 75
D) 75 to 100
E) >100

13. You are seeing a 24-month-old boy for a health maintenance visit. The parent reports that the child can kick and throw a ball, use a fork and spoon, remove simple clothing, and use two- and three-word phrases. Of the following, he most likely also can:
A) jump with two feet off the floor
B) use ≥100 words
C) use the words "I" and "me"
D) copy a circle
E) broad jump

14. You are seeing a 3-year-old girl for a health maintenance visit. She can tell you her name and gender and speaks in sentences five to eight words in length. Based on this information, you would expect to be able to understand at least:
A) 50% of her speech
B) 75% of her speech
C) 90% of her speech
D) 100% of her speech
E) none of the above

15. You are seeing a 4-year-old boy for a health maintenance visit. The child can balance on each foot for 3 seconds. He is excited to tell you about how he scored a goal in his soccer game. His mom reports that he can dress himself in simple clothing and put on his shoes, although he cannot yet tie them. He should be able to copy which of the following figures that you draw?
A) A straight line
B) A circle
C) A straight line and a circle
D) A circle and a cross
E) A straight line, a circle, and a cross

16. You are seeing a 5-year-old girl for a health maintenance visit. Her mother is concerned about the way she plays with other children. You remember that at this age, most developmentally normal children primarily engage in:
A) nonconnected play
B) side-by-side (but not interactive) play
C) solitary play
D) cooperative play
E) nonimaginative play

17. At what age would you expect a developmentally normal child to be able to write his or her name, identify written letters, know right from left, and ride a bicycle without training wheels?
A) 4 years
B) 5 years
C) 6 years
D) 7 years
E) 8 years

18. Which of the following scenarios is suggestive of an underlying condition that may be interfering with development?
A) A 15-month-old who primarily reaches for things with his left hand
B) A 4-month-old who rolls over both ways
C) A 5-year-old who skips with alternating feet
D) A 24-month-old who scribbles with his right hand only
E) A 12-month-old who walks well independently

19. The average weight of a full-term newborn born in the United States is closest to:
A) 2,500 g
B) 2,800 g
C) 3,000 g
D) 3,500 g
E) 4,000 g

20. Which of the following patients does not merit particular concern regarding growth?
A) A 14-month-old girl who weighs triple her birthweight
B) A 5-year-old girl whose height is double her birth length
C) A 6-month-old girl with a head circumference measurement that is consistently tracking the third percentile line
D) An infant whose head circumference went from 36 cm at birth to 42 cm at age 12 months
E) A breast-fed infant who loses 12% of her birth weight in the first 72 hours of life

21. A father brings his 18-month-old son to your office because he is concerned that the child "cannot do things that other children can do." In screening the child, you note that he can walk up stairs, although he needs to hold his father's hand to do so. He can build a

three-block tower. He can point to his eyes, nose, and mouth when asked to do so by his father. His father reports that his son likes to watch and play around other children but does not play with them. The child uses "mama" and "dada" appropriately and has three other words. You decide to refer the child for developmental testing. Given the information above, you expect his results to be most consistent with which of the following?
A) Global developmental delay
B) Isolated developmental delay
C) Atypical delay
D) Mental retardation
E) No delay

22. A full-term newborn has a weight of 3,400 g, a length of 19.5 cm, and a head circumference of 30 cm. Which of the following statements regarding the child's apparent microcephaly is TRUE?
A) The infant cannot have secondary microcephaly because he was born with a small head.
B) The infant has microcephaly because he is small for gestational age.
C) Cranial ultrasonography is the initial study of choice for determining the cause of this child's microcephaly.
D) The cause of the child's microcephaly is likely to have occurred only shortly before birth.
E) This infant has isolated microcephaly.

23. A 2-month-old infant who comes to your office for a health maintenance visit has a head circumference at the 98th percentile for age. He is at the 75th percentile for weight and height. At birth, his head circumference was slightly above the 95th percentile. His father and mother have large heads. The child has achieved appropriate developmental milestones for his age, and his physical examination is normal. When the parents ask you about his large head size, you tell them that:
A) the child needs a cranial ultrasound to rule out hydrocephalus
B) the child is likely to have subtle cerebral anomalies
C) the child is at risk for learning disabilities later in life
D) the child most likely has familial macrocephaly and needs no further workup
E) the child is at risk for craniosynostosis

24. Which of the following statements regarding the BMI value is FALSE?
A) BMI is not a reliable measurement of abnormal growth in children younger than 2 years of age.
B) BMI is calculated by dividing the patient's weight in kilograms by the patient's height in meters squared.
C) Stature is preferred to supine length for calculation of the BMI.
D) Gender does not affect the normal range for BMI.
E) A patient whose BMI falls at the 90th percentile is at risk for being overweight.

25. Secondary microcephaly may result from all of the following EXCEPT:
A) Down syndrome
B) Teratogen exposure
C) Congenital infection
D) Hypoxic encephalopathy
E) Meningitis

26. Isolated hearing impairment can affect early development by:
A) interfering with testing for delay in motor skills
B) interfering with social development
C) interfering with adaptive development
D) interfering with the ability to use consonants clearly
E) All of the above

27. Which of the following patients should receive further evaluation to rule out an abnormality that may be affecting his or her development?
A) A 2-month-old boy with a head lag
B) A 1-month-old boy who generally keeps his hands fisted
C) A 1-month-old boy who rolls back to front
D) A 15-month-old boy who uses jargon
E) A 3-year-old boy who cannot copy a triangle

28. Which of the following is not considered an example of atypical development?
A) Echolalia
B) Perseveration
C) Loss of skills previously achieved
D) Skipping skills
E) All are examples of atypical development.

ANSWERS

1. E
2. C
3. D
4. E
5. A
6. A
7. C
8. D
9. B
10. A
11. D
12. A
13. C
14. B
15. E
16. D
17. C
18. A
19. D
20. A
21. B
22. E
23. D
24. D
25. A
26. E
27. C
28. E

Nutrition and Nutritional Disorders

2

Good nutrition is essential for the optimal growth and development of infants, children, and adolescents. Sound eating behaviors early in life decrease the subsequent risk of developing heart disease, hypertension, and diabetes in adulthood. Infants and children are dependent on caregivers to meet their nutritional needs, and offering them a wide range of healthy foods influences their taste preferences and provides a positive example of beneficial dietary practices. Families' nutritional decisions are influenced by personal preferences, advice from extended family, cultural factors, media exposure, and availability (economic and geographic).

INFANT NUTRITION AND FEEDING

Healthy full-term neonates require about 120 kcal per kg per day to achieve the recommended 20 to 30 g of weight gain per day. By age 12 months, the same infants should be ingesting about 100 kcal per kg per day to gain 10 to 12 g of weight per day. Throughout the first year of life, 40% to 50% of dietary calories should consist of fat, 40% to 50% from carbohydrates, and 10% to 15% from protein.

The American Academy of Pediatrics recommends *exclusive breast-feeding* during the first 6 months of life in all infants and continuation of breast-feeding during the second 6 months. Commercially prepared infant formula is an acceptable alternative for the infant whose mother is unable to or chooses not to breast-fed. Cow milk should not be given to children younger than 12 months of age. The low iron content of cow milk, coupled with the possibility of gastrointestinal irritation and blood loss, may cause iron-deficiency anemia. Cow milk is also not nutritionally sufficient to meet an infant's specialized requirements. The infant's immature renal filtration system cannot handle the high solute load of cow milk, which may lead to dehydration in small infants. Goat milk, which has historically been used for infants with colic, should not be used as a substitution for human breast milk or formula. Goat milk is particularly low in folate, and ingestion of primarily goat milk leads to megaloblastic anemia in the young infant.

Full-term infants are born with adequate iron stores and do not need an additional source of iron until 4 to 6 months of age.

Breast-feeding

Breast-feeding affords demonstrable benefits to the infant and the mother. Breast milk is superior to formula with regard to infant nutrition, gastrointestinal performance, immunity, neurodevelopment, and psychological attachment (maternal–infant bonding). Mothers who breast-feed have a decreased risk of premenopausal breast and ovarian cancers. Other maternal advantages include more rapid weight loss, a longer infertile period, and decreased expense. Table 2-1 compares the composition of human breast milk with that of cow milk–based infant formulas.

Human milk changes in composition over time, providing specialized nutrition based on the needs of the infant at that age. Human milk *protein* is 70% whey and 30% casein. Cow milk protein is 82% casein and 18% whey, and formulas based on cow milk may be predominately casein or whey depending on the manufacturer. Whey is easier for the infant to digest and results in more rapid gastric emptying. In human milk, the whey protein contains α-lactalbumin, secretory immunoglobulin A, and other proteins that contribute to infant immunity. Infants who are breast-fed have significantly lower rates of otitis media, respiratory disease, and gastrointestinal illnesses. Human milk contains additional enzymes that are

TABLE 2-1
COMPARING HUMAN BREAST MILK AND COW MILK–BASED INFANT FORMULA

Component	Human Milk	Cow Milk–Based Infant Formula
Protein	1.0 g/dL	1.5 g/dL
Predominant protein type	Human whey protein	Casein or cow whey protein
Predominant whey protein	α-Lactalbumin	α-Lactoglobulin
Fat	50% composition	40% to 50% composition
Fat type	Human	Vegetable (with or without animal)
Primary carbohydrate	Lactose	Lactose
Caloric density	20 kcal/oz	20 kcal/oz

beneficial to the growth and function of the gastrointestinal system; for example, breast-fed infants are less likely to develop necrotizing enterocolitis. Although human milk has a lower concentration of protein than formula, this amount is sufficient to meet the infant's protein needs.

Human milk is 50% *fat*, mostly in the form of milk fat globules composed of fatty acids surrounding a base triglyceride molecule. Human milk fat is better absorbed than fat sources in formulas. Arachidonic acid and docosahexaenoic acid are two fats found in human milk that are involved in the formation of retinal and brain phospholipid membranes. As a group, babies who are breast-fed demonstrate enhanced cognitive development that persists beyond the infant years.

Lactose is the primary *carbohydrate* in breast milk and cow milk–based formulas. Breast milk has smaller amounts of calcium and phosphorus than infant formula, but the minerals are more bioavailable and better digested. There is not enough iron in human milk to meet the infant's needs beyond 6 months of age. Human milk is low in vitamin K; however, infants in developed countries are given an intramuscular dose at birth to prevent possible *hemorrhagic disease of the newborn*. Human milk is also low in vitamin D, and, although rare, rickets may develop in dark-skinned infants or those who are not exposed to adequate sunlight. Supplementation with 200 IU per day of vitamin D beginning in the first 2 months after birth is indicated for exclusively breast-fed infants.

Breast-feeding is initiated as soon after delivery as possible, preferably in the delivery room. Neonates should be nursed on demand, about every 2 to 3 hours (and not >4 hours apart), with 8 to 12 feedings per day in the first few weeks after birth. Newborns typically produce urine and stool within the first 24 hours of life, progressing to several wet diapers a day and a seedy yellow stool with each feeding. Supplements and pacifiers should be avoided until breast-feeding is progressing well. Inverted or retracted nipples may make breast-feeding more challenging but respond to simple interventions. Nipple fissuring and painful breast engorgement are not uncommon; local measures provide relief. Mothers who develop *acute mastitis* are encouraged to continue breast-feeding. Women who have undergone reduction mammoplasty may be unable to successfully breast-feed due to disruption of the milk duct system. Significant psychological stress (e.g., preterm birth, infant illness) may interfere with milk production in the mother. Frequent skin-to-skin contact between mother and infant promotes lactation and attachment.

The intake of the mother, in terms of food, supplements, and drugs, affects the intake of her breast-fed infant. For example, medicines that cause sedation in the mother may also result in significant lethargy in her infant. Certain drugs are contraindicated or should be avoided if possible during breast-feeding (Table 2-2). Breast-feeding is contraindicated in infants with galactosemia, and women in developed countries who have a safe source of infant formula should not breast-feed if they have human immunodeficiency virus, human T-cell lymphotropic virus, herpetic lesions of the breast, or active untreated tuberculosis. Mothers who wish to breast-feed infants with certain metabolic diseases may need to radically alter their diets, and such infants must be closely monitored.

TABLE 2-2
DRUGS AND MEDICATIONS THAT ARE CONTRAINDICATED DURING BREAST-FEEDING

Contraindicated (medications)
Amantadine
Amiodarone
Bromocriptine
Chloramphenicol
Cyclosporine
Ergotamine
Metronidazole
Most chemotherapeutic agents (including cyclophosphamide, doxorubicin, methotrexate, and others)

Contraindicated (substances of abuse)
Alcohol
Amphetamine
Cocaine
Heroin
Marijuana
Nicotine
Phencyclidine

Avoid If Possible
Benzodiazepines
Clonidine
Estrogen
Ethosuximide
Fluoxetine
Lithium
Nitrofurantoin
Phenobarbital
Quinolones

Infant Formula

Infant formula is an adequate alternative to human breast milk if this option is not available to the infant. Formula, rather than cow milk, should be offered if a breast-feeding mother decides to reduce or stop feeding at any time before the age of 12 months. Formula may also be given as supplemental nutrition in a breast-fed infant who is not gaining appropriate weight. Low-iron formulas, which contain ≤6.7 mg of iron per 100 kcal, are not appropriate substitutes for iron-fortified infant formulas. Infants fed primarily low-iron formulas cannot replenish their iron stores and may develop iron-deficiency anemia.

Soy formulas have been formulated for infants who are intolerant of milk protein or lactose. Soy formulas are appropriate for vegetarian families and infants with galactosemia or hereditary lactase deficiency; however, soy milk formulas do not provide sufficient nutrition for preterm infants. *Lactose intolerance* presents with irritability, abdominal cramping, and occasionally diarrhea. Infants with *cow milk protein allergy* usually present 2 to 6 weeks after they begin to ingest cow milk protein with irritability, rash, vomiting, and diarrhea. Stools typically test positive for reducing substances and occult blood and may be frankly bloody. Severely allergic infants may develop colitis even when they are breast-fed if the mother is ingesting dairy products; maternal dietary restriction should result in symptom resolution. The diagnosis is usually evident on history and physical examinaiton; however, questionable, persistent, or severe cases may require confirmation with flexible sigmoidoscopy and biopsy. Soy formulas are not an alternative for infants with suspected cow milk protein allergy; many of these infants (particularly those with enterocolitis) are also allergic to soy protein.

The protein in *protein hydrolysate formulas* consists of free amino acids and shortened peptide chains, which presumably are not large enough to elicit an immunologic response. These formulas are the preferred choice for infants with allergy or intolerance to cow and/or soy protein. Most are also free of lactose. If symptoms do not resolve with hydrolysate formula, an elemental formula may need to be substituted. Protein hydrolysate formulas are also beneficial for infants with malabsorption or pancreatic insufficiency (e.g., cystic fibrosis) because these contain medium-chain triglycerides that are well absorbed in these patients. Protein hydrolysate formulas are costly compared with other infant formulas.

Infants with poor growth due to underlying chronic disease may require fortification of breast milk or formula to obtain sufficient calories for growth (up to 30 kcal/oz). Human breast milk fortifiers contain additional protein, carbohydrates, fats, and minerals. Infant formulas can be concentrated with additional formula powder to 25 kcal per oz. Thereafter, special formula additives containing only carbohydrate and lipid sources should be added to avoid an excessive solute load due to too much protein. Adverse effects of fortification include diarrhea (from increased caloric density) and vomiting (due to prolonged gastric emptying).

Preterm Infants

Preterm infants have specialized nutritional needs that often necessitate the use of human milk fortifiers and/or preterm infant formulas. The goal is to stimulate growth patterns that approximate in utero development. Preterm infants need about 120 to 160 kcal per kg per day, including 3.5 to 4 g per kg per day of protein. Preterm caloric requirements vary depending on the infant's environment, medical status, and enteral intake. Energy requirements rise when the child has to maintain body temperature and/or is not in a humidity-controlled environment. Enteral feeding requires more calories to digest and metabolize nutrients than parenteral feeding, and bolus enteral feeding more than continuous.

The mother's milk should be given if at all possible. Preterm human breast milk is higher in calories, fat, protein, and sodium than term milk, but lower in lactose, calcium, and phosphorus. Human milk fortifiers provide additional calories, protein, and vitamins. Most preterm formulas have a caloric density of 24 kcal per oz. About three fourths of the calcium and phosphorus present in the term infant accumulates during the third trimester, so preterm infants are vulnerable to mineral deficiency states. Human breast milk fortifiers and preterm formulas have higher levels of calcium and phosphorus to counteract this imbalance. Preterm infants may also need additional sodium supplementation in the first few days of life.

Preterm infants are relatively deficient in lipase and bile salts, so their ability to break down certain fats is limited. The saturated fat of the human milk globule is well absorbed by the preterm infant. Preterm formulas contain medium-chain triglycerides and vegetable oils rich in polyunsaturated long-chain triglycerides, which can be digested by the preterm infant. Preterm infants do not need vitamin D supplementation over and above what is recommended for term infants. However, they are at an increased risk for rickets given their relative deficiencies in phosphorus and calcium.

Complementary Feeding

Infants are often developmentally ready to accept solid food between 4 and 6 months of age. Younger patients risk choking on solid foods. In addition, complementary feeding before 4 months of age decreases the intake of human breast milk or infant formula, both of which are vastly superior in nutritional value. Iron-fortified cereal should be started by 6 months of age in breast-fed infants to meet their iron needs. Thereafter, foods may be added one at a time every 5 to 7 days while watching for signs of intolerance or allergy.

Parents may decide to prepare their own food at home. Although acceptable, certain precautions should be observed. Foods must be scrupulously cleaned, cooked (except very soft fruits), pureed, and used or frozen immediately. Commercially canned foods cannot be substituted due to added salt and sugar; similarly, parents should not add salt, sugar, or seasonings to the foods they prepare for their infant.

Vegetarian families with infants 6 to 12 months of age must be diligent in their efforts to provide adequate levels of vitamin B_{12} and essential fatty acids for their children. In addition, vegetarian diets are typically bulky to provide sufficient calories, so foods that are calorically dense must be incorporated for the infant to meet energy needs.

NUTRITION IN CHILDHOOD

Providing a nutritional diet for a child not only affects present growth and development, but also encourages life-long healthy eating habits and limits future risk of medical conditions such as obesity, hypertension, cardiovascular disease, diabetes, and stroke. Caregivers should:

- offer a nutritionally balanced variety of foods to their children
- facilitate regularly scheduled, structured family mealtimes that are relaxed and pleasant
- model appropriate eating behavior
- limit consumption of high-fat, high-sugar foods
- limit exposure to media in terms of content (food commercials) and amount (time in front of the television)

Left to their own preferences, children are better at regulating their amount of food intake than they are at choosing a well-balanced diet. In particular, children are susceptible to dietary deficiencies of *iron, calcium,* and *vitamin D.* Recommendations regarding intake of these micronutrients are provided in Table 2-3. Iron-deficiency anemia, the most common nutritional deficiency in the American pediatric population, is discussed in detail in Chapter 15. States of calcium and vitamin D deficiency are discussed below. Although vitamin and mineral supplements are usually unnecessary in children who receive adequate, nutritionally balanced diets, the American Academy of Pediatrics recognizes that such supplements may be beneficial for:

- children with failure to thrive (FTT)
- children with certain chronic diseases
- obese children in dietary management programs

TABLE 2-3
DIETARY REFERENCE INTAKES FOR CHILDREN AND ADOLESCENTS[a]

Nutrient	Children	Adolescents
Iron	7 mg/d (age 1 to 3 y)	8 to 11 mg/d (male)
	10 mg/d (age 4 to 8 y)	8 to 15 mg/d (female)
Calcium	500 mg/d (age 1 to 3 y) 800 mg/d (age 4 to 8 y)	1,300 to 1,500 mg/d
Phosphorus	460 to 500 mg/d	1,250 mg/d
Vitamin D	5 μg/d	5 μg/d

[a]According to the National Academy of Sciences, Institute of Medicine Food and Nutrition Board.

- vegetarian children who do not consume dairy products
- children who are not regularly exposed to sunlight, or who do not consume ≥500 mL of vitamin D–fortified milk (or a 200-IU supplement of vitamin D) every day

NUTRITION IN ADOLESCENTS

Adolescents have more opportunities than children to decide for themselves what, when, and whether to eat. Not surprisingly, adolescents are more likely than children to report substandard nutritional intake. Adolescence is a period of marked physical growth and development, and energy and nutrient needs outstrip those of the child and adult. Based on their increased needs and dietary practices, adolescents often require supplementation to obtain the recommended amounts of iron, calcium, and vitamins. Although universal calcium supplementation during adolescence is controversial, it is difficult for even the most conscientious adolescent to fulfill the recommended intake without mineral supplementation. Female adolescents should also ingest 0.4 mg per day of folic acid, which is recommended for all girls and women after menarche for the prevention of fetal neural tube defects.

Athletes have additional caloric and iron needs over and above those of their less active peers. Every 2 hours of athletic participation translates into an additional 800 to 1,700 cal required. These needs can generally be met through increased intake of food. However, patients who participate in sports that place them at risk for more disordered eating patterns (wrestling, dance, cheerleading, gymnastics) may be reluctant to increase their caloric intake. Because athletes lose iron in their sweat, and possibly through occult urinary and gastrointestinal blood loss, iron deficiency may develop. Menstruating female athletes and long-distance runners are at particular risk for iron-deficiency anemia.

Athletes need not increase their protein intake; the typical American diet provides protein in excess of what normoactive and athletic adolescents need. Additional nutritional management of athletes is provided in Chapter 25.

Fad diets limit consumption of one or more food types based on questionable (or no) scientific data. It is difficult for adolescents who are limiting their food intake to meet energy and nutritional needs. Patients who need to lose weight should attempt to do so under the direct guidance of a physician by increasing energy expenditure, moderately reducing caloric intake, and adjusting food choices to reflect nutritional guidelines.

NUTRITION IN VEGETARIAN PATIENTS

Semi-vegetarians are a heterogeneous group; some avoid red meat only, whereas others also avoid poultry. *Lacto-ovo vegetarians* eat eggs and dairy products and may also eat fish.

Vegans eat no foods derived from animal products. Because vitamin B_{12} is found only in foods of animal origin, vegans require vitamin B_{12} supplementation. Vegans who do not get adequate sun exposure should also be supplemented with vitamin D. Children on any of the vegetarian diets listed above are more likely than their meat-eating peers to develop iron deficiency. This can be addressed by offering them iron-fortified grains and other foods and iron supplementation if indicated.

STATES OF EXCESS AND DEFICIENCY

Kwashiorkor and Marasmus

The Western diet is replete with protein, so *kwashiorkor* (clinically evident protein deficiency) in developed countries is usually due to an underlying chronic disease that interferes with protein absorption (diarrheal states), synthesis (liver disease), or retention (proteinuria). Clinical manifestations of kwashiorkor include irritability progressing to lethargy, edema (which may partially mask the weight loss), protuberant abdomen, scant muscle tissue, dermatitis, liver enlargement, and increased susceptibility to infections. In contrast, *marasmus* due to inadequate caloric intake results in cachexia and wasting but no edema or dermatitis. Chronic malnourishment is associated with suppressed T-cell function.

Protein-losing enteropathy is a clinical syndrome of edema, diarrhea, and abdominal pain that accompanies significant ongoing gastrointestinal protein loss. Protein-losing enteropathy may result from:

- infection of the gastrointestinal tract (*Giardia, Clostridium difficile, Salmonella, Shigella*)
- immune-mediated gastrointestinal disease (celiac disease, inflammatory bowel disease)
- ischemic disease of the bowel (necrotizing enterocolitis)
- general or localized vasculitis (hemolytic-uremic syndrome, Henoch-Schönlein purpura)

Vitamins

The signs and symptoms of hypervitaminosis A and hypervitaminosis D are listed in Table 2-4.

Vitamin B_9 (folate) is present in many foods of plant and animal origin and is absorbed from the small intestine. Folate deficiency may result from removal or dysfunction of the small bowel or from conditions of malabsorption (celiac disease, inflammatory bowel disease, chronic gastrointestinal infection, bowel fistulas). Patients at risk for folate deficiency may need supplementation to prevent the development of megaloblastic anemia.

Vitamin D deficiency is more common in people who avoid dairy products, are dark-skinned, and live at extreme geographic latitudes. Inadequate sunlight exposure combined

TABLE 2-4
CLINICAL MANIFESTATIONS OF EXCESSIVE VITAMIN A AND VITAMIN D

Hypervitaminosis A	Hypervitaminosis D
Symptoms (due to development of pseudotumor cerebri)	**Symptoms (develop within 3 mo)**
Severe headache	Irritability
Diplopia	Anorexia/nausea/vomiting
Signs	Constipation (or diarrhea)
Papilledema	Polydipsia
Laboratory/Radiologic Results	Polyuria/noctiuria
Increased intracranial pressure	**Signs**
Hyperostosis of the long bones	Poor growth/weight loss
If Prolonged and Severe	Hypotonia
Irritability	Hypertension
Fatigue/malaise	**Laboratory/Radiologic Results**
Anorexia/poor weight gain	Hypercalcemia
Pruritis	Hypercalciuria
Bone swelling, tenderness	Osteopenia
Liver enlargement/cirrhosis	**If Prolonged and Severe**
Seborrheic skin lesions	Nephrocalcinosis
Alopecia	Retinopathy/corneal clouding
Skin fissuring at corners of mouth	Multiorgan/soft tissue calcification

TABLE 2-5
CLINICAL AND LABORATORY MANIFESTATIONS OF RICKETS

Craniotabes (thinning of the outer skull layer)
Rachitic rosary (enlargement of the costochondral junctions)
Epiphyseal enlargement at the wrists and ankles
Delayed closure of abnormally large fontanelle
Bow legs
Delayed walking
Normal-to-low serum calcium
Low serum phosphorus
Elevated serum alkaline phosphatase
Low serum 25-hydroxycholecalciferol

with dietary insufficiency result in *rickets*, a condition in which developing bone fails to mineralize due to inadequate 1,25-dihydroxycholecalciferol. Rickets in nonsupplemented breast-fed infants becomes clinically and chemically evident in late infancy. The presentation of rickets is provided in Table 2-5. Rickets attributable solely to vitamin D deficiency begins to respond to supplementation within weeks.

Vitamin D deficiency may also present with symptomatic hypocalcemia and hypophosphatemia. In adolescents and adults, deficiency of vitamin D leads to demineralization of bone, osteomalacia, bone pain, and increased susceptibility to fractures.

Vitamin K is involved in the synthesis of prothrombin (factor II) and factor VII, which contribute to coagulation. Patients who take antibiotics that disrupt the normal flora of the intestine and those with disorders that interfere with vitamin K absorption (chronic diarrhea, cystic fibrosis, hepatitis, celiac disease) may develop vitamin K deficiency, resulting in prolonged bleeding or spontaneous hemorrhaging. Infants born at home and breast-fed infants who do not receive prophylactic vitamin K at birth are at risk for *hemorrhagic disease of the newborn*. This disorder is characterized by intracranial, gastrointestinal, and/or nasal bleeding and prolonged bleeding from sites of trauma (e.g., circumcision). Hemorrhagic disease of the newborn generally occurs within the first week of life. The condition responds quickly to vitamin K; more severe cases require infusion of plasma.

Minerals

Calcium and phosphorus comprise the mineral content of bone. Phosphorus is found in plant and animal foods. Calcium is present in dairy products, vegetables (particularly dark greens), and fortified grains and juice. Bone mineralization in children depends on adequate dietary intake of calcium and phosphorus. Preterm infants who do not receive enough calcium and/or phosphorus are at risk for *osteopenia of prematurity* (poor bone mineralization), which may progress to frank rickets. This is particularly true of infants who are supported primarily on parenteral nutrition, because these minerals may precipitate in solution if used in large amounts. Adolescents who do not achieve maximal peak bone mass are at increased risk for osteoporosis later in life. Disorders of calcium and phosphate *metabolism* are discussed in Chapter 11.

Zinc deficiency may result from chronic malabsorption or from *acrodermatitis enteropathica*, an autosomal recessive disorder involving a transport protein responsible for zinc absorption from the intestines. Breast-fed infants with this disorder do well until they are weaned because human breast milk contains a protein that encourages absorption. Clinical manifestations include irritability; hair loss and crusting of the scalp; symmetric, eczematous, or psoriatic red, moist lesions around the mouth and perineum and on the cheeks, elbows, and knees; stomatitis; nail dystrophies; chronic intermittent diarrhea; FTT; impaired wound healing; and decreased immunocompetency. Oral zinc supplementation results in rapid improvement.

NUTRITIONAL SUPPORT

Enteral Nutrition

Enteral feeding involves using a nasogastric tube or, for a more long-term solution, gastrostomy or a gastrojejunal tube or low-profile gastronomy "button." Patients who are unable to ingest sufficient calories orally, because of neurologic or gastrointestinal disease, food aversion, or growth failure, are candidates for enteral nutrition. Using the gut rather than parenteral feeding is preferred, if possible, because it helps to maintain normal gastrointestinal flora and immunity and preserve function. It is also less expensive, requires less invasive monitoring, and has less severe complications (Table 2-6).

Most patients are begun on continuous feeds to evaluate tolerance. Continuous feeds are generally better tolerated and result in fewer complications. Children with malabsorptive

TABLE 2-6
COMPLICATIONS OF ENTERAL FEEDING

Diarrhea (most common)
Emesis
Mechanical complications (clogging)
Dumping syndrome[a]
Fluid/electrolyte imbalances
Refeeding syndrome (may also occur with parenteral nutrition)

[a]Syndrome of abdominal distention, diarrhea, sweating, tachycardia, and hypoglycemia, which results when the tip of the tube migrates and disperses feeds directly into the duodenum.

gastrointestinal abnormalities (e.g., Crohn disease, chronic diarrhea, short bowel syndrome) have better nutritional outcomes when feedings are administered continuously. However, for most patients the goal is progression to intermittent bolus feeds, which more closely mimic typical feeding patterns and stimulate pancreatic and biliary secretions. Increasing gastric residuals, vomiting, aspiration, and malabsorption indicate *intolerance* to bolus feeds.

Refeeding syndrome, which can occur with the initiation of oral, enteral, or parenteral nutrition, is characterized by electrolyte abnormalities (most notably *hypophosphatemia*) and fluid retention. Affected patients present with edema and muscle weakness; cardiac arrhythmias are not uncommon. Refeeding syndrome is less likely to occur when feeds are initiated at low rates and advanced to full caloric requirements over 5 to 7 days. Daily monitoring of serum electrolytes, glucose, calcium, phosphorus, and magnesium is recommended during this time.

Parenteral Nutrition

Intestines that are too short (short bowel syndrome), inflamed (Crohn disease, necrotizing enterocolitis), or nonperistaltic (postoperative, severe burns) cannot support adequate nutrition and growth. In these circumstances, parenteral nutrition is a viable option. Parenteral nutrition consists of glucose, lipid, and amino acid sources of calories, with added vitamins and minerals. The relative amounts of each can be changed based on the patient's specific needs. Electrolyte and mineral levels are monitored daily until stable, with even more frequent glucose checks. Phosphorus in particular must be checked at least weekly thereafter. Albumin, liver function tests, and triglyceride levels are assessed weekly or as needed. Complications of parenteral nutrition can be significant and include electrolyte imbalance, infection, catheter occlusion, and intrahepatic cholestasis.

FAILURE TO THRIVE

FTT (also called pediatric undernutrition) is a term used to describe poor growth in children, particularly those who:

- are at less than the third percentile for weight or for weight-for-height, OR
- have weight curves that have crossed two percentile lines on the growth chart

FTT may be primarily organic, primarily nonorganic, or a mixture of the two. *Organic FTT* results from an identified medical condition such as chronic disease, malabsorption, increased energy expenditure, swallowing dysfunction, genetic syndromes, neurodevelopmental abnormalities, or endocrine disorders. *Nonorganic FTT* is poor growth due to inadequate intake that is not associated with any specific medical disorder. Most cases of FTT are nonorganic in origin. Inadequate caloric intake may result from:

- improper formula preparation
- breast-feeding problems
- improper feeding techniques (stopping a feed when the child is still hungry)
- poor transition to solid foods
- excessive caloric intake from juice
- consistently stressful/unpleasant mealtimes
- parental neglect
- parental avoidance of perceived "bad" or "harmful" foods
- inadequate parental education regarding nutritional needs

The evaluation of FTT includes a detailed history of the child's diet (food types and quantity), eating behaviors, perinatal course, and past growth. The social history may reveal sources of stress within the family. It is important to determine who feeds the child and how formula and/or other foods are prepared. The physician may note signs that the caregiver is depressed, poorly attached, or unresponsive to the child. The growth chart is essential for assessing the trajectory of growth in multiple areas. Unless FTT is due to underlying brain abnormalities, weight curves generally decelerate first, followed by height, and then head circumference. A partial differential diagnosis for FTT is listed in Table 2-7.

TABLE 2-7
DIFFERENTIAL DIAGNOSIS OF FAILURE TO THRIVE

Nonorganic/Psychosocial (most common)
Neglect
Abuse
Inadequate amount fed, due to improper food preparation, diet, or feeding techniques

Cardiac
Congenital heart malformations

Gastrointestinal
Malabsorption
Milk protein intolerance/allergy
Gastroesophageal reflux
Pyloric stenosis
Inflammatory bowel disease
Celiac disease
Hirschsprung disease

Pulmonary
Cystic fibrosis
Bronchopulmonary dysplasia
Chronic aspiration
Respiratory insufficiency

(continued)

TABLE 2-7
(continued)

Infectious
Human immunodeficiency virus
Tuberculosis
Chronic gastroenteritis
Intestinal parasites
Urinary tract infection
Neonatal
Prematurity
Low birth weight
Congenital or perinatal infection
Maternal drug or alcohol use/teratogens
Endocrine
Diabetes mellitus
Hypothyroidism
Hyperthyroidism
Adrenal insufficiency or excess
Growth hormone deficiency
Hypophosphatemic rickets
Neurologic
Cerebral palsy
Mental retardation
Degenerative disorders
Oral-motor dysfunction
Renal
Renal tubular acidosis
Chronic renal insufficiency
Other
Inborn errors of metabolism
Genetic syndromes
Malignancy
Chronic disease
Cleft palate
Immunodeficiency syndromes
Collagen vascular disease
Food aversion behavior

Exhaustive initial laboratory evaluation is neither informative nor cost-effective. Routine laboratory tests consist of review of the newborn screen in infants and possibly a complete blood cell count, electrolyte panel, urinalysis, and screens for iron deficiency and lead poisoning in older infants and toddlers. The decision to pursue other studies should be guided by significant elements of the history, growth chart, and physical examination. Widespread, low-yield testing should be limited to cases in which a concerted outpatient dietary intervention has failed to achieve growth. Hospitalization is reserved for treatment failures, cases of suspected abuse or neglect, or the discovery of a serious underlying medical condition.

Children who have FTT in the first 2 years of life are at increased risk for developmental delay, poor school performance, and behavioral problems.

OBESITY

Obesity may be *primary (exogenous)* or due to endocrine disease or genetic syndromes. Risk factors for obesity are listed in Table 2-8. Most patients with primary obesity are tall for their age; the obese patient who is short for age is more likely to have an underlying disorder such as Cushing syndrome, hypothyroidism, or Prader-Willi syndrome. Patients who are obese should be examined and/or screened for known complications, including:

- obstructive sleep apnea, Pickwickian syndrome, asthma
- slipped capital femoral epiphysis, Blount disease (bowing of the legs secondary to disordered tibial growth, presumably due to excess weight)
- gallbladder disease, steatohepatitis (fatty inflammation of the liver)
- polycystic ovarian syndrome

Metabolic syndrome is the combination of obesity, hypertension, insulin resistance, and dyslipidemia (increased triglycerides, decreased high-density lipoprotein levels, and abnormally dense low-density lipoprotein particles). Clinical and laboratory criteria for the diagnosis of metabolic syndrome are described in Table 2-9. Weight loss is the most effective treatment for metabolic syndrome; medication to decrease insulin resistance is second-line therapy if lifestyle changes prove insufficient. Metabolic syndrome is associated with high rates of type 2 diabetes, cardiovascular disease, and fatty liver disease.

TABLE 2-8
RISK FACTORS FOR DEVELOPMENT OF OBESITY

Genetic
Family history of obesity
Genetic tendency/heritability
Environmental
Obese parents
Poverty
Easy availability of fast foods, high-fat foods
Fewer family meals
Individual/Behavioral
Early childhood obesity
Sedentary lifestyle
Excessive time spent watching television

TABLE 2-9
INTERNATIONAL DIABETES FEDERATION CRITERIA FOR DIAGNOSIS OF METABOLIC SYNDROME (ADAPTED TO CHILDREN)

Body mass index or waist circumference >85th percentile for age, PLUS any two of the following:
- Fasting triglyceride concentration >150 mg per dL
- High-density lipoprotein cholesterol concentration <40 to 50 mg per dL
- Blood pressure >85th percentile for age and height
- Evidence of insulin resistance or type 2 diabetes (fasting blood glucose >100 mg/dL)

Fasting triglyceride and cholesterol levels and fasting blood glucose should be obtained in patients at increased risk for metabolic syndrome, particularly those with obesity and hypertension.

Obesity in adolescents is particularly troubling, because the later in childhood a person becomes or remains obese, the more likely that person is to become an obese adult. In addition to increasing the life-long risks for cardiovascular disease, hypertension, and type 2 diabetes (which may even present during adolescence), obesity can lead to low self-esteem, teasing from peers, and social isolation. Obsession with weight and disordered eating patterns may emerge. Depression is not uncommon.

Obesity is a chronic condition, and management depends on modification of environmental and behavioral factors under the patient's control. In other words, the patient and family must agree that the child's weight is a problem and be willing to effect necessary changes. Successful intervention programs include the elements of diet alteration, increased physical activity, and changes in eating and exercise habits. Educating moderately obese children about food choices based on a traffic signal model involves teaching them which foods are "red" (STOP: consume very rarely if at all), "yellow" (CAUTION: consume in limited quantities), and "green" (GO: no limits on consumption). In most obese children, the goal is to keep weight stable while height increases, rather than weight loss. Weight reduction is recommended for morbidly obese patients and those with significant complications. Limiting caloric intake to 300 to 400 kcal per day below maintenance needs should result in steady but safe weight loss. Aerobic exercise and promotion of a more active lifestyle (i.e., taking the stairs instead of the elevator) increase caloric expenditure and lean muscle mass. Behavioral modification therapy involving the patient and the family should occur at regular intervals to evaluate progress and offer encouragement. At present, bariatric surgery and anorectic medications have no role in the management of pediatric obesity.

SOURCES

American Academy of Pediatrics Committee on Nutrition. Kleinman RE, ed. *Pediatric nutrition handbook.* 5th ed. Elk Grove Village, IL: American Academy of Pediatrics; 2003.

Gahagan S. Failure to thrive: a consequence of undernutrition. *Pediatr Rev.* 2006;27:e1–e11.

Miller JL, Silverstein JH. The metabolic syndrome: growing challenge in pediatric care. *Contemp Pediatr.* 2006;23:32–45.

Ostrea EM, Mantaring JB, Silvestre MA. Drugs that affect the fetus and newborn infant via the placenta or breast milk. *Pediatr Clin North Am.* 2004;51:539–580.

Schneider MB, Brill SR. Obesity in children and adolescents. *Pediatr Rev.* 2005;26:155–162.

QUESTIONS

1. A 16-year-old menstruating girl comes to your office for a sports physical. On dietary history, you discover that she does not drink milk, but does have calcium-fortified orange juice at breakfast and usually has cheese or yogurt at least once a day. Her diet is carbohydrate-heavy, and she avoids red meat. Which of the following is the most appropriate course of action regarding her nutritional status?

A) Screen for iron-deficiency anemia and supplement if indicated.
B) Counsel the patient to increase her calcium intake through diet or supplements.
C) Counsel the patient to supplement her diet with folate.
D) Counsel the patient to increase her caloric intake 800 to 1,700 cal for every 2 hours that she participates in organized sports.
E) All of the above

2. You are seeing a 6-month-old infant in your office for a health maintenance visit. The review of systems is significant for frequent loose, runny stools. His weight curve demonstrates growth deceleration. A screening hemoglobin level is consistent with anemia. The mother admits that she weaned the child from breast milk to goat milk at age 2 months on the advice of her mother. Additional laboratory tests demonstrate megaloblastic anemia and a low reticulocyte count. This child's findings are most consistent with a deficiency in which of the following?

A) Folate
B) Vitamin D
C) Vitamin B_{12}
D) Zinc
E) Niacin

3. You are seeing a mother and infant in the hospital for a newborn examination. The mother is planning on breast-feeding exclusively for the first 6 months and is adamant about not giving her baby any "unnatural supplements." You review the nutritional benefits of breast milk and discuss with the parents the American Academy of Pediatrics' recommendation that:

A) exclusively breast-fed neonates need 3 to 6 mg per kg per day of iron to meet their iron needs
B) exclusively breast-fed neonates should be supplemented with 200 IU per day of vitamin D beginning within the first 2 months after delivery
C) exclusively breast-fed neonates are at increased risk of osteopenia given the low content of calcium and phosphorus in human breast milk
D) exclusively breast-fed neontes need 200 IU of vitamin K after the first week of life to prevent hemorrhagic disease of the newborn
E) no supplementation is recommended for exclusively breast-fed in infants in the first 6 months of life

4. Which of the following statements regarding human breast milk and cow milk–based infant formula is TRUE?
A) The principal protein of human breast milk and formula is α-lactalbumin.
B) The principal fat component of breast milk and formula is medium-chain triglycerides.
C) The principal carbohydrate in breast milk and formula is lactose.
D) Human breast milk has more iron than standard cow milk–based infant formulas.
E) Human breast milk has more calcium and phosphorus than standard cow milk–based formulas.

5. Which of the following conditions of the breast is most likely to result in the mother's inability to successfully breast-feed her infant?
A) Inverted nipples
B) Fissured nipples
C) Retracted nipples
D) Reduction mammoplasty
E) Breast engorgement

6. Breast-feeding is not contraindicated for which of the following mothers in developed countries?
A) A mother with acute mastitis
B) A mother with active untreated tuberculosis
C) A mother who is positive for human immunodeficiency virus
D) A mother who is infected with human T-cell lymphotropic virus
E) A mother with herpetic lesions of the breast

7. You are seeing a 2-month-old infant in your office for a complaint of bloody stools. The mother tells you that the infant was exclusively breast-fed for 1 month and then switched to a cow milk–based infant formula. For the past 2 weeks, the infant has become increasingly more irritable with feeding and has begun to vomit after feeds. Today, she noted blood mixed with his stool. The growth chart demonstrates slight deceleration in the child's growth. There are no significant findings on physical examination. The stool is guaiac-positive. Which of the following is the most appropriate next step in the management of this infant?
A) Advise the mother to change to a soy-based formula.
B) Advise the mother to change to a protein hydrolysate formula.
C) Advise the mother to change to folate-fortified goat milk.
D) Advise the mother to feed through the episodes.
E) Schedule the child for an upper gastrointestinal series to evaluate for significant reflux.

8. At a prenatal visit, a mother asks you about the benefits of breast-feeding over formula feeding. You are correct in relating each of the following EXCEPT:
A) The composition of breast milk changes based on the age of the infant.
B) Breast milk contains immunoglobulins and other proteins that contribute to infant immunity.
C) Breast milk has a higher concentration of protein than cow milk–based formula.
D) Breast milk contains arachidonic acid and docosahexaenoic acid, which are involved in the formation of retinal and brain phospholipids.
E) Breast milk has lower concentrations of calcium and phosphorus than cow milk–based formulas, but the minerals are more bioavailable and better absorbed from breast milk.

9. A 2-week-old breast-fed infant presents to the emergency room with fever, irritability, jaundice, and hepatomegaly. Pertinent laboratory findings include an elevated white blood cell count and a total serum bilirubin level of 6.8 mg per dL. The patient's urine is positive for reducing substances, and a blood culture becomes positive for *Escherichia coli* the next day. In addition to treating the patient's infection and underlying illness, this patient should be switched from breast milk to an exclusive diet of:
A) elemental formula
B) breast milk with fortifier
C) cow milk–based formula
D) soy-based formula
E) protein hydrolysate formula

10. Soy-based formula is the most appropriate nutritional choice for which of the following infants?
A) A premature infant weighing ≤1,800 g
B) A premature infant weighing >1,800 g

C) An infant with known hereditary lactase deficiency
D) An infant with enterocolitis resulting from cow milk allergy
E) An infant with eczema resulting from cow milk allergy

11. Mothers who breast-feed their infants should, if possible, avoid intake of which of the following medications?
A) Metronidazole
B) Estrogen
C) Lithium
D) Phenobarbital
E) All of the above

12. You are lecturing first-year pediatric residents about infant formulas. In regard to protein hydrolysate formulas, you are correct in telling them all of the following EXCEPT:
A) Protein hydrolysate formulas contain only free amino acids as their protein source.
B) Most protein hydrolysate formulas are lactose-free.
C) Protein hydrolysate formulas are an appropriate choice for infants with pancreatic insufficiency.
D) Protein hydrolysate formulas are an appropriate choice for infants with malabsorption.
E) Protein hydrolysate formulas are an appropriate choice for infants with cow milk allergy.

13. A 4-month-old infant with bronchopulmonary dysplasia is discharged from the neonatal intensive care unit on 24 kcal per oz of fortified formula. The infant was born at 28 weeks of gestation. When you see the infant for a follow-up visit 7 days later, the child has gained no weight. Upon consultation with the patient's nutritionist, you instruct the mother in how to fortify the formula to 28 kcal per oz and caution her that the increased caloric density may lead to which of the following?
A) Lethargy
B) Diarrhea and vomiting
C) Fat wasting
D) Rickets
E) Hypoalbuminemia

14. Which of the following, if available, is the most appropriate nutritional option for a neonate born at 30 weeks of gestation?
A) The mother's milk
B) The mother's milk with added human milk fortifier
C) Cow milk–based low-iron formula
D) Preterm cow milk–based formula
E) Soy-based formula

15. A multivitamin/mineral supplement is recommended for each of the following pediatric patients EXCEPT:
A) A 2-year-old with organic FTT
B) A 14-year-old obese patient in a dietary management program
C) A 5-year-old vegan child
D) A 17-year-old patient hospitalized for anorexia nervosa
E) An 8-year-old boy who plays competitive ice hockey

16. Current calcium recommendations state that adolescent patients should be ingesting how much calcium per day?
A) 200 to 400 mg
B) 600 to 800 mg
C) 1,000 to 1,200 mg
D) 1,300 to 1,500 mg
E) 1,750 to 2,000 mg

17. A 16-year-old female patient is brought to the emergency room by her mother complaining of a severe headache and double vision. The girl has no history or family history of migraine headaches. The examination is significant for papilledema. Computed tomogram of the head is normal. The patient admits that she has been taking some supplements she found at a nutrition store for her skin, and that she has been taking them at four times the recommended dose. Her clinical picture is most consistent with excessive intake of which of the following?
A) Vitamin A
B) Vitamin B complex
C) Vitamin C
D) Vitamin D
E) Vitamin E

18. A 6-month-old breast-fed infant is brought to the emergency room with irritability, vomiting, and hypotonia. A complete blood cell count is normal, and a toxicology screen is negative. The electrolyte panel is significant for an elevated blood calcium level and a slightly depressed phosphorus level. The mother went back to work in the mornings only 3 months ago; because the infant is asleep when she leaves, the maternal grandmother, who cares for the child, gives the infant her daily supplementation while the mother is at work. This child's condition is most consistent with which of the following?
A) Early rickets
B) Vitamin D deficiency
C) Osteopenia of infancy
D) Hypervitaminosis D
E) Severe iron-deficiency anemia

19. An infant born at home is brought to the emergency room with the mother and transferred to Labor and Delivery for further management. There are no complications or signs of infection in the child or the mother, who had good prenatal care. Breast-feeding progresses well. The baby is circumcised in the hospital on day of life 3 and develops prolonged bleeding from

the circumcision site. Within hours, the child has begun bleeding in the stools and from the nose. A review of the admission orders suggests the diagnosis. This child's clinical picture is most consistent with which of the following?
A) Factor IX deficiency
B) Thrombocytopenia
C) von Willebrand disease
D) Severe cow milk protein allergy
E) Hemorrhagic disease of the newborn

20. Which of the following preterm infants born at 30 weeks of gestation is most likely to develop rickets?
A) An exclusively breast-fed infant
B) An infant fed breast milk with added human milk fortifier who receives 200 IU per day of vitamin D supplementation
C) An infant fed with preterm infant formula who receives 200 IU per day of vitamin D supplementation
D) An infant fed breast milk with added human milk fortifier who does not receive vitamin D supplementation
E) An infant fed with preterm infant formula who does not receive vitamin D supplementation

21. A 9-month-old male infant is brought to your office with a 4-week history of a rash that is not responsive to hydrocortisone cream and is getting progressively worse. The child has also developed diarrhea and is quite irritable. The child was breast-fed exclusively for the first 6 months of life and was then switched to soy-based formula and complementary foods. The examination is significant for crusting of the scalp area and symmetric psoriatic lesions around the mouth, buttocks, elbows, and knees. There are also several erosive lesions in the mouth. Screening laboratory results are noncontributory. Which of the following represents the best next course of action based on the patient's physical findings?
A) Recommending that the child be switched to a protein hydrolysate formula
B) Initiation of zinc supplementation
C) Prescribing a stronger steroid cream for the lesions
D) Sending blood samples to the laboratory for quantitative immunoglobulin levels
E) Sending blood samples to the laboratory for qualitative immunoglobulin studies

22. A 2-year-old African-American boy with mental retardation comes to the clinic for his regular health maintenance visit with his grandmother, his sole caretaker. The woman is an elderly brittle diabetic who lives in a row house in a crime-ridden section of town. She confides that she finds caring for the child frustrating; she cannot let him play outside because he wanders away, and he refuses to eat anything except canned spaghetti and apple juice. On physical examination, the child appears bow-legged and has palpable enlargement of the costochondral junctions. All of the following laboratory abnormalities are consistent with the child's condition EXCEPT:
A) Elevated serum alkaline phosphatase
B) Depressed serum phosphorus
C) Normal to low serum calcium
D) Depressed serum 25-hydroxycholecalciferol
E) Elevated serum 1,25-hydroxycholecalciferol

23. An 18-month-old girl with a history of significant head trauma is transferred to your rehabilitation facility on full gastrostomy tube feeds. On her 14th day in the unit, she suddenly develops tachycardia, abdominal distention, and sweating during feeding. A dextrose-stick demonstrates hypoglycemia. Which of the following complications of enteral feeding best explains her symptoms?
A) Obstruction of the gastrostomy tube
B) Kinking of the gastrostomy tube
C) Elevated serum phosphorus levels
D) Dumping syndrome
E) Refeeding syndrome

24. Which of the following is the most common cause of FTT in the United States?
A) Inadequate caloric intake
B) Chronic disease
C) Malabsorption
D) Organic failure to thrive
E) None of the above

25. A 2-month-old patient has a weight below the third percentile, a length at the third percentile, and microcephaly. Which of the following is LEAST likely to be the principal contributor to this patient's FTT?
A) Perinatal infection
B) Teratogen exposure
C) Genetic syndrome
D) Cerebral palsy
E) Chronic aspiration

26. Children who develop FTT within the first 2 years of life are at increased risk for which of the following?
A) Developmental delay
B) Poor school performance
C) Behavioral problems
D) A and C
E) A, B, and C

27. You are lecturing a group of residents about obesity in the pediatric population. All of the following increase the risk of developing obesity EXCEPT:
A) Regular, family-centered meals in the home
B) A family history of obesity
C) Living with an obese parent

D) Excessive time spent watching television
E) Sedentary lifestyle

28. A 9-year-old boy has a body mass index well above the 95th percentile for his age and gender. His height is at the 15th percentile. Which of the following statements regarding this child's weight condition is TRUE?
A) This child most likely has primary obesity.
B) This child most likely has exogenous obesity.
C) This child should be screened for underlying genetic and endocrine conditions that may be the primary cause of his obesity.
D) This child's obesity is probably caused by metabolic X syndrome.
E) This child's obesity is probably caused by insulin resistance.

29. All of the following are known complications of obesity in children and adolescents EXCEPT:
A) Obstructive sleep apnea
B) Type 1 diabetes
C) Steatohepatitis
D) Polycystic ovarian syndrome
E) Blount disease

30. Metabolic syndrome includes all of the following features EXCEPT:
A) Insulin resistance
B) Elevated triglyceride levels
C) Hypertension
D) Type 2 diabetes
E) Decreased high-density lipoprotein levels

31. Which of the following interventions is likely to be the most effective at resulting in long-term weight loss?
A) Educating overweight children about placing foods into categories based on a traffic signal (RED/YELLOW/GREEN)
B) Limiting caloric intake to expected caloric expenditure minus 300 to 400 cal per day
C) A month away at weight-loss "boot camp" with the support of obese peers
D) Involvement of a personal trainer to help the patient increase caloric expenditure and build lean muscle mass
E) A physician-supervised program of diet alteration, increased physical activity, and behavioral therapy

32. Which of the following is not a recommended for management of pediatric obesity?
A) Family therapy
B) Bariatric surgery
C) Behavioral therapy
D) Nutritional therapy
E) Increased physical activity

33. Which of the following statements regarding initiating parenteral nutrition is FALSE?
A) Parenteral nutrition should be considered for patients who cannot absorb sufficient calories through the gut to meet their energy and growth needs.
B) A patient's serum electrolyte levels should be measured daily until stable.
C) A patient's phosphorus level should be measured at least weekly.
D) A patient's glucose level should be measured daily during initiation of parenteral nutrition.
E) Baseline serum albumin levels will assist in calculating a patient's protein needs.

34. All of the following antibiotics should be avoided in the mother if possible during breast-feeding EXCEPT:
A) Quinolones
B) Nitrofurantoin
C) Metronidazole
D) Chloramphenicol
E) Doxycycline

35. Healthy full-term neonates require about how many kilocalories per kilogram per day to achieve the recommended 20 to 30 g of weight gain per day?
A) 80
B) 120
C) 140
D) 175
E) 200

36. Cow milk should not be given to infants before 12 months of age for all of the following reasons EXCEPT:
A) Cow milk is not sufficient to meet the nutritional needs of the infant.
B) Cow milk may irritate the intestinal lining and result in blood loss.
C) Cow milk is low in iron and may predispose to iron-deficiency anemia.
D) The solute load of cow milk is too high for immature neonatal kidneys.
E) Cow milk is low in folate and may predispose to megaloblastic anemia.

37. Which of the following components of breast milk is involved in the formation of retinal and brain phospholipid membranes?
A) Arachidonic acid
B) α-lactalbumin
C) α-lactoglobulin
D) Whey
E) Casein

38. Infants 6 to 12 months of age who are fed an exclusively vegan diet require supplementation with which of the following to meet their nutritional needs?
A) Vitamin B_6
B) Vitamin B_{12}
C) Folate

D) Niacin
E) Vitamin C

39. You are providing a lecture to pediatric interns regarding protein-losing enteropathy. You would be correct in telling them that protein-losing enteropathy:
A) is a clinical syndrome of edema, diarrhea, and abdominal pain
B) results when protein loss occurs primarily from the gastrointestinal system
C) may be the result of vasculitis the gastrointestinal tract
D) may be the result of inflammatory bowel disease
E) All of the above

40. Which of the following patients with pediatric undernutrition is most likely to tolerate and benefit from bolus enteral feeds rather than continuous feeds?
A) A 10-year-old with extensive Crohn disease
B) A 3-year-old with oral–motor dysfunction
C) A 4-month-old with short bowel syndrome
D) A 6-year-old with protein-losing enteropathy
E) A 2-year-old with increasing gastric residuals on low-rate continuous enteral feeds

41. A 12-year-old girl in your office for her regular health maintenance visit has a body mass index >95th percentile for age and a blood pressure at the 90th percentile for age. Which of the following groupings of laboratory tests is most appropriate in evaluating this patient for metabolic syndrome?
A) Two-hour glucose tolerance test, total cholesterol
B) High-density lipoprotein cholesterol, fasting triglycerides, fasting blood glucose
C) Serum fibrinogen, C-reactive protein
D) Islet cell autoantibodies, insulin antibody assays
E) Urinalysis for glucose, ketones, red blood cells

42. A 16-year-old girl with a body mass index of 33 kg per m^2 (>95th percentile for age) is in the office for a repeat blood pressure measurement. Her blood pressure today is 130/82 mm Hg; two previous measurements were similarly elevated. Her cholesterol concentration is 210 mg per dL, with a high-density lipoprotein cholesterol concentration of 45 mg per dL and a fasting triglyceride value of 165 mg per dL. Her fasting blood glucose level is 112 mg per dL. A 2-hour postoral glucose blood glucose level is 160 mg per dL. This clinical and laboratory scenario is most consistent with a diagnosis of which of the following?
A) Type 1 diabetes
B) Type 2 diabetes
C) Metabolic syndrome
D) Hypercortisolism
E) Hypothyroidism

43. A 16-year-old African-American boy presents to your office in January with a chief complaint of tingling and numbness in his extremities. His vital signs and physical examination are within normal limits. Pertinent screening laboratory results include a total serum calcium concentration of 5.2 mg per dL, a serum phosphorus concentration of 2.2 mg per dL, and a serum magnesium concentration of 2.0 mg per dL. Which of the following conditions is the most likely cause of this patient's symptoms?
A) Vitamin D deficiency
B) Primary hypoparathyroidism
C) Secondary hypoparathyroidism
D) Hypomagnesemia
E) Liver disease

ANSWERS

1. E
2. A
3. B
4. C
5. D
6. A
7. B
8. C
9. D
10. C
11. E
12. A
13. B
14. B
15. E
16. D
17. A
18. D
19. E
20. A
21. B
22. E
23. D
24. A
25. E
26. E
27. A
28. C
29. B
30. D
31. E
32. B
33. D
34. E
35. B
36. E
37. A
38. B
39. E
40. B
41. B
42. C
43. A

Preventive Pediatrics

3

IMMUNIZATIONS

Table 3-1 contains a simplified version of the 2007 immunization schedules currently recommended by the Centers for Disease Control and Prevention, Department of Health and Human Services, and American Academy of Pediatrics. Guidelines are amended periodically; updated recommendations are available through the Centers for Disease Control and Prevention Web site (http://www.cdc.gov/vaccines/recs/acip/default.htm). Catch-up schedules for patients who are inadequately immunized are detailed in Table 3-2. The Advisory Committee on Immunization Practices (ACIP) has recently recommended that two additional vaccines become standard practice in the pediatric age group:

- In August of 2006, the ACIP recommended that infants receive the oral rotavirus vaccine at ages 2, 4, and 6 months (must be started before age 12 weeks and completed before age 32 weeks).
- In June of 2006, the ACIP recommended that the quadrivalent human papillomavirus vaccine be administered to all girls at age 11 to 12 years and to all girls 12 to 18 years of age who have not previously been vaccinated. Three doses are required for completion of the series.

Some vaccines are only recommended for use in certain patient populations; others are indicated for all patients but may be administered at different times for specific patient subgroups.

- The trivalent inactivated influenza vaccine is recommended for all patients 6 to 59 months of age and close contacts of children 0 to 59 months of age. The influenza vaccine is also indicated for *any* patient ≥6 months of age who has a condition that compromises respiratory function (e.g., asthma, cystic fibrosis) or predisposes to aspiration of respiratory secretions. Children at risk for the development of severe influenza (i.e., patients with cardiac, metabolic, hematologic, renal, or immunosuppressive diseases, among others), their close contacts, and patients on long-term aspirin therapy should also be vaccinated yearly. The virus undergoes frequent antigenic shifts, so patients need to be inoculated yearly with a vaccine preparation matching the most significant current antigenic strains. The inactivated (killed-virus) injectable form of the vaccine causes local irritation in a third of patients; about 5% develop mild systemic symptoms. An aerosolized, live, attenuated influenza vaccine is available for healthy children ≥5 years of age.
- The heptavalent pneumococcal conjugate vaccine (PCV7) is recommended for children 24 to 59 months of age who have sickle cell disease, splenic dysfunction, human immunodeficiency virus, chronic illness, or conditions that result in immunocompromise. Two doses of the conjugate vaccine should be administered 2 months apart, followed by one dose of the 23-valent pneumococcal polysaccharide vaccine. Invasive pneumococcal disease can still occur in vaccinated patients but is much less likely.
- The 23-valent pneumococcal polysaccharide vaccine should also be administered to children in the above risk groups who completed their initial PCV7 series before age 2 years. The 23-valent pneumococcal polysaccharide vaccine has limited immunogenicity in children younger than 24 months of age and therefore is not indicated for this age group.
- Vaccination against meningococcal disease is recommended for patients with terminal complement deficiencies or anatomic or functional asplenia and people who are traveling to areas where meningococcal disease is endemic. Vaccination is also used to control outbreaks with serotypes contained in available vaccines. The tetravalent meningococcal conjugate vaccine (MCV4) is approved for use in patients ≥11 years of age; the tetravalent meningococcal polysaccharide vaccine MPSV4 must be used in children 2 to 10 years of age, although it may be substituted for MCV4 in older children if the conjugate vaccine is not available. Both vaccines afford protection against disease serotypes A, C, Y, and W-135. Neither is effective versus *Neisseria meningitidis* serogroup B.

Premature infants should be vaccinated on the same schedule as their full-term peers according to their chronological age, regardless of how early they were born or how little they weighed. The initial hepatitis B vaccine (HBV1) is an exception. Premature infants weighing <2,000 g born to mothers negative for the hepatitis B surface antigen (HBsAg) should receive HBV1 at age 1 month or when they achieve 2,000 g in weight. Premature infants born to HBsAg-positive (or HBsAg-status unknown) mothers should receive HBV1 and hepatitis B immunoglobulin within 12 hours of birth. If these infants weigh <2,000 g at HBV1, then this first dose does not count toward completion of their three-dose series.

TABLE 3-1
CHILDHOOD IMMUNIZATION SCHEDULES

Vaccine	Age: Birth	1 mo	2 mo	4 mo	6 mo	12 mo	15 mo	18 mo	24 mo	4 to 6 y	11 to 12 y	13 to 14 y	15 y	16 to 18 y
Hepatitis B	HBV(1)[a]	HBV(2)			HBV(3)									
Diphtheria, tetanus, pertussis[b]			DTaP(1)	DTaP(2)	DTaP(3)		DTaP(4)[c]			DTaP(5)	Tdap(6)[d]	[Tdap(6) if not received at 11 to 12 y]		
Haemophilus influenzae type b[e]			Hib(1)	Hib(2)	Hib(3)	Hib(4)								
Poliovirus[f]			IPV(1)	IPV(2)	IPV(3)					IPV(4)				
Pneumococcal			PCV7(1)	PCV7(2)	PCV7(3)	PCV(7), PCV7(4)								
Hepatitis A						HAV(1) [HAV(2) ≥6 mo later]								
Measles, mumps, rubella						MMR(1)[g]					MMR(2)[h]			
Varicella						VAR(1)				VAR(2)[i]	[VAR(1) and VAR(2) if no history of vaccination or clinical disease			
Meningococcal											MCV4(1)[j], MCV(1)]		[MCV4(1)[j], MCV(1) if not received at 11 to 12 y]	
Influenza					Indicated yearly for all children 6 to 59 mo[k] (children ≥5 y of age may receive the intranasal vaccine)									

[a]Infants born to mothers positive for hepatitis B surface antigen (HBsAg) should receive HBV(1) and hepatitis B immunoglobulin within 12 hours of birth. Infants born to mothers of unknown HBsAg status should receive HBV(1) within 12 hours of birth, followed by hepatitis B immunoglobulin by 1 week of age if the maternal screening obtained at delivery demonstrates that she is HBsAg-positive.

[b]Children younger than 7 years of age who have a contraindication to receiving the acellular pertussis vaccine may receive the pediatric diphtheria-tetanus combination DT. The adult formulation (dT) is not appropriate for use in this population.

[c]DTaP(4) may be administered as early as 12 months of age or 6 months after the third dose if the child is unlikely to return for reimmunization at age 15 to 18 months.

[d]After Tdap (an adolescent formulation that serves as the sixth immunization in the diphtheria-tetanus-pertussis series), the tetanus and diphtheria toxoids booster (Td) should be administered every 10 years, or at the time of a "dirty" injury if the last tetanus vaccination occurred >5 years previously.

[e]Five different polysaccharide conjugate Hib vaccines are available in the United States: HbOC (HibTITER): three-dose primary series with a booster dose at 12 to 15 months; PRP-T (ActHIB): three-dose primary series with a booster dose at 12 to 15 months; PRP-OMP (Pedvax HIB): two-dose primary series (2 and 4 months of age) with a booster dose at 12 to 15 months; TriHIBit (DPaP-Hib combinations vaccine): should not be used in the primary series but is appropriate as a booster; Comvax (hepatitis B-Hib combination vaccine): may be used to fulfill primary series requirements for both components of the vaccine as long as the doses are administered at ages older than 6 weeks. *No conjugate or combination Hib vaccine should be administered to any infant <6 weeks of age under any circumstances.*

[f]Poliovirus is acquired through fecal–oral transmission. Wild poliovirus has been eradicated from the United States and many parts of the world. Three doses of IPV confer life-long immunity to poliovirus in 99% of recipients. Vaccine-associated paralytic poliomyelitis (VAPP) is an exceedingly rare complication of the oral poliovirus vaccine (which is no longer used in the United States). No serious reactions to IPV, including VAPP, have been reported.

[g]Any child who received MMR(1) before 12 months of age may not be adequately protected against measles.

[h]MMR(2) may be administered anytime beginning 4 weeks after the administration of MMR(1), but typically is administered at the 4- to 6-year visit.

[i]VAR(2) may be administered anytime beginning 4 weeks after the administration of VAR(1), but typically is administered at the 4- to 6-year visit.

[j]MCV(4) is indicated for adolescents at the routine 11- to 12-year health maintenance visit. The American Academy of Pediatrics also recommends MSV(4) vaccination for any 15-year-old adolescent entering high school or any college student living in a dormitory who was not inoculated at the 11- to 12-year health maintenance visit as described above.

[k]Children who are younger than 8 years of age who have not previously been vaccinated require two doses of the influenza vaccine (a minimum of 4 weeks apart) to be fully protected.

HBV, hepatitis B vaccine; DTaP, diphtheria and tetanus toxoids and acellular pertussis vaccine; Tdap, tetanus and diphtheria toxoids and acellular pertussis vaccine (adolescent preparation); Hib: *Haemophilus influenzae* type b conjugate vaccine; IPV, inactivated poliovirus vaccine; PCV(7), heptavalent pneumococcal conjugate vaccine (effective against serotypes 4, 6B, 9V, 14, 18C, 19F, and 23F); HAV, hepatitis A vaccine; VAR, varicella vaccine; MCV(4), meningococcal conjugate vaccine (effective against serotypes A, C, Y, and W-135, which cause about 75% of meningococcal disease in adolescents).

TABLE 3-2
IMMUNIZATION CATCHUP SCHEDULES

	Minimum Age at First Dose	Minimum Interval Between Doses 1 and 2	Minimum Interval Between Doses 2 and 3	Minimum Interval Between Doses 3 and 4	Minimum Interval Between Doses 4 and 5
Hepatitis B[a]	Birth	4 wk	8 wk (with a minimum of 16 wk between doses 1 and 3)		
Diphtheria, tetanus, pertussis (ages 4 mo to 6 y)	6 wk	4 wk	4 wk	6 mo	6 mo[b]
Diphtheria, tetanus, pertussis (ages 7 to 18 y)		4 wk	6 mo	6 mo (if DTaP1 administered before 1 y of age and patient is currently ≥11 y old; otherwise 5-y minimum interval)	
Haemophilus influenzae type b[c] (if first dose is given at younger than 12 mo of age)	6 wk; unnecessary in children older than 5 y of age	4 wk	4 wk if younger than 12 mo of age; 8 wk if given as final dose	8 wk (only necessary if Hib1, 2, and 3 all given when child is younger than 12 mo of age)	
Haemophilus influenzae type b (if first dose is given at 12 to 24 mo of age)		8 wk			
Poliovirus (inactivated)	6 wk	4 wk	4 wk	4 wk	
Pneumococcal[d]	6 wk	4 wk, or 8 wk if second dose is final dose	4 wk, or 8 wk if third dose is final dose	8 wk	
Measles, mumps, rubella	12 mo	4 wk			
Varicella	12 mo	4 wk			
Meningococcal conjugate	One dose needed; if not administered at age 11 to 12 y, should be given at entry to high school (15 y); should be administered to college freshmen living in dormitories if not previously vaccinated				

[a]A two-dose hepatitis B virus vaccination series has been approved for use in patients 11 to 15 years of age.
[b]If DTaP4 is administered after the child turns 4 years old, a fifth dose is not needed.
[c]Once a dose of Hib has been administered when the child is ≥15 months of age, no further doses are needed.
[d]Once a dose of pneumococcal conjugate vaccine has been administered when the child is ≥24 months of age, no further doses are needed.
HBV, hepatitis B vaccine; DTaP, diphtheria and tetanus toxoids and acellular pertussis vaccine; Hib: *Haemophilus influenzae* type b conjugate vaccine.

In general, live vaccines (measles, mumps, rubella and varicella vaccines) are contraindicated in patients who are severely immunocompromised (particularly those with inherited or acquired cell-mediated/T-cell immunodeficiencies), on long-term, high-dose corticosteroid therapy, or pregnant. The risk of congenital vaccine-associated rubella syndrome is merely theoretical and has never been reported. An exception is that patients with human immunodeficiency virus who are not severely compromised, even if they are symptomatic, should receive measles, mumps, rubella and varicella vaccines. Patients who are immunocompromised may have suboptimal responses to other vaccinations.

There is no reliable way to determine whether a child adopted from a foreign country has been adequately immunized short of revaccination or serologic studies. Written documentation is supportive and often correct but not definitive. In most cases, it is less expensive to vaccinate the child in the United States according to the catchup schedule listed in Table 3-2. Hepatitis B vaccination is an exception; serologies are preferred.

TABLE 3-3
VACCINATION CONTRAINDICATIONS AND PRECAUTIONS

Absolute Contraindications	Precautions (relative contraindications)
Severe allergic reaction (e.g., anaphylaxis) after previous vaccine dose	Shock/hyporesponsive episode ≤48 h after previous dose of DTaP[a]
Severe allergic reaction to a known component of a vaccine	Fever >40.5°C within 48 h of previous dose of DTaP[a]
Encephalopathy within 7 d of administration of a previous dose (DTaP)[a]	Seizure ≤3 d after previous dose of DTaP[a]
Pregnancy (MMR; varicella)	Moderate-to-severe acute illness with or without fever

[a]Contraindication or precaution pertains only to DTaP. Administering a decreased volume of the DTaP vaccine is never appropriate; rather, a decision should be made to administer or withhold the vaccine based on information listed in the table.
DTaP, diphtheria, tetanus, and acellular pertussis vaccine.

Information regarding vaccination recommended before foreign travel can be found listed by country at the Centers for Disease Control and Prevention's Web site (www.cdc.gov). True contraindications to vaccination are rare (Table 3-3). Of note, patients with severe sensitivity to egg protein should not receive the inactivated influenza vaccine. Other egg-based vaccines, such as measles and mumps, are believed to be safe for these patients.

SCREENING PROCEDURES

Screening involves testing apparently healthy individuals or populations for disease. Screening tests are generally chosen as such because:

- The disease they are testing for is relatively serious.
- The disease they are testing for is relatively common.
- The disease they are testing for has a preclinical stage that may be affected by early treatment.
- The test is easy and inexpensive to perform.
- The test has a low risk-to-benefit ratio.
- The test results are clear and not subject to interpretation.

Examples of disorders that are screened for in the pediatric population include hypertension, anemia, lead poisoning, hearing loss, vision impairment, and elevated cholesterol/lipid levels. Screening studies recommended in adolescents are discussed in Chapter 24.

Blood Pressure

The American Academy of Pediatrics recommends that routine blood pressure measurement be performed in all children ≥3 years of age at every health maintenance visit. Measurement should be undertaken after several minutes of rest in a patient sitting with the arm at the level of the heart. The cuff bladder width should cover about 70% to 80% of the acromian–olecranon distance, with the bladder completely encircling the arm. Patients with systolic and diastolic measurements that average <90th percentile for age, gender, and height have "normal" blood pressure. That is, their blood pressure does not place them at any increased risk for atherosclerosis, diabetes, coronary and cerebrovascular diseases, or end-stage renal disease. Patients who have measurements that average between the 90th and 95th percentiles are considered "borderline." Readings in the >95th percentile signify "significant" hypertension, and those in the >99th percentile are termed "severe." At least three separate reliable blood pressure measurements should be assessed before the patient is given the diagnosis of *hypertension*.

Hematocrit

Iron-deficiency anemia is the most common nutritional deficiency in the United States, occurring most frequently in children 1 to 3 years of age. Iron deficiency adversely affects cognitive development, so diagnosis is particularly important in infants and young children. Currently, the American Academy of Pediatrics recommends screening patients for anemia once between 9 and 12 months of age, with additional screening for "at-risk" patients (e.g., those with high milk intakes) 1 to 5 years of age. An alternative approach would be to limit the first screening to infants who are not on iron-fortified formula, with additional testing for all patients at ages 2 and 3 years. Screening hemoglobin (or hematocrit) levels will reveal children who have anemia (iron deficiency or otherwise) but cannot identify the child who is iron deficient but not yet anemic.

Healthy full-term infants are born with high hemoglobin levels that decrease to a *physiologic nadir* of about 9.5 g per dL at 10 to 12 weeks before climbing to typical childhood levels. This is a normal process that neither requires nor responds to iron therapy. Hemoglobin levels in preterm infants decrease further and faster than those of their full-term peers and may require intervention.

Lead

Lead poisoning is an ideal condition for which to screen given its lack of early symptoms, its harmful effect on cognitive development at preclinical levels, and its amenability to treatment. *The great majority of affected children are asymptomatic.* Early symptoms of lead poisoning can include irritability, hyperactivity, apathy, decreased play, anorexia, intermittent abdominal pain, constipation, and occasional vomiting. Children with mild, chronically elevated lead levels may manifest only developmental delay, behavioral problems, attention disorders, or poor school performance. *Acute encephalopathy*, characterized by increased intracranial pressure, vomiting, ataxia, confusion, seizures, and coma, is the most serious complication of severe lead poisoning. The principal source of lead exposure is the presence of lead-based paint in older homes; children may eat the flaking paint but more commonly ingest lead-contaminated household dust or soil.

Children ages 9 months to 6 years should be assessed for an increased risk of lead exposure with a questionnaire developed by the Centers for Disease Control and Prevention (2001). Current recommendations vary depending on practice location, with most areas under "universal screening" coverage, which involves testing all children at the ages of 12 and 24 months. Research is underway to determine how to better define and target high-risk groups and decrease the number of tests performed on the general population. New recommendations are due in late 2007.

Many offices screen for elevated blood lead levels by performing a capillary micro-lead measurement. Any capillary blood level ≥10 μg per dL must be confirmed by a venous blood lead test due to a relatively high false-positive rate. Although there is no direct correlation between blood levels and morbidity, levels of 10 to 19 μg per dL are considered borderline, and the term "lead poisoning" is reserved for levels ≥20 μg per dL. Cognitive effects may result from levels <10 μg per dL; lead is not naturally present in the human body, and no lead level has even been defined as "safe."

The management of increased blood lead levels is provided in Table 3-4. Symptomatic children should be removed to a lead-free environment and treated with chelation therapy immediately. Children with levels between 45 and 69 μg per dL may be treated with inpatient intravenous calcium-disodium ethylenediaminetetra-acetic acid or outpatient oral succimer (DMSA). Intramuscular dimercaprol (BAL) is added to ethylenediaminetetra-acetic acid for the inpatient (required) treatment of children with levels >70 μg per dL. A rebound increase in blood lead levels occurs even in the absence of lead exposure, due to the release of lead from bone stores. Although the direct benefits in lead poisoning are unproven, many treatment centers recommend optimizing the patient's iron and calcium intake through diet and/or supplementation. All children with elevated blood lead levels should receive neurodevelopmental screening.

TABLE 3-4
MANAGEMENT OF ELEVATED BLOOD LEAD LEVELS IN ASYMPTOMATIC CHILDREN

Venous Lead Level	Recommendations
10 to 14 μg per dL	Risk reduction and nutritional education
15 to 19 μg per dL	Risk reduction and nutritional education, plus repeat test in 1 to 3 mo
	Coordinate home inspection and other services with local lead poisoning prevention programs
	If still elevated at 3 mo, consider abdominal radiography and bowel decontamination
20 to 44 μg per dL	As above, plus consider abdominal radiography/decontamination at initial elevation
45 to 69 μg per dL	As above, plus chelation therapy within 48 h
	Consider obtaining free erythrocyte protoporphyrin or zinc protoporphyrin level to help assess response to treatment
≥70 μg per dL	As above, with immediate inpatient chelation therapy

Vision

In pediatrics, detection of strabismus and other conditions leading to amblyopia and vision impairment is the goal of vision screening. Children ≥3 years of age should be examined for ocular alignment (using the unilateral cover test) and tested for visual acuity (Snellen chart, or modified for younger children) at every health maintenance visit. Ophthalmoscopic examination of the retina is also recommended at each visit. Ocular alignment may be evaluated in younger children by comparing left and right corneal light reflexes. Photoscreening techniques permit the screening of children younger than 3 years of age and may improve detection of subtle abnormalities in older children. Indications for referral are discussed in Chapter 22.

Hearing

The American Academy of Pediatrics recommends universal newborn screening for hearing loss before hospital discharge and intervention, if necessary, before 6 months of age. Tests appropriate for newborn screening are described in Chapter 5. The American Speech-Language-Hearing Association recommends hearing screens be performed upon entry into school (kindergarten) and yearly through third grade, with additional screens conducted in grades 7 and 11. Hearing impairment is discussed in detail in Chapter 23.

Cholesterol/Lipids

Atherosclerosis, the accumulation of vascular fatty plaques that lead to coronary artery disease, begins in childhood. Low-density lipoproteins (LDLs) are the principal component of atherosclerotic plaques. Figure 3-1 provides an algorithm for screening children at increased risk for elevated cholesterol

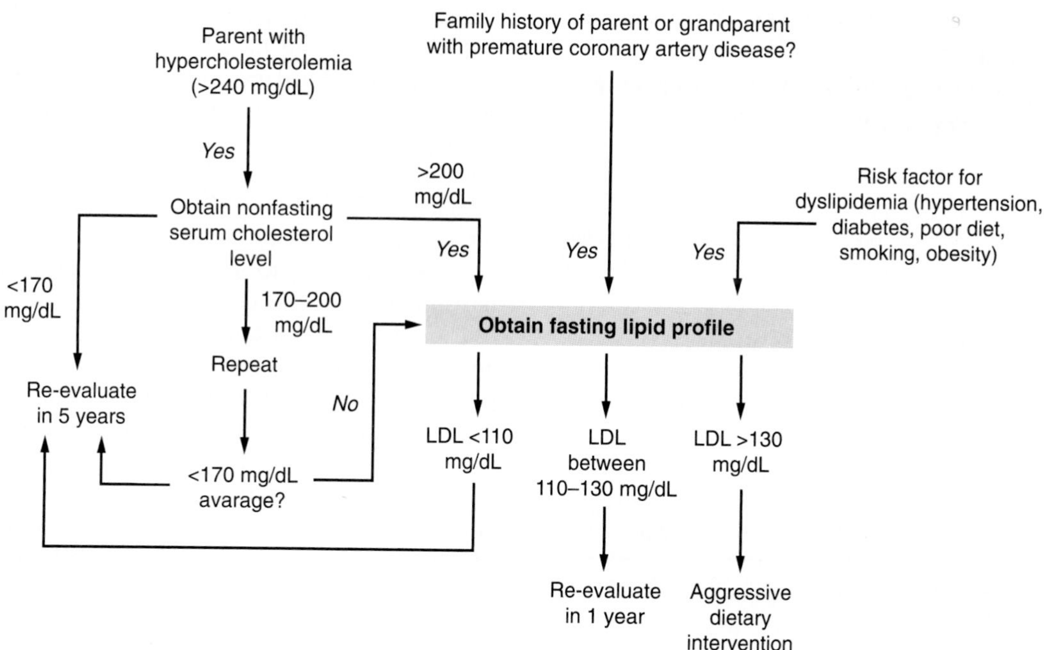

Figure 3-1 Evaluation of patients at risk for elevated cholesterol/lipid levels.

and/or lipid levels. A nonfasting cholesterol level alone is an appropriate initial screen in patients without a family history of premature coronary artery disease (PrCAD). Those with a family history of PrCAD or familial disorders associated with extremely high cholesterol levels should receive a fasting lipid profile, which allows fractionation of LDL, high-density lipoprotein (HDL), and triglycerides to identify dyslipidemias (e.g., low HDL, high triglyceride levels) in children with normal total cholesterol levels.

Aggressive dietary therapy is recommended in patients with LDL levels >130 mg per dL. Medication is reserved for older patients with a high risk of PrCAD in whom dietary therapy has failed.

Patients with extremely high cholesterol levels (>300 mg/dL) may have an underlying genetic abnormality such as *familial hypercholesterolemia* (FH), an autosomal dominant condition. FH and other genetic conditions that interfere with lipoprotein metabolism greatly increase a patient's risk of death from PrCAD. Clinical manifestations of FH are uncommon but may include tendinous (most common), cutaneous, or palpebral xanthomas and arcus corneae, a gray-white ring of cholesterol deposition at the corneal margin. Cholesterol levels are elevated even in the first year of life, and dietary and pharmacologic interventions should begin as soon as the hypercholesterolemia is diagnosed.

DISEASE PREVENTION

Counseling regarding disease prevention involves educating the patient and family about how they can lower the child's future risk of developing heart disease, osteoporosis, respiratory tract illnesses, and skin cancer. Risk factors associated with the development of coronary artery disease are listed in Figure 3-1. Appropriate dietary choices and regular weight-bearing exercise modify the risk of heart disease and osteoporosis. As a group, children who are exposed to cigarette smoke in the home have more frequent and severe episodes of respiratory illness than their peers in nonsmoking households. Respiratory irritation may also be caused by animal dander, wood-burning stoves, and aerosol sprays. Cumulative sun exposure increases the risk of skin cancer. Infants younger than 6 months of age should be kept out of the sun, their skin covered by hats or clothing, and a small amount of sunscreen applied to exposed areas. Parents should limit their children's exposure between 10:00 a.m. and 4:00 p.m. and apply sunscreen with a sun protection factor of ≥15, even on cloudy days.

ANTICIPATORY GUIDANCE

Injury

Traumatic injury is the most significant cause of morbidity and mortality in the pediatric population. Parents should be counseled regarding ways they can lower the risk of injuries and death from head trauma, motor vehicle accidents, falls, recreational sporting injuries, burns, drowning, and firearms.

Traumatic injuries sustained as an occupant in motor vehicle crashes are the number one cause of death in children and adolescents. Children ≤12 years of age should be properly restrained in the back seat, in a safety seat if

TABLE 3-5
RECOMMENDATIONS FOR THE PROPER USE OF CHILD SAFETY SEATS

Age	Birth to 12 mo[a]
Weight	<20 lb[a]
Recommendation	Infant-only seat in the rear-facing position and the infant at approximately 45° angle
Age	≥12 mo
Weight	20 to 40 lb
Recommendation	Forward-facing safety seat with harness straps at or above the shoulders
Age	4 to 8 y
Weight	40 to 80 lb
Recommendation	Forward-facing booster seat with lap belt low and tight across lap and shoulder belt across chest and shoulder

[a]Infant should be 12 months of age AND weigh 20 lb before the safety seat is turned to the front-facing position.

indicated based on age and weight (Table 3-5). Infants born before 37 weeks of gestation undergo a 1- to 2-hour period of observation in their car safety seats before discharge to monitor for episodes of apnea, bradycardia, or oxygen desaturation related to positioning.

Falls result in more preadolescent pediatric emergency department visits than any other injury. Parents should be advised about stair safety, gating, and avoiding the use of walkers.

Injuries sustained in accidents involving bicycles, scooters, rollerblades, and skateboards are a significant cause of head trauma, disability, and death in pediatric patients. Children on bicycles may collide with automobiles or other objects, or the rider may lose control and fall. Overall, proper helmet use decreases the risk and severity of head trauma. Helmets should also be considered for other recreational activities as listed above.

Residential fires are a preventable source of pediatric accidental death. Families should be counseled about smoking cessation and maintenance of functional smoke detectors (e.g., changing batteries every 6 months). Scald injuries can be prevented by setting hot water heaters to ≤120°F and keeping hot liquids on the back stove burner or otherwise out of a child's reach.

Drowning is a regrettably frequent cause of mortality in the pediatric population. Incidence peaks in the older infant/toddler age group and again in adolescence. Rates are twice as high in blacks and three times higher in boys. Bathtubs are the most common site of drowning in the first year of life. Large buckets and residential pools are particularly dangerous for toddlers, whereas natural water sources account for most adolescent injuries. Toddlers and young children must be supervised at all times while in the bathtub or around pools or other bodies of water. Residential and commercial swimming pools should be fenced in (with unscalable fences) and have locked gates. Isolation fencing (fencing limited to the immediate pool area) is more effective than perimeter property fencing. Each person participating in boating activities should wear a personal flotation device, with alcohol use prohibited. Cardiopulmonary resuscitation training is available to parents through the American Heart Association and many area hospitals. Learning to swim is an important preventive measure but does not take the place of close supervision.

Almost half of all homes in the United States contain guns. Although many gun owners say that they have a gun primarily to protect themselves and their families, the presence of a gun in the home actually increases the risk of firearm death in family members. Family members in homes with guns are three times as likely to die of homicide and five times as likely to commit suicide by shooting themselves. Many of these guns used for "protection" are kept loaded and within easy reach, where they may be found by young children. Families should be made aware of their increased risk. If they still choose to own a gun, the gun should have a trigger lock and must be kept unloaded and locked away separate from ammunition.

Poisoning

Physicians should discuss poisoning at the 6-month health maintenance visit, before infants gain mobility. All poisonous substances should be stored in their original containers in locked cabinets or otherwise out of reach of children. Parents should request and purchase medications with child-resistant caps whenever possible and post the telephone number of their poison control center in a prominent place. Syrup of ipecac is no longer recommended for the management of poisonings at home. The presentations, identification, and management of poisonings that occur in the pediatric population are discussed in Chapter 4.

Bites and Stings

Animal bites are most common in children younger than 10 years of age. The majority of children are bitten by a dog that is familiar to them. Pit bulls and Rottweilers account for about half of all dog bites, and male dogs are more likely to bite than female ones. Programs that educate children about how to tell if a dog should be avoided (growling, feeding, etc.) are of questionable benefit. If the family chooses to own a dog, they can lower their risk by choosing a breed that is less likely to be aggressive.

Parents should be reminded to check their children for ticks after playing, walking, or camping in grassy or wooded areas. Virtually every parent will have to remove a tick from their child at one time or another. The tick should be grasped firmly in a pair of tweezers and lifted directly up off the skin with slow, steady pressure. Excessive pressure can result in the regurgitation of the tick's infected body fluids into the site of attachment. Scratching the tick off the site rather than lifting up may separate the tick, leaving mouth parts behind in the skin break. Burning and suffocation of the tick should also be avoided.

Insect stings are painful and may result in marked swelling. Some patients are highly allergic to stings by certain insects. Honeybees, yellow jackets, hornets, wasps, and fire ants are responsible for most Hymenoptera stings.

- Honeybees (native and africanized) are not aggressive. They will sting if trapped or stepped on. They are attracted to sweet substances and sweat. They sting only once before they die and may leave the stinger behind.
- Yellow jackets have characteristic yellow and black stripes. They are most aggressive in late summer and early fall, particularly if their ground nest is disturbed, and can sting multiple times.
- Hornets nest in trees or bushes and are extremely aggressive if the nest is disturbed or even shaken by vibrations from a mower or power tool.
- Fire ants are found mostly in the Southeast and South Central states. They move quickly, can sting multiple times, and are aggressive if their hill is disturbed.

After removing the patient to a safe place, the stinger (if present) should be removed by scraping it out with a plastic edge or card. The area should then be cleaned. A cool compress may provide symptomatic relief. Topical antihistamines are best avoided. Emergency medical personnel should be summoned for any person who develops difficulty breathing, widespread hives, or systemic skin flushing in response to a sting. The patient with a history of anaphylaxis to stings should wear a medical alert bracelet and carry an epinephrine autoinjector, even if skin and in vitro antibody testing are negative. The EpiPen is suitable for patients who weigh >30 kg; the EpiPen Jr. is reserved for patients weighing 15 to 30 kg. The patient and caretakers should know where (anterolateral area of the thigh) and how to use the injector.

SOURCES

Advisory Committee on Immunization Practices. *Recommended vaccination schedules*. 2007. Available at: www.cdc.gov/nip/acip.

American Academy of Pediatrics Committee on Practice and Ambulatory Medicine, Section on Ophthalmology. Vision screening guidelines. *Pediatrics*. 1996;98:156.

Belay B, Belamarich P, Racine AD. Pediatric precursors of adult atherosclerosis. *Pediatr Rev*. 2004;25:4–15.

Centers for Disease Control and Prevention. Managing elevated blood lead levels among young children: recommendations from the Advisory Committee on Childhood Lead Poisoning Prevention. *Pediatrics*. 1998;101:1072–1078.

Howard J, Loiselle J. A clinician's guide to safe and effective tick removal. *Contemp Pediatr*. 2006;23:36–41.

Johnston BD, Rivara FP. Injury control: new challenges. *Pediatr Rev*. 2003;24:111–118.

Krakowski AC, Golden DB. Hymenoptera stings: a practical guide to prevention and management. *Contemp Pediatr*. 2006;23:30–37.

Laraque D, Trasande L. Lead poisoning: successes and 21st century challenges. *Pediatr Rev*. 2005;26:435–443.

Norwood VF. Hypertension. *Pediatr Rev*. 2002;23:197–209.

Segel GB, Hirsh MG, Feig SA. Managing anemia in pediatric office practice: part 1. *Pediatr Rev*. 2002;23:75–84.

Sokol J, Hyde M. Hearing screening. *Pediatr Rev*. 2002;23:155–162.

QUESTIONS

1. You are seeing an 11-year-old girl for her first regular health maintenance visit since the age of 9 years. She has received four diphtheria-tetanus-pertussis (DTaP) vaccines, four poliovirus vaccines, and three measles-mumps-rubella vaccines. She was vaccinated against hepatitis A due to foreign travel at the age of 10 years by the health department. She has no reliable history of chicken pox and has not been vaccinated against varicella. This patient should be offered which of the following vaccines at this visit?

A) Hepatitis B, DTaP, meningococcal conjugate, human papillomavirus
B) Hepatitis B, DTaP, meningococcal polysaccharide, human papillomavirus
C) Hepatitis B, DTaP, meningococcal conjugate, human papillomavirus, varicella
D) Hepatitis B, DTaP, meningococcal polysaccharide, human papillomavirus, varicella
E) Hepatitis B, tetanus-diphtheria, meningococcal conjugate, human papillomavirus, varicella

2. A woman with no prenatal care delivers a female term newborn weighing 3.2 kg. The baby transitions well and has no anomalies. No maternal prenatal laboratory results are available. By 12 hours of age, this neonate should receive which of the following?

A) Hepatitis B vaccine and hepatitis B immune globulin
B) Hepatitis B vaccine, with hepatitis B immune globulin to follow by 1 week of age if the mother is found to be HBsAg-positive
C) Hepatitis B vaccine and interferon
D) Hepatitis B vaccine and gancyclovir
E) Hepatitis B immune globulin, with hepatitis B vaccine to follow at 1 month of age

3. A preterm infant weighing 1,200 g is born at 28 weeks of gestation to an HBsAg-positive mother. The infant receives the hepatitis B vaccine and hepatitis B immune globulin within 12 hours of birth. What is the most appropriate schedule for completion of the hepatitis B vaccination series in this infant?

A) A second dose at 2,000 g OR 4 weeks after the first and a third dose 12 weeks after the second.

B) A second dose 4 weeks after the first and a third dose 12 weeks after the second.
C) A second dose at 2,000 g, a third dose 4 weeks after the second, and a fourth dose 12 weeks after the third.
D) A second dose 4 weeks after the first, a third dose 4 weeks after the second, and a fourth dose 12 weeks after the third.
E) This child does not need another hepatitis B vaccine because the first vaccine was given in conjunction with hepatitis B immune globulin.

4. A 3-year-old patient is referred to your office from the emergency department after stitches for a facial injury sustained at his brother's baseball game. Before removing the stitches, you review the patient's immunization records and note that he has had two hepatitis B vaccines, three DTaP vaccines, three *Haemophilus influenzae* type b (Hib) vaccines, three poliovirus vaccines, and one measles-mumps-rubella vaccine. The patient received an additional DTaP vaccine in the emergency department. Which of the following collections of vaccinations is most appropriate for the patient at this visit?
A) Hepatitis B, Hib, hepatitis A, and measles-mumps-rubella
B) Hepatitis B, Hib, hepatitis A, and poliovirus
C) Hepatitis B, Hib, measles-mumps-rubella, and varicella
D) Hepatitis B, Hib, hepatitis A, and varicella
E) Hepatitis B, hepatitis A, and varicella

5. A 15-year-old female patient is up-to-date with all her immunizations, except that she has never been vaccinated against varicella and has no clinical history of disease. She agrees to receive a varicella vaccination today. You are correct in informing her of which of the following?
A) She is now up-to-date on all her vaccinations.
B) The soonest that she can return for her next varicella vaccination is 16 weeks from today.
C) The soonest that she can return for her next varicella vaccination is 12 weeks from today.
D) The soonest that she can return for her next varicella vaccination is 8 weeks from today.
E) The soonest that she can return for her next varicella vaccination is 4 weeks from today.

6. Which of the following patients who has never had a meningococcal vaccine should not receive the meningococcal conjugate vaccine?
A) A 2-year-old boy with functional asplenia
B) A 15-year-old boy who is entering high school this year
C) An 18-year-old man who is entering college and will be living in a dormitory
D) A 13-year-old boy who has a close friend with invasive infection due to serotype Y *Neisseria meningitidis*
E) A 12-year-old boy in the office for his regular health maintenance visit

7. You are seeing a 15-month-old former full-term infant for her regular health maintenance visit. She is due to be vaccinated against DTaP, poliovirus, measles-mumps-rubella, and hepatitis A. The soonest that she can receive her next hepatitis A vaccine is at which of the following ages?
A) 18 months
B) 21 months
C) 24 months
D) 36 months
E) 4 to 5 years

8. You are seeing a 15-month-old male patient for a regular health maintenance visit. The child and his family have recently moved to your area and missed their 12-month well-child care visit. The toddler has received two doses of the Hib vaccine. After administering an additional dose at today's visit, you note in the child's chart that he can receive his final Hib dose at which of the following ages?
A) 18 months
B) 21 months
C) Today's Hib vaccination is the final dose needed for this patient.
D) 24 months
E) 36 months

9. Which of the following is an absolute contraindication to receiving the DTaP vaccine?
A) Fever >40.5°C after administration of a previous DTaP vaccine
B) Development of a hyporesponsive episode <48 hours after administration of a previous DTaP vaccine
C) Development of shock <48 hours after administration of a previous DTaP vaccine
D) Encephalopathy within 7 days of administration of a previous dose of DTaP
E) Seizure 2 days after a previous DTaP vaccine

10. A 9-month-old female infant who has been hospitalized twice due to wheezing and respiratory distress presents to your office for an influenza vaccination. Which of the following statements regarding this patient is FALSE?
A) She should return for a second dose in 1 month.
B) She should receive vaccination against influenza yearly until age 6 years or until she is no longer at increased risk for more severe disease (whichever occurs later).
C) She will only require a single dose of influenza vaccine to be fully protected next year.
D) Close contacts of this patient should be vaccinated against influenza.
E) The intranasal influenza vaccine is an appropriate option for this patient.

11. Vaccination against influenza is recommended for all of the following patients EXCEPT:

A) A 5-month-old with sickle cell disease
B) The primary caretaker of a healthy 4-month-old former full-term infant
C) A healthy male 6-month-old former full-term infant
D) A healthy female 4-year-old infant
E) A 9-month-old with bronchopulmonary dysplasia

12. The 23-valent pneumococcal vaccine is recommended at the present visit for all but which of the following patients?

A) A 2-year-old with sickle cell disease who has completed her initial PCV7 vaccine series
B) A 15-month-old who has received three doses of pneumococcal vaccine
C) A 2-year-old with splenic dysfunction who has completed her initial PCV7 vaccine
D) A 24-month-old with human immunodeficiency virus who has received one dose of PCV7 vaccine
E) A 5-year-old with chronic nephritis who has completed her initial PCV7 vaccine series

13. A 5-year-old boy adopted from Guatemala is brought to your office for his initial postadoption visit. According to the child's vaccination records, he is up to date on his hepatitis B, DTaP, poliovirus, and measles-mumps-rubella vaccinations; however, the 2-month, 4-month, and 6-month visits each occurred on the 31st day of the month in April, June, and August. Which of the following is the most appropriate vaccination for which to check titers before automatic revaccination?

A) Measles-mumps-rubella
B) Poliovirus
C) Hepatitis B
D) Pertussis
E) Diphtheria-tetanus

14. A 15-month-old Hispanic male patient is leaving the country with his parents who are being deported to Ecuador. He is currently up to date on his vaccinations. If he receives his first measles-mumps-rubella vaccination today, when can receive a second dose?

A) At age 4 years
B) At age 5 years
C) At age 24 months
D) In 4 weeks
E) In 8 weeks

15. An 18-year-old patient tells you that she is considering having a child with her boyfriend. After counseling her about the risks of teenage pregnancy to herself and the child, you review her immunization records and note that she has never been vaccinated against varicella and has no clinical history of disease. Which of the following is your best advice to this patient regarding varicella vaccination?

A) To wait until after delivery before considering vaccination
B) To wait to see if she conceives before considering varicella vaccination
C) To receive one dose of the varicella vaccine today and one dose in 6 months before discontinuing birth control the following month
D) To receive one dose of the varicella vaccine today and wait one month before discontinuing birth control
E) To receive one dose of the varicella vaccine today and one dose in 4 weeks before discontinuing birth control the following month

16. With the exception of the hepatitis B vaccine, preterm infants should be vaccinated on a schedule that is:

A) based on their chronological age
B) based on their gestational age
C) based on their weight
D) based on their chronological age and weight
E) based on their gestational age and weight

17. Vaccination against varicella should be avoided in all the following patients EXCEPT:

A) A 12-month-old who is severely immunocompromised.
B) A 12-month-old with human immunodeficiency virus who is symptomatic but not significantly compromised
C) A 5-year-old on chronic oral steroid therapy
D) A 17-year-old girl pregnant with her second child
E) Vaccination against varicella should be avoided in all of the above patients.

18. Which of the following statements regarding patients with egg protein allergy is correct?

A) These patients should not receive the hepatitis A vaccine.
B) These patients can receive the trivalent inactivated influenza vaccine even though it is egg-based.
C) These patients can receive the measles-mumps-rubella vaccine even though it is egg-based.
D) These patients should be tested for allergies to other vaccine components before being vaccinated.
E) These patients should be retested for egg protein allergy before each set of vaccinations.

19. Which of the following is not a characteristic of screening tests?

A) They test for a disease that is relatively common.
B) They test for a disease that is relatively serious (or has relatively serious complications).
C) They are relatively inexpensive.
D) They are sensitive and specific based on individual interpretation of the results.
E) They have a low risk-to-benefit ratio.

20. A 9-year-old obese female patient in the office for her regular health maintenance visit has a diastolic blood pressure at the 95th percentile for age, height, and gender. Which of the following is the most appropriate course of action at this time?

A) Referral to a cardiologist
B) A prescription for nifedipine
C) A prescription for hydralazine
D) Counseling regarding healthy diet and weight-bearing exercise and rechecking the blood pressure in 1 year
E) Rechecking the blood pressure in 1 week

21. All of the following are true for a male adolescent with normal blood pressure for age, height, and gender EXCEPT:

A) Systolic and diastolic measurements are between the 85th and 95th percentiles.
B) The patient's blood pressure does not place him at increased risk for atherosclerosis.
C) The patient's blood pressure does not place him at increased risk for cerebrovascular disease.
D) The patient's blood pressure does not place him at increased risk for diabetes.
E) The patient's blood pressure does not place him at increased risk for end-stage renal disease.

22. Which of the following statements regarding iron deficiency and anemia is TRUE?

A) Physiologic anemia of infancy is normal and does not need to be treated, but theoretically would respond to iron supplementation.
B) Iron-deficiency anemia is the most common nutritional deficiency of childhood.
C) A screening hemoglobin level at 9 to 12 months of age will reveal children who are deficient in iron.
D) Patients should be screened for iron deficiency anemia at age 9 to 12 months and again as needed at ages 1 to 5 years if they are considered "at risk."
E) As a group, adolescents have the highest incidence of iron-deficiency anemia.

23. A 24-month-old male patient in your office for his regular health maintenance visit has the following results on screening tests: hemoglobin 9.6 g per dL, capillary blood lead level 16 μg per dL. He lives in Section 8 housing in poor repair built before 1960. Which of the following is the most appropriate next course of action?

A) Counsel the family regarding lead removal and recheck the level in 6 months.
B) Refer the family to the local governmental lead management agency.
C) Obtain a venous lead level for confirmation.
D) Start the patient on oral succimer on an outpatient basis.
E) Obtain neurodevelopmental testing for the patient.

24. A 5-year-old patient with mental retardation and pica begins accompanying his father to work at an outdoor shooting range in the summer. Three months later his father brings him to your office with acute-onset vomiting and "not making sense." The father has also noticed that the patient has been unsteady on his feet for the past few days. The child's hemoglobin is 8.8 g per dL, and the red blood cells are hypochromic and microcytic. The blood lead level is 72 μg per dL. Which of the following represents the most appropriate treatment for this patient?

A) Inpatient oral succimer
B) Calcium disodium ethylenediaminetetra-acetic acid (EDTA)
C) Intramuscular dimercaprol
D) EDTA and dimercaprol
E) EDTA and hemodialysis

25. Which of the following complaints is most common in children with elevated blood lead levels?

A) Constipation
B) Pallor
C) Attention-deficit disorder
D) Poor school performance
E) No symptoms

26. Physicians who do not live in areas with high rates of lead poisoning use questionnaires developed by the American Academy of Pediatrics and the Centers for Disease Control and Prevention to screen children for increased risk of lead exposure. Which of the following screening questions identifies the most children at increased risk for elevated blood lead levels?

A) Does your child spend a significant amount of time in a home built before 1960, or in a home built before 1980 with recent or ongoing renovation?
B) Does your child frequently come in contact with someone who works with or has a hobby involving exposure to lead?
C) Does your child live near a heavily traveled street or highway?
D) Does your child have pica behavior?
E) Does your child exhibit any of the following symptoms more than three times a week: constipation, irritability, behavior problems, difficulties in school?

27. Which of the following is not a specifically recommended vision screening test for all children older than 3 years of age at every health maintenance visit?

A) Unilateral cover test
B) Corneal light reflex test
C) Visual acuity testing with Snellen chart
D) Ophthalmoscopic examination of the retina
E) All of the above are recommended for vision screening of children ≥3 years of age.

28. You are visiting a new 17-year-old mother in the hospital. She had good prenatal care and has delivered a healthy full-term infant. She does not have insurance for the infant and is interested in postponing the newborn hearing screen until she is sure that the baby will be covered by his father's insurance. In educating the mother about this screening test, you tell her that the American Academy of Pediatrics recommends which of the following in all infants?

A) Completion of a newborn hearing screen within the first month of life and intervention in cases of hearing impairment before the infant is 3 months of age
B) Completion of a newborn hearing screen before discharge and intervention in cases of hearing impairment before the infant is 3 months of age
C) Completion of a newborn hearing screen before discharge and intervention in cases of hearing impairment before the infant is 6 months of age
D) Completion of a newborn hearing screen before discharge and intervention in cases of hearing impairment before the infant is 9 months of age
E) Completion of a newborn hearing screen before discharge and intervention in cases of hearing impairment before the infant is 12 months of age

29. A female newborn has failed a hearing test in the newborn nursery. Which of the following is considered an appropriate second test for this infant?

A) Automated auditory brainstem response
B) Transient evoked otoacoustic emissions
C) Distortion product otoacoustic emissions
D) Visual reinforcement audiometry
E) All of the above are appropriate for a second test.

30. For which of the following patients is a nonfasting serum cholesterol concentration a sufficient screen for hypercholesterolemia?

A) A 15-year-old obese boy
B) A 15-year-old male smoker
C) A 15-year-old boy with type 2 diabetes
D) A 15-year-old boy whose maternal grandfather died of a heart attack at age 43 years but whose parents have normal serum cholesterol levels
E) A 15-year-old boy with no family history of premature coronary artery disease whose father has a serum cholesterol measurement of 250 mg per dL

31. A 13-year-old girl seen in your office this week for a health maintenance visit has a total nonfasting serum cholesterol level of 185 mg per dL. There is no family history of premature coronary artery disease, and she has no risk factors for dyslipidemia. A repeat cholesterol level is 190 mg per dL. Which of the following is the most appropriate next step in the management of this patient?

A) Obtain a fasting lipid profile and base further management on the LDL level.
B) Obtain a fasting lipid profile and base further management on the LDL:HDL ratio.
C) Provide counseling regarding diet and exercise and re-evaluate in 3 months.
D) Provide counseling regarding diet and exercise and re-evaluate in 6 months.
E) Provide counseling regarding diet and exercise and re-evaluate in 1 year.

32. A 16-year-old Caucasian male who was adopted at birth has a fasting serum cholesterol level of 427 mg per dL. Which of the following conditions is most consistent with this presentation?

A) Metabolic syndrome
B) Familial hypercholesterolemia
C) Body mass index at the 97th percentile
D) Smoking a pack of cigarettes a day
E) Essential hypertension

33. A 14-year-old girl with a questionable diet has a serum LDL level of 138 mg per dL on initial assessment. Which of the following is the most appropriate next course of action?

A) Recheck the fasting lipid profile in 6 months.
B) Recheck the fasting lipid profile in 1 year.
C) Aggressive dietary management
D) Pharmacologic management
E) Renal angiography

34. When present during adolescence, all of the following conditions increase the risk of coronary artery disease EXCEPT:

A) Hypertension
B) Type 2 diabetes
C) Obesity
D) Non–weight-bearing exercise
E) Smoking

35. The father of a 2-month-old healthy former full-term girl has recently been diagnosed with melanoma. While discussing this source of stress on the family with the girl's mother, she asks you what she can do to reduce her daughter's chances of developing skin cancer later in life. All of the following behaviors will help limit her daughter's risk EXCEPT:

A) Significantly limiting her daughter's exposure to sun before the age of 6 months
B) Covering her daughter's skin with a hat and clothing and applying sunscreen to exposed areas before the age of 6 months

C) Limiting her daughter's exposure to sun between the hours of 10:00 a.m. and 4:00 p.m. after the age of 6 months
D) Applying sunscreen with sun protection factor (SPF) of ≥15 daily, even on cloudy days
E) Yearly referral to a dermatologist beginning at puberty to evaluate moles for irregularity in color and size

36. Counseling regarding disease prevention involves educating the patient and family about how they can lower the child's future risk of developing heart disease, osteoporosis, respiratory tract illness, and skin cancer. Which of the following statements regarding disease prevention is FALSE?
A) Parents should apply sunscreen daily with an SPF of ≥30 on sunny days and sunscreen with an SPF of ≥15 on cloudy days.
B) Appropriate dietary choices and regular weight-bearing exercise modify the risk of developing heart disease and osteoporosis.
C) Risk factors associated with the development of coronary artery disease include dyslipidemia, hypertension, and obesity.
D) Respiratory irritation may be caused by animal dander, wood-burning stoves, and aerosol sprays.
E) As a group, children exposed to cigarette smoke at home have more episodes of respiratory illness than their peers from nonsmoking homes, and the respiratory illnesses they have are more severe.

37. Which of the following statements regarding injury in the pediatric population is TRUE?
A) Pedestrian injury is the most significant cause of morbidity and mortality in the pediatric population.
B) Helmet use is not required in most states for children who are participating in rollerblading and skateboarding activities.
C) Maintaining a gun in the home decreases the risk that a family member will die of homicide.
D) Hot water heater thermostats should be set at ≤140°F to prevent scald burn injuries in children.
E) Learning to swim is the most important preventive measure that can be taken to prevent pediatric accidental drowning.

38. Which of the following statements regarding pediatric drowning is INCORRECT?
A) Drowning rates are three times higher in boys than in girls.
B) The incidence of drowning peaks in the older infant/toddler age group and again in adolescence.
C) Perimeter fencing is more effective at preventing drowning death than isolation fencing.
D) Bathtubs are the most common site of drowning in the first year of life.
E) Patients who are pulled from the water with a pulse have a better prognosis than those who are initially pulseless.

39. All of the following are reliable predictors of patient outcome in cases of near drowning EXCEPT:
A) Water temperature
B) Time of submersion
C) Degree of aspiration
D) Presence of a pediatric tertiary care center <30 minutes away
E) Response to initial cardiopulmonary resuscitation efforts

40. All of the following statements regarding gun ownership by families with children are true EXCEPT:
A) Almost half of all homes in the United States contain guns.
B) Family members in homes with guns are three times more likely to die of homicide.
C) Family members in homes with guns are five times more likely to commit suicide with a gun.
D) Guns should be kept locked away rather than within easy access of family members.
E) Only handguns with a trigger lock may be kept locked and loaded; all other guns should be stored separately from ammunition.

41. First-time parents have brought their 6-month-old son to your office for his regular health maintenance visit. You note that the standard 6-month form used by your office lists "poisoning prevention" under anticipatory guidance. These parents should be educated about all of the following EXCEPT:
A) Keeping syrup of ipecac in the home for initial management of ingestions in children
B) Leaving all poisonous substances in their original containers
C) Purchasing medications and vitamins with child-resistant caps whenever possible
D) Keeping all poisonous substances in locked cabinets or otherwise out of reach of the child
E) Posting the number for the poison control center in a prominent place for easy access

42. You are seeing 5-year-old twin girls in your office for their regular health maintenance visits. Their father tells you that the family is considering getting a dog and asks you if you have any advice on breeds. All of the following regarding dog bites in children are true EXCEPT:
A) Male dogs are more likely to bite than female dogs.
B) Most children are bitten by dogs that they do not know.
C) Animal bites are most common in children younger than 10 years of age.

D) Pit bulls and Rottweilers account for about half of all dog bites.
E) Dogs should not be approached while they are growling or feeding.

43. Which of the following methods for tic removal is most effective for removing a tic without increasing the risk of injury or infection?
A) Burning the tic with a hot, extinguished match and allowing it to detach on its own after death
B) Grasping the tic firmly in a pair of tweezers and squeezing underneath the body before lifting up with gentle, steady pressure
C) Grasping the tic firmly in a pair of tweezers and lifting directly up with gentle, steady pressure
D) Suffocating the tic with petroleum jelly and allowing it to detach on its own after death
E) Scratching the tic off the skin with a plastic card such as a credit card

44. You are serving as the camp doctor at a summer program in North Carolina for pediatric leukemia survivors. An 11-year-old girl is brought to the office after being stung on the left forearm by "some big thing that was flying." She is teary but has no difficulty breathing, hives, or systemic flushing. Appropriate management of this patient includes all of the following EXCEPT:
A) Removing the stinger (if present) by scraping it out with a plastic card such as a credit card
B) Cleaning the area thoroughly
C) Applying a cool compress
D) Applying a topical antihistamine
E) Checking the patient's medical form for information regarding significant medical history, medications, and allergies

45. You are seeing a 9-year-old boy for his regular health maintenance visit. He weighs 33 kg. The child has a history of an anaphylactic reaction to a hornet sting. He has an EpiPen Jr. that he carries with him at all times, as do his parents and his school. The last time he renewed his EpiPen Jr. prescription was at his 8-year visit 14 months ago. At this visit, the patient:
A) should be switched to an EpiPen based on his weight
B) should be issued a new prescription for EpiPen Jr. based on the shelf life of the product
C) should be switched to an EpiPen based on his age
D) should have blood drawn to see if he is still allergic to hornet venom
E) should be referred to an allergist for testing for other allergies

ANSWERS

1. A	16. A	31. A
2. B	17. B	32. B
3. C	18. C	33. C
4. D	19. D	34. D
5. E	20. E	35. E
6. A	21. A	36. A
7. B	22. B	37. B
8. C	23. C	38. C
9. D	24. D	39. D
10. E	25. E	40. E
11. A	26. A	41. A
12. B	27. B	42. B
13. C	28. C	43. C
14. D	29. A	44. D
15. E	30. E	45. A

4

Poisonous Ingestions and Environmental Exposures

INGESTIONS: IDENTIFICATION AND MANAGEMENT

About 85% of pediatric poisonings occur in children younger than 5 years of age. These ingestions are usually *accidental* (but occasionally result from abuse) and typically involve only one substance. Adolescents account for the remaining 15%. Adolescent ingestions are usually *intentional* (e.g., suicide attempt or gesture) and may involve multiple substances. Intentional ingestions require medical intervention and have a significantly higher rate of death. The possibility of a toxicologic ingestion should be considered in any patient presenting with acute-onset illness involving multiple organ systems, including acute behavior changes, vomiting, respiratory compromise, seizures, arrhythmias, altered mental status, and/or coma.

Poison control centers are invaluable partners in the identification and management of poisonous ingestions. These organizations have access to component lists for household products and medications. They are also knowledgeable in the area of plant toxins and illegal substances. Parents should be instructed to call their local poison control center (or 911) in the event of ingestion. Administration of ipecac in the home is no longer recommended; it does not appear to improve patient outcome and in fact may lead to vomiting, which precludes the use of more effective products in the emergency department.

Patients who present in unstable condition should be evaluated and treated in accordance with the "ABCDE" primary survey (Airway, Breathing, Circulation, Disability, Exposure) discussed in detail in Chapter 29. In regard to ingestions, the "D" in the mnemonic may also allude to dextrose (because several agents commonly ingested result in hypoglycemia), drug treatment (e.g., antidotes), and decontamination. The clinical manifestations and treatments of specific pediatric poisonings are detailed in Table 4-1.

TABLE 4-1
SIGNS, SYMPTOMS, AND TREATMENT OF SPECIFIC PEDIATRIC POISONINGS

Substance	Clinical Manifestations	Suggested Laboratory Tests[b]	Antidote/Treatment
Acetaminophen[a]	Nausea/vomiting, anorexia; may progress over days to jaundice, abdominal pain, liver failure	Serum acetaminophen level 4 to 24 h after ingestion[c]; (late) serum hepatic transaminases (↑), prothrombin time (↑)	Antidote: Oral *N*-acetylcysteine (most effective within 8 to 10 h of ingestion) 140 mg/kg PO × 1 dose, 70 mg/kg PO q4h × 17 doses Treatment: Gastric emptying (within 1 h); activated charcoal (within 4 h)
Anticholinergic agents[a] (atropine, scopolamine, first-generation antihistamines)	"Mad as a hatter, red as a beet, blind as a bat, hot as a hare, dry as a bone"; drowsiness, delirium, hallucinations, seizure; skin flushing; fixed dilated pupils; fever, cardiac dysrhythmias; dry mouth, speech and swallowing difficulties, nausea, vomiting	Drug screen	Antidote: Physostigmine in select cases of severe anticholinergic signs and symptoms Treatment: Gastric emptying (early), activated charcoal/cathartic; whole bowel irrigation for sustained-release preparations; cardiorespiratory support, seizure control; benzodiazepines/haloperidol for agitation

(*continued*)

TABLE 4-1
(continued)

Substance	Clinical Manifestations	Suggested Laboratory Tests[b]	Antidote/Treatment
Carbon monoxide[a]	Lethargy, irritability, confusion, dizziness, headache; nausea; irregular breathing, cyanosis; palpitations; progression to coma, death	Blood carboxyhemoglobin levels; blood gas (metabolic acidosis with normal PaO_2); urine dipstick (myoglobinuria); ECG	Antidote: Oxygen Treatment: Normobaric oxygen 100% until asymptomatic and carboxyhemoglobin level ≤5%; hyperbaric oxygen if available for severe poisoning
Ethanol[a,d] (wine/beer/liquor; also found in cold preparations and mouthwash)	Lethargy, CNS depression, nausea/vomiting, ataxia, respiratory depression, coma, hypotension, hypothermia (in young children)	Serum ethanol level, blood glucose (↓), electrolytes (↓ potassium), blood pH (↓), ↑ osmolal gap	Antidote: None Treatment: Supportive care, glucose if needed, correction of electrolytes, parenteral fluids
Ethylene glycol (radiator fluid, deicing solution)	Anorexia, vomiting, lethargy, respiratory/cardiovascular collapse	Serum ethylene glycol level; serum ammonia (↑); arterial blood gas monitoring (metabolic acidosis); serum electrolytes (↑ anion gap); ↑ osmolal gap; serum calcium (↓); urinalysis (calcium oxalate crystals)	Antidote: None Treatment: Fomepizole (preferred) or ethanol to prevent metabolism; sodium bicarbonate to correct metabolic acidosis; hemodialysis; respiratory and cardiovascular support
Hydrocarbons (in fuels, household cleaners, polishes, and other solvents)	Tachypnea, coughing, respiratory distress, cyanosis, fever (aspiration); nausea/vomiting, gastrointestinal discomfort (oral ingestion); mental status changes	Arterial blood gas monitoring, chest radiography (initial and 4 to 6 h after exposure)	Antidote: None Treatment: Avoid gastric emptying[e]; prevent aspiration, which results in chemical pneumonitis and possibly proliferative alveolar thickening and chronic lung function abnormalities; supportive respiratory care
Ibuprofen	Nausea/vomiting, anorexia, stomach pain; gastrointestinal bleeding (obvious or occult) Massive ingestion: mental status changes/stupor/coma; seizures	Serum ibuprofen level 4 h after ingestion[f]; serum transaminase levels (↑), alkaline phosphatase (↑); metabolic acidosis with ↑ anion gap	Antidote: None Treatment: Gastric lavage (early); activated charcoal/cathartic; respiratory support/seizure control
Iron[a]	Nausea/vomiting, diarrhea, gastrointestinal blood loss, acute liver failure, seizures, shock, coma	Serum iron level (3 to 5 h after ingestion), serum pH (↓), glucose (↑), bilirubin and liver function tests (↑), PT (prolonged), WBC count (↑); abdominal radiograph (radiopaque material)	Antidote: Deferoxamine chelation Treatment: Gastric lavage (early); whole bowel irrigation; dialysis (late, severe)

(continued)

TABLE 4-1
(continued)

Substance	Clinical Manifestations	Suggested Laboratory Tests[b]	Antidote/Treatment
Methanol (in windshield washer fluid; toxic in very small amounts; toxicity related to formation of formic acid)	Nausea/vomiting, inebriation; ↑ minute ventilation to offset metabolic acidosis as methanol is metabolized; ocular findings 18 to 24 h after ingestion (blurred vision, optic disc hyperemia/edema)	Serum methanol level; arterial blood gases; severe metabolic acidosis; ↑ osmolal gap	Antidote: None Treatment: Ethanol to block metabolism; sodium bicarbonate for metabolic acidosis; folate to hasten formic acid elimination; hemodialysis in severe cases
Organophosphates[a] (insecticides)	SLUDGE; small but reactive pupils; sweating; muscle fasciculations; confusion; coma	Plasma or red blood cell cholinesterase activity (↓)	Antidote: Atropine sulfate followed by pralidoxime chloride Treatment: Gastric lavage (early), activated charcoal (if ingested)
Opiates	Bradycardia, hypotension, decreased respiratory rate, pinpoint pupils, somnolence, coma	Toxicologic screen (urine and serum)	Antidote: Naloxone[g] Treatment: Gastrointestinal decontamination if appropriate; respiratory support
Salicylates (aspirin, antidiarrheal medications	Hyperpnea/tachypnea (respiratory alkalosis/metabolic acidosis), fever, nausea, vomiting, dehydration, tinnitus, agitation, seizures	Blood gas (↑ pH, ↓ PCO_2, ↓ bicarbonate), glucose (↑), electrolytes (↓ potassium), PT and PTT (prolonged), serum salicylate level	Antidote: None Treatment: Gastric emptying/activated charcoal,[h] alkalinization of the serum to increase renal excretion and prevent entry into CNS; correct hypokalemia which inhibits salicylate excretion; fluid/electrolyte management; hemodialysis in severe cases
Sympathomimetic agents (decongestants[a]; also amphetamines, cocaine)	Tachycardia, hypertension, fever, large but reactive pupils, sweating, agitation, delirium/psychosis, seizures	Electrolytes (↓ potassium), blood glucose (↑), ECG	Antidote: None Treatment: Gastric lavage/activated charcoal/cathartics; sedatives for severe agitation; cardiorespiratory support
Theophylline	Tachycardia, hypotension, tachypnea, vomiting, agitation, seizures	Serum theophylline level (every 2 to 4 h), blood glucose (↑), potassium (↓), pH (↓), calcium (↑), phosphate (↓), ECG	Antidote: None Treatment: Activated charcoal/whole bowel decontamination; hemodialysis in severe ingestions
Tricyclic antidepressants	Anticholinergic effects as above; tachycardia, hypertension progressing to hypotension, confusion, drowsiness, dry mucous membranes,	ECG (prolonged PR interval, widened QRS complex, prolongation of the QT interval, AV	Antidote: None[j] Treatment: Gastric lavage/activated charcoal[k]; sodium bicarbonate (blood alkalinization) for conduction abnormalities;

(continued)

TABLE 4-1
(continued)

Substance	Clinical Manifestations	Suggested Laboratory Tests[b]	Antidote/Treatment
	dilated but responsive pupils, agitation, seizures, coma, dysrhythmias[i]	block, ventricular arrhythmias); these effects may be delayed	all patients with tricyclic antidepressant ingestions should be admitted and monitored in an intensive care unit

[a]These substances represent the most common pediatric toxicologic emergencies.
[b]All patients with suspected ingestions should receive serum and urine toxicologic screens because ingestion of multiple substances is common, especially in intentional poisonings.
[c]An accepted nomogram exists for predicting the severity of the toxicity based on a blood acetaminophen measurement taken ≥4 hours after ingestion.
[d]Physicians should have a high suspicion of co-ingestions in adolescents with ethanol intoxication. The clinical manifestations of co-ingestion of a CNS stimulant may be attenuated, whereas ingestion with a depressant may potentiate the effects of the alcohol.
[e]Some specific exceptions.
[f]An accepted nomogram exists for predicting the severity of the toxicity based on a blood ibuprofen measurement taken 4 hours after ingestion.
[g]Naloxone administration may result in withdrawal symptoms (tachypnea, tachycardia, sweating, agitation, seizures) in chronic users.
[h]Aspirin ingestions causes delayed gastric emptying, so gastrointestinal decontamination plays a significant role.
[i]Although extremely rare, fatal dysrhythmias have occurred up to several days after ingestion.
[j]Despite the anticholinergic effects of tricyclic antidepressants, physostigmine is *contraindicated* in these ingestions.
[k]Tricyclic antidepressant ingestions causes delayed gastric emptying, so gastrointestinal decontamination plays a significant role.
PO, per oral; PaO_2, partial pressure of oxygen, arterial; ECG, electrocardiography; CNS, central nervous system; PT, prothrombin time; WBC, white blood cell; SLUDGE, salivation, lacrimation, urination, defecation, gastric cramping, emesis; PCO_2, partial pressure of carbon dioxide; PTT, partial thromboplastin time; AV, atrioventricular.

Gastric evacuation may be achieved through induced vomiting or gastric lavage, but is effective only if performed within 1 hour of ingestion. Induction of vomiting is *contraindicated* under certain circumstances (Table 4-2). If a large amount of a highly toxic substance (calcium channel blockers, digoxin, iron) has been ingested within the previous hour, gastric lavage may be of benefit and is preferable to inducing vomiting. Gastric lavage allows dilution of the stomach contents and may recover pill fragments to aid in diagnosis. Some substances (aspirin, tricyclic antidepressants) slow gastric emptying time; the window of time during which gastric evacuation can provide benefit may be lengthened in such cases. In young children, the small bore of the nasogastric tube limits the usefulness of lavage.

Activated charcoal, cathartics, and whole bowel irrigation are methods of achieving gastrointestinal decontamination. All are contraindicated in the presence of bowel obstruction or ileus.

- Activated charcoal by mouth or nasogastric tube minimizes absorption by binding the substance. Activated charcoal does not bind heavy metals, iron, lithium, hydrocarbons, or alcohols, so it is not useful in ingestions with these substances.
- Cathartics may be added to the first dose of activated charcoal to hasten elimination of the substance.
- Whole bowel irrigation is an option for ingestions that are not cleared with activated charcoal. It may also be initiated after activated charcoal in ingestions with extended-release preparations.

The results of screening laboratory studies are often extremely helpful in the diagnosis and management of ingestions. Such tests include serum electrolytes, metabolic panel, electrocardiography, and blood and urine tox-

TABLE 4-2
CONTRAINDICATIONS TO INDUCTION OF EMESIS

Vomiting[a]
Ingestion of a corrosive substance[a]
Ingestion of a hydrocarbon[a]
Ingestion of an agent that may lead to neurologic depression[a]
Known bleeding diathesis
Age younger than 6 mo
Depressed arousal (gastric lavage may be used in these patients if they are intubated with a protected airway)

[a]Also a contraindication to gastric lavage.

icology screens, which vary among hospitals but generally consist of barbiturates, amphetamines, marijuana, cocaine, opiates, ethanol, tricyclic antidepressants, salicylates, and acetaminophen. If a specific substance is suspected, the laboratory may be able to obtain a blood level of the agent.

Caustics

Caustic (corrosive) agents include strong acids, bases (alkalines), and oxidizers. Examples of common caustic household solutions include laundry detergents, bleaches, stain/mildew removers, ammonia, disinfectants, and a myriad of cleaners (floor, window, bathroom/toilet, oven, all-purpose).

- Acids begin to burn superficial skin layers almost immediately, which tends to limit their ingestion. The most severe involvement is usually in the stomach (rather than the mouth or esophagus).
- Bases (alkalines) cause liquefaction necrosis of the squamous epithelium in the mouth and esophagus. These substances penetrate farther than acids and may result in more extensive injury.

Clinical manifestations include signs and symptoms of gastrointestinal and/or respiratory system injury (drooling, dysphagia, nausea, vomiting, hematemesis, wheezing, stridor, hoarseness, chest pain). Burns may be evident on the lips and in the mouth, but their absence does not rule out ingestion or severe internal injury. Induced vomiting and gastric lavage are contraindicated in patients with corrosive ingestions. Evaluation includes an electrolyte panel and blood gases to monitor the patient's acid–base status and a chest radiograph to assess for evidence of aspiration or injury. Endoscopy is performed when the patient's condition stabilizes and the injury is fully developed (≥12 hours after ingestion). Significant strictures require dilatation.

Coins and Batteries

Ingestion of coins is most common between the ages of 9 months and 3 years. Evaluation varies depending on symptoms and length of time since ingestion. Children who are asymptomatic after swallowing a coin and remain so can be observed at home for 3 to 4 days while waiting for the coin to pass as long as they are swallowing and eating well. Another option in these patients is localizing the coin to the stomach (by metal detector or radiograph), because 99% of stomach coins will pass without incident. If the coin has not passed within several days, the asymptomatic child should undergo radiography to make sure the coin is not in the esophagus. Any symptoms of choking or gagging, drooling, pain with swallowing, vomiting, stridor, or respiratory distress demand immediate evaluation. Coins that have lodged in the esophagus can usually be removed by endoscopy. Surgery may be required in rare cases.

The management of ingestion of a disk or "button" battery merits special mention. Although almost any object lodged in the esophagus can cause esophageal perforation if not removed, disk batteries result in rapid liquefaction necrosis and perforation and should be removed as soon as possible after diagnosis. Batteries that progress to the stomach without incident generally cause no problems. However, if the battery is relatively large (diameter >2 cm) or remains in the stomach for >48 hours, retrieval is recommended.

Foreign bodies that lodge in the airway are discussed in Chapter 13.

Toxic Plants

Houseplants and outdoor plants may contain toxins that are harmful when ingested.

- Houseplants: dieffenbachia (dumbcane), philodendron, alocasia, caladium, peace lily, colocasia (elephant ears)
- Outdoor plants: nightshade, pokeweed, evergreen bittersweet, yew, wisteria, milkweed, mistletoe, and black locust

Local poison control centers can be of great assistance in identification of the ingested plant, expected complications, and management. The most common symptom of toxic plant ingestion is persistent vomiting. Management typically involves gastric emptying (depending on how long ago the ingestion occurred), activated charcoal, and supportive care. The presentation and management of allergic contact dermatitis due to plant contact are discussed in Chapter 20.

EXPOSURE TO ENVIRONMENTAL TOXINS

Environmental Contaminants

Toxic environmental substances include ambient air pollution, contaminants in drinking water and food, pesticides, and industrial waste. Infants and children are more vulnerable to the toxic effects of many environmental substances because:

- They put their hands and other objects in their mouths more frequently than adults.
- They absorb certain toxins more efficiently than adults.
- They ingest more food and water per unit of body weight than adults.
- Their developing brains and lungs are more susceptible to insult.

- The child has a higher minute ventilation than the adult.
- Children spend more time outdoors than adults.
- The potential lifespan of the child results in a longer period for latent illnesses related to exposure to become symptomatic.

Significant air pollutants include:

- ozone (formed when sunlight reacts with gases emitted by automobiles and factories); parents of small children and patients with asthma should make a habit of checking the ozone alert status daily and limiting exposure on peak days.
- particulate matter (from diesel engines, burning wood, and industry emissions)
- automobile exhaust emissions

All of the above are associated with decreased lung function, increased respiratory disease, and asthma exacerbations in children.

Organisms (*Escherichia coli, Giardia lamblia, Cryptosporidium*) and chemicals (nitrogen from fertilizer runoff, mercury, lead, trichlorethylene and perchlorethylene from factory/industrial emissions) may contaminate drinking water. Food may become contaminated with *E. coli* or other bacteria. Fish obtained from polluted lakes or streams and long-lived, predatory sea fish (tuna, swordfish, mackerel, shark) in particular are associated with elevated concentrations of mercury, which should limit their ingestion by pregnant women and developing children. Children who are exposed to asbestos or lead during the renovation of older houses are at risk for lung disease and neurodevelopmental abnormalities, respectively.

The patient history regarding exposure to environmental toxins involves information regarding:

- prenatal history (the mother's diet and water sources; exposure to radiation)
- the area where the child lives (inner city, suburb, sparsely populated)
- the age of the child's house
- area industrial plants
- the source of the child's water (well vs. city) and whether the home has a septic tank
- food sources (organic, nonorganic/pesticide-treated, fish, meat from animals raised with supplemental hormones/antibiotics)
- the use and storage of pesticides by the family
- underlying respiratory disease

Exposure Related to Chemical or Biological Terrorism

Chemicals that have been released (or successfully prevented from being released) for terrorist purposes include sarin, chlorine, and ricin. Sarin, a nerve agent, is dispersed in the air and causes loss of consciousness, paralysis, and respiratory failure leading to death. Chlorine is an irritant that burns the skin and eyes and affects the lungs if inhaled. Skin decontamination is the first step to aiding a victim of chemical exposure. First responders and health care workers must protect themselves from exposure through the air or victims' clothing.

In contrast to chemical agents, signs and symptoms related to exposure to biological weapons may not become evident until a variable time after exposure, giving the organism time to spread and making the illness more difficult to recognize initially. *Bacillus anthracis* (anthrax) is a bacterium that causes a severe flulike illness, often progressing to shock and death. Cutaneous anthrax occurs as a result of direct contact of nonintact skin with anthrax spores. An itchy papule develops around the skin break, which then blisters and forms a large black ulcer surrounded by marked swelling. The organism may spread to the bloodstream, resulting in the severe disease mentioned above. Ciprofloxacin is the antibiotic of choice. Anthrax does not spread person to person.

Smallpox is another potential biological agent, one with airborne droplet and contact person-to-person spread. Smallpox was eradicated from the world population in 1977; most adults and all children are currently susceptible to the illness. In addition, many physicians practicing now have never seen smallpox lesions, which may easily be mistaken for varicella. Smallpox sores develop first on the oropharyngeal mucosa, face, and arms and then spread to the trunk and legs. Two days after they appear, the lesions become vesicular with umbilicated centers. These progress to round, tense, pustules that become crusted after 8 to 9 days and result in severe scarring. Of note, skin lesions on any particular body part are in the same stage of development, unlike varicella. Smallpox has a high mortality rate (30%). Cidofovir is the treatment of choice.

SOURCES

American Academy of Pediatrics Committee on Environmental Health. Ambient air pollution: health hazards to children. *Pediatrics*. 2004;114:1699–1707.

American Academy of Pediatrics Committee on Environmental Health and Committee on Infectious Disease. Chemical-biological terrorism and its impact on children: a subject review. *Pediatrics*. 2000;105:662–670.

Balk SJ, Forman JA, Johnson CL, et al. Safeguarding kids from environmental hazards. *Contemp Pediatr*. 2007;24:64–81.

Barry JD. Diagnosis and management of the poisoned child. *Pediatr Ann*. 2005;34:936–946.

Cordero B, Savage RR. Corrosive ingestions. *Pediatr Rev*. 2006;27:154–155.

Henry K, Harris CR. Deadly ingestions. *Pediatr Clin North Am*. 2006;53:293–316.

Kind T. In brief: carbon monoxide. *Pediatr Rev*. 2005;26:150–151.

Lanphear BP, Wright RO, Dietrich KN. Environmental neurotoxins. *Pediatr Rev*. 2005;26:191–198.

McGuigan ME. Poisoning potpourri. *Pediatr Rev*. 2001;22:295–301.

Metzel K. Coin ingestion. *Pediatr Rev*. 2003;24:395.

QUESTIONS

1. In which of the following nonintubated patients is gastric lavage an appropriate management option if the patient presents within 1 hour of ingestion?

A) A 3-year-old who has ingested nortriptyline
B) A 3-year-old who has ingested an ammonia cleaning solution
C) A 3-year-old who has ingested a hydrocarbon-based polish
D) A 3-year-old who has ingested radiator fluid
E) A 3-year-old who has ingested a narcotic

2. In which of the following patients is activated charcoal an effective management option?

A) A 30-month-old who has ingested iron
B) A 30-month-old who has ingested baby aspirin
C) A 30-month-old who has ingested lithium
D) A 30-month-old who has ingested windshield de-icing solution
E) A 30-month-old who has ingested methanol

3. Which of the following statements regarding pediatric ingestions is FALSE?

A) Most poisonings in the pediatric population occur in children younger than 5 years of age.
B) Ingestions in children younger than 5 years of age usually involve only one substance.
C) Accidental ingestions are more likely to result in death than intentional ingestions.
D) Ingestions in adolescents are usually intentional.
E) Ingestions in adolescents are more likely than those in younger children to involve multiple substances.

4. Which of the following substances is not routinely reported on either blood or urine toxicologic screens?

A) Amphetamines
B) Barbiturates
C) Cocaine
D) Ibuprofen
E) Acetaminophen

5. A 3-year-old boy is brought to the emergency department by ambulance after drinking fluid out of a soda can stored beneath the sink. The emergency medical technicians have brought the can, which is now empty but smells sharply like disinfectant or an all-purpose cleaner. The child is drooling and has a stridorous cry; no obvious lesions are noted in the perioral region. Which of the following statements about this patient is TRUE?

A) This patient cannot have significant internal injuries because there is no evidence of burns on the hands, face, or lips.
B) This patient has probably ingested an alkaline substance because there is no evidence of burns on the hands, face, or lips.
C) This patient should have received syrup of ipecac at home immediately after the ingestion.
D) This patient should have upper endoscopy within 6 hours.
E) Gastric lavage is contraindicated in this patient.

6. You are called by the school nurse of one of your 7-year-old patients because he has swallowed a quarter on a dare and she cannot reach his parents. You would be correct in telling her all of the following EXCEPT:

A) The patient should undergo chest radiography if he has any symptoms of coughing or choking at the present time.
B) If symptoms of choking or gagging were initially present but have resolved, the parents can wait 3 to 4 days to see if the coin passes before further evaluation.
C) A metal detector can be used to localize the coin to the stomach.
D) Ingested coins that do not pass within several days should be localized by radiograph to make sure they are not in the esophagus.
E) Ingested coins that are localized to the stomach almost always pass through the rest of the gastrointestinal tract without incident.

7. A 4-year-old mentally challenged girl is brought to the emergency department with persistent vomiting. Her mother found her outside with red berries in her mouth before the vomiting started. She was unable to find the source of the berries and does not know how many the child may have ingested. The child is slightly tachycardic, but otherwise her vital signs and temperature are stable. All of the following statements regarding this patient are true EXCEPT:

A) Gastric emptying is an appropriate initial treatment in the management of this patient.
B) The local poison control will probably be helpful in identifying possible plants ingested and suggesting management strategies.
C) The patient's persistent vomiting is consistent with toxic plant ingestion.
D) Activated charcoal is recommended in the management of patients with toxic plant ingestion.
E) An intravenous line may be required in the management of this patient.

8. Two teenage boys are dropped off at the front door of the emergency room by a friend. The three of them broke into an indoor municipal water park nearby and upended several containers onto the floor and into the pool before they were overcome with stinging eyes and intense red skin lesions. One of the teens is complaining of chest pain and has started to wheeze. Which of the following is the most important initial step in the management of these patients?

A) Inhaled humidified room air
B) Inhaled humidified 100% oxygen

C) Skin and eye decontamination
D) Application of cold compresses to the skin
E) Instillation of tetracaine drops into the eyes

9. Which of the following statements regarding smallpox lesions is FALSE?
A) They develop first on the oropharyngeal mucosa, face, and arms.
B) The next stage of development involves the trunk and legs.
C) Each lesion becomes vesicular with an umbilicated center about 2 days after first appearing.
D) Each involved body part typically has lesions in multiple stages of development.
E) The lesions become tense pustules that crust over about 8 to 9 days after they first appear.

10. While providing mobile medical care to migrant farm workers, you are asked to look at a lesion on a 16-year-old boy's hand. Through the interpreter, the youth tells you that he cut his hand on a barbed-wire fence about 6 days ago. A few days later the scratch began itching, and he noticed a bump that eventually blistered and broke. His hand is markedly swollen, and a 3-cm–diameter black ulcer has developed at the site of the original injury. The patient is afebrile, and there is no discharge from the site, streaking, or associated lymphadenopathy. Which of the following is the most appropriate treatment of the patient at this time?
A) Isolation
B) Debridement
C) Cidofovir
D) Ceftriaxone
E) Ciprofloxacin

11. A 14-year-old patient familiar to the emergency room staff due to multiple visits in the previous 3 months is brought in by her mother for ingestion of an unknown number of acetaminophen tablets. The mother states that she keeps all the medicines in the house locked up because "this is just the sort of thing my daughter would do to me." She saw the girl stuffing something into her bedside drawer while she was passing the girl's room and discovered a bottle marked "acetaminophen, 250 tablets." Only four tablets remained in the bottle. The mother did not believe that the daughter took the tablets until she began vomiting about an hour later. The girl refuses to speak in her mother's presence but eventually admits that she took "many tablets" at about 4:00 p.m. (3 hours ago). Oral *N*-acetylcysteine should be administered in this patient:
A) immediately after activated charcoal
B) immediately after gastric emptying
C) immediately after whole bowel irrigation
D) immediately after a toxicologic screen that is positive for acetaminophen
E) immediately after the 4-hour serum acetaminophen level

12. A 16-year-old boy with a known prior suicide attempt is brought to the emergency department by ambulance after telling his parents that he swallowed an entire bottle of acetaminophen tablets 4 days previously. The parents tell you that he was given an antidote the last time he took acetaminophen. You remember that oral *N*-acetylcysteine:
A) is most effective if given within the first hour after ingestion
B) is most effective if given within the first 8 to 10 hours after ingestion
C) is ineffective if given >2 hours after ingestion
D) is ineffective if given >4 hours after ingestion
E) is effective in reversing early liver damage

13. A 2-year-old girl is brought to the emergency department with hallucinations resulting in intermittent screaming and shaking. She has a rectal temperature of 103.2°F, with flushed skin and a dry mouth. Her pupils are dilated. She vomits in the emergency room. Her grandmother arrives and tells you that she found an unmarked bag of what appear to be seeds scattered about her nephew's room in her home. The substance appears to be jimson weed seeds. This patient's hallucinations and agitation would probably respond to which of the following?
A) Anticholinergic medication
B) Naloxone
C) Benzodiazepine
D) Atropine sulfate
E) Pralidoxime chloride

14. You are moonlighting in the pediatric emergency department when a 10-year-old boy arrives by ambulance with lethargy, confusion, dizziness, and a severe headache. His parents and maternal grandmother are in the adult emergency room with less severe but similar symptoms. The emergency medical technicians report that they were called by the police who found the family sleeping in their car with the engine running at their Christmas tree stand. Which of the following should be the first step in the evaluation and management of this patient?
A) Obtain an electrocardiogram
B) Draw an arterial blood gas
C) Draw a blood carboxyhemoglobin level
D) Administer normobaric 100% oxygen
E) Stabilize the patient for transfer to a hyperbaric oxygen chamber

15. A 3-year-old boy is brought to the emergency department by his grandmother who states that "he got into my pills" at home. She is on nortriptyline and verapamil. Her daughter fills her pillbox, so she has no idea what or how much medication might be missing. The child appears sleepy and confused. He is afebrile on examination, with a heart rate of 144 beats per minute, respirations of 26 breaths per minute, and blood pressure that is elevated above the 95th percentile. On examination, he has dry mucous membranes, and his pupils are dilated but responsive. If electrocardiographic abnormalities are present, you are most likely to see which of the following?

A) Torsades de pointes
B) Significant Q waves in leads I, II, V_5, and V_6
C) Runs of multifocal premature ventricular contractions
D) Flattened P wave, widened QRS complex, and peaked T wave
E) Prolonged PR interval, widened QRS complex, and QTc prolongation

16. A 15-year-old boy is brought to the emergency department by ambulance after police raided an illegal concert at a liquor house. The patient is in restraints and is struggling and delirious. The patient's vitals show a temperature of 101.7°F (temporal artery), respiratory rate of 40 breaths per minute, heart rate of 160 beats per min, and blood pressure of 155/90 mm Hg. On examination, the patient is sweating and has large but reactive pupils. Pertinent laboratory values include a serum potassium level of 3.2 mEq per L and a glucose level of 132 mg per dL. This clinical picture is most consistent with ingestion of which of the following?

A) Cocaine
B) Ethanol
C) Heroin
D) Phencyclidine
E) Theophylline

17. A 3-year-old girl presents to the emergency department with a presumed ingestion of her mother's iron tablets within the previous 2 hours. She is vomiting, but the emesis is nonbloody. Which of the following tests is the best indicator of toxicity?

A) Serum pH on admission to the emergency room
B) Serum iron level 3 to 5 hours after ingestion
C) Serum glucose on admission to the emergency room
D) Serum liver function test results 3 to 5 hours after ingestion
E) Serum prothrombin time results 3 to 5 hours after ingestion

18. Which of the following toxic substances is a component of windshield washer fluid?

A) Ethanol
B) Ethylene glycol
C) Methanol
D) Hydrocarbons
E) Organophosphates

19. An unresponsive adolescent patient is brought to the emergency department with suspected ingestion of an unknown substance. Emergency medical service received a call from the hotel room where the youth was found, but no one else was there when they arrived. The patient is on 100% inspired oxygen and has required several bouts of positive pressure ventilation in the ambulance. On examination, the patient has a heart rate of 55 beats per minute, blood pressure of 85/50 mm Hg, pinpoint pupils, and track lines on his left arm. Along with ongoing cardiovascular and respiratory support, which of the following should be administered to this patient?

A) Pralidoxime chloride
B) Haloperidol
C) Atropine sulfate
D) Naloxone
E) Desferrioxamine

20. Which of the following metabolic abnormalities is most consistent with acute salicylate poisoning?

A) Elevated serum bicarbonate
B) Hyperkalemia
C) Hypoglycemia
D) Respiratory acidosis/metabolic alkalosis
E) Respiratory alkalosis/metabolic acidosis

21. A 17-year-old boy who works for his father in the pest control business is brought to the emergency department complaining of vomiting, sweating, confusion, and twitching muscles. Which of the following is the most effective antidote regimen for this patient's presumed toxic exposure?

A) Atropine sulfate followed by pralidoxime chloride
B) Fomepizole followed by sodium bicarbonate
C) Physostigmine
D) Scopolamine
E) Diphenhydramine

22. A 16-year-old girl is brought to the emergency department by her parents who found her unresponsive on the front lawn at 3:00 a.m. The girl smells strongly of alcohol. Which of the following laboratory profiles is most consistent with alcohol poisoning?

A) Elevated serum alcohol level, hyperglycemia, hyperkalemia, alkalosis
B) Elevated serum alcohol level, hypoglycemia, hyperkalemia, alkalosis
C) Elevated serum alcohol level, hypoglycemia, hypokalemia, alkalosis
D) Elevated serum alcohol level, hypoglycemia, hypokalemia, acidosis

E) Elevated serum alcohol level, hypoglycemia, hyperkalemia, acidosis

23. Which of the following is the primary component of radiator fluid?
A) Ethylene glycol
B) Ethanol
C) Methanol
D) Hydrocarbons
E) Scopolamine

24. Gastric emptying is contraindicated in patients with hydrocarbon ingestion due to the risk of aspiration and subsequent chemical pneumonitis. Which of the following is a known long-term complication of chemical pneumonitis?
A) Asthma
B) Proliferative alveolar thickening
C) Cystic malformation
D) Bronchial narrowing and obstruction
E) None of the above; there are no long-term complications of chemical pneumonitis.

ANSWERS

1. A
2. B
3. C
4. D
5. E
6. B
7. A
8. C
9. D
10. E
11. A
12. B
13. C
14. D
15. E
16. A
17. B
18. C
19. D
20. E
21. A
22. D
23. A
24. B

Infant Medicine 5

FETAL ASSESSMENT

Obstetricians employ a variety of tests to assess the well-being of the fetus before and during delivery. Understanding the results can help pediatricians prepare for complications that may arise in the delivery room or thereafter.

- *Nonstress test* (NST) measures fetal heart rate reactivity in response to spontaneous fetal movement. NST results reflect fetal autonomic nervous system integrity. Results may be reactive (reassuring) or nonreactive (concerning). Nonreactive studies require further evaluation (i.e., ultrasonography).
- *Stress test* (ST) measures fetal heart rate reactivity in response to induced uterine contractions. The ST detects placental insufficiency and predicts fetal tolerance to labor. The study is considered "positive" when decelerations that begin during contractions and persist thereafter are detected.
- *Biophysical profile* includes results of the NST and a prenatal ultrasound to assess amniotic fluid volume, fetal movement and tone, and fetal heart rate. The lower the profile score, the higher the risk to the fetus.
- *Fetal heart rate monitoring* during delivery: The normal fetal heart rate at term is 120 to 160 beats per minute. Variability of the fetal heart rate is reassuring. Repetitive late decelerations indicate fetal compromise.

DELIVERY ROOM MANAGEMENT

Temperature Control

Temperature control in the delivery room is critical because the relatively high surface area-to-body mass ratio in the newborn results in significant *evaporative* heat loss. Neonates subjected to cold stress use valuable fat and glycogen energy stores and consume more oxygen. Rapid drying followed by placing the infant skin-to-skin with the mother keeps the infant warm and encourages bonding and breast-feeding. Healthy newborns who have successfully transitioned may then be swaddled with hats on their heads and placed in open bassinets. Unstable infants should be dried and placed under a servo-controlled radiant warmer for evaluation and/or resuscitation. Radiant warmers minimize energy expenditure by providing a thermo-controlled environment, and their open design facilitates easy access to neonates who need close observation or additional intervention. However, use of a radiant warmer increases the infant's insensible water losses and may result in volume depletion if weight and fluid intake/output are not properly monitored. Radiant warmers can also cause hyperthermia if a skin probe falls off. Core body temperature should be measured routinely in infants under warmers to detect central temperature instability, which might be a first sign of illness (e.g., sepsis).

Apgar Assessment

Apgar scores (Table 5-1) are assessed at 1 and 5 minutes of life (and again at 10 minutes if the second Apgar is low). The 1-minute Apgar score is reflective of the newborn's intrauterine environment and tolerance of delivery. Newborns with 1-minute Apgar scores ≤4 are more likely to be acidotic than those with higher values. The 5-minute Apgar score is indicative of the infant's adjustment to the extrauterine environment. Apgar scores suggest which infants will transition successfully and which will need sustained support; however, decisions regarding intervention and resuscitation *should be based on the patient's condition, not on Apgar scores.* The longer the Apgar score remains ≤3, the more likely the child is to develop multiorgan damage and long-term neurologic impairment due to *perinatal asphyxia*. In contrast, the newborn with low initial Apgar scores who rapidly recovers and goes on to have a normal neonatal course and physical examination is at no greater risk of subsequent cognitive impairment than infants with higher Apgar scores.

Meconium-stained Amniotic Fluid

Fetal passage of meconium in utero is uncommon before 37 weeks of gestation but occurs with some frequency in term and (especially) post-term infants. Meconium can be a sign of fetal difficulty and/or hypoxia; as the fetus becomes distressed, it passes meconium that may then be aspirated into the large airways by gasping behavior before or after delivery. Once in the lungs, meconium results in airway obstruction and inactivation of lung surfactant and may also cause pneumonitis.

If meconium is present in the amniotic fluid, the infant's mouth and pharynx should be suctioned before delivery of the shoulders and the rest of the body (or immediately

TABLE 5-1
APGAR SCORING SYSTEM

	0	1	2
Heart rate	Pulseless	<100 beats/min	≥100 beats/min
Respiratory effort	None	Slow/irregular	Strong/crying
Muscle tone	Limp	Some flexion of extremities	Active motion
Reflex irritability	None	Grimace	Cough or sneeze
Color	Blue/pale	Body pink/blue extremities[a]	Body and extremities pink

[a]Cyanosis that is limited to the distal extremities (acrocyanosis) is a common finding in healthy term newborns during the first 24 to 48 hours of life and is not indicative of disease.

after delivery of the head in a child born in the breech position). The vigorous, crying newborn needs no further intervention. However, an infant who is depressed at birth requires visualization of the larynx, intubation, and tracheal suctioning, preferably before the first breath (especially if the meconium is thick or particulate). If meconium is recovered from the trachea, the child should be intubated and suctioned again.

Meconium aspiration syndrome is discussed later in this chapter.

Resuscitation in the Delivery Room

Newborns should establish regular respirations by 1 minute of age. If the infant has cyanosis beyond that of the distal extremities but has adequate respirations and a heart rate ≥100 beats per minute, blow-by oxygen is provided. The newborn with a heart rate <60 beats per minute requires positive pressure ventilation by face mask and bag breaths with 100% oxygen at a rate of 40 to 60 breaths per minute. Because the fetal lung is filled with fluid, the inflation pressure required for the initial breath is greater than that needed for subsequent breaths. If the chest is not inflating, the infant must be repositioned ("sniffing" position) to obtain a patent airway. Once the alveoli are inflated, surfactant assists in maintaining residual lung volume. Infants born before 34 weeks of gestation may be surfactant-deficient; these infants will require increased inflation pressures and/or positive end-expiratory pressure until exogenous surfactant is administered.

Most newborns with bradycardia and ineffective respirations respond to positive pressure ventilation and oxygen. However, if the heart rate remains depressed (<60 beats per minute) after 15 to 30 seconds of positive pressure ventilation, external cardiac massage must be initiated. This involves encircling the infant's chest with both hands and using the thumbs to depress the distal third of the sternum. Compressions should depress the chest about one third of the anterior-posterior diameter at a rate of 100 compressions per minute, with one breath for every three compressions. Compressions can be discontinued when the heart rate reaches 60 beats per minute. Those infants whose heart rates do not respond to external cardiac massage and coordinated breaths within 30 to 60 seconds require intubation and endotracheal epinephrine.

Infants with inadequate perfusion develop hypoxia and acidosis, leading to constriction of the pulmonary vascular bed (hypertension) and right-to-left shunting. In addition, hypoxia at the cellular level results in the release of inflammatory mediators, tissue necrosis, and multiorgan system damage and dysfunction.

MATURITY AND GROWTH ASSESSMENT

Evaluation of the newborn includes review of the patient's prenatal and delivery history, the mother's laboratory results, the infant's gestational age (based on date of the last menstrual period), growth percentiles, and vital signs.

Gestational Age

Date of last menstrual period, prenatal ultrasound results, and postnatal Ballard and/or Dubowitz scores should be considered in assigning a gestational age. Infants may be:

- preterm (gestation <37 weeks)
- near-term (gestation 35 to 36 6/7 weeks)
- term (gestation 37 to 41 6/7 weeks)
- post-term (gestation ≥42 weeks)

Table 5-2 notes some of the physical characteristics of preterm, term, and post-term infants.

The growth and development of preterm infants should be assessed based on gestational age, not on chronologic age. For instance, an infant born at 32 weeks who is now 12 weeks old would have the growth parameters and

TABLE 5-2
PHYSICAL CHARACTERISTICS OF PRETERM, TERM, AND POST-TERM INFANTS

Preterm	Term	Post-term
Abundant vernix, decreased subcutaneous fat, thin pink skin, decreased tone, immature reflexes	Pink, chubby, normal muscle tone and reflexes	Dry, cracked, peeling or wrinkled skin; decreased subcutaneous tissue; sparse hair; possibly meconium staining

developmental milestones compared with those of the average 4-week-old.

As stated in Chapter 2, preterm infants need more calories per kilogram of body weight than full-term infants. They also require more fluid per kilogram than their full-term cohorts due to an even larger surface area-to-mass ratio.

Prenatal Growth Assessment

The infant's weight, height, and head circumference measurements must be assessed in relation to the child's gestational age. For example, a newborn weighing 1,850 g has a birth weight at the third percentile if the gestational age is $35^{3}/_{7}$ weeks, whereas the same weight would be at the 50th percentile for a 32-week-old infant.

- *Large-for-gestational age* (LGA): An infant whose weight and/or length are at the >97th percentile for gestational age (or greater than two standard deviations above the mean)
- *Appropriate-for-gestational age* (AGA): An infant with growth within two standard deviations of the mean. Some practitioners consider infants at the >90th or 95th percentile LGA, and those at the <10th or 5th percentile SGA, with all other infants labeled AGA by default.
- *Small-for-gestational age* (SGA): An infant whose weight and/or length are less than the third percentile for gestational age (or greater than two standard deviations below the mean)
- *Intrauterine growth retardation* (IUGR): Implies abnormally delayed accumulation of growth that may involve weight, height, and head circumference (symmetric IUGR) or growth retardation that is head-sparing (asymmetric IUGR)
- *Low birth weight* (LBW): birth weight <2,500 g
- *Very low birth weight* (VLBW): birth weight <1,500 g

LGA growth is usually constitutional, but maternal diabetes, maternal obesity, transposition of the great vessels, and Beckwith-Wiedemann syndrome may also result in LGA babies. LGA babies are disproportionately affected by hypoglycemia, polycythemia, jaundice, and pulmonary hypertension, but the most frequent complication of an LGA delivery is birth trauma (clavicular fracture, brachial plexus injury).

Infants who are SGA may be constitutionally small or may have experienced inadequate growth secondary to maternal, placental, or fetal conditions.

- Maternal contributions include chronic illness (diabetes mellitus; autoimmune disorders; hypertension; chronic cardiac, pulmonary, or renal disease), malnutrition, smoking, substance use/abuse, pre-eclampsia, twin pregnancies.
- Placental contributions consist of placental insufficiency, abruption, infarction, or placenta previa (note: poor growth due primarily to placental abnormalities is typically asymmetric).
- Fetal contributions include chromosomal or metabolic disorders; syndromes; infection (note: these are more likely to result in symmetric retardation of intrauterine growth).

As a group, SGA infants have increased morbidity and a higher neonatal mortality rate than their AGA peers. Intrauterine distress, perinatal asphyxia, persistent fetal circulation, and polycythemia are more common in SGA infants. SGA infants are susceptible to hypoglycemia, especially if placental insufficiency was the cause of their poor growth, because they do not have adequate liver glycogen stores and are inefficient at gluconeogenesis. Hypothermia is also a problem in many SGA infants, who lose heat faster than AGA babies because of less substantial subcutaneous adipose tissue. Conversely, SGA infants are less likely to develop respiratory distress syndrome.

Newborns with IUGR have poor growth resulting in anthropomorphic values that are inconsistent with the expected prenatal growth pattern. The term "intrauterine growth retardation" is often reserved for cases in which growth parameters are asymmetric (e.g., when weight is more severely affected than length and/or head circumference). These infants often lack significant subcutaneous adipose tissue and may appear alert, anxious, and/or wide-eyed. Newborns with IUGR are at risk for problems related to decreased caloric reserves, increased metabolic requirements, poor feeding, hypothermia, polycythemia, and hypoglycemia. Perinatal asphyxia is more common in IUGR deliveries, although the asphyxia is generally related more to the condition that caused the IUGR (pre-eclampsia, placental insufficiency) rather than the delayed growth itself.

All LGA and SGA/IUGR newborns should be screened for hypoglycemia within 2 hours of birth (see Screening).

The great majority of VLBW newborns are preterm; in fact, 1,500 g is at the 50th percentile for fetal weight at 30 weeks of gestation. The initial management of VLBW infants includes maintenance of a thermoneutral environment, monitoring blood glucose and arterial oxygen concentrations, and evaluation for sepsis if appropriate. Delivery and transition deplete the newborn's already limited energy stores, predisposing the infant to hypoglycemia, which is damaging to the developing nervous system. VLBW infants cannot consume enough calories by the enteral route to meet their basal metabolic needs. This dilemma is exacerbated by cold stress, respiratory distress, sepsis, or other illnesses. Providing these newborns with glucose (in the form of 10% dextrose in water at 5 to 7 mg per kg per minute) supplies the energy substrates necessary to meet metabolic demands without resulting in fluid overload. Once initial volume contraction has taken place (by days of life 1 to 3), saline is added to maintenance solution.

VLBW infants usually transition poorly and are at great risk for significant perinatal asphyxia. Arterial oxygen measurement is essential in the management of VLBW infants during the initial evaluation and subsequent period of assisted ventilation.

VLBW infants who survive often have extended stays in the neonatal intensive care unit (NICU). The earlier the gestational age at birth, the more likely the child is to develop significant long-term morbidity. Other factors associated with a poor outcome include severity of disease/complications during the NICU course, presence of a significant intracranial hemorrhage, and development of retinopathy of prematurity. Positive prognostic factors include normal brain growth, normal findings on neurologic examination, and normal oral–motor progression. VLBW infants who survive may need long-term care for bronchopulmonary dysplasia, gastroesophageal reflux, feeding problems, and poor weight gain. In addition, these children are at risk for early developmental delay.

ROUTINE CARE OF THE NEWBORN

Infant feeding is discussed in detail in Chapter 2.

Prophylaxis

Infants born in the United States receive prophylactic *vitamin K* (1 mg intramuscularly) as part of routine neonatal care. Vitamin K administration prevents *classic hemorrhagic disease of the newborn* (Table 5-3). Classic hemorrhagic disease of the newborn responds rapidly to infusion of vitamin K. Bleeding due to vitamin K deficiency that occurs within the first 24 hours of life is due to maternal medications that interfere with the absorption or function of the vitamin (anticoagulants, some antibiotics, numerous anticonvulsants). Routine vitamin K administration does not prevent this early-onset disorder.

Perinatal ocular prophylaxis against *ophthalmia neonatorum* (conjunctivitis in the neonatal period) is administered to all infants born in the United States. Neonates may develop conjunctivitis secondary to maternal *Chlamydia trachomatis* or *Neisseria gonorrhoeae* infections. Silver nitrate drops are effective against *N. gonorrhoeae* but do not protect against chlamydia, and there is a fairly high incidence

TABLE 5-3
PRESENTATION OF CLASSIC HEMORRHAGIC DISEASE OF THE NEWBORN

Clinical Manifestations (onset days of life 2 to 7)
Oozing from the umbilical stump
Oozing from circumcision site
Oozing from venipuncture, injection, or heel stick sites
Gastrointestinal bleeding
Enlarging cephalohematomas
Signs of intracranial hemorrhage

Laboratory Values
Normal platelet count
Prolonged PT/PTT
Depressed levels of factors II, VII, IX, and X, and proteins C and S
Normal levels of vitamin K–independent factors (V, VIII, and fibrinogen)

PT, prothrombin time; PTT, partial thromboplastin time.

of associated chemical conjunctivitis. Erythromycin ophthalmic ointment is effective against both pathogens and does not cause chemical irritation. Povidone iodine is an acceptable alternative. Ocular prophylaxis should be supplied and dispensed in single-dose packaging to avoid cross contamination within the nursery.

Screening

Vitals signs (including temperature, respiratory rate, heart rate, and pain assessment) should be monitored frequently in the first few hours after birth until stable. Blood pressure monitoring is reserved for infants who are ill or transitioning poorly. The normal range of blood pressure varies with gestational age and birth weight.

Table 5-4 lists groups of infants who are at risk for *hypoglycemia*. These patients should be screened within 2 hours of birth and, if needed, before each feed for the first 24 hours of life.

The normal ranges of hemoglobin and hematocrit levels in the healthy full-term infant are as follows:

- Hemoglobin: 13.7 to 20.1 g per dL (mean 16.5 g per dL)
- Hematocrit: 40% to 64% (mean 51%)

Term infants typically reach a mean hemoglobin nadir of 11.5 g per dL at 8 to 12 weeks of age (*physiologic anemia of infancy*). Hemoglobin levels in the fetus increase throughout gestation, so preterm infants have lower hemoglobin/hematocrit values than their term peers. *Physiologic anemia of prematurity* occurs sooner (4 to 8 weeks) and results in lower minimum hemoglobin levels. Preterm infants may require intervention (erythropoietin and/or transfusion) as they reach their physiologic nadirs. Because they have lower total body stores of iron, and these iron stores are depleted more

TABLE 5-4
SCREENING INFANTS AT HIGH RISK FOR EARLY HYPOGLYCEMIA

Infants who should be screened with bedside dextrose stick[a] within 2 h of birth:

- Preterm infants
- Post-term infants
- SGA/IUGR infants
- LBW/VLBW infants
- LGA infants
- Infants who require resuscitation in the delivery room
- Infants with respiratory distress, tachypnea, apnea, or cyanosis
- Infants being evaluated for sepsis
- Hypothermic infants
- Jittery/irritable/lethargic/comatose infants
- Infants who have hypotonia
- Infants with seizure activity
- Infants of diabetic mothers (gestational or insulin dependent)
- Infants of mothers with toxemia
- Infants whose mothers received no prenatal care

Infants who should be screened with a bedside dextrose stick[a] before each feed for the first 24 h of life:

- Preterm infants
- SGA infants
- LBW/VLBW infants
- LGA infants
- Infants of diabetic mothers
- Infants with feeding problems
- Infants with an initial glucose ≤45 mg/dL

[a]Glucose oxidase strip testing is rapid and simple but may yield false results (reads too low if the blood sample is not left on the strip long enough, does not cover the reagent pad entirely, or is too thin in areas on the pad; reads too high if the sample is contaminated with a glucose-containing intravenous fluid). Questionable test results should be confirmed by a central glucose test.
SGA, small for gestational age; IUGR, intrauterine growth retardation; LBW, low birth weight; VLBW, very low birth weight; LGA, large for gestational age.

rapidly, preterm infants should begin iron supplementation or iron-fortified formula by age 2 months (sooner if birth weight doubles).

Of note, infants with ABO or Rh incompatibility may present with severe anemia at 4 to 6 weeks of age due to persistence of maternal antibodies. The hemoglobin concentration in these infants is significantly lower than that expected for physiologic anemia of infancy.

Disorders identified by the *newborn screen* vary from state to state. Currently, all states screen newborns for *phenylketonuria* and congenital hypothyroidism. The phenylketonuria screen detects increased blood levels of phenylalanine. However, levels in affected patients may not become elevated until days of life 2 to 3, so if the specimen is obtained too early, the normal result will be equivalent to a "false negative." False-positive results can also occur in the infant with an increased phenylalanine level but no genetic defect. Testing for known genetic variations that result in phenylketonuria should take place as soon as possible after confirmation of a positive screen result.

Untreated *congenital hypothyroidism* results in mental retardation and poor growth and development. Newborns who are severely affected may be lethargic and have puffy faces and large tongues; however, most have normal physical examinations. The screening test for congenital hypothyroidism measures thyroxine (T_4) levels with the addition of thyroid-stimulating hormone (TSH) analysis if T_4 is low. If the sample is gathered within the first 24 hours of life, false-negative findings can occur. Signs of congenital hypothyroidism are nonspecific but include prolonged jaundice, delayed passage of meconium, poor feeding, and hypothermia; older children develop coarse facial features, dry skin, umbilical hernias, and severe constipation with abdominal distention. Infants who develop such symptoms should have T_4 and TSH levels drawn even if the newborn screen was negative. Additional testing recommended for neonates with positive screens and the conditions that lead to decreased T_4 levels in the newborn are outlined in Figure 5-1. T_4 therapy should be initiated before results are confirmed. Patients subjected to severe hypothyroidism in utero and those who remain undiagnosed in the first 3 months of life develop permanent cognitive impairment. Infants who are identified shortly after birth and appropriately treated remain developmentally intact.

Because fetal T_4 production increases throughout gestation, preterm infants usually have T_4 levels that are lower than the "normal" range. The same is true for LBW infants. If TSH is in the normal range, no intervention is necessary. Infants who are sick, preterm, and/or LBW and have elevated TSH levels may have primary hypothyroidism but should also be evaluated for iodine exposure and receptor blockade (elevated urinary iodine levels). All infants (preterm, term, LBW, etc.) with depressed T_4 and elevated TSH levels should receive L-thyroxine after bone age studies to look for delayed maturity. Infants born to mothers with autoimmune hypothyroidism may have transient hypothyroidism due to antibody transfer across the placenta.

The American Academy of Pediatrics recommends universal newborn screening for *hearing loss* before hospital discharge and intervention, if necessary, by age 6 months. Infants should be tested in a quiet room (to limit external noise) and while asleep, if possible. Acceptable automated screening tests include:

- *automated auditory brainstem response* (ABR), which detects an electrical waveform generated by auditory nerve pathways in response to sound; intact cortical function is necessary to obtain a reliable test
- *transient evoked otoacoustic emissions* (OAEs) and *distortion product* OAEs, in which standardized sounds generated

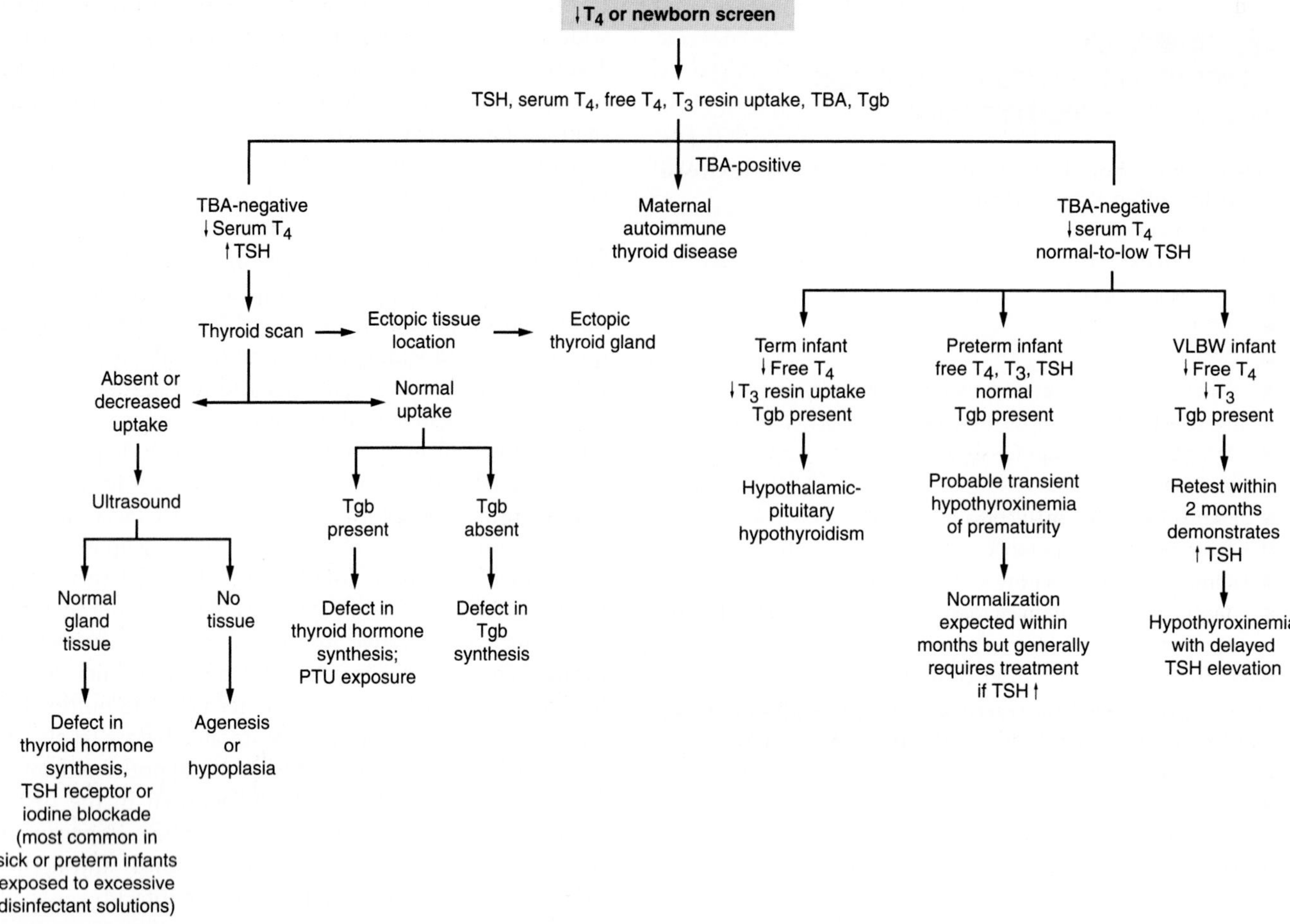

Figure 5-1 Evaluation of the infant with low T_4 on the neonatal screen. T_3, triiodothyronine; T_4, thyroxine; TBA, thyroid-blocking antibodies; Tgb, thyroglobulin; TSH, thyroid-stimulating hormone.

in the external canal "echo" back from the inner ear and are recorded. This test does not evaluate the adequacy of auditory nerve or central auditory function

A "pass" on the newborn hearing screen does not rule out hearing impairment. Moreover, delayed hearing impairment due to a congenital infection (cytomegalovirus) or infections acquired after birth (meningitis) will not be detected by newborn screening. False-positive results are most likely to occur on the first day of life, with the incidence decreasing on subsequent days. ABR is considered more reliable than OAEs; neonates who fail an initial screen (OAEs or ABR) should be rescreened with ABR. Referral for full audiologic assessment is indicated for infants who fail this second test.

Urination and Passage of Meconium

Most infants void by 12 hours of age and stool by 48 hours of age. If urination is delayed beyond 24 hours after birth:

- Review obstetric history, including results of any prenatal sonograms and exposure to drugs or medications.
- Review family history for renal disease.
- Review vital sign trends and assess the infant for signs of perinatal asphyxia or sepsis.
- Check intake and hydration status.
- If intake is sufficient, repeat the abdominal, flank, and genital examinations and look for evidence of edema or congenital anomalies consistent with Potter sequence.
- If repeated examinations are normal, catheterize the infant to see if urine is present in the bladder. Any urine obtained should be sent for urinalysis, culture, and urinary electrolyte and creatinine levels.
- Check serum urea nitrogen and creatinine levels, calculate the fractional excretion of sodium, and obtain a sonogram of the kidneys, ureters, and bladder.

If the infant then voids spontaneously and continues to do so, the evaluation need not be completed. However, the infant who does not void requires urgent urology referral.

Delayed passage of meconium virtually always results from anatomic (imperforate anus) or functional (meconium ileus, Hirschsprung disease) colonic obstruction. After checking that the patient is feeding well and hydrated, the abdomen and rectum should be re-examined for evidence of obstruction (distention) or anatomic abnormalities. The presentation, evaluation, and management of congenital colonic obstruction are provided later in this chapter.

As the meconium clears, breast-fed infants begin to have loose, seedy, yellow stools after every feeding. By 2 months of age, however, breast-fed infants may go as long as 7 days between stools, as long as they are soft and pass without evidence of discomfort. Formula-fed infants generally have one or more stools daily but may go 2 to 3 days with no stool.

Physiologic Jaundice

Clinical jaundice results when a large quantity of unconjugated and/or conjugated bilirubin is present in the extracellular fluid space. It is often noted in healthy term infants, and even more preterm infants develop jaundice. Bilirubin forms as a product of the breakdown of heme-containing proteins from senescent red blood cells and other sources. Hemoglobin is split into heme and globin within the tissue macrophages. The heme ring is then broken down to produce free iron and another molecule that is broken down into carbon monoxide and biliverdin. Biliverdin is altered by the enzyme biliverdin reductase to form free bilirubin, which is released into the plasma and binds to albumin for transport to the hepatic cells. There the majority of bilirubin is conjugated to form bilirubin glucuronide, a water-soluble molecule that can be excreted with bile salts. Most conjugated bilirubin is eventually excreted in the feces, although some is converted into urobilinogen (which is then eliminated in the urine or, after conversion, in the stool). A small amount of bilirubin is reabsorbed and undergoes enterohepatic circulation.

Bilirubin levels in full-term infants with physiologic jaundice typically peak on days of life 3 to 5 at a level ≤12 mg per dL. Similarly affected preterm infants peak later (days of life 5 to 7) and develop higher levels (up to 15 mg/dL). Even though these higher levels are "physiologic" (i.e., they occur in the absence of any abnormalities in bilirubin metabolism), treatment should be initiated at lower levels in preterm infants because they develop neurologic consequences at lower bilirubin measurements. These neonates have lower albumin levels than full-term infants, so free bilirubin levels may be higher. Acidosis, sepsis, and the use of certain antibiotics, all relatively common in preterm infants, result in further displacement of bilirubin from albumin. The serum bilirubin level should not be allowed to exceed the infant's weight in kilograms multiplied by 10 (e.g., 15 mg/dL in a 1.5-kg patient). Hyperbilirubinemia due to pathologic processes is discussed later in the chapter.

Cord Care

The two goals of cord care are prevention of infection and facilitation of drying and separation. Most hospitals use a plastic cord clamp that is then retained on the end of the umbilical stump. No one form of conventional cord care has been shown to be clearly superior. Many programs recommend that parents use isopropyl alcohol to lightly clean the area during each diaper change.

Physiologic Breast Hypertrophy

Infants of either gender may develop physiologic breast hypertrophy due to maternal estrogen exposure. This presents as uni- or bilateral painless enlargement under the nipple area and is accompanied by swelling of the external genitalia in female infants. The condition is nonpathologic, requires no therapy, and resolves spontaneously.

Hospital Discharge

Healthy term infants are generally discharged at 48 hours of life for vaginally delivered infants and 72 to 96 hours of life for cesarean section deliveries. Earlier discharge (before 48 hours of age) may be appropriate for some babies if the parents so desire (Table 5-5). Although early discharge might improve bonding and minimize risks associated with hospitalization, it also removes the baby and the mother from direct medical supervision. Premature termination of breast-feeding and delayed detection of treatable diseases are possible risks associated with early discharge.

TABLE 5-5
EARLY DISCHARGE: CRITERIA THAT MUST BE MET

Both parents desire early discharge
Uncomplicated prenatal course
Uncomplicated vaginal delivery
Infant is full-term
Infant is appropriate for gestational age
Uncomplicated postnatal course
Infant appears healthy
Infant has normal examination
Vital signs stable for at least the past 12 h
Infant has urinated and passed meconium
Infant is feeding well
All screening tests have been completed
Infant has been evaluated for jaundice
Parental education has been completed and competency demonstrated
Follow-up with a medical professional has been scheduled within 2 d of discharge
No family risk factors (adolescent and/or single parent; mother who did not seek prenatal care)

ABNORMAL CONDITIONS IN THE NEONATE

Perinatal Asphyxia and Hypoxic–Ischemic Encephalopathy

In the neonate, hypoxic–ischemic encephalopathy (HIE) refers to cerebral dysfunction brought on by significant *perinatal asphyxia* (inadequate oxygenation, blood flow, and gas exchange). Perinatal asphyxia is more common in infants who are preterm, IUGR, and breech. It should be anticipated when Apgar scores remain low (≤3), positive pressure ventilation is required for >1 minute, and cord blood acidosis is confirmed. The vast majority of cases result from intrapartum placental insufficiency, but infants may also become hypoxic after delivery due to cardiac, respiratory, or neurologic abnormalities. Significant and/or prolonged asphyxia is associated with multisystem organ damage, most notably involving the kidneys, brain, intestines, liver, heart, and lungs.

The Sarnet staging system categorizes HIE severity based on clinical manifestations and the presence or absence of seizure activity:

- Stage 1 (mild HIE): Infant is irritable, with exaggerated primitive reflexes, a weak suck, and dilated pupils. Muscle tone and electroencephalogram are normal, and there is no seizure activity. The neurologic signs and symptoms resolve within 24 hours, and there are no associated long-term deficits.
- Stage 2 (moderate HIE): Infant is obtunded but arousable, with proximal muscle hypertonia, constricted pupils, and occasional apnea and bradycardia. Focal or multifocal seizures typically begin within the first 24 hours of life; in fact, *HIE is the most common cause of neonatal seizures in the full-term infant.* These seizures may be associated with hypoxia and hypercapnea, and they require treatment. Phenobarbital is the initial medication of choice, with addition of fosphenytoin and a benzodiazepine if the seizures are difficult to control. Symptoms last up to 14 days. Although the majority of infants with stage 2 HIE have no long-term neurodevelopmental sequelae, a number develop seizure disorders, cerebral palsy, hearing loss, and/or visual impairment.
- Stage 3 (severe HIE): Infant is comatose, with generalized muscle flaccidity and intermittent posturing. Seizures are uncommon in this stage. The majority of patients die; those who survive remain critically ill for days to weeks and are severely compromised for life.

The differential diagnosis of seizures in the neonate includes bacterial meningitis, intracranial hemorrhage, metabolic abnormalities (hypoglycemia, hypocalcemia, hyper- or hypomagnesemia, hypernatremia), and benign familial seizure disorder. Lethargy and coma are associated with moderate and severe HIE, respectively, but other conditions such as hypothermia, infection, birth trauma, genetic syndromes, structural anomalies, intracranial hemorrhage, and metabolic abnormalities (inherited and acquired) also should be considered.

Respiratory Distress

Reliable signs of respiratory distress in the newborn include nasal flaring, retractions, tachypnea (normal respiratory rate in the neonate 30 to 60 breaths per minute), and grunting. *Cyanosis* may be due to inadequate gas exchange, poor perfusion, or abnormal blood flow. The normal arterial blood gas values for a newborn infant are listed in Table 5-6. Respiratory distress in the newborn may be due to perinatal asphyxia, transient tachypnea of the newborn, hyaline membrane disease (HMD), pneumonia, meconium aspiration syndrome, tension pneumothorax, structural anomalies (e.g., diaphragmatic hernia), or congenital heart defects (Table 5-7). HMD, formerly called respiratory distress syndrome, results from inadequate surfactant levels in the fetal lung. If phosphatidylglycerol is present in amniotic fluid (obtained by amniocentesis), the fetus can be expected to have sufficient surfactant levels, and the risk of developing HMD is low.

Because HMD and *neonatal pneumonia* cannot reliably be differentiated based on clinical presentations, management of respiratory distress that develops in the first day of life must include intravenous antibiotic treatment effective against bacterial pathogens commonly responsible for infectious pneumonia in this age group (*Escherichia coli*, group B streptococci, group D streptococci, anaerobic organisms, *Haemophilus influenzae*, *Streptococcus pneumoniae*, and *Listeria monocytogenes*). Blood, urine, and cerebrospinal fluid specimens should be obtained for laboratory evaluation and culture before the initiation of antimicrobial medications.

Pulmonary blood flow is low in the fetus due to high pulmonary vascular resistance. After delivery, pulmonary vascular resistance falls below systemic vascular resistance, resulting in increased pulmonary blood flow. In *persistent pulmonary hypertension of the newborn* (PPHN), pulmonary vascular resistance remains high, leading to marked hypoxemia and right-to-left shunting. PPHN may accompany meconium aspiration syndrome or lung hypoplasia (e.g., diaphragmatic hernia). Response to inhaled nitric oxide is the most helpful diagnostic tool for evaluating PPHN.

TABLE 5-6
ARTERIAL BLOOD GAS MEASUREMENTS FOR A TYPICAL HEALTHY, FULL-TERM NEWBORN

pH	7.35 to 7.45
PaO_2	60 to 90 mm Hg
$PaCO_2$	35 to 45 mm Hg
HCO_3	~24 mEq/L

PaO_2, partial pressure of oxygen, arterial; $PaCO_2$, partial pressure of carbon dioxide, arterial.

TABLE 5-7
RESPIRATORY DISTRESS IN THE NEWBORN

	Transient Tachypnea of the Newborn	HMD	Pneumonia	Meconium Aspiration Syndrome
Definition	Transient pulmonary edema resulting from delayed clearance of fetal lung fluid	Newborn respiratory distress syndrome resulting from insufficient surfactant	Lung infection acquired before, during, or after birth	Aspiration of meconium resulting in obstructive lung disease, chemical pneumonitis, and inactivation of surfactant
Epidemiology	Occurs in term and preterm infants; more common in infants delivered by cesarean section (especially if delivery takes place before onset of labor)	More common in preterm infants	Varies depending on etiology (in utero infection, group B *Streptococcus*, bacterial pneumonia)	Uncommon before 37 wk of gestation; more common in post-term pregnancies and infants with perinatal asphyxia
Presentation	Presents shortly after birth with tachypnea and occasionally grunting and nasal flaring	Presents shortly after birth with progressive tachypnea and respiratory distress	Signs of respiratory distress and/or sepsis; presentation may be virtually identical to that of HMD	Presents at birth with tachypnea, flaring, grunting; rales/rhonchi on chest examination; "barrel" chest
Arterial blood gas changes	Respiratory acidosis (↓ pH, ↑ $PaCO_2$), mild-to-moderate hypoxemia (↓ PaO_2)	Respiratory acidosis (↓ pH, ↑ $PaCO_2$), hypoxemia (↓ PaO_2)	Respiratory acidosis, hypoxemia	Hypoxemia
Chest radiograph	Prominent perihilar streaking, increased interstitial markings, fluid in the interlobar fissures	"Ground-glass" appearance of lung fields due to air bronchograms superimposed on widespread atelectasis	Localized, patchy, or widespread consolidation; possibly pleural effusions; chest radiograph of pneumonia due to group B *Streptococcus* virtually identical to that for HMD	Areas of atelectasis, coarse, irregular densities interspersed with areas of overinflation
Treatment	O_2 therapy; continuous nasal positive airway pressure, if needed	Prevention (antenatal steroids); exogenous surfactant[a] administration at birth (prophylactic) or within 6 h of birth (rescue therapy); respiratory support (e.g., mechanical ventilation) as needed	Empiric intravenous antibiotic therapy with ampicillin and cefotaxime until culture and sensitivity results are known; to complete a 10- to 21-d course	Prevention (see "Meconium Delivery" above); mechanical ventilation with high concentration O_2 and high mean airway pressures
Complications/ long-term prognosis	Spontaneous recovery within days with no long-term complications	Generally minimal when recognized and treated	Prognosis depends more on whether infection is present at other sites (CNS)	Prognosis depends more on degree and duration of ventilatory support required; chronic lung disease is a known sequelae of severe meconium aspiration

[a]Pulmonary hemorrhage is an uncommon complication of surfactant administration.
HMD, hyaline membrane disease; $PaCO_2$, partial pressure of carbon dioxide, arterial; PaO_2, partial pressure of oxygen, arterial; CNS, central nervous system.

Nitric oxide causes prompt dilation of the pulmonary vessels and significantly improves the oxygenation of most infants with PPHN. PPHN due to lung hypoplasia does not respond to inhaled nitric oxide.

Respiratory distress resulting from a *tension pneumothorax* is typically accompanied by inadequate chest excursions, unequal breath sounds, abnormally shifted heart sounds, and a chest radiograph demonstrating mediastinal shift. Tension pneumothorax should also be suspected in any infant undergoing mechanical ventilation who suddenly develops respiratory acidosis and hypoxemia, especially if any of the above signs are present. Administration of surfactant in preterm infants decreases the incidence of pneumothorax and other pulmonary air leaks.

Congenital diaphragmatic hernia (CDH) is herniation of contents of the abdominal cavity into the chest cavity due to a developmental defect in the diaphragm. Most occur on the left side through the foremen of Bochdalek. The classic presentation involves a newborn with severe respiratory distress, a scaphoid abdomen, shifted heart sounds, and breath sounds limited to one side of the chest. A small minority of affected patients present beyond the newborn period with recurrent pneumonia, vomiting, or chronic abdominal pain. When present, CDH is often discovered on a prenatal sonogram, along with associated polyhydramnios. Newborns with CDH decompensate rapidly due to lung hypoplasia and *pulmonary hypertension*. Initial stabilization consists of intubation immediately after birth, mechanical ventilation, and gastric decompression. Bag–mask ventilation should be avoided. Surgical repair is necessary but cannot address the many complications of CDH, including persistent pulmonary hypertension, poor growth, and gastroesophageal reflux. A significant minority of patients die in infancy despite maximal intervention.

Cyanotic congenital heart disease often presents with tachypnea and cyanosis and may be difficult to distinguish from primary pulmonary disease, especially PPHN. The physical examination and radiograph provide clues to the diagnosis. Infants with cyanotic congenital heart disease are more likely to have abnormal cardiac findings and may have enlarged hearts or decreased pulmonary markings on chest radiographs. Although neonates with respiratory disease may have a splitsecond heart sound, the predominant examination irregularities are respiratory in nature (e.g., retraction, grunting), and the heart size is virtually always normal in infants with isolated pulmonary involvement. The partial pressure of arterial carbon dioxide is increased in respiratory disease but usually normal or decreased with cardiac disease. The hyperoxygenation test measures the response of the partial pressure of arterial oxygen (PaO_2) produced from increasing inspired oxygen to 100% for 20 minutes. The PaO_2 in infants with cyanotic congenital heart disease does not rise above 150 mm Hg, whereas infants with hypoxemia due to pulmonary processes are able to increase PaO_2 to >150 mm Hg. *Echocardiography* is the definitive diagnostic study for confirming congenital heart disease.

The newborn with severe respiratory failure that is unresponsive to intubation and maximal mechanical ventilatory support may require inhaled nitric oxide, high-frequency ventilation, or extracorporeal membrane oxygenation.

Bronchopulmonary Dysplasia

Bronchopulmonary dysplasia (BPD) is the term for characteristic lung changes resulting from persistent dependence on oxygen therapy. BPD is the most common cause of chronic respiratory disease during infancy. BPD is discussed in detail in Chapter 13.

Intracranial Hemorrhage

Although intracranial hemorrhage is more likely to occur in certain subsets of infants (preterm, significant hypoxia/asphyxia, birth trauma), the condition should be suspected in any patient who develops irritability, decreased consciousness, apnea, seizures, or focal neurologic deficits. Rapid, large bleeds present with signs of increased intracranial pressure (bulging fontanelle, vomiting, bradycardia, coma) and/or vascular compromise (rapid decrease in hematocrit, acidosis, hypotension, shock). In the neonate, intracranial hemorrhaging can occur in the subdural, subarachnoid, or epidural (rare) spaces; in the brain parenchyma; and/or in the ventricles.

A lumbar puncture is indicated in infants with suspected intracranial hemorrhage to rule out meningitis (unless there are signs of increased intracranial pressure or thrombocytopenia). Cerebrospinal fluid that contains many red blood cells (which do not clear), elevated protein levels, and depressed glucose is consistent with intracranial bleeding. Diagnostic testing in unstable infants is limited to bedside cranial ultrasonography, which is sensitive for intraventricular bleeds. Subdural and subarachnoid hemorrhages are more easily detected by computed tomography unless the blood is within the cerebellum or posterior fossa; magnetic resonance imaging is superior for assessing these abnormalities. Serial studies may be necessary to evaluate evolving lesions and detect the development of ventricular dilatation and/or *posthemorrhagic hydrocephalus*.

The goals of treatment are twofold:

- First and most immediately, life-threatening complications must be addressed. Mechanical ventilation and cardiovascular support may be necessary for severely compromised infants. Coagulation studies should be obtained to assess for a bleeding diathesis. Phenobarbital and other antiepileptic medications (fosphenytoin, lorazepam) are indicated for seizures.
- Second, posthemorrhagic hydrocephalus must be detected and treated with serial lumbar punctures, medication to decrease cerebrospinal fluid production, and/or surgical placement of a ventricular access device or permanent ventriculoperitoneal shunt.

Polycythemia

Polycythemia, defined as a central venous hematocrit in excess of 65%, is associated with a variety of conditions including maternal diabetes, maternal toxemia, placental insufficiency, delayed clamping of the cord, and babies who are SGA, LGA, or post-term. The increased viscosity caused by polycythemia results in poor oxygen transport and, when extreme, the formation of microthrombi. Up to 40% of infants with polycythemia develop hypoglycemia; hyperbilirubinemia is another known complication. Most newborns with polycythemia are asymptomatic. Possible clinical manifestations of polycythemia include lethargy or tremulousness; poor feeding; seizures; cyanosis or tachypnea; tachycardia or signs of congestive heart failure; and renal vein thrombosis and/or hematuria. Partial exchange transfusion is indicated for the infant with a venous hematocrit >65% who develops symptoms or complications related to polycythemia; saline is the diluent of choice.

Nonphysiologic Jaundice

Jaundice due to a pathologic process does not appear any different on physical examination than physiologic jaundice. However, identification of infants with nonphysiologic jaundice is critical to preventing morbidity due to toxic bilirubin levels and complications of the underlying disease process (e.g., severe anemia from cell lysis). Nonphysiologic jaundice is suggested by any of the following:

- Evidence of jaundice prior to 24 hours of age (suspect hemolytic disease)
- Rise in serum bilirubin level >0.5 mg per dL per hour
- Total serum bilirubin level ≥75th percentile for age in hours
- Jaundiced infant with history of traumatic delivery
- Need for phototherapy
- Persistent jaundice (>8 days in a term infant or >14 days in a preterm infant)
- Jaundice in an ill-appearing infant
- Jaundice in an infant with microcephaly or petechiae
- Jaundice in an SGA infant
- Jaundice in an infant born to Mediterranean or Asian parents
- Family history of hemolytic anemia, liver disease, or sibling with nonphysiologic jaundice as a neonate

A simplified schematic for the diagnosis of infants with presumed nonphysiologic jaundice is presented in Figure 5-2. Potential causes of nonphysiologic unconjugated (indirect) and conjugated (direct) hyperbilirubinemia in the neonate are listed below.

Unconjugated hyperbilirubinemia:

- Increased lysis of red blood cells: blood group incompatibility (ABO or Rh incompatibility, the latter being extremely rare in a first-born child); red blood cell enzyme defects (glucose-6-phosphate dehydrogenase deficiency); red blood cell structural defects (spherocytosis); sequestered blood (cephalohematoma, intracranial hemorrhage); polycythemia
- Decreased hepatic conjugation of bilirubin: Gilbert or Crigler-Najjar syndromes; hypothyroidism

Direct hyperbilirubinemia:

- Hepatitis from congenital infection
- Bacterial infections (*E. coli*, urinary tract infection, sepsis)
- Erythroblastosis fetalis
- Metabolic disorders (galactosemia)
- Congenital biliary tree abnormalities/obstruction

In July 2004, the American Academy of Pediatrics Subcommittee on Hyperbilirubinemia published extensive and extremely helpful clinical practice guidelines regarding the management of hyperbilirubinemia and prevention strategies. The article (listed under Sources) also included nomograms that could be used to place infants into low-, intermediate-, or high-risk zones based on serum bilirubin levels and postnatal age in hours. Additional nomograms provide phototherapy and exchange transfusion treatment guidelines for infants in each risk group. Treatment decisions should be based on *total* serum levels, even though conjugated bilirubin does not cross an intact blood–brain barrier. Of course, the underlying disease process should be specifically addressed, if possible.

Special blue fluorescent tubes are the most effective light source for providing *intensive phototherapy*. The light source is placed as close to the infant as practical, with lighting above and below if possible. The infant should be virtually naked and wearing eye protection. Adequate hydration is critical for preventing significant enterohepatic circulation and increasing urine and bile output. If possible, the infant should be allowed to breast-feed. Phototherapy may cause "bronzing" of the skin in infants with elevated direct bilirubin measurements and is of limited usefulness in infants with cholestasis.

Exchange transfusion is recommended for infants with levels directed in the practice guideline nomograms mentioned above and any infant with a total serum bilirubin level ≥25 mg per dL or clinical manifestations of acute bilirubin encephalopathy. Infants with isoimmune hemolytic disease may respond to early intervention with intravenous γ-globulin therapy and avoid exchange transfusion.

Acute bilirubin encephalopathy (ABE) refers to central nervous system signs and symptoms caused by bilirubin toxicity seen in the first few weeks after birth. ABE is divided into clinical stages based on symptomatology.

- Early ABE: lethargy, poor suck, hypotonia
- Intermediate ABE: fever, irritability, high-pitched cry, moderate stupor, hypertonia (retrocollis, opisthotonos)
- Advanced ABE: pronounced hypertonia, apnea, deep stupor to coma, seizures, and death

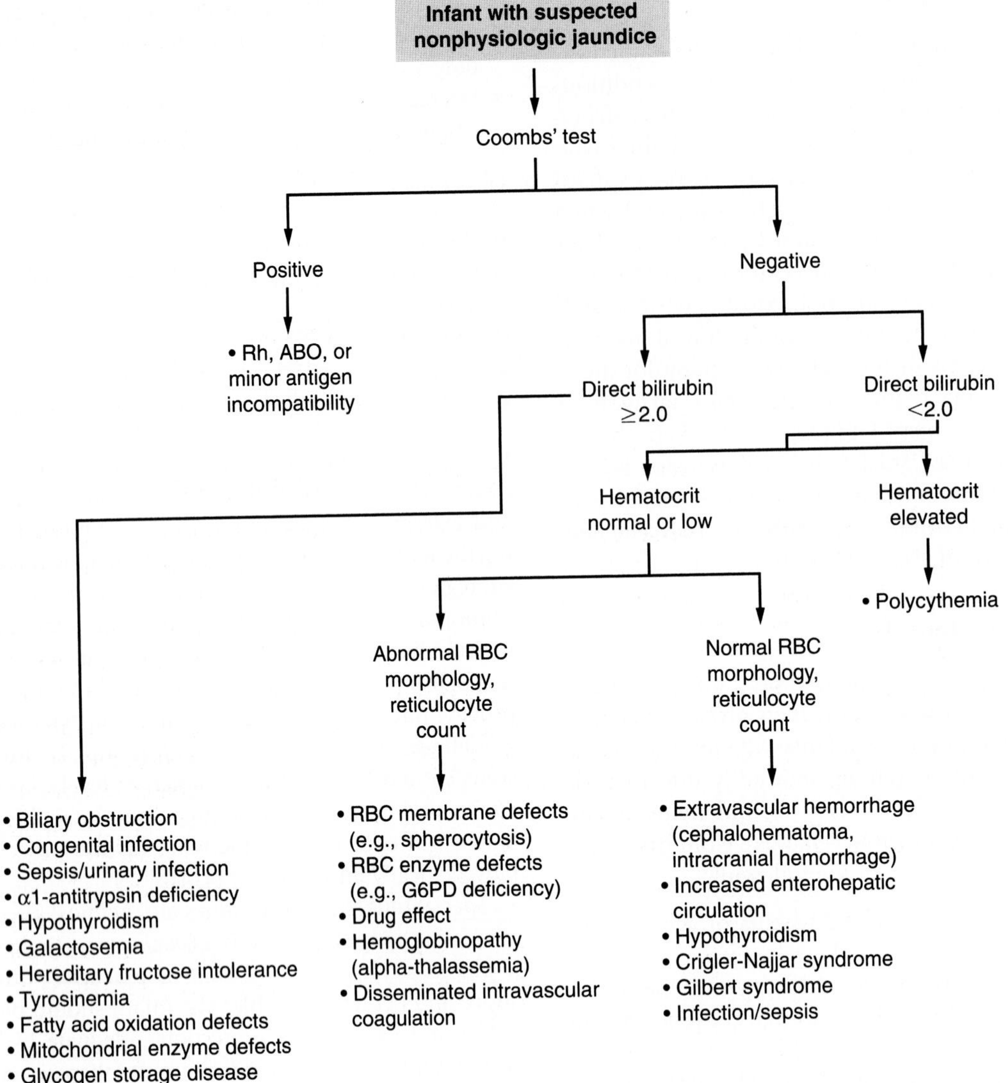

Figure 5-2 Evaluation of the infant with suspected nonphysiologic jaundice. G6PD, glucose-6-phosphate dehydrogenase; RBC, red blood cell.

In contrast, *kernicterus* describes the irreversible clinical effects of bilirubin toxicity to the basal ganglia, hippocampus, cerebellum, and various additional brainstem neurons. These include:

- athetoid cerebral palsy/extrapyramidal movement disorders
- paralysis of upward gaze and problems with visual focusing and recognition
- auditory dysfunction, especially isolated auditory neuropathy (a form of sensorineural hearing loss)
- dysplasia of the enamel of the deciduous teeth

The previously mentioned American Academy of Pediatrics policy statement lists ten "key elements" with the collective goal of reducing the incidence of severe hyperbilirubinemia and bilirubin encephalopathy, including:

- encouraging and supporting breast-feeding
- establishing nursery protocols for the detection and evaluation of hyperbilirubinemia (which includes screening mothers/infants for blood incompatibilities, assessment for jaundice every 8 to 12 hours, etc.)
- measuring total serum or transcutaneous bilirubin in infants who become jaundiced at younger than 24 hours of age
- understanding that visual estimation of jaundice based on level of skin involvement can lead to errors
- interpreting bilirubin results with regard to the infant's age in hours

- understanding that infants born <38 weeks of gestation are at increased risk for hyperbilirubinemia, especially if breast-fed, and require closer monitoring
- assessing infants using a systematic approach for the risk of severe hyperbilirubinemia before discharge (jaundice in first 24 hours, blood group incompatibility, preterm gestational age, cephalohematoma, etc.)
- providing written and verbal instructions for parents regarding neonatal jaundice
- assuring appropriate follow-up based on assessed risk and age at discharge (within 3 to 5 days)
- treatment with phototherapy or exchange transfusion when indicated

Sepsis

Early-onset neonatal sepsis (within the first week of life) should be at or near the top of the differential whenever a neonate appears ill. Most infected newborns become symptomatic within 24 hours of birth. Signs include respiratory distress, temperature instability, apnea, poor feeding/vomiting, irritability, lethargy, bradycardia, poor perfusion, and cardiovascular compromise. Neonates may not manifest fever as a sign of infection due to immaturity of the thermoregulatory center of the hypothalamus. Sepsis may be accompanied by pneumonia and/or meningitis. Bacterial sepsis is the most common cause of thrombocytopenia in the neonate. At a minimum, complete blood cell counts and blood cultures should be obtained from asymptomatic infants who are at increased risk for neonatal sepsis; empiric treatment considerations are based on the patient's degree of risk and initial laboratory results. Lumbar puncture should be performed in all symptomatic infants before treatment (if possible) and all asymptomatic infants with positive blood cultures. Maternal and infant characteristics that increase the neonate's likelihood of developing early-onset sepsis include:

- maternal factors: prolonged rupture of membranes (>18 hours); intrapartum fever ≥101°F; chorioamnionitis (abdominal tenderness, foul-smelling amniotic fluid)
- infant factors: preterm birth; LBW

Possible causative organisms include group B *Streptococcus* (GBS), *E. coli*, *L. monocytogenes*, *H. influenzae*, and enterococci. Cefotaxime (or ampicillin) and gentamicin in combination are appropriate empiric therapy until culture and sensitivity results are known.

GBS bears particular mention due to specialized practice parameters designed to decrease the incidence of perinatal infection. Expectant mothers are screened at 35 to 37 weeks of gestation for GBS by rectovaginal culture. Mothers who test positive, have documented GBS bacteriuria during pregnancy, or have tested positive during previous pregnancies should be treated during labor with ampicillin. The newborn is considered adequately treated if the maternal ampicillin is administered ≥4 hours before delivery. Adequate intrapartum therapy decreases the rate of early-onset infection but has no effect on the incidence of late-onset infections.

Organisms implicated in the development of nosocomial sepsis among infants in the NICU include coagulase-negative staphylococci, *Staphylococcus aureus*, enterococci, *Pseudomonas aeruginosa*, and *Enterobacter* species. The presence of intravascular catheters (e.g., umbilical vessel, central lines), extensive use of antibiotics, and prolonged intubation, all common interventions in preterm LBW infants, increase the likelihood that a neonate will become infected with a nosocomial pathogen.

Tracheoesophageal Fistula

The majority of infants with esophageal atresia (EA) also have associated tracheoesophageal fistula. A prenatal ultrasound that demonstrates maternal polyhydramnios and the absence of a stomach bubble in the fetus is consistent with EA. The condition is more common in preterm, VLBW, and SGA newborns. Patients present with excessive oral secretions and frothing and bubbling at the mouth and nose; frequent episodes of coughing, choking, and/or cyanosis; and respiratory distress that is exacerbated by feeding. EA is suggested when there is an inability to pass a catheter into the stomach confirmed by radiograph (catheter coiled in a blind pouch). If questions remain regarding the diagnosis, flexible bronchoscopy with methylene blue and fiberoptic endoscopy permit further evaluation. Surgical repair is necessary but may have to be delayed if the patient is unstable.

Diaphragmatic Hernia

The newborn with herniation of the abdominal contents through the diaphragm and into the chest cavity presents with a scaphoid abdomen, severe respiratory distress, and cyanosis. Breath sounds will be absent on the side of the herniation, and cardiac beats are displaced to the opposite side of the chest. Less severe cases result in only mild respiratory symptoms and vague feeding difficulties. A chest radiograph will reveal the abnormality.

Necrotizing Enterocolitis

Necrotizing enterocolitis (NEC) is a potentially devastating disease consisting of acute intestinal necrosis, most commonly involving the terminal ileum and ascending colon. NEC occurs disproportionately in infants who are preterm, VLBW, and/or exposed to cocaine in utero. The vast majority of affected neonates have begun enteral feeds. Physicians who care for high-risk infants must maintain a high degree of vigilance regarding NEC because early detection and prompt treatment positively affect outcome.

The clinical manifestations of NEC may be enteric or systemic in nature; usually there is a mixture of both. Signs include:

- irritability, lethargy; temperature instability; apnea, bradycardia; poor perfusion, acidosis, shock
- abdominal distention, tenderness, and guarding; increasing gastric residuals, vomiting; bloody stools; abdominal erythema, ascites; persistent abdominal mass

Pneumatosis intestinalis (PI), the presence of gas within the wall of the bowel on an abdominal plain radiograph, is the radiologic hallmark of NEC. PI is not detected in all infants with NEC. The degree of PI does not correlate with the severity of the disease, and its disappearance does not necessarily signify improvement. Nonspecific radiographic signs include generalized bowel distention, a persistently dilated loop of bowel, bowel wall thickening, and intraperitoneal fluid. Gas in the portal venous system is an ominous development.

When NEC is suspected, enteral feeds must be stopped immediately and a nasogastric tube with suction placed to decompress the bowel. Ampicillin and gentamicin (or zosyn) afford the appropriate broad-spectrum coverage. Abdominal films should be obtained every 6 to 8 hours until the disease process and the patient have stabilized. Once sepsis has been ruled out, a central line is placed for parenteral nutrition (if necessary). Resection of the involved segment of bowel is indicated for patients with perforation, full-thickness necrosis, or worsening clinical status despite maximal medical therapy.

Stricture formation is the most common long-term gastrointestinal complication of NEC. Most are located in the large bowel and may be asymptomatic. Multiple strictures are not uncommon. Short bowel syndrome and gastrointestinal malabsorption may result from surgical intervention.

Congenital Intestinal Obstruction

Nonbilious vomiting and spitting-up are not uncommon in the healthy infant but may also result from overfeeding, feeding intolerance, or pyloric stenosis. In contrast, bilious emesis in the neonate is considered a medical emergency. *Malrotation with or without midgut volvulus* is the most urgent obstructive condition encountered in the infant population; delay in diagnosis results in massive bowel necrosis. Plain films typically demonstrate gastric or duodenal distention with paucity of gas in the distal bowel. The upper gastrointestinal series is the radiographic study of choice. Surgical management is required.

Other congenital intestinal obstructions that present with bilious emesis include duodenal, jejunal, ileal, or colonic atresia; duodenal stenosis or web; annular pancreas; and Hirschsprung disease. Abdominal distention may be generalized (distal obstruction) or localized to the left upper quadrant (proximal obstruction). Duodenal obstruction may result in no distention at all. Small bowel obstructions usually manifest earlier than those of the distal gastrointestinal tract.

An obstructive lesion located in the small intestine typically presents with bilious vomiting that occurs shortly after the initial feeding. Duodenal atresia is more common in newborns with Down syndrome or a history of maternal polyhydramnios. Radiographic studies reveal an enlarged duodenal air bubble or a "double-bubble" and absence of air the in the remainder of the abdomen.

The signs and symptoms of *Hirschsprung disease* are consistent with congenital large bowel obstruction. In this case, the obstruction is functional in nature, resulting from the absence of ganglion cells in the distal colon and associated disordered motility. Classic symptoms of Hirschsprung disease include bilious emesis, marked abdominal distention, and failure to pass meconium. Radiographs demonstrate multiple dilated loops of air-filled bowel but no air in the rectum. A contrast enema will show a normal-size rectum with a transitional zone to the distended bowel, often located in the rectosigmoid area. Diagnosis is confirmed by rectal biopsy.

Patients with congenital bowel obstruction are made *non per oral* and started on intermittent gastric suction. Optimization of fluid and electrolyte status should take place in addition to consultation of the pediatric surgical team.

Meconium ileus is a form of intestinal obstruction that results from obstruction of the distal small bowel by thick, inspissated meconium. The clinical presentation is identical to that of Hirschsprung disease. Characteristic radiographic findings include multiple dilated loops of bowel, with a "ground-glass" appearance and/or small bubbles noted in the area of the obstruction; intraluminal calcifications also may be present. A contrast enema with hypertonic solution is diagnostic (microcolon) and may also prove to be therapeutic. Cases that do not resolve with repeated enemas or are complicated by perforation require surgical management. Meconium ileus is virtually pathognomonic for *cystic fibrosis*, although sporadic cases occasionally occur.

Abdominal/Intestinal Wall Defects

An *omphalocele* is a defect in the abdominal wall that results in herniation of the midgut within a translucent peritoneal sac that may or may not be intact. Associated congenital anomalies are common. If the sac is ruptured or there is vascular compromise, urgent surgical repair is indicated. Patients with intact sacs may be stabilized before surgery. In *gastroschisis*, there is no peritoneal sac covering the intestines, which are outside the abdominal cavity. Surgical intervention is necessary. Gastroschisis is not usually accompanied by other anomalies.

MATERNAL CONDITIONS THAT AFFECT THE FETUS AND/OR NEONATE

Congenital/Perinatal Infections

Several important congenital and/or neonatal infections are detailed in Table 5-8. Whenever a congenital infection is suspected, serum should be collected from the infant and the mother when possible. Titers are obtained from the patient as soon as possible and repeated every 2 to 4 weeks. In the infant, maternally derived immunoglobulin G (IgG) is nondetectable by 6 to 12 months of age; significant elevation in specific IgG beyond 4 months of age or a greater than fourfold increase in IgG concentration is consistent with congenital infection. Ophthalmologic examination is indicated in children with suspected congenital infections due to the high incidence of ophthalmologic complications and subsequent visual impairment.

TABLE 5-8
IMPORTANT CONGENITAL AND PERINATAL INFECTIONS

Cytomegalovirus

Transmission

Congenital: Transmission may occur at any time during the pregnancy. Transmission rate significantly higher if the mother acquires the disease during pregnancy. Transmission possible even when the primary maternal infection occurred years before the pregnancy. Risk and severity of complications not related to stage of pregnancy in which the infection occurred.

Acquired: Transmission through exposure to organism in maternal genital tract, breast milk, urine, respiratory secretions, or blood transfusion.

Presentation

Congenital: Asymptomatic (90%), OR combination of any of the following: preterm birth, IUGR, microcephaly, poor feeding, lethargy, petechiae/purpura, "blueberry muffin" spots, jaundice, hepatosplenomegaly, elevated liver transaminases, anemia, thrombocytopenia, intracranial (particularly periventricular) calcifications, seizures, chorioretinitis.

Acquired: Term infants generally remain asymptomatic.

Diagnosis: CMV detected in the urine (saliva, blood) within the first 2 weeks of life is consistent with congenital infection. Organism is demonstrable in urine of infants with perinatal transmission by 4 to 8 weeks of age.

Treatment: Supportive care; ongoing trials with gancyclovir.

Long-term sequelae

Congenital: Congenital CMV is the most common infectious cause of sensorineural hearing loss. Seventy-five percent of infants with symptomatic congenital CMV will develop hearing loss. Hearing is often normal at birth, with progressive impairment over the first year. Other possible long-term complications include developmental delay, mental retardation, cerebral palsy (motor spasticity), and dental defects (abnormal enamel production).

Acquired: None, unless extremely premature/low-birth weight

Screening/prevention: Antibody testing before or early in pregnancy to document prior infection. Ongoing research into whether antiviral medication may prevent long-term sequelae in infants with congenital CMV.

HSV

Transmission: Perinatal infection acquired through exposure to organism in maternal genital tract during delivery. Transmission rate significantly higher if the mother contracts primary infection during pregnancy (up to 50% vs. <5% for infants born to mothers with recurrent infections). That being said, *most infants with neonatal HSV are born to women who have never experienced symptoms and do not know that they are infected.* Infants may also become infected through contact with herpetic breast lesions while feeding or from maternal oral secretions after birth.

Presentation: Neonatal HSV presents in the first 4 wk of life with any of the following three distinct clinical pictures

Isolated mucocutaneous lesions [skin, eye (see Chapter 22), and/or mouth], including keratoconjunctivitis

Encephalitis

Disseminated disease involving multiple organs (lungs, liver, often CNS)

Infants with encephalitis and/or disseminated HSV disease may not manifest the characteristic vesicular skin lesions, leading to a delay in diagnosis.

Diagnosis: Viral culture or direct fluorescent antibody testing of vesicular scrapings. If no lesions present, virus also demonstrable in nasopharynx, conjunctivae, and urine. CSF infection: pleocytosis, increased protein; virus detected on PCR testing; electroencephalogram shows periodic epileptiform discharges; magnetic resonance imaging demonstrates hyperintensity of the periventricular white matter.

Treatment: Intravenous acyclovir. Any neonate with vesicular lesions is presumed to have HSV, and acyclovir should be started pending laboratory confirmation. Early initiation of acyclovir therapy in neonatal HSV significantly improves outcome. Consultation with a pediatric ophthalmologist is required in infants with ocular involvement.

(continued)

TABLE 5-8
(continued)

Long-term sequelae

Local disease: Recurrent mucocutaneous lesions

Encephalitis: Cataracts/blindness; microcephaly; developmental delay/learning disabilities

Disseminated disease: Severe neurologic impairment, death (50%)

Screening/prevention: Deliver infants by cesarean section if genital lesions are present at start of labor. If maternal lesions are found after delivery, culture infant and treat with acyclovir if culture-positive or symptoms develop. Although it should still be performed, cesarean section delivery is not as effective at preventing neonatal HSV when membranes have been ruptured >6 h.

Parvovirus

Transmission: Congenital infection with vertical transmission.

Presentation: Hydrops fetalis (risk increased if mother becomes infected during the first trimester).

Diagnosis: Maternal IgM, IgG levels.

Treatment: Intrauterine blood transfusions; supportive care.

Long-term sequelae: None, if fetus survives pregnancy and perinatal interventions.

Screening/prevention: None routine

HIV

Transmission

Congenital: Transmission may occur at any time during the pregnancy. Likelihood of vertical transmission increases with increasing maternal viral load.

Acquired: Transmission through exposure to the organism in maternal genital tract or breast milk.

Presentation: Most infected infants are asymptomatic. Clinical manifestations that may develop over time include lymphadenopathy/hepatosplenomegaly; failure to thrive; developmental delay; encephalopathy; frequent bacterial infections; opportunistic infection (*Pneumocystis jiroveci*); lymphoid interstitial pneumonitis.

Diagnosis: HIV culture; PCR.

Treatment: Antiretroviral therapy (see Chapter 10).

Long-term sequelae: All of the above listed under "Presentation"; death.

Screening/prevention: Antibody testing before or early in pregnancy to document infection. Zidovudine administered to the infected mother throughout pregnancy and delivery, and zidovudine in the infant for the first 6 wk of life. This protocol decreases the rate of transmission from 25% to <2%. Breast-feeding is contraindicated.

Varicella Zoster Virus

Transmission

Congenital: Transmission may occur at any time during the pregnancy. Rash developing within the first 10 d of life is due to in utero infection.

Neonatal acquired: Infants with mothers who develop varicella lesions anytime from 5 d before delivery to 2 d after delivery are at high risk for severe (fatal) disease.

Acquired: Transmission through exposure to the organism in vesicular fluid, mucosa, or infected respiratory secretions.

Presentation

Congenital: Congenital varicella syndrome includes any combination of the following: IUGR, cutaneous "zig-zag" scarring, limb atrophy, ocular abnormalities (cataracts, chorioretinitis).

Neonatal acquired: Widespread cutaneous lesions, pneumonia, hepatitis; death in up to a third of affected infants.

Acquired: Mild clinical disease.

Diagnosis: Generally clinical; immunofluorescent antibody testing of vesicular scrapings is confirmatory.

Treatment: Intravenous acyclovir for infants at risk for severe disease.

Long-term sequelae: Early death (congenital varicella syndrome and about one third of patients with neonatal-acquired varicella); otherwise minimal.

Screening/prevention: Vaccination before pregnancy; acyclovir for the mother if she develops primary disease during the pregnancy.

Rubella

Transmission: Congenital infection may occur at any time during pregnancy. Cases in which the fetus is infected before 20 wk of gestation are particularly devastating. The virus crosses the placenta during maternal viremia, which may be asymptomatic.

Presentation: Fetal demise, premature delivery, and/or *congenital rubella syndrome*, a constellation of any of the following: cataracts, sensorineural hearing loss (the most common impairment associated with congenital rubella syndrome), congenital cardiac defects, developmental delay (may be accompanied by IUGR, hepatosplenomegaly, thrombocytopenic purpura).

(*continued*)

TABLE 5-8
(continued)

Diagnosis: Maternal antibody titers during pregnancy; after birth, the infant may be tested for the virus, rubella-specific IgM, or persistently elevated rubella-specific IgG.

Treatment: No specific treatment. Infants with congenital rubella syndrome shed the virus for up to 1 y and can transmit the infection to susceptible hosts.

Long-term sequelae: Hearing impairment, glaucoma, mental retardation.

Screening/prevention: All women of child-bearing age should have documented evidence of appropriate vaccination or immunity. Immunity should be confirmed with serology in all women who are considering becoming pregnant. In nonimmune women, pregnancy should be delayed until ≥1 mo after vaccination. Although vaccine-associated rubella virus has been reported in extremely rare cases in infants born to mothers inadvertently vaccinated during pregnancy, receiving the vaccine during pregnancy is not an indication for terminating the pregnancy.

Syphilis

Transmission: Congenital infection results from transplacental transmission of spirochetes and may occur at any time during pregnancy. Transmission rates are extremely high if the mother is in the primary or secondary stage during pregnancy.

Presentation: Fetal demise; premature delivery; infants may be asymptomatic at birth but develop typical skin lesions, anemia, thrombocytopenia, jaundice, "snuffles," hepatosplenomegaly, elevated liver enzymes, and skeletal abnormalities, such as osteochondritis (inflammation of the cartilage and bone around a joint) and periostitis. A significant number of infected neonates are identified by routine screening; others may not develop clinical symptoms such as failure to thrive or neurologic complications until the second year of life.

Diagnosis: All pregnant women should be screened for syphilis. Those in high-risk categories should be screened again at delivery. Confirmation of infection requires treatment with penicillin. Testing should be carried out in all symptomatic infants and asymptomatic infants of mothers with positive screens whose treatment occurred within 1 mo of delivery, was inadequate or undocumented, or did not result in a reduction in nontreponemal titers. If the neonatal nontreponemal titer is not ≥4 times the maternal titer, the infant is unlikely to be infected.

Treatment: Penicillin G. All infants should be presumed to have neurosyphilis and be treated with aqueous crystalline penicillin G (intravenously) or procaine penicillin (intramuscularly) for 10 to 14 d. Serial titers document resolution of infection.

Long-term sequelae: Neurosyphilis, deafness.

Screening/prevention: Routine maternal nontreponemal testing confirmed by a treponemal test; treatment of maternal disease during pregnancy.

Toxoplasmosis

Transmission: Transmission may occur at any time during pregnancy. Fetal infection rates are lowest in the first trimester and highest in the third; conversely, disease severity is highest in the first trimester and lowest in the third.

Presentation: Intracranial calcifications and chorioretinitis; anemia, jaundice, hepatosplenomegaly, lymphadenopathy; infants may be asymptomatic at birth.

Diagnosis: Toxoplasma-specific antibody testing in the infant.

Treatment: Multidrug therapy of the infant.

Long-term sequelae: Blindness, developmental delay.

Screening/prevention: Keep cats indoors and change litter frequently; avoid eating undercooked meats; limit exposure to contaminated soil.

IUGR, intrauterine growth retardation; CMV, cytomegalovirus; HSV, herpes simplex virus; CNS, central nervous system; CSF, cerebrospinal fluid; PCR, polymerase chain reaction; IgM, immunoglobulin M; IgG, immunoglobulin G; HIV, human immunodeficiency virus.

Maternal Illness

Infants of mothers with insulin-dependent diabetes (IDM) are at risk for complications in multiple systems. The most common is *hypertrophic cardiomyopathy,* although this disorder is usually clinically silent and resolves within several months of birth. Symptoms, when they occur, are consistent with obstructive left heart failure. Neonatal *small left colon syndrome* also occurs more frequently in IDMs and may rarely result in colonic obstruction, although usually the disorder is asymptomatic and resolves spontaneously. Polycythemia is present in about one fourth of IDMs, often leading to hyperbilirubinemia and jaundice. Hypocalcemia and hypomagnesemia are more common in these patients. Infants of diabetic mothers have pulmonary function consistent with earlier gestational ages due to the delayed appearance of mature phospholipids in fetal surfactant, even at 36 to 38 weeks. There is an increased incidence of congenital anomalies in IDMs, particularly *caudal regression,* which is characterized by hypoplasia or agenesis of the lower vertebrae and sacrum. Depending on the extent of involvement, lower extremity motor deficits and abnormalities of bowel and bladder function may result.

Maternal hyperglycemia leads to fetal hyperglycemia, which results in fetal hyperinsulinemia due to islet cell hypertrophy and β-cell hyperplasia. When the maternal supply of glucose is interrupted at birth, this insulin in excess of needs precipitates hypoglycemia in the infant. Infants born to diabetic mothers typically develop hypoglycemia (blood glucose level <45 mg/dL) 1 to 4 hours after birth. Most remain asymptomatic, but cases of significant, prolonged hypoglycemia do occur. Prolonged in utero hyperinsulinemia also results in *macrosomia* and visceromegaly, although some of these infants develop IUGR.

Management of infants born to diabetic mothers is the same as that for other newborns at increased risk of neonatal hypoglycemia. Infants are screened within the first 2 hours of life, even if asymptomatic. Thereafter, a bedside dextrose stick is obtained before each feed (for 12 to 24 hours) and whenever the neonate becomes symptomatic. Asymptomatic hypoglycemic infants may be given oral glucose solution. Symptomatic infants who cannot feed are started on parenteral glucose. Glucose checks should be performed within 30 to 60 minutes to document normalization.

Another maternal illness with known consequences for the fetus is *systemic lupus erythematosus* (SLE). Infants of mothers with SLE may develop *neonatal thrombocytopenia*, which can last up to a week, due to placental transmission of LE factor. Another complication of maternal SLE is *congenital heart block*, which occurs despite the presence of a structurally normal heart.

Maternal Medications During Labor

Tocolytic agents are often given to the mother in preterm labor to inhibit uterine contractions. *Magnesium sulfate* may result in neonatal lethargy, hypotonia, respiratory depression, and decreased serum calcium. *Terbutaline*, a β-adrenergic drug, has been associated with fetal tachycardia, hyperinsulinemia, and hypoglycemia. *Ritodrine* is a β_2-receptor agonist that can cause hypoglycemia, hyperinsulinemia, hypocalcemia, and hypotension in the newborn.

Narcotic analgesics commonly administered during labor include mepivacaine, bupivacaine, meperidine, butorphanol, and nalbuphine. Any of these can result in apnea and hypotension in the neonate. When meperidine in particular is given, these effects may last for a few days. Butorphanol and nalbuphine have been known to result in fetal heart rate changes that mimic those of hypoxia.

Maternal Substance Use

Table 5-9 presents the neonatal withdrawal syndromes associated with maternal use of various substances. Substances used by the mother during pregnancy may also have teratogenic potential and result in congenital anomalies. For example, *fetal alcohol syndrome* consists of characteristic facial anomalies, growth retardation, and cognitive impairment with or without behavior problems. This preventable condition is the leading cause of mental retardation in the United States. Table 5-9 lists the potential teratogenic effects of each substance when known.

TABLE 5-9
MATERNAL SUBSTANCE USE: ASSOCIATED FETAL ABNORMALITIES/NEONATAL WITHDRAWAL SYNDROMES

	Fetal Abnormalities	Increased Future Risks	Neonatal Withdrawal Syndromes	Management of Neonatal Abstinence Syndromes
Alcohol (onset 6 to 12 h after birth)	Growth retardation[a] Microcephaly Short palpebral fissures[a] Midface hypoplasia Smooth philtrum[a] Thin, smooth upper vermillion border[a] Joint anomalies Altered palmar creases Small distal phalanges Hypoplastic nails Fifth-finger clinodactyly Hirsutism Congenital (septal) heart defects	Mental retardation[a] Impaired linear growth Sensorineural hearing loss Strabismus Developmental delay[a] (motor, speech) Learning disorders[a] Behavior problems (ADHD, conduct disorder)	Newborns with fetal alcohol syndrome are irritable and tremulous, regardless of whether they were exposed after the first trimester. If the mother is intoxicated at delivery, the infant may be lethargic and hypoglycemic. Withdrawal is uncommon but may include sweating, irritability, jitteriness, tachypnea, tremors, hypertonia, and seizures.	None required

(continued)

TABLE 5-9 (continued)

	Fetal Abnormalities	Increased Future Risks	Neonatal Withdrawal Syndromes	Management of Neonatal Abstinence Syndromes
Amphetamines	No known organ teratogenicity Reduced birth weight Encephalopathy Poor feeding Increased arousal Increased tone Tachycardia Hypertension	None known	No significant withdrawal syndrome; possibly irritability, sneezing, high-pitched cry	None required
Barbiturates (within 2 wk)	No known organ teratogenicity	Under investigation	Irritability, tremors, exaggerated startle, excessive crying, vasomotor instability, diarrhea, restlessness, increased tone, hyperphagia, vomiting, disturbed sleep	Usually none required
Cocaine	Intracranial hemorrhage Seizures Limb reduction defects Intestinal atresia Gastroschisis Urinary tract abnormalities	Increased incidence of sudden infant death syndrome; subtle abnormalities in attention/concentration	Irritability; otherwise none recognized	Usually none required
Hallucinogens (LSD, PCP, psilocybin, mescaline)	No known organ teratogenicity	Under investigation	Jitteriness, exaggerated startle response	None required
Marijuana	No known organ teratogenicity	Under investigation; possibly measurable effects on IQ	Uncommon and mild; fine tremors, amplified Moro reflex	None required
Opiates: short-acting narcotics[b] (onset within 1 to 4 d)	No known organ teratogenicity Impaired fetal growth	Developmental delay Behavioral problems	Hyperirritability, gastrointestinal dysfunction, respiratory distress, vague autonomic symptoms (yawning, sneezing, mottling, fever), tremulousness, jitteriness, high-pitched cry, increased muscle tone, irritability, loose stools	Avoid naloxone administration; symptomatic care (tight swaddling, rocking, minimizing stimulation); administer oral neonatal morphine solution or paregoric q4h with a 10% wean per day
Opiates: methadone[b] (onset within 3 wk)	No known organ teratogenicity Impaired fetal growth	Developmental delay Behavioral problems	Any combination of the above	
Tobacco	No known organ teratogenicity Intrauterine growth restriction Low birth weight Preterm labor Late fetal demise	Sudden infant death syndrome Developmental delay Asthma Otitis media	Fine tremors, hypertonia	None required

[a]Characteristic findings of fetal alcohol syndrome.
[b]Requires medical intervention with paregoric, phenobarbital, or methadone and assistance with feeding.
ADHD, attention-deficit/hyperactivity disorder; LSD, lysergic acid diethylamide; PCP, phencyclidine.

Maternal smoking continues to be common despite the clear association with negative effects on the fetus and infant. IUGR and LBW are common in newborns of mothers who smoke, and a dose–response relation is well-documented; women who smoke the most during pregnancy have the smallest newborns. Complications related to the placenta (abruption, insufficiency, and placental previa) occur at a higher rate in pregnancies affected by tobacco use. Infants of mothers who smoke during pregnancy are three times as likely to die of sudden infant death syndrome as infants of mothers who abstain from smoking. They are also more likely to develop asthma and have frequent otitis media. Research into whether tobacco use during pregnancy increases the risk of certain birth defects is ongoing.

SOURCES

Aly H. Respiratory disorders in the newborn: identification and diagnosis. *Pediatr Rev.* 2004;25:201–208.

American Academy of Pediatrics Subcommittee on Hyperbilirubinemia. Clinical practice guideline: management of hyperbilirubinemia in the newborn infant 35 or more weeks of gestation. *Pediatrics.* 2004; 114:297–316.

Apgar V. A proposal for a new method of evaluation of the infant. *Res Anesth Analg.* 1953;32:260.

Boyle RJ. Effects of certain prenatal drugs on the fetus and newborn. *Pediatr Rev.* 2002;23:17–24.

Bhutani VK, Johnson L, Sivieri EM. Predictive ability of a predischarge hour-specific serum bilirubin for subsequent significant hyperbilirubinemia in healthy term and near-term newborns. *Pediatrics.* 1999;103:6–14.

Das UG, Sysyn GD. Abnormal fetal growth: intrauterine growth retardation, small for gestational age, large for gestational age. *Pediatr Clin North Am.* 2004;51:639–654.

Friedman MA, Spitzer AR. Discharge criteria for the term newborn. *Pediatr Clin North Am.* 2004;51:599–618.

Hoyer A. Effects on the fetus of maternal drugs during labor. *Pediatr Rev.* 2002;23:256–257.

Kates EH, Kates JS. Anemia and polycythemia in the newborn. *Pediatr Rev.* 2007;28:33–34.

Leuthner SR, Das UG. Low Apgar scores and the definition of birth asphyxia. *Pediatr Clin North Am.* 2004;51:737–746.

Maisels MJ. Jaundice a newborn: Answers to questions about a common clinical problem. *Contemp Pediatr.* 2005;25:1–7.

Sasidharan P. An approach to diagnosis and management of cyanosis and tachypnea in term infants. *Pediatr Clin North Am.* 2004;51:999–1022.

Stellwagen L, Boies E. Care of the well newborn. *Pediatr Rev.* 2006;27: 89–98.

QUESTIONS

1. A 42-year-old woman is expecting her first child and has had an uneventful pregnancy. At 37 weeks of gestation, she calls her obstetrician and reports that she thinks the baby is moving much less than before. An NST is nonreactive. Which of the following options is the most appropriate next step?

A) Fetal ultrasound
B) Fetal stress testing
C) Fetal heart rate monitoring
D) Induction of labor with oxytocin
E) Emergency cesarean section

2. Which of the following is not evaluated by a fetal biophysical profile?

A) Fetal heart rate reactivity in response to fetal movement
B) Fetal heart rate reactivity in response to uterine contractions
C) Amniotic fluid volume
D) Fetal movement
E) Fetal heart rate

3. A 6-week-old male infant born at 29 4/7 weeks of gestation has been maintained in an open bassinet with swaddling and a hat for the past 10 days. However, he develops apnea and bradycardia and is placed under a servo-controlled radiant warmer for evaluation and management. Which of the following statements is FALSE?

A) Use of a radiant warmer is appropriate in this situation given the infant's need for further evaluation and close monitoring.
B) Use of a radiant warmer will increase this infant's insensible water loses.
C) Use of a radiant warmer will increase this infant's energy expenditures.
D) Core body temperature should be measured routinely to detect temperature instability.
E) Careful attention to fluid "ins and outs" and patient weight will assist in the management of fluid status while under the radiant warmer.

4. Which of the following statements regarding Apgar scoring is FALSE?

A) The 1-minute Apgar is reflective of the newborn's intrauterine environment.
B) The 5-minute Apgar indicates the infant's adjustment to the extrauterine environment.
C) The 1-minute Apgar is reflective of the newborn's tolerance of delivery.
D) Decisions regarding intervention and resuscitation should be based on the patient's 5-minute Apgar score, not the 1-minute Apgar score.
E) Apgar scores suggest which infants will transition successfully and which will need sustained support.

5. A 27-year-old woman is in labor at 41 weeks of gestation. Particulate meconium is noted in the amniotic fluid upon rupture of membranes at the onset of delivery. When the infant's head is delivered, the mouth, nares, and pharynx are suctioned by the obstetrician. After delivery of the rest of the infant, no respiratory effort or spontaneous movement is noted. When the infant is placed under the radiant warmer, which of the following should take place FIRST?

A) Vigorous stimulation
B) Blow-by oxygen

C) Positive pressure ventilation
D) Drying and warming
E) Visualization of the larynx, intubation, and tracheal suctioning

6. A 17-year-old woman is admitted from the emergency department in active labor. She received no prenatal care and does not know the date of her last menstrual period. Meconium-stained amniotic fluid is noted, but the variability of the fetal heart rate is reassuring. The mouth and pharynx are suctioned after delivery of the head. The infant responds to clamping of the cord with a strong cry and vigorous movement. Which of the following is the most appropriate course of action?
A) The infant should be dried and placed under the radiant warmer for further evaluation.
B) The infant's larynx should be visualized.
C) The infant's trachea should be suctioned.
D) The infant should receive blow-by oxygen regardless of clinical status.
E) The infant should be intubated.

7. A newborn infant is delivered by elective cesarean section at $40\frac{0}{7}$ weeks of gestation after an uneventful pregnancy. The infant is depressed at birth, with a heart rate of 55 beats per minute and central cyanosis at 1 minute of age despite vigorous stimulation. The patient has a weak cry and appears to be struggling to breathe. Which of the following resuscitation measures is the most appropriate at this time?
A) Blow-by oxygen
B) Positive pressure ventilation by face mask and bag breaths
C) External cardiac massage
D) Intubation and mechanical ventilation
E) Endotracheal epinephrine

8. A newborn infant is delivered to a 15-year-old with no history of prenatal care who is $32\frac{5}{7}$ weeks of gestation based on dates. The infant is unresponsive at birth and does not respond to vigorous stimulation and drying. After 30 seconds of positive pressure ventilation with face mask and bag breaths, the patient has no spontaneous respirations, and the heart rate is 50 beats per minute. Which of the following is the most appropriate next course of action?
A) Placement of an intraosseous line and administration of epinephrine
B) Intubation and instillation of epinephrine
C) External cardiac massage at 100 compressions per minute
D) Emergency transport to the neonatal intensive care unit for extracorporal membrane oxygenation
E) Emergency transport to the neonatal intensive care unit for exogenous surfactant administration

9. A newborn infant is born at 38 weeks of gestation after an uncomplicated pregnancy. The infant has a heart rate of 50 beats per minute despite vigorous stimulation. Positive pressure ventilation does not result in inflation of the chest. Which of the following is the most appropriate next step in the management of this patient?
A) Intubation and high-pressure ventilation
B) Intubation and administration of surfactant
C) Increasing inflation pressure
D) Repositioning of the infant's head into the "sniffing" position
E) External cardiac massage

10. Which of the following statements regarding resuscitation in the delivery room is TRUE?
A) If indicated, chest compressions should depress the chest about half of the anterior-posterior diameter.
B) If indicated, chest compressions should depress the chest at a rate of 60 compressions per minute.
C) The recommended ratio of breaths-to-compressions is 1 to 4.
D) If the infant's heart rate is <100 beats per minute after 30 seconds of positive pressure ventilation, the infant should receive external cardiac massage.
E) The inflation pressure required for the initial breath is greater than that needed for subsequent breaths.

11. A 1-month-old infant born at 35 weeks of gestation has persistent microcephaly. Computed tomography reveals periventricular calcifications, and cytomegalovirus (CMV) is detected in the patient's urine. Which of the following statements regarding this clinical scenario is FALSE?
A) Fluorescent antigenic testing can be used to differentiate congenital CMV from acquired CMV.
B) This patient may have congenital CMV.
C) This patient may have perinatally acquired CMV.
D) Infants with acquired CMV are not at risk for sensorineural hearing loss.
E) Infants with symptomatic congenital CMV have an increased risk of cerebral palsy.

12. Which of the following pairs denote by when a typical newborn has urinated and passed meconium, respectively?
A) 8 hours; 24 hours
B) 12 hours; 48 hours
C) 12 hours; 24 hours
D) 18 hours; 48 hours
E) 24 hours; 48 hours

13. Which of the following pairs of answers denote the weight cutoffs for LBW and VLBW newborns, respectively?
A) 2,000 g; 1,200 g
B) 2,000 g; 1,500 g
C) 2,500 g; 1,500 g
D) 2,800 g; 1,500 g
E) 2,800 g; 1,800 g

14. LGA growth is constitutional in the majority of cases. However, maternal and fetal conditions can result in the birth of an LGA infant. Which of the following conditions is not associated with LGA birth weight?
A) Maternal obesity
B) Gestational diabetes
C) Beckwith-Wiedemann syndrome
D) Maternal steroid use
E) Transposition of the great vessels

15. You are discussing the care of LGA infants with a senior medical student who is rotating through the NICU. He is already aware that the most frequent complication of an LGA birth is birth trauma (e.g., clavicular fracture). You are correct in informing him that all of the following are additional conditions that are disproportionately encountered in LGA infants EXCEPT:
A) Hypoglycemia
B) Polycythemia
C) Jaundice
D) Pulmonary hypertension
E) Persistent fetal circulation

16. You are discussing the care of SGA infants with an intern rotating through the newborn nursery. You are correct in informing her that all of the following conditions are disproportionately encountered in SGA infants EXCEPT:
A) Respiratory distress syndrome
B) Hypothermia
C) Perinatal asphyxia
D) Hypoglycemia
E) Persistent fetal circulation

17. Which of the following statements regarding iron stores and supplementation in the preterm infant is TRUE?
A) Preterm infants have total body iron stores equivalent to those of full-term infants.
B) The iron stores of preterm infants are depleted more rapidly than those of their full-term peers.
C) Preterm infants should begin iron supplementation or iron-fortified formula by the age of 6 months or sooner if birth weight doubles.
D) Physiologic anemia of prematurity results in equivalent minimum hemoglobin levels to those found during physiologic anemia of infancy in full-term infants.
E) Physiologic anemia of prematurity occurs at 8 to 12 weeks of age.

18. A full-term infant with unremarkable prenatal history and perinatal course has not urinated by 24 hours of age. Which of the following is the most appropriate first step in evaluation of the infant?
A) Bladder catheterization of the infant
B) Obtain a renal sonogram.
C) Evaluate hydration status and review the infant's intake history.
D) Obtain serum blood urea nitrogen and creatinine levels.
E) Request an urgent urology referral.

19. A mother brings her 2-month-old infant to your office because he has not stooled in 5 days. The patient is a former full-term infant with no significant pre- or perinatal history. His birth weight was at the 50th percentile, and his growth has continued to parallel that line. He is exclusively breast-fed and continues to feed well. His mother is concerned that the time between his stools has become progressively longer. In the first 3 weeks of life, he stooled after every feed. Now, several days may pass between his stools, which remain yellow, soft, and easy for him to pass. The physical examination, including the abdominal and external rectal portions, is normal. Which of the following is the most appropriate next step in the management of this patient?
A) Schedule a consultation with a pediatric surgeon.
B) Obtain a barium enema.
C) Obtain an upper gastrointestinal series with small bowel follow-through.
D) Reassure the mother that the infant's stool pattern is normal for a 2-month-old breast-fed infant.
E) Obtain an abdominal radiograph.

20. A 5-day-old female infant born at 34 weeks of gestation has a serum total bilirubin level of 14 mg per dL. She requires no supplemental oxygen or respiratory support, and there is no clinical evidence of intraventricular hemorrhage or infection. Which of the following statements regarding this infant's condition (physiologic jaundice) is true?
A) This patient does not require phototherapy because the preterm brain is less affected by elevated bilirubin levels.
B) This patient should be started on phototherapy immediately because her level exceeds 12 mg per dL, the upper limit of physiologic jaundice in the preterm infant.
C) Subsequent evaluation of this infant's bilirubin levels may be undertaken by estimating the level of jaundice of the infant's skin.
D) This infant probably will not require intervention for her elevated bilirubin level because she is 5 days old and past the time of "peak" elevation.
E) This infant should be started on phototherapy because her peak level has likely not yet occurred, and preterm infants are known to develop neurologic consequences at lower bilirubin levels than full-term infants.

21. The mother of a 1-week-old full-term infant is concerned about a bump she found beneath the girl's right nipple. The physical examination reveals a 0.75-cm firm nodule directly beneath the right nipple. Palpation does not appear to cause the patient pain or discomfort. She continues to feed well and has no history of fever or any other symptoms. As you discuss the infant's condition with the mother, you are correct in telling her which of the following?

A) The condition is physiologic, requires no therapy, and resolves spontaneously.
B) The condition is nonphysiologic but should resolve spontaneously within 6 months.
C) The condition will require excision of the nodule if it persists >12 months.
D) The condition should be evaluated by ultrasound as soon as possible.
E) The nodule is likely a benign cyst.

22. Which of the following conditions is the most common cause of neonatal seizures in full-term infants?

A) Hypoglycemia
B) HIE
C) Hypoxic-ischemic encephalopathy
D) Hypocalcemia
E) Inborn errors of metabolism

23. A full-term LGA infant of a diabetic mother develops isolated hematuria. The infant's venous hematocrit is 69%. Which of the following is the most appropriate next step in the management of this patient?

A) Hydration with 20-mL per kg boluses of normal saline, one per hour, until the hematuria clears
B) Partial exchange transfusion with albumin as the diluent
C) Partial exchange transfusion with saline as the diluent
D) Renal ultrasonography
E) Ultrasonography of the cranial contents

24. The presence of nonphysiologic jaundice is suggested by which of the following conditions?

A) Jaundice before 24 hours of age
B) Increase in serum bilirubin concentration >0.5 mg per dL per hour
C) Total serum bilirubin level ≥75th percentile for age in hours
D) Jaundice in an infant with a history of a traumatic birth
E) All of the above

25. An 8-hour-old AGA male infant born at 35 weeks of gestation has fed poorly and develops temperature instability and bradycardia. His mother had an intrapartum fever to 101.5°F. After collection of specimens for laboratory evaluation, which of the following treatment regimens is most appropriate for this patient?

A) Ampicillin and sulbactam
B) Cefotaxime and piperacillin
C) Cefotaxime and oxacillin
D) Ampicillin and gentamicin
E) Vancomycin, with or without gentamicin

26. An infant born at 30 weeks of gestation requires mechanical ventilation for respiratory distress that developed shortly after birth. Current ventilator settings include a positive end-expiratory pressure of 4 cm H_2O, a peak inspiratory pressure of 24 cm H_2O, a ventilator respiratory rate of 40 breaths per minute, and a fraction of inspired O_2 of 0.7 to maintain a PaO_2 of 60 mm Hg. A portable chest radiograph demonstrates low lung volumes with a "ground-glass" appearance of the lung fields. The decision is made to administer endotracheal surfactant. Which of the following is most likely to occur within the next 4 hours?

A) Reduced O_2 requirement
B) Increased partial pressure of arterial carbon dioxide
C) Decreased PaO_2
D) Bradycardia
E) Pneumothorax

27. A 3-week-old neonate born at 26 weeks of gestation is undergoing enteral feeds. He develops increasing residuals, irritability, and abdominal distention. Blood cultures and a complete blood cell count are drawn and sent to the laboratory. A portable abdominal radiograph demonstrates generalized bowel distention, a limited area of gas within the wall of the intestine, but no free air. Which of the following is the most important first step in the management of this patient?

A) Obtain a surgical consultation.
B) Stop all enteral feeds and place a nasogastric tube to intermittent suction to decompress the bowel.
C) Begin broad-spectrum antibiotics.
D) Place a central line for parenteral alimentation.
E) Obtain another abdominal radiograph in 4 to 6 hours.

28. A 12-month-old infant born at 26 weeks of gestation required medical treatment for NEC while in the NICU. He has been undergoing occupational therapy for oromotor dysfunction since his discharge from the hospital. His mother reports that he is gaining appropriate weight on his enteral feeds and beginning to tolerate some oral intake. She asks you if there are any long-term gastrointestinal complications to be expected based on his neonatal course. You are correct in telling her which of the following?

A) The most common long-term complication of NEC is gastrointestinal reflux.
B) The most common long-term complication of NEC is gastrointestinal malabsorption.
C) The most common long-term complication of NEC is intestinal stricture formation.
D) The most common long-term complication of NEC is hepatic failure.
E) No long-term complications are to be expected in this patient because his NEC did not require surgical management.

29. A 26-year-old primagravida develops preterm labor at 21 weeks of gestation. She is discharged on oral terbutaline, which she continues for 12 weeks despite repeated attempts at withdrawal. Long-term exposure to terbutaline places her fetus at risk for the development of which of the following complications?
A) Bradycardia
B) Respiratory depression
C) Hypotension
D) Hypertrophic cardiomyopathy
E) Placental abruption

30. A 36-year-old woman with no prenatal care delivers an infant shortly after arriving in the emergency department. A urine toxicology screen is positive for multiple illicit drugs, including opiates. She admits that she has been using narcotics throughout her pregnancy. The infant requires no resuscitation and is judged to be full-term based on physical findings. Opiate withdrawal in this infant is most likely to present with which of the following?
A) Sedation, depression of the respiratory drive
B) Hyperactivity, crying, sweating
C) Hypoglycemia, lethargy
D) Bradycardia, thermoregulatory problems
E) Tremors, jitteriness, feeding problems, loose stools

31. A full-term infant is born to a mother in a methadone treatment program who has been managed on progressively lower doses throughout her pregnancy. Which of the following statements regarding treatment of opiate withdrawal in this infant is correct?
A) An oral narcotic solution may be used to treat withdrawal symptoms should the infant become symptomatic.
B) Symptoms of withdrawal, if they are to occur, should present within the first 3 days of life.
C) This infant will not experience symptomatic opiate withdrawal because his mother used methadone rather than heroin.
D) This infant will not experience symptomatic opiate withdrawal because his mother has been on a decreasing methadone dose throughout her pregnancy.
E) None of the above are correct.

32. An infant born at 37 weeks of gestation has excessive oral secretions, frothing at the nose, and choking spells when attempting to feed. The prenatal course was complicated by polyhydramnios. The physical examination is significant for moderate abdominal distention. Which of the following diagnostic procedures is most likely to reveal the diagnosis?
A) Attempting to pass a catheter through both nares in succession
B) Attempting to pass a nasogastric tube into the stomach
C) Real-time chest ultrasonography
D) Upper gastrointestinal series with small bowel follow-through
E) Barium swallow

33. Which of the following radiographic signs is most specific for NEC in the neonate?
A) Persistently dilated loop of bowel
B) Generalized bowel distention
C) Pneumatosis intestinalis
D) Bowel wall thickening
E) Intraperitoneal fluid

34. A 9-day-old female former full-term infant presents to the emergency department after 2 hours of vomiting, irritability, and progressive lethargy. The patient's vital signs include a temperature of 36.8°C, a respiratory rate of 60 breaths per minute, a heart rate of 150 beats per minute, and a blood pressure of 60/30 mm Hg. The physical examination is significant for green staining of the tongue, marked abdominal distention, and hypoactive bowel sounds. A plain radiograph demonstrates gastric distention with a paucity of gas in the distal bowel. This presentation is most likely to result from which of the following conditions?
A) Congenital large bowel obstruction
B) Duodenal atresia
C) Hirschsprung disease
D) Malrotation with midgut volvulus
E) NEC

35. Prolonged rupture of membranes is an important risk factor for infection in the newborn infant. Prolonged rupture of membranes is defined as which of the following?
A) Rupture of membranes without the onset of labor within 4 hours
B) Rupture of membranes without the onset of labor within 8 hours
C) Rupture of membranes ≥8 hours before delivery
D) Rupture of membranes ≥12 hours before delivery
E) Rupture of membranes ≥18 hours before delivery

36. What is the most common significant complication of intratracheal surfactant therapy?
A) Pneumothorax
B) Hypotension
C) Temperature instability
D) Bradycardia
E) Endotracheal colonization with *Pseudomonas*

37. A 6-hour-old infant has persistent acrocyanosis. His hands and feet feel cool to the touch. He is breast-feeding well and has a stable internal temperature. Examination of the cardiac and pulmonary systems reveals no abnormalities. Capillary refill is within normal limits. Which of the following is the most appropriate next step in the management of this patient?
A) Hyperoxia test
B) No further evaluation is required

C) Four-extremity blood pressures
D) Complete blood count and blood cultures
E) Echocardiography

38. An infant born at 30 weeks of gestation after preterm labor develops tachypnea, expiratory grunting, nasal flaring, and retractions within 2 hours of birth. There is no history of maternal illness, intrapartum fever, or uterine tenderness. Intrapartum prophylaxis against GBS was initiated ≥8 hours before delivery. The child required only blow-by oxygen in the delivery room. A portable chest radiograph is most likely to demonstrate which of the following?
A) Cadiomegaly
B) "White-out" of the lung fields
C) Diffuse reticulogranular pattern over the lung fields
D) Right-sided pneumothorax
E) Hyperaeration

39. All of the following conditions occur more frequently in infants of diabetic mothers EXCEPT:
A) Hypertrophic cardiomyopathy
B) Neonatal small left colon syndrome
C) Polycythemia
D) Hypercalcemia
E) Caudal regression

40. A 40-year-old woman with poorly controlled SLE is pregnant. If she is able to carry the pregnancy to term, which of the following complications is most likely to occur in her infant?
A) Potter syndrome
B) Pulmonary hypertension
C) Persistent fetal circulation
D) Coloboma of the iris
E) Congenital heart block

41. You are on call at the hospital when you are paged to the emergency department to evaluate an infant born by precipitous vaginal delivery to a woman who did not receive prenatal care. The infant has dry, cracked, peeling skin that is stained yellow; decreased subcutaneous tissue; and sparse hair. Based on physical characteristics alone, this infant's gestational age is closest to which of the following?
A) Post-term
B) Full-term
C) Preterm
D) Late second trimester
E) Unable to determine gestational age based on physical characteristics

42. Which of the following laboratory results is not consistent with classic hemorrhagic disease of the newborn?
A) Normal fibrinogen level
B) Thrombocytopenia
C) Prolonged prothrombin time
D) Decreased serum levels of proteins C and S
E) Normal factor V levels

43. With regard to screening infants at high risk for early-onset hypoglycemia, which of the following groups of infants should be screened with bedside dextrose sticks within 2 hours of birth?
A) Infants who exhibit temperature instability
B) Infants who require resuscitation in the delivery room
C) Infants who are hypotonic
D) Infants who develop seizure activity
E) All of the above

44. Which of the following full-term healthy infants should not be approved for early discharge (i.e., younger than 48 hours of age)?
A) Infant born into a stable home with two parents who desire early discharge
B) Infant who is feeding well
C) Infant with stable vital signs for the past 12 hours
D) Infant who has a follow-up appointment scheduled with his pediatrician within 5 days of discharge
E) Infant of an uncomplicated vaginal delivery

45. An infant born at 35 weeks of gestation has IUGR, microcephaly, hepatosplenomegaly, and "blueberry muffin" spots. Periventricular intracranial calcifications are noted on computed tomogram. CMV is detected in the infant's urine on the fourth day of life. This child is at high risk for development of which of the following complications due to his congenital infection?
A) Cataracts
B) Keratoconjunctivitis
C) Sensorineural hearing loss
D) Cutaneous "zig-zag" scarring
E) Congenital heart defects

46. Which of the following statements regarding neonatal herpes simplex virus (HSV) infection is FALSE?
A) Most patients with neonatal HSV infection are infected in utero.
B) The transmission rate is significantly higher if the mother experiences her primary HSV infection while she is pregnant.
C) Most infants who develop neonatal HSV are born to women who have never experienced symptoms due to HSV and do not know that they are infected.
D) Infants may become infected with HSV through contact with herpetic maternal breast lesions while breast-feeding.
E) Infants of mothers with herpetic genital lesions at the time of labor should be delivered by caesarean section.

47. A woman positive for human immunodeficiency virus (HIV) is treated with zidovudine throughout pregnancy and delivery. She delivers a healthy full-term infant without

complications. Which of the following options is the most appropriate for initial management of this patient?

A) The infant should be started on zidovudine if enzyme-linked immunosorbent assay and western blot are positive for HIV.
B) The infant should be treated with zidovudine for the first 6 weeks of life.
C) The infant should be treated with nevirapine for the first 12 weeks of life.
D) The infant should be treated with a protease inhibitor for the first 6 months of life.
E) The infant has received adequate prophylaxis against HIV in utero.

48. A woman develops primary varicella zoster infection 2 days after delivering a full-term healthy infant. She is resistant to allowing the infant to be treated with varicella zoster immunoglobulin because it is a blood product. In discussing the risks associated with varicella zoster infection in the neonate, you are correct in informing her of all the following complications EXCEPT:

A) Pneumonia
B) Hepatitis
C) Sensorineural hearing loss
D) Death
E) Widespread cutaneous lesions

49. You are performing the initial physical examination on a full-term infant born at 36 weeks of gestation. The infant has bilateral congenital cataracts, hepatosplenomegaly, and a heart murmur. You suspect congenital rubella syndrome. Which of the following laboratory tests would be most helpful in determining if the infant's condition is due to congenital rubella infection?

A) Culture of rubella virus from the infant's urine
B) The mother's rubella-specific IgM
C) The mother's rubella-specific IgG
D) The infant's rubella-specific IgM
E) The infant's rubella-specific IgG

50. Which of the following antibiotic courses is indicated for the treatment of an infant with congenital syphilis?

A) Intramuscular procaine penicillin for 10 to 14 days
B) Oral penicillin VK for 10 to 14 days
C) Intramuscular ceftriaxone for 7 to 10 days
D) Intravenous cefotaxime for 7 to 10 days
E) Intravenous imipenem for 5 to 7 days

51. A woman who uses cocaine regularly discovers that she is pregnant. She is concerned about the effect of her cocaine use on the fetus. Which of the following fetal anomalies is associated with regular maternal cocaine use?

A) Short palpebral fissures
B) Midface hypoplasia
C) Fifth-finger clinodactyly
D) Hirsutism
E) Gastroschisis

52. A 2-day-old full-term male infant with unremarkable pre- and perinatal histories has failed his newborn hearing screen (automated auditory brainstem response). Which of the following is the most appropriate next course of action in this patient?

A) Arrange for the patient to undergo repeat automated auditory brainstem response testing soon after discharge.
B) Arrange for the patient to undergo repeat screening with transient evoked OAE testing soon after discharge.
C) Arrange for the patient to undergo repeat screening with distortion product OAE testing soon after discharge.
D) Arrange for the patient to undergo full audiologic assessment soon after discharge.
E) Repeat automated auditory brainstem response testing at age 6 months.

53. You are preparing a lecture for medical students regarding the use of screening tests in newborn infants. You would be correct in informing the students of all of the following regarding universal newborn screening for hearing loss EXCEPT:

A) Intact cortical function is required to obtain a reliable result from automated auditory brainstem response testing.
B) Intact cortical function is required to obtain a reliable result from OAE testing.
C) Automated auditory brainstem response testing is more reliable than OAE testing.
D) False-positive results are more likely to occur when newborn hearing screens are conducted on the first day of life rather than on subsequent days.
E) If possible, the infant should be screened for hearing loss while asleep.

54. An infant born at 33 weeks of gestation is found to have microcephaly and hepatosplenomegaly. CMV is detected in the urine. A medical student who is working with you asks you what you are planning to tell the mother about the consequences of this child's congenital infection. Which of the following statements regarding long-term sequelae of symptomatic congenital CMV infection is CORRECT?

A) Twenty-five percent of neonates with clinically evident congenital CMV infection will eventually develop sensorineural hearing loss.
B) Seventy-five percent of neonates with clinically evident congenital CMV infection will eventually develop conductive hearing loss.
C) A normal newborn hearing screen does not preclude the development of significant hearing impairment by 1 year of age.
D) Congenital CMV is the most common cause of conductive hearing loss in the pediatric population.

E) Hearing loss is common in patients with asymptomatic congenital CMV infection.

55. A married couple expecting their first child is in your office for their prenatal visit. While gathering information about the parents, you find out that the mother smoked before her pregnancy and has continued to do so. In providing information about the effects of maternal smoking on the fetus, you would be correct in telling them all of the following EXCEPT:

A) Smoking is harmful to the fetus.
B) Fetuses of mothers who smoke are at increased risk for late fetal demise.
C) Infants born to mothers who smoke are three times more likely to die from sudden infant death syndrome than infants born to nonsmokers.
D) Infants of mothers who smoke during pregnancy are at increased risk for congenital intestinal malformations.
E) Mothers who smoke less during pregnancy typically have larger babies on average than women who smoke more.

56. You are examining a full-term 1-week-old neonate in your office. The pregnancy was uncomplicated. Apgar scores at birth were 3 at 1 minute, 7 at 5 minutes, and 9 at 10 minutes. The remainder of the perinatal course was unremarkable, and the patient was discharged 48 hours after birth. Although the patient is "doing well at home" according to his mother, she is concerned that the child may develop mental retardation because of his low Apgar score. You would be correct in telling the mother which of the following?

A) This child is likely to have deficits in adaptive skills.
B) This child is likely to have mild mental retardation.
C) This child may have an IQ 5 to 10 points lower than average, but it is unlikely that the boy will be labeled "mentally retarded."
D) This child will have normal intelligence but is at increased risk for social developmental delay.
E) Given the remainder of the infant's clinical course, it is unlikely that the initial low Apgar score has any bearing on potential cognitive achievement in this child.

ANSWERS

1. A	20. E	39. D
2. B	21. A	40. E
3. C	22. B	41. A
4. D	23. C	42. B
5. E	24. E	43. E
6. A	25. D	44. D
7. B	26. A	45. C
8. C	27. B	46. A
9. D	28. C	47. B
10. E	29. D	48. C
11. A	30. E	49. D
12. B	31. A	50. A
13. C	32. B	51. E
14. D	33. C	52. A
15. E	34. D	53. B
16. A	35. E	54. C
17. B	36. A	55. D
18. C	37. B	56. E
19. D	38. C	

Genetic Disorders and Congenital Anomalies

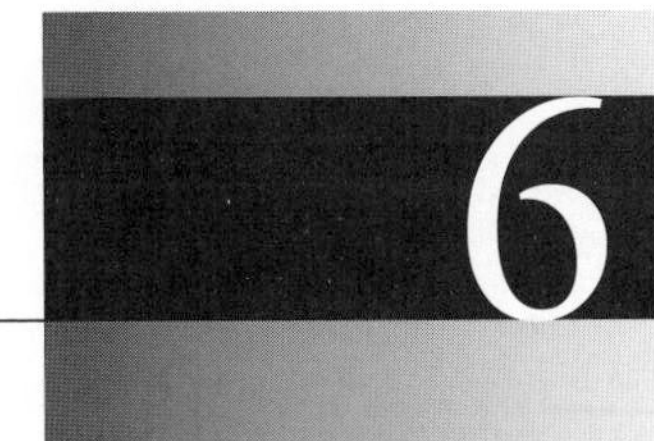

PRENATAL DIAGNOSIS

Maternal serum α-fetoprotein (AFP) levels are routinely measured in all pregnant women at 16 to 18 weeks of gestation. Maternal serum AFP levels are elevated in women carrying fetuses with *open neural tube defects* and/or anencephaly. Folate supplementation before and during the first trimester of pregnancy decreases the incidence of neural tube defects. Other fetal conditions that may result in an increased maternal serum AFP value include omphalocele, congenital nephrosis, multiple gestation pregnancy, and fetal demise. Incorrect dating of the pregnancy is the most common cause of a falsely elevated maternal serum AFP level. Thus, women with a positive screening test result should undergo prenatal ultrasonography to more closely ascertain the gestational age of the fetus and look for anomalies. If the maternal serum AFP is still high given the gestational age of the fetus and no abnormalities are discovered on sonogram, the mother is offered amniocentesis to evaluate the AFP level of the amniotic fluid. Amniocentesis is not typically performed until ≥14 weeks of gestation and is associated with a 1:250 risk of miscarriage.

A depressed maternal serum AFP level is associated with an increased risk of Down syndrome in the fetus. When combined with the results of two other maternal serum markers, the *triple screen* (maternal serum AFP, human chorionic gonadotrophin, and unconjugated estriol) identifies the majority of Down syndrome pregnancies (although ≥25% are still missed). The prenatal sonogram can detect certain physical characteristics of the fetus consistent with Down syndrome, but definitive diagnosis relies on chromosomal analysis of amniotic fluid. *Chorionic villus sampling* offers the same information and can be performed as early as 9 to 10 weeks; however, it is associated with a higher rate of miscarriage (about 1%).

Sickle cell disease is another example of a disorder that can be diagnosed in the prenatal period. Polymerase chain reaction testing of fetal DNA obtained by chorionic villus sampling or amniocentesis will detect the single gene mutation.

In addition to evaluating the maturity of the fetus (i.e., gestational age), prenatal ultrasonography can detect many major congenital anomalies such as hydrocephalus, open neural tube defects, congenital heart defects, and hydronephrosis. Table 6-1 lists some of the more common abnormalities noted on prenatal sonograms. Serial ultrasonographic studies are useful for assessing intrauterine growth.

TABLE 6-1
COMMON ABNORMAL FINDINGS ON PRENATAL ULTRASONOGRAPHY

Hydronephrosis
Recommended postnatal studies: renal ultrasound, voiding cystourethrography
Infants with vesicoureteral reflux should be discharged from the newborn nursery on prophylactic antibiotics
Infants with severe disease or bladder outlet obstruction should be referred to a urology specialist

Echogenic Bowel
Most infants with this finding have no associated abnormalities
Also can occur in association with an abnormality in the number of chromosomes (aneuploidy), cystic fibrosis, and congenital cytomegalovirus infection

Choroid Plexus Cysts
Of no significance unless associated with other fetal anomalies

GENETIC DISORDERS

Genetic defects may be inherited or spontaneous in nature. When a *de novo* mutation is the cause of the disorder, the risk of having a subsequent child who is affected with the disorder is not increased over that of the general population. Abnormalities resulting from genetic aberrations fall into three categories:

- *Single-gene mutations* that follow a Mendelian pattern of inheritance (Table 6-2)
- *Non-Mendelian* single-gene mutations (Table 6-3)
- *Multifactorial disorders,* which occur when an individual who has inherited a genetic susceptibility to the disorder is exposed to environmental factors that then result in disease

In general, single-gene mutations that follow a Mendelian pattern of inheritance have the highest rate of recurrence in future pregnancies (25% for autosomal recessive traits and 50% for

TABLE 6-2
MENDELIAN SINGLE-GENE MUTATIONS

AD Disorders

Expression: The disorder is expressed when a normal allele is paired with a mutant allele.

Characteristics

Vertical transmission (the disorder appears in successive generations)

Male and female individuals are equally affected.

Affected children have an affected parent (except in cases of spontaneous mutation).

Affected parents transmit the disorder to 50% of their children on average.

Affected men can transmit the disease to sons and daughters.

Nonaffected parents do not transmit the disorder to their children.

Examples: achondroplasia, Marfan syndrome, neurofibromatosis, tuberous sclerosis, von Willebrand disease, Treacher-Collins syndrome

Special points

Some AD disorders are *variably expressive*, i.e., individuals with the mutant allele may be affected to a greater or lesser extent.

Some AD disorders may not be fully *penetrant*, i.e., some individuals with the mutant gene will appear to be unaffected with the disorder.

If two individuals each have a mutant allele, it may appear as though two-thirds of their offspring have the disorder, when in fact fetuses that are homozygous for the mutant allele are nonviable.

Autosomal Recessive Disorders

Expression: The disorder will not be expressed unless mutations are present in both alleles.

Characteristics

Horizontal clustering (the disorder tends to appear in siblings within a generation)

Male and female individuals are equally affected.

Affected children usually have two unaffected parents.

A pair of affected parents transmits the disorder to 25% of their children on average.

Affected men can transmit the disorder to sons and daughters.

Consanguinity increases the likelihood of expression

Examples: cystic fibrosis, sickle cell anemia, Tay-Sachs disease

Special points

Unaffected carriers may have biochemical abnormalities associated with the product of the mutant gene (can aid in diagnosis).

X-Linked Dominant Disorders

Expression: The mutant gene is on the X chromosome. The presence one X chromosome with a mutant allele results in expression of the disease.

Characteristics

The disorder is at least two times more common in female individuals.

All daughters of affected men express the disorder; none of the sons of affected men express the disorder.

Affected female individuals transmit the disorder to half their daughters and half their sons.

Examples: incontinentia pigmenti

X-linked Recessive Disorders

Expression: The mutant gene is on the X chromosome. The presence of an X chromosome with a normal allele prevents expression of the disease.

Characteristics

Male individuals are disproportionately affected.

Men cannot transmit the disorder to their sons.

All daughters of affected men are carriers.

Female carriers transmit the disorder to half their sons and the carrier status to half their daughters.

Examples: hemophilia A, muscular dystrophy

AD, autosomal dominant

TABLE 6-3
NONTRADITIONAL SINGLE-GENE MUTATIONS

Mitochondrial Inheritance
All offspring of affected women are affected with the disorder.
No offspring of affected men is affected with the disorder.
Most disorders resulting from mitochondrial inheritance involve muscle weakness or dysfunction.

Trinucleotide Repeats
The genetic defect results from repetition of a trinucleotide sequence within the gene.
The length of the repetition expands with successive generations, resulting in more severe disease.
Example: fragile X syndrome (see "Additional Syndromes and Sequences of Importance")

autosomal dominant traits). Birth defects with multifactorial inheritance (e.g., clubfoot, neural tube defects, cleft palate) typically have a recurrence rate of 2% to 4% in subsequent pregnancies.

CHROMOSOMAL DISORDERS

Chromosomal abnormalities may be numerical (aneuploidy) or structural in nature. The defect may come from a parent or arise *de novo*.

Aneuploidy

Aneuploidy is the condition of having more or fewer than 46 chromosomes. Numerical defects typically result from meiotic (or less commonly mitotic) disjunction. When a gamete with an additional chromosome combines with a normal gamete, chromosomal trisomy is the result. Viable trisomies include those of chromosomes 21, 13, and 18 (Table 6-4). The recurrence risk for having an additional child with trisomy is equal to the mother's age-related risk of having a child with trisomy plus 1%. For example, a 40-year-old woman has about a 1% chance of having a child with trisomy 21; if she already has one child with the disorder, her risk for bearing a subsequent child with Down syndrome is 2% (1% + 1%). Parents with Robertsonian translocations are exceptions (see "Structural Defects").

Abnormal disjunction of sex chromosomes also occurs. *Turner syndrome* (45,X) results from the absence of one set of genes on the short arm of the X chromosome. It should be suspected in the newborn girl who presents with loose neck skin and nonpitting edema of the lower extremities. However, many patients are not diagnosed until late childhood or adolescence due to high variance in phenotypic presentation. Before adolescence, short stature due to growth retardation may be the only clinical evidence of Turner syndrome. Signs of ovarian dysgenesis and failure (e.g., no breast development or menstruation) are present in virtually all female adolescents with Turner syndrome. Other physical characteristics include webbed neck, broad

TABLE 6-4
VIABLE TRISOMIES: PHYSICAL CHARACTERISTICS, ASSOCIATED MEDICAL PROBLEMS, AND PROGNOSES

Trisomy 21 (Down syndrome; most common viable trisomy)
Physical characteristics (newborn)
Hypotonia
Microcephaly
Flat occiput
Midfacial hypoplasia
Brushfield spots
Epicanthal folds
Upslanting palpebral fissures
Protuberant tongue
Simian creases
Short phalanges
Dysplasia of the midphalanx of the fifth finger
Redundant skin at the nape of the neck
Widening of space between first and second toes
Associated medical problems
Mental retardation

(continued)

TABLE 6-4
(continued)

Developmental delay
Strabismus/cataracts/glaucoma/refractive errors
Autoimmune disorders (i.e., hypothyroidism, diabetes, celiac disease)
Duodenal atresia/Hirschsprung disease
Leukemia (risk elevated to 20 times that of age-matched peers)
Cardiac septal defects (particularly atrioventricular canal) or other congenital heart defects
Atlantoaxial instability
Prognosis: shortened life span (average mid-50s)

Trisomy 13
Physical characteristics
Holoprosencephaly
Microcephaly
Sloping forehead
Microphthalmia
Coloboma of the iris
Cleft lip/palate
Abnormally formed, low-set ears
Polydactyly
Cryptorchidism
Associated medical problems
Congenital heart defects
Seizures
Apnea
Prognosis: death typically occurs within days of birth

Trisomy 18
Physical characteristics
Narrow biparietal diameter with occipital prominence
Short palpebral fissures
Micrognathia
Malformed, low-set ears
Hypoplastic nails
Overlapping fingers
Rocker-bottom feet
Cryptorchidism
Associated medical problems
Central nervous system malformations
Failure to thrive
Congenital heart defects
Thrombocytopenia
Prognosis: Average survival into the second year of life.

chest with widely spaced nipples, cubitus valgus (outward turning of the elbows), lymphedema, and small, cupped ears. Cardiac and/or renal abnormalities (coarctation of the aorta, bicuspid aortic valve, horseshoe kidney) are found in a significant minority of patients. Although elevated luteinizing and follicle-stimulating hormone levels are suggestive of Turner syndrome, definitive diagnosis requires peripheral blood chromosome analysis. Affected patients are treated with growth hormone and estrogen replacement therapy; medical complications of Turner syndrome such as hypertension, cardiac abnormalities, and hypothyroidism are also addressed when present.

The most common karyotype in patients with *Klinefelter syndrome* is 47,XXY. Klinefelter syndrome results in hypogonadism (primary testicular failure), infertility, pubertal gynecomastia, developmental delay, and behavior problems.

Most cases remain undiagnosed until the patient reaches puberty.

Of note, all the conditions described above can also result from mosaicism or unbalanced structural defects (discussed below).

Structural Defects

Structural defects occur when chromosomal breakage leads to disordered repair. Repair that results in genetic content equivalent to that of 46 normal chromosomes is *balanced.* Repair that results in additional or missing genetic content is *unbalanced.* Individuals who obtain a balanced rearrangement from one parent and a normal set of genes from the other parent are usually unaffected (unless the breakage occurs within a gene). Individuals who obtain an unbalanced rearrangement are likely to express phenotypic abnormalities. When a structural chromosomal abnormality is detected in an infant or child, chromosomal analysis should be performed for both parents to determine if the defect is familial.

Robertsonian translocation is the rearrangement of segments between two (usually nonhomologous) acrocentric chromosomes. The most common translocation occurs between chromosomes 14 and 21. Women who are carriers of a 14/21 translocation have a 10% to 15% chance of having a child with Down syndrome compared with a <5% chance for men with the 14/21 translocation and about 0.1% to 0.2% chance for women who do not carry a 14/21 translocation.

Other examples of abnormal chromosomal structure include inversions, deletions, and duplications. A group of disorders termed *contiguous gene syndromes* results from microdeletion of multiple gene loci that are adjacent to one another. A consistent feature of contiguous gene syndromes is the presence of multiple, distinct, and apparently unrelated abnormalities. Table 6-5 provides information about the constellations of abnormalities and managements of DiGeorge, Angelman, Prader-Willi, and Beckwith-Wiedemann syndromes. Although major deletions may be evident on routine chromosome analysis, fluorescent in situ hybridization testing is more sensitive for these defects.

Chromosomal analysis detects numerical and major structural abnormalities and should be considered for:

- any newborn with multiple congenital abnormalities, dysmorphic features, hypotonia, and growth retardation
- any older child with unexplained mental retardation or autism

ADDITIONAL SYNDROMES, SEQUENCES, AND ASSOCIATIONS OF IMPORTANCE

Treacher-Collins syndrome is a rare autosomal dominant disorder with variable expressivity. Affected patients may have any of the following: severe micrognathia, facial bone hypoplasia, eyelid coloboma, cleft palate, microtia, and hearing impairment. Most have typical cognitive development. Treacher-Collins syndrome is associated with abnormalities on chromosomes 5 or 19.

Robin anomalad (formerly called Pierre-Robin syndrome) may be autosomal recessive or X-linked. The sequence consists of severe micrognathia, retroglossoptosis (downward displacement or retraction of the tongue), and cleft palate. Infants may have severe respiratory distress leading to cor pulmonale and feeding problems. Many patients with Robin anomalad also have associated cardiac defects.

Fragile X syndrome is the most common inherited cause of mental retardation. The underlying genetic defect, which occurs on the X chromosome, is the repetition of a three-nucleotide sequence. The severity of disease parallels the number of repetitions, and the number of repetitions increases with subsequent generations. Patients with >50 but <200 repeats are said to have a premutation; those with >200 repetitions have the full mutation. Patients with fragile X syndrome have mental retardation or significant developmental delay, which usually becomes evident in the second year of life. Associated conditions include attention-deficit/hyperactivity disorder, autistic behaviors, and behavior problems. Physical characteristics are usually subtle and consist of a long, thin face with prominent forehead and nasal bridge; protuberant ears; high, arched palate or cleft; and joint laxity. Postpubertal men virtually always develop macro-orchidism. Female patients with the full mutation may manifest some aspects of the syndrome, including mental retardation. Molecular genetic testing (i.e., Southern blot or polymerase chain reaction) allows definitive diagnosis. It is estimated that at least half of patients with fragile X syndrome remain undiagnosed. Identification of affected patients is rare before late childhood.

Malformations that occur in known groupings for which no etiology has been elucidated are referred to as multiple congenital anomaly associations. Two examples include VATER (or VACTERL) association and CHARGE association (Table 6-6).

TERATOGENS

Congenital anomalies are structural defects that are present at birth. They may be genetic or teratogenic and may occur in isolation or as part of a syndrome. Congenital anomalies are categorized as major or minor.

- *Major anomalies* impair function or result in significant cosmetic deformity. Most require surgical intervention.
- *Minor anomalies* have no functional or cosmetic significance.
- *Normal phenotypic variants* are heritable traits found throughout the population and have no association with syndromes or dysfunction.

TABLE 6-5
CONTIGUOUS GENE SYNDROMES

DiGeorge Syndrome
Cause: hemizygous deletion of 22q11.2; dysmorphogenesis of the third and fourth pharyngeal pouches

Characteristics: Phenotypic severity varies and may include any of the following:

Facial dysmorphism (hypertelorism, short philtrum, micrognathia, ear anomalies, cleft palate)

Thymic dysplasia (T-cell dysfunction and deficient cellular immunity)

Parathyroid hypoplasia (hypocalcemia, seizures)

Aortic arch anomalies

Heart defects (tetralogy of Fallot, ventricular septal defect, truncus arteriosus)

Management

Calcium and vitamin D supplementation

Management of immunodeficiency; possible early thymic transplantation

Surgical correction of aortic arch and cardiac defects

Angelman Syndrome
Cause: hemizygous deletion of maternal 15q11.2–q13 region

Characteristics

Microcephaly

Mental retardation or developmental delay

Speech impairment

Gastroesophageal reflux, oromotor dysfunction

Ataxia or tremulousness of the limbs

Seizures

Consistently (inappropriately) happy demeanor

Management

Medical/surgical treatment of reflux

Oromotor/feeding occupational therapy

Anticonvulsant medication

Speech therapy

Prader-Willi Syndrome
Cause: hemizygous deletion of paternal 15q11.2–q13 region

Characteristics

Neonatal hypotonia, poor suck, weak cry, genital hypoplasia

Developmental delay (especially motor); mental retardation

Behavior problems

Hyperphagia progressing to obesity

Short stature

Cryptorchidism/hypogonadism

Management

Gavage feedings in infancy

Dietary management of obesity

Management of complications of obesity (e.g., obstructive sleep apnea)

Growth hormone therapy

Beckwith-Wiedemann Syndrome
Cause: hemizygous (functional) deletion of 11p15.5

Characteristics

Large-for-gestational age infant with hypoglycemia

Macroglossia

Anterior abdominal wall defects/abdominal tumors

Management

Management of hypoglycemia

Surgical management of abdominal defects/tumors

TABLE 6-6
MULTIPLE CONGENITAL ANOMALY ASSOCIATIONS

VATER Association
Vertebral anomalies
Anal atresia
Tracheo**e**sophageal fistula
Renal (and **r**adial limb) dysplasia

VACTERL Association
Same as above, with the inclusion of **c**ardiac anomalies and **l**imb dysplasia in the acronym

CHARGE Association
Coloboma
Heart defects
Choanal **a**tresia
Retardation of growth and developmental delay
Genital anomalies
Ear abnormalities

A *teratogen* is any in utero exposure that results in postnatal abnormalities. The list of potential teratogens includes congenital infections, maternal disease, drugs and chemicals, and mechanical forces. Typically, teratogens only result in anomalies if the exposure occurs during a specific period of the pregnancy (usually between 2 weeks after conception and the end of the first trimester), and not all exposed fetuses develop abnormalities. Congenital infections, maternal diseases, and substance use which may affect the fetus are discussed in Chapter 5. A partial list of the more commonly prescribed medications with teratogenic potential is provided in Table 6-7.

Amniotic rupture sequence (amniotic band syndrome) is thought to result from entanglement of the fetus in strands of amniotic tissue after rupture that occurs before 12 weeks of gestation. Amniotic bands that form constriction rings cause limb reduction defects and digit amputation, and adhesions can lead to asymmetric facial clefts, encephaloceles, and thoracoabdominoschisis. Severe *oligohydramnios* from any cause results in a characteristic sequence ("Potter syndrome") consisting of facial dysmorphism (flattened nose, recessed chin, prominent epicanthal folds, and abnormal, low-set ears), pulmonary hypoplasia, and urinary tract anomalies. Infants who have facial features consistent with oligohydramnios sequence merit detailed radiographic evaluation of the genitourinary tract to assess for renal dysgenesis and other potential abnormalities.

Deformation sequences are composed of characteristic anomalies related to mechanical forces acting on the fetus due to compression or positioning within the uterus. They may include any combination of facial asymmetry, deviation of the nose to one side; overfolded pinnae; small chin; craniosynostosis; torticollis; congenital hip dysplasia; and clubfoot. Malformations associated with abnormal positioning occur more frequently in the breech infant.

TABLE 6-7
MATERNAL MEDICATIONS WITH TERATOGENIC POTENTIAL

Angiotensin-Converting Enzyme Inhibitors (e.g., captopril)
Renal tubular dysgenesis
Fetal compression syndrome (oligohydramnios with pulmonary hypoplasia, limb defects)

Anticonvulsants
Carbamazepine
- Small, short nose
- Small fingernails
- Neural tube defects

Phenytoin
- Intrauterine growth retardation
- Facial dysmorphia: arched eyebrows; widely spaced eyes; short, upturned nose; cleft lip and palate
- Hypoplasia of the distal digits and nails
- Cardiac defects
- Mental retardation

Valproate
- Facial dysmorphia: short palpebral fissures; epicanthal folds; anteverted nostrils; long philtrum; cleft lip; straight contour to the upper vermillion border with small mouth
- Heart defects
- Long, thin digits with hyperconvex nails
- Neural tube defects
- Mental retardation

Isotretinoin
Microphthalmia, ocular hypertelorism
Hypoplastic ears (severe ear anomalies)
Cleft palate
Conotruncal heart defects
Thymic abnormalities
Microcephaly, hydrocephalus, spina bifida
Mental retardation

Lithium
Ebstein anomaly (malformed tricuspid valve with associated abnormalities of the right atrium and ventricle)

Warfarin
Low birth weight
Severe nasal hypoplasia
Stippling of the epiphyses
Shortened fingers with nail hypoplasia
Mental retardation

SOURCES

Boyle RJ. Effects of certain prenatal drugs on the fetus and newborn. *Pediatr Rev.* 2002;23:17–24.
Hudgins L, Cassidy SB. Congenital anomalies. In: Fanaroff JS, Martin JO, eds. *Diseases of the fetus and infant.* 8th ed. St. Louis: Elsevier/Mosby Publishing; 2005:561–581.
Phalen JA. In brief: fragile X syndrome. *Pediatr Rev.* 2005;26:181–182.
Schwartz S. Genetic aspects of perinatal disease and prenatal diagnosis. In: Fanaroff JS, Martin JO, eds. *Diseases of the fetus and infant.* 8th ed. St. Louis: Elsevier/Mosby Publishing; 2005:561–581.

QUESTIONS

1. A maternal serum AFP level screen is drawn in a first-time mother at 18 weeks of gestation by dates. The result is labeled "elevated." Which of the following fetal conditions is unlikely to result in an elevated maternal serum AFP level?
A) Down syndrome
B) Neural tube defect
C) Anencephaly
D) Omphalocele
E) Twin pregnancy

2. A woman who is 17 weeks' pregnant has a triple screen suggestive of Down syndrome in the fetus. Which of the following is the most appropriate study for definitive diagnosis of Down syndrome in the fetus?
A) Prenatal ultrasonography
B) Amniocentesis with chromosomal analysis of fluid
C) Chorionic villus sampling
D) Polymerase chain reaction
E) Southern blot

3. The amniotic fluid concentration of which of the following substances correlates with fetal lung maturity?
A) Sphingomyelin
B) AFP
C) Phosphatidylglycerol
D) Cholesterol
E) Unconjugated estriol

4. Which of the following conditions has no specific associated findings on prenatal ultrasonography?
A) Hydrocephalus
B) Down syndrome
C) Renal agenesis
D) Fragile X syndrome
E) Hydronephrosis

5. A patient is afflicted with disorder X, which is also found in several members of his extended family. His father and a paternal aunt have disorder X, as do the aunt's daughter and the patient's paternal grandfather. The patient's mother, an additional paternal aunt and uncle, paternal grandmother, and the remainder (two) of the patient's paternal cousins do not have disorder X. Disorder X is most likely inherited in what fashion?
A) Mitochondrial
B) X-linked recessive
C) X-linked dominant
D) Autosomal recessive
E) Autosomal dominant

6. A patient is afflicted with disorder Y, which is also found in her brother. None of her other extended family members have the disorder. The patient also has six siblings who are not affected with disorder Y. Assuming that disorder Y is an inherited disorder, the mode of inheritance for this disorder is most likely which of the following?
A) Autosomal recessive
B) Autosomal dominant
C) X-linked recessive
D) X-linked dominant
E) Mitochondrial

7. A patient is afflicted with disorder Z, as are several other male members in his extended family. One of the patient's two sisters has one son with disorder Z and one son without the disorder. The patient's daughter has a son with the disorder. None of the patient's son's children have the disorder. The inheritance pattern of disorder Z is most consistent with which of the following?
A) Autosomal recessive
B) X-linked recessive
C) Autosomal dominant
D) X-linked dominant
E) Y-linked dominant

8. A patient is afflicted with disorder M. All the patient's sons (three) and daughters (two) are afflicted with disorder M. All of her daughters' children are affected with the disorder, but none of her sons' children are. Disorder M is most likely passed on through which of the following modes of inheritance?
A) X-linked dominant
B) X-linked recessive
C) Mitochondrial
D) Autosomal dominant
E) Autosomal recessive

9. Which of the following inherited diseases is NOT considered a multifactorial (genetic susceptibility combined with environmental exposure creates disease) disorder?
A) Hypertension
B) Cardiovascular disease
C) Hypercholesterolemia
D) Tay-Sachs disease
E) Type 2 diabetes

10. A full-term infant born to a 42-year-old woman is hypotonic. On physical examination, the infant has microcephaly, a flat occiput with redundant skin at the nape of the neck, epicanthal folds, and upslanting palpebral fissures. Which of the following syndromes is most consistent with the infant's presentation?
A) Beckwith-Wiedemann syndrome
B) Angelman syndrome
C) Trisomy 13
D) Trisomy 18
E) Trisomy 21

11. An infant born at 37 weeks of gestation to a 39-year-old woman has coloboma of the right iris, polydactyly, and holoprosencephaly. The infant requires mechanical ventilation due to profound apnea. This infant's presentation is most consistent with which of the following?
A) Trisomy 13
B) Trisomy 18
C) Trisomy 21
D) Angelman syndrome
E) Beckwith-Wiedemann syndrome

12. You are seeing a 2-week-old infant in the clinic for a health maintenance visit. The child has poor weight gain due to feeding difficulties related to severe micrognathia. He has a striking facial appearance, with a narrow biparietal diameter, occipital prominence, short palpebral fissures, and low-set, malformed ears. Examination of the patient's extremities shows hypoplastic nails and rocker-bottom feet. This clinical picture is most consistent with which of the following inherited disorders?
A) Trisomy 21
B) Trisomy 18
C) Trisomy 13
D) Prader-Willi syndrome
E) Treacher-Collins syndrome

13. The parents of a 2-week-old male infant with Down syndrome have questions for you regarding which medical problems are more common in children with trisomy 21. You are correct in counseling them that Down syndrome places their child at increased risk for all of the following EXCEPT:
A) Hypothyroidism
B) Celiac disease
C) Thrombocytopenia
D) Leukemia
E) Glaucoma

14. A 14-year-old girl with short stature has pubic and axillary hair but no breast development, and she has never menstruated. Luteinizing and follicle-stimulating hormone levels are elevated. Which of the following conditions is most likely to be responsible for this patient's amenorrhea?
A) Cystic fibrosis
B) Poor nutrition
C) Klinefelter syndrome
D) Turner syndrome
E) Celiac disease

15. A 15-year-old boy with developmental delay and behavior problems presents with increasing bilateral gynecomastia of 18 months' duration. His testicles measure 2.5 cm in diameter. Which of the following conditions is most consistent with this patient's clinical presentation?
A) Fragile X syndrome
B) Angelman syndrome
C) Treacher-Collins syndrome
D) Turner syndrome
E) Klinefelter syndrome

16. An 8-year-old girl with short stature and a history of bicuspid aortic valve has a webbed neck, a broad chest with widely spaced nipples, outward turning of the elbows, and low-set ears. The patient has streak gonads in place of ovaries, and her luteinizing and follicle-stimulating hormone levels are elevated. This patient would benefit from which of the following medications?
A) Growth hormone therapy and estrogen replacement therapy when indicated
B) Growth hormone therapy and alendromate
C) Growth hormone therapy alone
D) Estrogen replacement therapy alone when indicated
E) Growth hormone therapy and progesterone replacement therapy

17. A 22-year-old married woman has a full-term child with Down syndrome. Chromosomal analysis is performed on both parents, and the mother is found to have a 14/21 Robertsonian translocation. This woman's risk for having a subsequent child with Down syndrome is closest to which of the following?
A) 3% to 5%
B) 10% to 15%
C) 20% to 25%
D) 33%
E) 50%

18. A 2-day-old infant with truncus arteriosus develops seizures due to hypocalcemia. There is no thymic shadow on chest radiograph. This patient's clinical picture is most consistent with which of the following microdeletion syndromes?
A) Angelman syndrome
B) Prader-Willi syndrome
C) DiGeorge syndrome
D) Beckwith-Wiedemann syndrome
E) Cri-du-chat syndrome

19. Which of the following disorders is not typically associated with mental retardation?
A) Fetal alcohol syndrome
B) Angelman syndrome
C) Prader-Willi syndrome
D) Treacher-Collins syndrome
E) Fragile X syndrome

20. Chromosomal analysis is recommended for all of the following patients EXCEPT:

A) A newborn with multiple congenital anomalies of unknown origin
B) A newborn with dysmorphic features of unknown origin
C) A newborn with hypotonia of unknown origin
D) A child with unexplained mental retardation
E) Chromosomal analysis is indicated for all of the above patients.

21. A 13-year-old boy with mental retardation has a 10-year-old sister with an IQ of 80 and behavior problems at home and at school. The boy has a long, thin face with a prominent forehead, prognathia, and protuberant ears. Which of the following laboratory results is diagnostic of fragile X syndrome?

A) An expanded sequence >200 CGG repetitions on the X chromosome
B) Microdeletion of 21q11.2
C) Microdeletion of 14p15.5
D) Microdeletion of 7q13
E) 47,XXY

22. A 36-week–gestation infant is delivered to a 37-year-old woman. The infant has a transverse facial cleft, a constriction band around the left lower calf, and amputation of the third, fourth, and fifth digits of the right hand. This patient's clinical picture is most consistent with which of the following?

A) VATER association
B) Amniotic rupture sequence
C) In utero lithium exposure
D) In utero phenytoin exposure
E) In utero valproate exposure

23. A 19-year-old woman with severe bipolar disorder discovers that she is pregnant. A prenatal ultrasound dates the pregnancy at 16 weeks of gestation. The woman takes lithium daily to control her bipolar symptoms. She asks you how her use of lithium during the first trimester might have affected her baby. You are confident in counseling her that her infant is at increased risk for

A) intrauterine growth retardation
B) mental retardation
C) ebstein anomaly
D) polydactyly
E) hypoplasia of the distal digits and nails

24. A 27-year-old woman with a seizure disorder wants to have a baby. Her disorder is well controlled with valproic acid. She resists advice to alter her antiepileptic medication because she has experienced break-through seizures on other medications in the past and her job requires that she be able to drive. If she continues to use valproate during her pregnancy, this woman places her infant at increased risk for which of the following?

A) Mental retardation
B) Congenital heart defects
C) Neural tube defects
D) A, B, and C
E) A and B only

25. Which of the following disorders carries the greatest risk of recurrence in a subsequent pregnancy?

A) Neural tube defect
B) Down syndrome, neither parent with 14/21 Robertsonian translocation
C) Down syndrome, father with 14/21 Robertsonian translocation
D) Down syndrome, mother with 14/21 Robertsonian translocation
E) Galactosemia

ANSWERS

1. A	10. E	19. D
2. B	11. A	20. E
3. C	12. B	21. A
4. D	13. C	22. B
5. E	14. D	23. C
6. A	15. E	24. D
7. B	16. A	25. E
8. C	17. B	
9. D	18. C	

Fluid and Electrolyte Disorders

7

REGULATION OF OSMOLALITY AND INTRAVASCULAR VOLUME

Total body water (TBW) as a percentage of body weight varies according to age and body composition (Table 7-1). TBW is the sum of intracellular (ICF) and extracellular fluid compartments (ECF). The ECF is distributed between the interstitial space and the plasma (Fig. 7-1).

Movement of water between the interstitial space and the intravascular (plasma) space is governed by three factors (Starling forces):

- *Hydrostatic pressure* (provided by the pumping heart; pushes fluid out of the intravascular space)
- *Oncotic pressure* (results from the higher albumin concentration in the intravascular space; draws fluid into the intravascular space)
- *Permeability of the capillary membrane*

TABLE 7-1
TOTAL BODY WATER AS A PERCENTAGE OF BODY WEIGHT BASED ON AGE, BODY COMPOSITION

Age	TBW
24-week gestation fetus	85%
Full-term infant	70%
Toddlers and young children	65%
Older children, adolescents, and adults	60%

During gestation and at birth, intracellular fluid volume exceeds extracellular fluid volume. The compartments equalize by 3 to 4 months of age, with adult proportions being obtained by age 5 years.

Body Composition
Since adipose tissue contains virtually no water, TBW is a lower percentage of body weight in obese individuals.

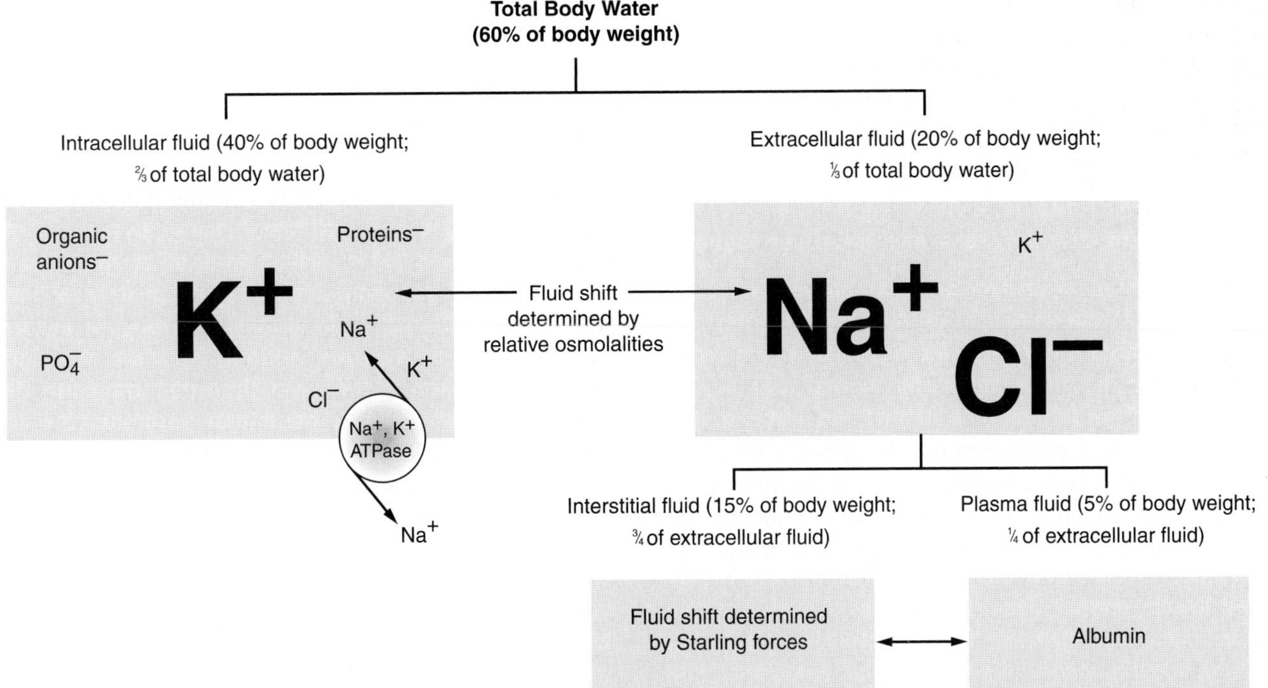

Figure 7-1 Distribution of total body water and principal cations/anions.

TABLE 7-2
DISEASE STATES WHICH ALTER STARLING FORCES/MEMBRANE PERMEABILITY

Decreased Hydrostatic Pressure
- Example: dehydration

Increased Hydrostatic Pressure
- Example: heart failure
- Example: acute glomerulonephritis

Decreased Oncotic Pressure
- Results in generalized edema due to increase in interstitial fluid volume
- Results in reduction of plasma, circulatory volume
- Hypoalbuminemia (liver failure, nephrotic syndrome)
- Hypoproteinemia (Kwashiorkor)

Increased Vascular Permeability
- Exacerbated when albumin leaks into the interstitial space, altering oncotic gradient
- Capillary leak syndromes

TABLE 7-3
WHEN SERUM ELECTROLYTE CONCENTRATIONS DO NOT REFLECT TOTAL BODY CONTENT: EXAMPLES

Sodium
Patients with isonatremic dehydration may have a normal serum sodium level, but since total body water is decreased, the total body sodium level must have also decreased to maintain a normal serum value.

Potassium
In diabetic ketoacidosis, intracellular potassium is shifted into the ECF, resulting in normal or elevated serum potassium levels in spite of significant potassium loss.

Calcium
The majority of the body's calcium is contained within bone. Release of calcium from the bone occurs when serum calcium concentrations fall. The serum calcium concentration may remain relatively constant in the normal range despite significant calcium loss from bony deposits.

In the proximal (arteriolar) capillary bed, hydrostatic pressure exceeds oncotic pressure, and fluid moves out of the vascular space. In the distal (venous) capillary bed, hydrostatic pressure is lower relative to oncotic pressure, resulting in transfer of fluid into the intravascular compartment. Disease states which alter any of the above parameters affect intravascular volume (Table 7-2).

The predominant electrolytes in the ECF are sodium (Na^+) and chloride (Cl^-). The predominant cation in the ICF is K^+, balanced on the negative side by phosphate, proteins, and organic anions.

Movement of water between the ICF and ECF is determined by osmolality. Since the cell membrane is freely permeable to water, a change in the solute load of one compartment is rapidly followed by fluid shifts to equalize ICF and ECF osmolalities. Serum osmolality can be estimated using the following formula:

$$[2 \text{ X } Na^+(\text{mEq/L})] + [\text{BUN(mg/dL)}/2.8] + [\text{Glucose(mg/dL)}/18] = \text{estimated serum osmolality}$$

Under normal circumstances, sodium is the main determinant of ECF osmolality. The estimated serum osmolality is usually slightly lower than the measured serum osmolality (within 10 mOsm/kg of the normal 285 to 295 mOsm/kg). This difference is termed the osmolal gap. A gap of >10 mOsm/kg indicates the presence of an unmeasured osmole (e.g., ethanol, ethylene glycol, methanol).

Substances which move readily across cell membranes (urea, ethanol) are not osmotically active. That is, although an increase in total body urea results in an increase in TBW (and thereby serum) osmolality, it does not result in net movement of fluid between the ICF and ECF; intravascular volume remains intact, albeit at a higher osmolality. Substances which are confined to the ECF space are osmotically active and do result in fluid shifts. In diabetic ketoacidosis, the osmotic effect of hyperglycemia draws a significant amount of water out of the ICF into the ECF, effectively diluting serum Na^+ concentration. This is an example of the fact that the measured serum concentration of an electrolyte is not always reflective of the total body content of that substance. Additional examples are provided in Table 7-3. The corrected serum Na^+ is the measurement that would be obtained if the serum glucose was normal and can be calculated using the following formula:

$$Na^+_{\text{corrected}} = Na^+_{\text{measured}} + 1.6 \text{ X } [(\text{glucose}) - 100 \text{ mg/dL}]/100$$

The corrected serum sodium is more reflective of the total body sodium content when hyperglycemia is present.

Total body water determines osmolality; total body sodium content determines volume status. A drop in serum osmolality triggers increased hypothalamic secretion of antidiuretic hormone (ADH), which binds to receptor sites in the kidney and stimulates concentration of urine to limit water losses. Although ADH secretion is primarily dictated by osmolality, intravascular volume depletion stimulates ADH secretion even in the face of decreased osmolality. The syndrome of inappropriate antidiuretic hormone (SIADH) and diabetes insipidus (DI), two disorders that result in water imbalance, are discussed later in the chapter.

As stated above, sodium is the main determinant of intravascular volume status (along with its predominant anion, chloride). Chronic sodium depletion results in intravascular volume contraction. The kidney regulates sodium balance by altering sodium reabsorption along the nephron. This variable retention is under the influence of intrarenal co-transporters, the renin-angiotensin-aldosterone system, and atrial natriuretic peptide. Disorders which impact sodium balance (e.g., renal disease, primary hyperaldosteronism, cystic fibrosis) are discussed in detail in their respective chapters.

DISORDERS OF WATER BALANCE

Syndrome of Inappropriate Antidiuretic Hormone

The underlying abnormality in the syndrome of inappropriate antidiuretic hormone (SIADH) is the continued secretion of ADH despite low plasma osmolality. The excess ADH prevents excretion of free water through dilution of the urine. SIADH is uncommon in pediatric patients (Table 7-4) but may complicate cases of head trauma or bacterial meningitis. The diagnosis of SIADH in a child with hyponatremia and no evidence of volume depletion (weight loss, tachycardia) is essentially one of exclusion. Edema and hypertension are not present on exam. Urinary sodium concentration is elevated (>50 mEq/L), and urinary osmolality remains greater than 1.5 times plasma osmolality (or 500 mOsm/L) despite a decrease in serum osmolality. SIADH is generally self-limited; fluid restriction attenuates the effects of the disorder. Fluid intake should be restricted to half to one third of the patient's maintenance requirement per day, with an iso-osmolar fluid composition providing at least 3 to 4 mEq per kg per day of sodium (maintenance needs). Children with severe, refractory hyponatremia or cardiac/neurologic complications may benefit from demeclocycline, which interferes with ADH secretion.

Diabetes Insipidus

Diabetes insipidus results from either inadequate ADH secretion (central DI) or renal tubular insensitivity (nephrogenic DI). Table 7-5 lists potential causes of each. The predominant clinical manifestations are impressive polyuria and polydipsia. The diagnosis is suggested by hypernatremia, volume depletion (weight loss), low urinary sodium (<20 mEq/L), and urinary osmolality <300 mOsm per L (or <1.2 times serum osmolality) in the setting of elevated serum osmolality.

Central DI is managed with oral or intranasal DDAVP, a long-acting vasopressin analog, or synthetic aqueous vasopressin in hospitalized patients. Nephrogenic DI responds to resolution of the underlying disorder, if possible. Treatment of congenital nephrogenic DI is aimed at preventing dehydration and providing adequate calories for growth. Pharmacologic intervention has proven less successful.

TABLE 7-4
CAUSES OF SIADH

Iatrogenic
Vasopressin administration
Post-operative complication of hypothalamic-pituitary surgery
Antiepileptic medication (carbamazepine)
Chemotherapeutic agents (vinblastine, vincristine)

Central Nervous System Abnormality
Infection
Tumor
Trauma

Pulmonary Disease
Mechanical ventilation
Lung disease

TABLE 7-5
CAUSES OF CENTRAL AND NEPHROGENIC DIABETES INSIPIDUS

Central DI
Inherited (autosomal dominant)
Acquired
Central nervous system disorder (trauma, malformation, neoplasm, infection)
Idiopathic

Nephrogenic DI
Inherited (X-linked, autosomal dominant, autosomal recessive)
Acquired
Hypokalemia
Hypercalcemia
Kidney disease (ureteral obstruction, chronic renal failure)
Drug effect (amphotericin, methicillin, rifampin)

Electrolyte Abnormalities

The normal ranges and daily requirements of several physiologically important electrolytes are listed in Table 7-6.

Hypernatremia

Hypernatremia is defined as serum sodium concentration in excess of 145 mEq per L. Hypernatremia results from free water loss, excess sodium intake, or both. Mild hypernatremia may occasionally be observed in children who are dehydrated due to infectious gastroenteritis. Otherwise,

TABLE 7-6
NORMAL SERUM ELECTROLYTE RANGES AND MAINTENANCE REQUIREMENTS

Electrolyte	Normal Range	Maintenance Requirement
Sodium (Na^+)	135 to 145 mEq/L	2 to 3 mEq/kg/day
Potassium (K^+)	3.5 to 5.0 mEq/L	1 to 2 mEq/kg/day
Chloride (Cl-)	96 to106 mEq/L	Paired with above cations in diet and solution

TABLE 7-7
CAUSES OF HYPERNATREMIA

Dehydration (usually mild imbalance)
Ineffective breastfeeding
Extensive burns
Excessive sweating in cystic fibrosis
Renal disease
Hyperaldosteronism
Diabetes insipidus
Iatrogenic (infusion of hypertonic parenteral solution; complication of high-solute enteral feeds)

pediatric hypernatremia is an uncommon occurrence (Table 7-7). Signs and symptoms include muscle weakness, irritability, and lethargy. As fluid shifts from the ICF to the ECF to compensate for the increase in ECF osmolality, the acute decrease in brain cell volume can lead to intracranial hemorrhaging, evidenced by loss of consciousness and seizures. Hemorrhaging is even more likely if the patient is dehydrated. A diagnostic algorithm for the evaluation of hypernatremia is provided in Figure 7-2.

Initial treatment goals are two-fold: normalization of the serum sodium concentration without precipitating brain edema, and restoration of intracellular fluid volume. It is difficult to accurately quantitate free water deficits in patients with hypernatremic dehydration because the bulk of the water loss occurs in the ICF, while most of the signs and symptoms used to evaluate water deficit are related to depletion of the ECF (which is relatively spared). Correction must occur over at least 48 to 72 hours, with a drop in serum sodium of no more than 1 mEq per L per hour. Hypernatremia which is corrected too rapidly causes cerebral edema; if mental status changes or seizures occur during correction, infusion of hypertonic solution may be necessary to temporarily raise the serum sodium slightly.

Hyponatremia

Hyponatremia is defined as serum sodium <135 mEq per L. The presence of hyponatremia does not necessarily mean that total body sodium is decreased. Rather, hyponatremia is an indication that the overall water-to-sodium proportion is elevated. Figure 7-3 provides an algorithm which is useful for differentiating the causes of hyponatremia based on serum osmolality, urine osmolality, and volume status.

Patients with hyponatremia may complain of muscle cramps and weakness. Severe hyponatremia which results in rapid fluid shift may manifest as vomiting, lethargy, mental status changes, altered sensorium, headache, seizures, and coma. Brainstem herniation is a potentially catastrophic complication.

The treatment strategy is dictated by the presence or absence of CNS symptoms and the volume status of the patient:

- If symptoms of CNS compromise are present, hypertonic (3% sodium chloride) saline is infused to rapidly increase the serum sodium (and thereby serum osmolality), drawing fluid from the ICF into the ECF. As with hypernatremia, overly rapid correction can lead to neurological complications.
- If the patient is dehydrated, correction of intravascular volume status should suppress ADH secretion, and the serum sodium level will normalize through excretion of excess free water.
- If the patient has hypervolemic hyponatremia, treatment involves fluid restriction, sodium restriction, diuretics,

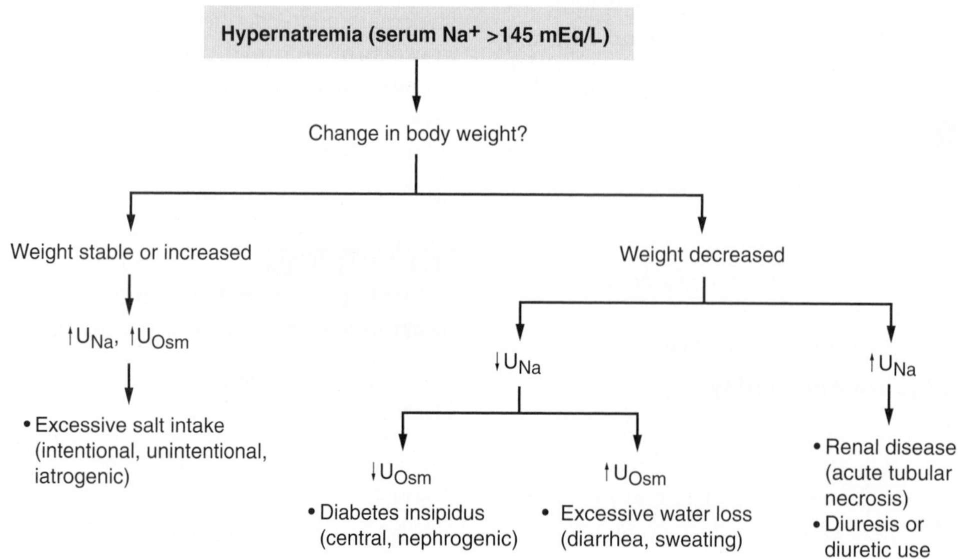

Figure 7-2 Diagnostic algorithm for the evaluation of hypernatremia. U_{Na}, urinary sodium concentration; U_{Osm}, urinary osmolality.

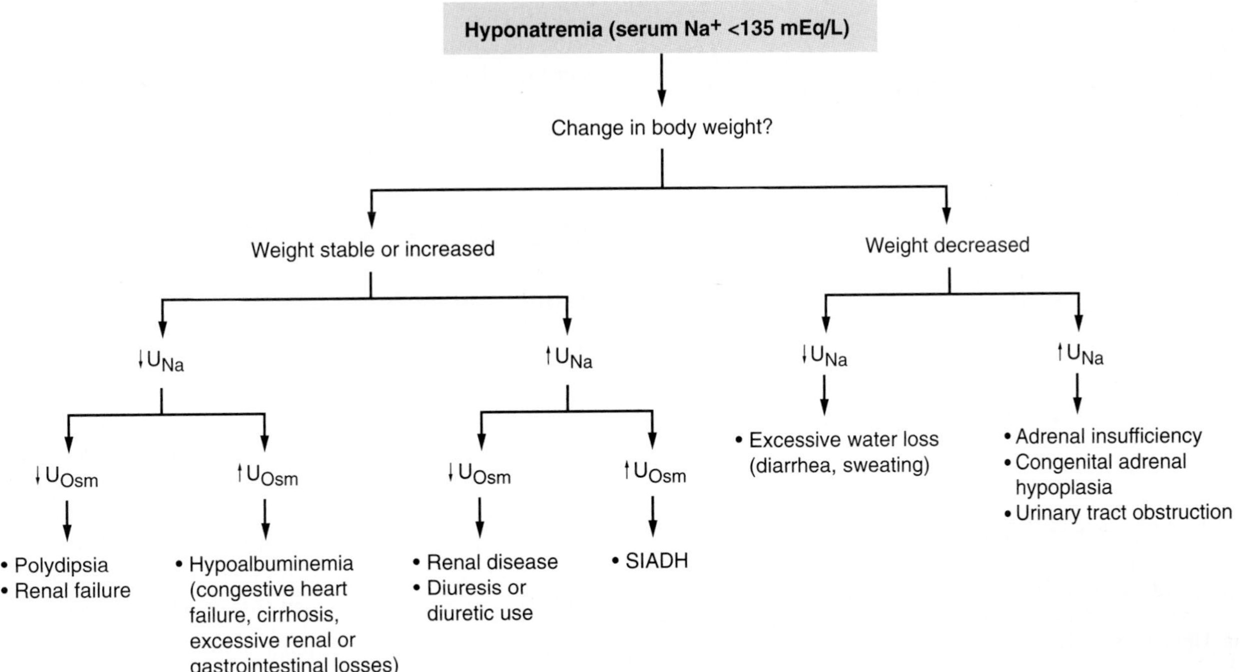

Figure 7-3 Diagnostic algorithm for the evaluation of hyponatremia. U_{Na}, urinary sodium concentration; U_{Osm}, urinary osmolality.

and correction of the underlying disorder (e.g., hypoalbuminemia, cardiac failure).

- If the patient is isovolemic, fluid restriction is the cornerstone of treatment.

The reported serum sodium may be falsely depressed (*factitious hyponatremia*) in the setting of hyperglycemia, hyperlipidemia, or hyperproteinemia. As previously noted, every 100 mg per dL elevation of serum glucose above the normal range decreases the measured serum sodium by 1.6 mEq per L. Extremely high circulating levels of lipids or proteins displace plasma water. Although serum osmolality and sodium-to-serum water ratio remain the same, laboratories employing an indirect, dilutional method of calculating serum sodium will report lower values than labs which use ion-specific electrodes to measure the sodium concentration directly.

Hyperkalemia

A serum concentration of 5.5 mEq per L or greater is considered hyperkalemia. In children, the most frequent cause of an abnormally high potassium level is artifactual, due to hemolysis of red cells during sample collection. Causes of hyperkalemia in the pediatric patient are listed in Table 7-8. Transcellular shifts in hydrogen ions increase serum potassium without changing total body content; for every unit reduction in serum pH, plasma potassium increases 0.2 to 0.4 mEq per L. Disorders and medications that interfere with renal excretion of the electrolyte precipitate true hyperkalemia.

Paresthesias and weakness are the earliest symptoms; flaccid paralysis and tetany occur late. Cardiac involvement correlates with specific progressive ECG changes (Fig. 7-4). T-wave elevation ("peaking") is early and fleeting, followed by loss of P waves, widening QRS complexes, and ST segment depression. In some cases, wide QRS complexes noted on the cardiac monitor are the initial indication of life-threatening hyperkalemia. Ventricular fibrillation and cardiac arrest occur at serum levels >9 mEq per L.

Calcium gluconate protects the heart by stabilizing the cardiac cell membrane and should be administered emergently in all cases of hyperkalemia with associated ECG changes. Patients who do not have ECG changes are treated with infusion of sodium bicarbonate or insulin (and glucose), both of which drive potassium into the cells.

TABLE 7-8
HYPERKALEMIA: POSSIBLE CAUSES

Acidosis
Severe dehydration
Potassium-sparing diuretics (e.g., spironolactone)
Excessive parenteral infusion
Renal failure
Adrenal insufficiency (e.g., Addison disease, adrenal hemorrhage)
Renal tubular acidosis
Massive crush injury
Beta-blocker or digitalis toxicity
Excessive supplementation

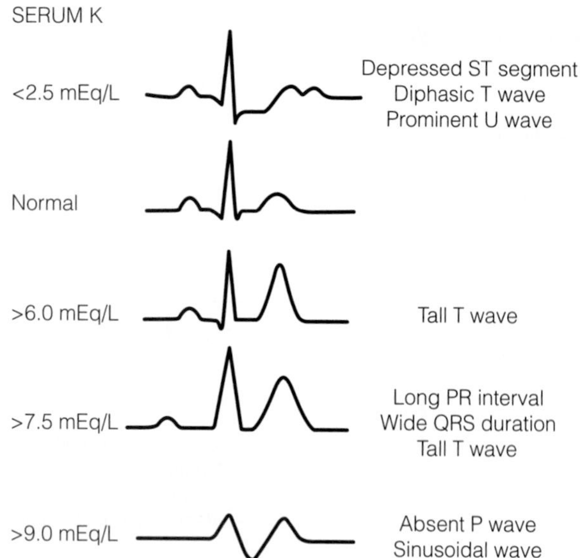

Figure 7-4 ECG findings consistent with hyperkalemia (lead II). (From Marino BS, Fine KS. *Blueprints Pediatrics*. 4th ed. Philadelphia: Lippincott Williams & Wilkins; 2006 with permission.)

Hypokalemia

Hypokalemia in the pediatric population is usually encountered in the setting of alkalosis secondary to vomiting, administration of loop diuretics (furosemide), or diabetic ketoacidosis. Signs and symptoms include weakness, tetany, constipation, polyuria, and polydipsia. Significant myoglobinuria resulting from muscle breakdown compromises renal function. ECG changes (prolonged QT interval, T wave flattening, appearance of U waves) are noted at levels ≤2.5 mEq per L; cardiac arrhythmias (ventricular tachycardia/fibrillation) can occur and are more likely if the patient is being treated with digitalis. Blood pressure changes and urine electrolyte content assist in diagnosis (Fig. 7-5). Treatment involves normalizing pH and replenishing potassium stores orally or intravenously.

ACID-BASE PHYSIOLOGY

Regulation of Body pH

Acids are substances that are capable of donating protons; bases accept protons. The pH is the negative logarithm of the hydrogen ion concentration. As the hydrogen ion concentration increases, the pH decreases; the two are inversely proportional. Acids are highly reactive with proteins, and are partially responsible for alterations in enzyme function when serum pH is low. Normal serum pH is 7.4, with an acceptable range of 7.35 to 7.45.

Acid-base balance is regulated through three mechanisms:

- *Extracellular and intracellular buffers* accept or donate protons to modulate pH changes. The predominant extracellular buffer is bicarbonate, which combines with hydrogen ions to reversibly produce carbon dioxide and water:

$$H^+ + HCO_3^- \leftrightarrow H_2CO_3 \leftrightarrow H_2O + CO_2$$

- *Changes in respiratory rate* cause alterations of the partial pressure of carbon dioxide (P_{CO2}). Increasing the respiratory rate decreases P_{CO2} and increases pH; decreasing the respiratory rate causes retention of CO_2 and a drop in serum pH.
- *Adjustments in renal acid secretion* cause alterations of the plasma bicarbonate concentration. Acid secretion increases

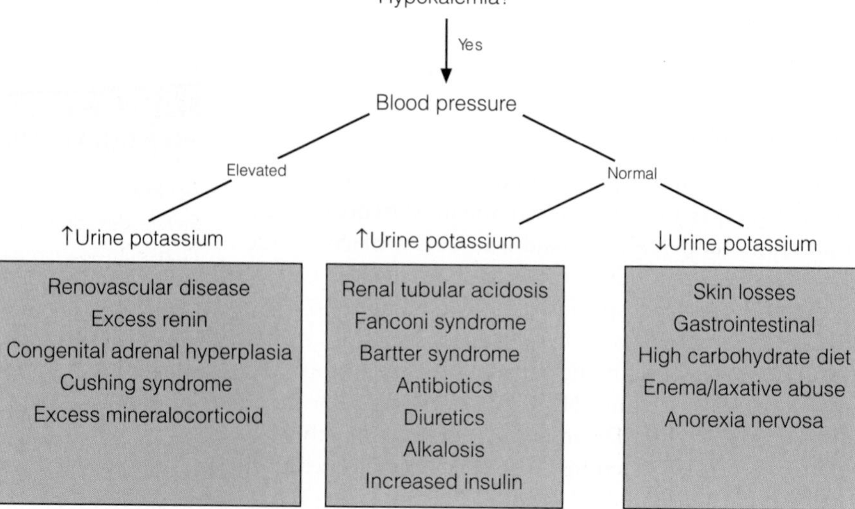

Figure 7-5 Diagnostic algorithm for the evaluation of hypokalemia. (From Marino BS, Fine KS. *Blueprints Pediatrics*. 4th ed. Philadelphia: Lippincott Williams & Wilkins; 2006 with permission.)

TABLE 7-9
EXPECTED COMPENSATORY SHIFTS IN ISOLATED ACID-BASE DISORDERS

Disorder	Expected Compensation
Metabolic acidosis	Each 1 mEq/L ↓ in serum HCO_3^- results in a 1.2 mm Hg ↓ in P_{CO2}
Metabolic alkalosis	Each 1 mEq/L ↑ in serum HCO_3^- results in a 0.7 mm Hg ↑ in P_{CO2}
Respiratory acidosis (acute)	Each 10 mm Hg ↑ in P_{CO2} results in a ↑ 1.0 mEq/L in serum HCO_3^-
Respiratory acidosis (chronic)	Each 10 mm Hg ↑ in P_{CO2} results in a ↑ 3.5 mEq/L in serum HCO_3^-
Respiratory alkalosis (acute)	Each 10 mm Hg ↓ in P_{CO2} results in a ↓ 2.0 mEq/L in serum HCO_3^-
Respiratory alkalosis (chronic)	Each 10 mm Hg ↓ in P_{CO2} results in a ↓ 4.0 mEq/L in serum HCO_3^-

Steady state serum HCO_3^-, 24 mEq/L (normal range 21 to 29 mEq/L); Normal P_{CO2}, 39 to 41 mm Hg

serum HCO_3^- and increases pH; acid retention decreases both serum HCO_3^- and pH.

When an acid-base disturbance is present, compensatory changes in the pulmonary or renal system act to bring the pH closer to normal, although neither can fully neutralize the primary process. Table 7-9 lists expected changes in HCO_3^- and P_{CO2} during compensation. If the secondary changes are more or less than expected, a *mixed* acid-base disorder is present. For example, a combined metabolic and respiratory acidosis would have both an underlying metabolic disorder (decreased renal acid secretion) and an underlying respiratory disorder (hypoventilation resulting in CO_2 retention). A patient with respiratory acidosis due to pulmonary edema may also develop metabolic alkalosis from the loop diuretic used to treat the volume overload.

Metabolic Acidosis

Metabolic acidosis is defined as a serum pH <7.35, which results from any of the following:

- Increased acid production
- Increased acid intake
- Decreased renal acid secretion
- Increased HCO_3^- loss from the gastrointestinal tract and/or kidney

Isolated metabolic acidosis always results in a decrease in serum bicarbonate. Causes of metabolic acidosis (Table 7-10) can be categorized based on whether the process results in a normal anion gap or an increased anion gap, according to the following formula:

$$Na^+ - (Cl^- + HCO_3^-)$$

If the sum is greater than 12 (or 16 in young children), elevated anion gap acidosis is present. Diagnosis is based on history of illness (acute vs. chronic), symptomatology, and laboratory measurements of pH, HCO_3^-, P_{CO2}, and serum osmolality.

If the acidosis is mild, the predominant signs and symptoms are related more to the underlying process than to the acidosis itself. An increase in the respiratory rate may be an early indication of compensation. Severe acidosis (pH ≤7.20) impairs contractility of the heart and predisposes to arrhythmias. Hyperkalemia, another complication of acidosis, may increase the severity of cardiac complications. Lethargy and coma are late sequelae. Chronic metabolic acidosis should be considered in the differential diagnosis of growth impairment and failure to thrive.

TABLE 7-10
COMMON CAUSES OF METABOLIC ACIDOSIS

Normal Anion Gap Metabolic Acidosis
Diarrhea
Renal tubular acidosis
Spironolactone (potassium-sparing diuretic)
Acetazolamide (carbonic anhydrase inhibitor)

Elevated Anion Gap Metabolic Acidosis
Acute or chronic renal failure
Diabetic ketoacidosis
Toxic ingestions (methanol, ethanol, ethylene glycol, salicylates)
Inborn errors of metabolism

Management consists of reversing the underlying process while preventing cardiac, respiratory, and central nervous system complications. Mild-to-moderate acidosis often responds to hydration alone once the causative factors are addressed. Patients with serum HCO_3^- levels <8 mEq per L and those with cardiac or central nervous system complications require controlled sodium bicarbonate infusion.

Metabolic Alkalosis

Metabolic alkalosis is defined by a serum pH >7.45, which is due to a pathological process causing any of the following:

- Loss of hydrogen ions from the ECF
- Increased intake of bicarbonate or decreased excretion of bicarbonate
- Volume contraction with no change in total serum HCO_3^- amount

Isolated metabolic alkalosis always results in an increase in serum HCO_3^-. In pediatric medicine, the two most common causes of metabolic alkalosis are loss of gastric secretions (via emesis or nasogastric suction) and diuretic use. Table 7-11 contains a list of disorders which should be considered in patients with metabolic alkalosis. Metabolic alkalosis which is secondary to chloride loss and subsequent volume depletion is termed "chloride-responsive," and should return to normal with appropriate hydration. Hydration alone will not normalize serum pH if the metabolic alkalosis is chloride-resistant. A urinary chloride level <15 mEq per L is consistent with chloride-responsive conditions; chloride-resistance is indicated by a level >20 mEq per L.

Most of the symptoms observed in patients with metabolic alkalosis result from the underlying disorder, volume depletion, and/or hypokalemia. Arrythmias are a complication of alkalosis, particularly in the presence of decreased potassium levels. Hypoventilation due to respiratory compensation can be significant and may precipitate hypoxia. Alkalemia also causes a decrease in the serum ionized calcium concentration, which may result in tetany and seizures.

Management depends on the underlying etiology. Mild metabolic alkalosis may not require treatment, especially if it results from diuretic use that prevents complications of more serious disease (heart failure). Potassium supplementation and switching to potassium-sparing diuretics can be helpful in many cases. Patients who are losing gastrointestinal fluids can be put on histimine$_2$-receptor blockers or proton pump inhibitors. Volume expansion is beneficial in patients with chloride-responsive disease who can tolerate this intervention. Acetazolamide or dialysis may be employed in cases of severe alkalosis.

TABLE 7-11
METABOLIC ALKALOSIS: CHLORIDE-RESPONSIVE VS. CHLORIDE-RESISTANT

Chloride-Responsive

Loss of upper gastrointestinal fluid (vomiting, pyloric stenosis, nasogastric suctioning)

Use of thiazide (hydrochlorothiazide) or loop (furosemide) diuretics

Cystic fibrosis

Chronic volume contraction

Chloride-Resistant

With hypertension

- Adrenal adenomas or adrenal hyperplasia
- Congenital adrenal hyperplasia
- Renovascular disease; renin secreting tumors
- Cushing syndrome

With normal blood pressure

- Bartter and Gitelman syndromes

TABLE 7-12
CAUSES OF RESPIRATORY ACIDOSIS

Abnormal respiratory drive (CNS depression, trauma, hemorrhage, stroke, or infection)

Alveolar hypoventilation (status asthmaticus, airway obstruction, pulmonary edema, pneumonia)

Abnormalities of the respiratory muscles (reversible or irreversible paralysis)

Space-occupying lesions of the thorax (pneumothorax, hemothorax)

Anatomic abnormalities of the chest (flail chest)

Respiratory Acidosis

Respiratory acidosis is defined as a serum pH <7.35 due to a pathological process which causes an increase in P_{CO2} due to ineffective ventilation (Table 7-12). Treatment centers on reversing the underlying disorder if possible, preventing electrolyte abnormalities, and providing respiratory support (supplemental oxygen, mechanical ventilation).

Respiratory Alkalosis

Respiratory alkalosis is defined as a serum pH >7.45 due to a pathological respiratory process which decreases the P_{CO2} (Table 7-13), typically by increasing the ventilatory

TABLE 7-13
CAUSES OF RESPIRATORY ALKALOSIS

Hypoxia

Mechanical ventilation

Medications/ingestions (salicylates, catecholamines)

CNS disease, which results in increased respiratory drive

Anxiety (hyperventilation)

drive. Treatment of the underlying disorder is usually sufficient.

Dehydration

Dehydration is defined as the loss of some combination of water and salt which produces signs and symptoms of volume depletion. The most common cause of dehydration in infants and young children is infectious gastroenteritis. Dehydration may be classified as isotonic, hypotonic, or hypertonic:

- In *isotonic (isonatremic) dehydration,* sodium chloride losses roughly parallel free water losses. A child with infectious diarrhea, normal kidneys, and access to fluid containing physiologic proportions of water, salt, and glucose will likely present with isonatremic dehydration.
- In *hypotonic (hyponatremic) dehydration,* sodium chloride losses exceed free water losses (serum sodium ≥130 mEq/L).The ICF is relatively preserved at the expense of the ECF, so signs and symptoms of dehydration manifest with less total fluid loss. An example would be an infant with significant diarrhea who is given only water to drink.
- In *hypertonic (hypernatremic) dehydration,* free water losses exceed sodium chloride losses (serum sodium ≥150 mEq/L). Since sodium and chloride are predominantly confined to the ECF space, intravascular volume is relatively preserved. Patients with vomiting and diarrhea who are unable to tolerate fluids may lose water in excess of sodium chloride. In general, however, hypernatremic dehydration is uncommon in the pediatric population.

The clinical manifestations of dehydration result primarily from reduction of the ECF. The earliest sign of dehydration is an increase in heart rate. As opposed to adults, hypotension is a late and ominous finding in children with dehydration and is usually preceded or accompanied by an altered level of consciousness. Table 7-14 details symptoms, signs, and laboratory values associated with varying degrees of (isotonic) dehydration. As noted, these changes will present with a smaller percentage of volume loss in hypotonic dehydration. Because ECF is less affected in hypertonic dehydration, clinical manifestations related to intravascular volume depletion occur rather late; instead, CNS abnormalities predominate, including altered sensorium, lethargy, seizures, and coma.

TABLE 7-14
CLINICAL ESTIMATION OF DEGREE OF DEHYDRATION

	Mild	Moderate	Severe
Weight loss	<5%	5% to 10%	>10%
Vital signs			
Heart rate	increased	increased	greatly increased
Respiratory rate	normal	normal	increased
Blood pressure	normal	normal (orthostasis)	decreased
Skin			
Capillary refill	<2 seconds	2 to 3 seconds	>3 seconds
Mucous membranes	normal/dry	dry	dry
Anterior fontanelle	normal	depressed	depressed
Eyes			
Tearing	normal/absent	absent	absent
Appearance	normal	sunken	sunken
Mental status	normal	altered	depressed
Lab values			
Urine osmolarity	600 mOsm/L	800 mOsm/L	maximal
Urine specific gravity	1.020	1.025	maximal
Blood urea nitrogen	<20	elevated	high
Blood pH	normal	mildly acidotic	moderate/profound acidosis
Stage of shock	not in shock	compensated shock	uncompensated shock

*Infants will exhibit greater weight loss per degree of dehydration (5% mild, 10% moderate, 15% severe), whereas adolescents will exhibit less weight loss per degree of dehydration (3% mild, 5% to 6% moderate, 7% to 9% severe).

TABLE 7-15
FLUID CHOICES FOR MAINTENANCE NEEDS, DEFICIT REPLENISHMENT, AND REPLACEMENT OF ONGOING LOSSES

Maintenance

Volume

100 mL/kg/day for the first 10 kg of body weight, plus 50 mL/kg/day for each additional kg of body weight up to 20 kg, plus 20 mL/kg/day for each kg of body weight thereafter, up to a maximum of 2,000 to 2,500 mL/day.

Composition

D_5 ¼ NS + 20 mEq/L KCl* (patients weighing ≤20 kg)

D_5 ½ NS + 20 mEq/L KCl* (patients weighing >20 kg)

Deficit Replenishment

Volume

Can be estimated based on clinical assessment and changes in patient weight

Composition

Normal saline 20 mL/kg boluses until intravascular volume is restored, followed by replacement of the deficit as per guideline in Table 7-16.

Replacement of Ongoing Losses

Volume

Can be estimated by careful recording of "ins and outs" and changes in the patient's weight

Composition

Stool—excessive sodium, potassium, and bicarbonate losses

Appropriate replacement fluid choice: D_5 ¼ NS + 15 mEq/L bicarbonate + 25 mEq/L KCl (replace mL for mL)

Gastric fluid (emesis, nasogastric suction)—excessive chloride, sodium, and potassium losses

Appropriate replacement fluid choice: D_5 ½ NS + 10 mEq/L KCL (replace mL for mL)

Renal tubular acidosis—bicarbonate (see Chapter 16)

*Potassium should not be added to fluids until urine output is assured.

TABLE 7-16
MANAGEMENT STRATEGIES FOR PEDIATRIC DEHYDRATION

Severe dehydration with hypovolemic shock

- Restoration of intravascular volume through IV administration of 20 mL/kg normal saline bolus (alternatives: 20 mL/kg 5% albumin followed by 20 mL/kg $D_{10}W$; 20 mL/kg normal saline followed by 20 mg/kg $D_{10}W$)
- Frequent clinical reassessment with additional boluses as needed
- Proceed as below, depending on which type of dehydration is present

Significant isotonic or hypotonic dehydration

- Calculate the fluid deficit based on clinical assessment. Estimate maintenance fluid needs over the next 24 hours. Add together and divide by 2. The first half is delivered over the first 8 hours, the second half over the next 16 hours.
- The appropriate parenteral fluid includes 5% glucose with ¼ to ½ normal saline with or without sodium bicarbonate depending on the makeup of ongoing fluid losses. Potassium is added at 20 mEq/L when the patient begins to urinate.

Significant hypertonic dehydration

- Calculate the fluid deficit based on clinical assessment and history. Estimate maintenance fluid needs over the next 48 to 72 hours (the deficit needs to be replaced more slowly due to the risk of cerebral edema and seizures with overly rapid correction, as noted earlier). Add together and divide to determine the hourly rate.
- The appropriate parenteral fluid includes 5% glucose with ¼ to ½ normal saline with or without sodium bicarbonate depending on the makeup of ongoing fluid losses. Potassium is added at 20 mEq/L when the patient begins to urinate.

Moderate dehydration

- Normal saline fluid boluses (20 mL/kg) with frequent reassessment until circulatory volume is normalized, followed by oral rehydration therapy (ORT)
- Oral rehydration therapy alone

Mild dehydration

- Oral rehydration therapy

Management of dehydration depends on both the degree and type of fluid loss (Table 7-15) *and* associated electrolyte and acid-base disturbances. Serum electrolytes (sodium, potassium, chloride; possibly calcium) and bicarbonate levels, BUN and creatinine, serum osmolality, and arterial blood gas measurements are all helpful in the evaluation of dehydration. Specific recommendations regarding management are provided in Table 7-16.

The World Health Organization recommends that oral rehydration solutions contain 90 mEq per L sodium, 20 mEq per L potassium, and 20 g per L glucose. Commercial preparations that approximate these concentrations are available. The presence of glucose in the solution enhances gastrointestinal sodium absorption. ORT is particularly labor intensive, requiring small volumes of fluid given very frequently. Administered correctly, it is extremely effective in the majority of children.

SOURCES

American Academy of Pediatrics Provisional Committee on Quality Improvement, Subcommittee on Acute Gastroenteritis. Practice parameter: The management of acute gastroenteritis in young children. *Pediatrics*. 1996;97:424.

Bender BJ, Skae CC, Ozuah PO. Oral rehydration therapy: The clear solution. *Contemp Pediatr.* 2005;22:72–76.

Finberg L. Dehydration in infancy and childhood. *Pediatr Rev.* 2002;23:277–282.

Moritz ML, Ayus JC. Disorders of water metabolism in children: Hyponatremia and hypernatremia. *Pediatr Rev.* 2002;23:371–380.

Roberts KB. Fluid and electrolytes: Parenteral fluid therapy. *Pediatr Rev.* 2001;22:380–387.

Ruth JL, Wassner SJ. Body composition: Salt and water. *Pediatr Rev.* 2006;27:181–188.

Schwaderer AL, Schwartz GJ. Acidosis and alkalosis. *Pediatr Rev.* 2004;25:350–357.

Wathen JE, MacKenzie T, Bothner JP. Usefulness of the serum electrolyte panel in the management of pediatric dehydration treated with intravenously administered fluids. *Pediatrics*. 2004;114:1227–1234.

QUESTIONS

1. A 5-year-old male presents to the emergency department with weakness and muscle cramping. He vomited non-bloody, non-bilious material twice 3 days ago and had a low-grade fever. Since then, the fever and vomiting have resolved, and the patient has developed eight to ten loose, foul-smelling stools per day. This patient's complaints of weakness and muscle cramping are most likely due which of the following electrolyte imbalances?
A) Hyponatremia
B) Hyperkalemia
C) Metabolic alkalosis
D) Hypochloremia
E) Hypomagnesemia

2. Movement of fluid between the extracellular space and the intracellular space is determined by which of the following?
A) Hydrostatic pressure
B) Relative osmolality
C) Oncotic pressure
D) Permeability of the capillary membrane
E) A, C, and D

3. Movement of fluid between the interstitial space and the plasma space is determined by which of the following?
A) Hydrostatic pressure
B) Relative osmolality
C) Oncotic pressure
D) Permeability of the capillary membrane
E) A, C, and D

4. A 6-year-old female with hyponatremia of unknown origin is transferred from a county hospital for further management. Upon admission, she has the following laboratory results: sodium 125 mEq per L, potassium 4.5 mEq per L, chloride 89 mEq per L, bicarbonate 22 mEq per L, blood urea nitrogen 28 mg per dL, glucose 72 mg per dL. This patient's estimated serum osmolality is closest to which of the following?
A) 125 mOsm per kg
B) 175 mOsm per kg
C) 220 mOsm per kg
D) 260 mOsm per kg
E) 320 mOsm per kg

5. A 15-year-old patient with altered mental status has an estimated serum osmolality of 285 mOsm per kg and a measured serum osmolality of 310 mOsm per kg. In this instance, the osmolal gap is most consistent with ingestion of which of the following?
A) Theophylline
B) Heroin
C) Ethanol
D) Iron
E) Tricyclic antidepressants

6. A 5-week-old former full-term male infant with a benign neonatal course presents with increasingly forceful vomiting over the past 3 weeks. He is judged to be moderately dehydrated based on physical examination, and an "olive" is noted on palpation of the mid-upper abdomen. Ultrasonography reveals hypertrophic pyloric stenosis. Which of the following sets of serum electrolyte results is most consistent with this diagnosis?
A) Sodium 125 mEq per L; potassium 3.9 mEq per L; chloride 86 mEq per L; bicarbonate 30 mEq per L
B) Sodium 145 mEq per L; potassium 3.9 mEq per L; chloride 86 mEq per L; bicarbonate 30 mEq per L
C) Sodium 125 mEq per L; potassium 5.4 mEq per L; chloride 86 mEq per L; bicarbonate 30 mEq per L
D) Sodium 125 mEq per L; potassium 3.9 mEq per L; chloride 115 mEq per L; bicarbonate 30 mEq per L
E) Sodium 125 mEq per L; potassium 3.9 mEq per L; chloride 86 mEq per L; bicarbonate 21 mEq per L

7. A 4-month-old female infant who was recently changed from ready-to-feed formula to powdered formula presents with vomiting and diarrhea of 3 days duration. Vital signs include a temperature of 99.9°F, heart rate 174 beats per minute, respiratory rate 47 breaths per minute, and blood pressure 60/30 mm Hg. She has dry mucous membranes, and sunken fontanelle, and a capillary refill time of 4 seconds. Serum laboratory results include sodium 168 mEq per L, potassium 5.0 mEq per L, chloride 144 mEq per L, and bicarbonate 8 mEq per L. No urine is obtained on catheterization of the bladder. Which of the following represents the most appropriate management of this child's condition?
A) Intravenous boluses of 20 mL per kg normal saline, repeated as needed to restore intravascular volume, followed by rehydration over 24 hours
B) Intravenous boluses of 20 mL per kg normal saline, repeated as needed to restore intravascular volume, followed by rehydration over 48 to 72 hours
C) Intravenous boluses of 20 mL per kg ½ normal saline, repeated as needed to restore intravascular volume, followed by rehydration over 24 hours
D) Intravenous boluses of 20 mL per kg ½ normal saline, repeated as needed to restore intravascular volume, followed by rehydration over 48 to 72 hours
E) Intravenous boluses of 20 mL per kg normal saline, repeated as needed to restore intravascular volume, followed by fluid restriction until electrolyte levels normalize

8. Which of the following dehydration states is associated with the greatest percentage of water loss in a child who is 5% dehydrated based on clinical assessment?
A) Hyponatremic
B) Isonatremic
C) Hypernatremic
D) Hypotonic
E) Hypoosmolar

9. A 17-year-old patient with known severe asthma presents in status asthmaticus. Arterial blood gas measurements are as follows: pH 7.1, PCO_2 55 mm Hg, HCO_3^- 15 mEq per L. This patient's blood gas values are most consistent with which of the following?
A) Respiratory acidosis with metabolic compensation
B) Respiratory acidosis without metabolic compensation
C) Metabolic acidosis with respiratory compensation
D) Combined metabolic and respiratory acidosis
E) Metabolic acidosis without respiratory compensation

10. A 7-month-old former full-term male presents with poor growth over the past 3 months. The patient's weight is below the third percentile, height is at the tenth percentile, and head circumference is at the tenth percentile. The respiratory rate is mildly elevated; otherwise the physical examination is generally unremarkable. Laboratory studies include: (serum) sodium 135 mEq per L, potassium 4.1 mEq per L, chloride 110 mEq per L, bicarbonate 14 mEq per L; normal blood urea nitrogen and creatinine levels; pH of 7.22, with PCO_2 26 mm Hg by venous blood gas analysis; urine pH 7.00, specific gravity 1.015, negative for leukocyte esterase, protein, and glucose. Which of the following is the most likely underlying cause of the child's poor growth?
A) Neglect (starvation)
B) Incorrect mixing of powdered formula
C) Cystic fibrosis
D) Inborn error of metabolism
E) Renal tubular acidosis

11. A 6-year-old male with mental retardation and cerebral palsy is admitted to the hospital with hypernatremic dehydration following several days of diarrhea. His initial serum sodium is 170 mEq per L. Following two 20 mL per kg boluses of normal saline to restore intravascular volume, the patient is started on D_5 ¼ normal saline at a rate calculated to meet maintenance needs and replace half of his deficit in the first 8 hours of therapy. Three hours into this regimen, the patient begins to seize. This patient's seizures are most likely related to which of the following?
A) Overly rapid correction of the serum sodium
B) His underlying central nervous system abnormalities
C) Hypokalemia
D) Hypophosphatemia
E) Hypercalcemia

12. A 12-month-old female presents to the emergency department with copious watery diarrhea of 4 days duration. While intravenous access is being obtained, she loses consciousness and becomes apneic, requiring mechanical ventilation. Her deterioration is most likely due to which of the following complications?
A) Brainstem herniation
B) Intracranial hemorrhage
C) Cerebral edema
D) Hypokalemia
E) Central hypoxia

13. An 8-year-old male is admitted to the hospital for elective surgery. He weighs 66 pounds. Which of the following is the most appropriate parenteral fluid choice for maintenance needs in this patient?
A) 5% dextrose with 0.20% normal saline + 20 mEq per L potassium chloride at 50 mL per hour
B) 5% dextrose with 0.20% normal saline + 40 mEq per L potassium chloride at 70 mL per hour
C) 5% dextrose with 0.20% normal saline + 20 mEq per L potassium chloride at 70 mL per hour
D) 5% dextrose with 0.20% normal saline + 40 mEq per L potassium chloride at 50 mL per hour
E) 10% dextrose with 0.20% normal saline + 20 mEq per L potassium chloride at 70 mL per hour

14. A patient in diabetic ketoacidosis presents with a serum sodium of 128 mEq per L and a serum glucose of 1,200 mg per dL. What is this patient's corrected serum sodium value?
A) 117 mEq per L
B) 128 mEq per L
C) 135 mEq per L
D) 145 mEq per L
E) 157 mEq per L

15. A 9-year-old male with seizures is maintained on carbamazepine. He develops hyponatremia. The patient is normotensive, and there is no evidence of volume depletion or edema on the physical examination. The urinary sodium concentration is >50 mEq per L, and urine osmolality is 500 mOsm per L. This clinical picture is most consistent with which of the following?
A) Cystic fibrosis
B) Adrenal insufficiency
C) Renal salt wasting
D) Diabetes insipidus
E) SIADH

16. The primary determinant of plasma oncotic pressure is
A) albumin
B) sodium
C) potassium
D) phosphate
E) organic anions

17. Which of the following progressions of ECG changes are consistent with increasing hyperkalemia?
A) Prolonged Q-T interval; T wave flattening; appearance of U waves
B) Peaked T waves; loss of P waves; wide QRS complexes; ST segment depression
C) Left axis deviation; bundle branch block; ventricular fibrillation
D) Right axis deviation; right ventricular strain; T wave inversion in Lead II
E) Premature ventricular contractions; ventricular trigeminy; ventricular fibrillation

18. Which of the following sets of ECG changes are consistent with worsening hypokalemia?
A) Left axis deviation; bundle branch block; ventricular fibrillation
B) Peaked T waves; loss of P waves; wide QRS complexes; ST segment depression
C) Prolonged Q-T interval; T wave flattening; appearance of U waves
D) Right axis deviation; right ventricular strain; T wave inversion in Lead II
E) Premature ventricular contractions; ventricular trigeminy; ventricular fibrillation

19. A 16-year-old male patient presenting with muscle weakness and constipation is found to have hypokalemia. His blood pressure is at the 50th percentile for age, height, and gender. His urinary potassium level is elevated. This clinical picture is most consistent with which of the following conditions?
A) Laxative abuse
B) High carbohydrate diet
C) Adrenal hyperplasia
D) Renal tubular acidosis
E) Renovascular disease

20. A 16-year-old male patient presenting with muscle weakness and constipation is found to have hypokalemia. His blood pressure is at the 50th percentile for age, height, and gender. His urinary potassium level is low. This clinical picture is most consistent with which of the following conditions?
A) Bartter syndrome
B) Renal tubular acidosis
C) Cushing syndrome
D) Renovascular disease
E) Laxative abuse

21. A 9-year-old female who is on steroids for dermatomyositis develops edema. Which of the following diuretics is least likely to cause hypokalemia is this patient?
A) Spironolactone
B) Bumetanide
C) Furosemide
D) Chlorothiazide
E) Hydrochlorothiazide

22. Which of the following is the earliest sign of dehydration in a young child?
A) An increase in respiratory rate
B) An increase in heart rate
C) A decrease in blood pressure
D) Tacky mucous membranes
E) Extended capillary refill

23. A 3-year-old female presents with a 2-day history of vomiting and diarrhea. She is alert and fussy but consolable, and she is able to tolerate fluids. She has urinated three times today. Her heart rate is 110 beats per minute, and she has lost about 3% of her body weight based on information from a health maintenance visit last month. Capillary refill is 2 to 3 seconds; there are no other abnormalities on exam. Which of the following is the most appropriate fluid choice for rehydration of this patient?
A) 5% dextrose with 0.20% normal saline
B) 5% dextrose with 0.45% normal saline
C) Oral rehydration therapy
D) Apple juice
E) Water and crackers

24. Which of the following combinations represents the correct daily maintenance requirements for sodium and potassium?
A) 3 to 4 mEq per kg sodium; 3 to 4 mEq/kg potassium
B) 3 to 4 mEq per kg sodium; 1 to 2 mEq per kg potassium
C) 4 to 5 mEq per kg sodium; 2 to 3 mEq per L potassium
D) 3 to 4 mEq per kg sodium; 2 to 3 mEq per kg potassium
E) 3 to 4 mEq per kg sodium; 2 to 3 mEq per kg potassium

25. In which of the following patients is the total body water the highest percentage of body weight?
A) An adolescent male
B) An adolescent female
C) A 5-year-old child
D) A full-term infant
E) A 28-week preterm infant

26. Which of the following conditions is most likely to result in a primary respiratory acidosis?
A) Guillain-Barre syndrome
B) Hypoxia
C) Mechanical ventilation
D) Salicylate ingestion
E) Anxiety

27. Which of the following conditions causes metabolic alkalosis, which is NOT responsive to hydration?
A) Nasogastric suctioning
B) Adrenal hyperplasia
C) Loop diuretic use
D) Cystic fibrosis
E) Thiazide diuretic use

28. When a patient presents with diabetic ketoacidosis,
A) the serum sodium measurement is not representative of the total body sodium content
B) the serum potassium measurement is not representative of the total body potassium content
C) the excess glucose is osmotically active
D) the excess glucose is primarily confined to the extracellular space
E) All of the above are true.

29. A 4-year-old male with no significant past medical history presents with polyuria and polydipsia. He has lost 2 kg in the past month. His serum sodium concentration is 160 mEq per L. Urinary studies reveal low urinary sodium and osmolality values. A trial of vasopressin does not affect urine output. This patient's hypernatremia is most likely due to which of the following?
A) Excessive salt intake
B) Craniopharyngioma
C) SIADH
D) Nephrogenic diabetes insipidus
E) Central diabetes insipidus

30. A patient with significant metabolic acidosis (serum HCO_3^- 8 mEq/L) develops widening QRS complexes on the cardiac monitor. Which of the following is the most appropriate next step in the management of this patient?
A) Urgent dialysis
B) Administer intravenous adenosine followed by insulin and glucose.
C) Administer intravenous calcium gluconate, followed by sodium bicarbonate.
D) Administer acetazolamide and admit to the pediatric intensive care unit.
E) Administer intravenous 3% sodium chloride.

ANSWERS

1. A	11. A	21. A
2. B	12. B	22. B
3. E	13. C	23. C
4. D	14. D	24. B
5. C	15. E	25. E
6. A	16. A	26. A
7. B	17. B	27. B
8. C	18. C	28. E
9. D	19. D	29. D
10. E	20. E	30. C

Metabolic Disease

GENERAL PRESENTATION, EVALUATION, AND MANAGEMENT

Genetic mutations which alter the structure or quantity of proteins involved in cellular biochemical processes are referred to as inborn errors of metabolism (IEM) (Table 8-1). Most IEMs are autosomal recessive. State-sponsored newborn metabolic screening tests often suggest the diagnosis of IEM before the neonate becomes symptomatic and are cost-effective for use in the population at large. However, IEMs can and do occur in children with negative newborn screens. Targeted prenatal diagnosis is offered to couples in high risk groups (e.g., consanguinity or a prior child with metabolic disease). Medical professionals who care for children must know when to suspect an IEM, how to proceed with the evaluation, and how to limit serious and irreversible complications.

IEMs may present in the newborn period or thereafter. The clinical presentations of metabolic disease are extensive and often nonspecific (Table 8-2). Table 8-3 provides a list of initial laboratory tests which will identify major abnormalities and assist in determining the direction of further

TABLE 8-1
INBORN ERRORS OF METABOLISM

Disorders of Protein Metabolism

Aminoacidopathies (phenylketonuria, homocystinuria, maple syrup urine disease)

Organic acidemias (isovaleric acidemia, propionic acidemia, methylmalonic acidemia)

Urea cycle defects (X-linked ornithine transcarbamylase deficiency; arginase deficiency)

Disorders of Carbohydrate Metabolism

Galactosemia

Glycogen storage diseases (von Gierke disease, Pompe disease, McArdle Disease)

Disorders of Fat Metabolism

Lysosomal storage disorders (Tay-Sachs disease, Gaucher disease, Niemann-Pick disease)

Mucopolysaccharidoses (Hurler syndrome, Hunter syndrome, Sanfilippo syndromes)

Fatty acid oxidation defects

Defects in carnitine transporters

TABLE 8-2
PRESENTATION OF INBORN ERRORS OF METABOLISM

Signs and symptoms of IEMs that typically present in the neonatal period:

Recurrent vomiting

Poor feeding

Jaundice (due to conjugated hyperbilirubinemia)

Lethargy with progressively depressed sensorium

Seizures unresponsive to glucose, calcium, anticonvulsants

Coma

Severe, persistent hypoglycemia

Abnormal odor to urine, other bodily fluids

Any of the above in an infant with no risk factors for sepsis

Any of the above presenting hours to days after birth in an infant who was initially well

IEMs that typically present in the neonatal period:

Urea cycle defects

Organic acidemias

Some aminoacidopathies

Galactosemia

Signs and symptoms of IEMs that typically present beyond the neonatal period:

Mental retardation

Motor deficits

Developmental delay or regression

Failure to thrive

Convulsions

Recurrent emesis with hepatic dysfunction

Recurrent episodes of unexplained hypoglycemia

Hepatomegaly

Muscle weakness or cardiomyopathy

Renal stones

Intermittent episodes of unexplained vomiting, acidosis, mental deterioration, or coma

Unusual odor during an acute illness

Asymptomatic periods alternating with episodes of acute deterioration

IEMs that typically present beyond the neonatal period:

Some aminoacidopathies

Lysosomal storage disorders

Mucopolysaccharidoses

Some fatty acid oxidation defects (medium-chain acyl CoA dehydrogenase deficiency)

TABLE 8-3
SUGGESTED LABORATORY EVALUATION OF THE PATIENT WITH SUSPECTED METABOLIC DISEASE

Initial studies
Complete blood count including differential cell count and cell morphology
Serum electrolytes, including calcium and magnesium
Blood gas analysis
Serum glucose
Plasma ammonia
Plasma lactate, pyruvate
Liver function tests
Urine reducing substances
Urine ketones
Additional tests to consider
Plasma amino acids
Urine organic acids

evaluation. It is important to note that these studies should be obtained prior to intervention if possible, while the patient is still symptomatic. Some conditions do not produce laboratory abnormalities unless the patient is under "metabolic stress" (e.g., fasting, infection). The specific presentations and laboratory results characteristic of each disorder are covered in Table 8-4. Suggested evaluation strategies for a few of the more common acute presentations of IEMs are provided in Figures 8-1, 8-2, and 8-3.

Metabolic acidosis with an increased anion gap is a classic presentation of a group of specific IEMs, which includes organic acidemias and fatty-acid oxidation defects. Many patients with metabolic acidosis will be tachypneic due to respiratory compensation measures. Some of these disorders also result in the accumulation of ammonia, which readily crosses the blood-brain barrier and is toxic to the central nervous system. Hemodialysis causes a rapid drop in plasma ammonia and should be considered for levels exceeding 300 mcmol per L. Severely acidotic patients require hydration and sodium bicarbonate administration (see Chapter 7).

Hypoglycemia is a frequent presentation of organic acidemias, disorders of carbohydrate metabolism, and fatty acid oxidation defects. Seizures and encephalopathy progressing to coma are encountered more frequently in patients with organic acidemias, urea cycle defects, maple-syrup urine disease, and fatty acid oxidation defects.

TREATMENT OF ACUTE METABOLIC DECOMPENSATION

Patients in acute metabolic crisis require intravenous hydration with glucose-containing fluids. They should be given nothing by mouth until stabilization (and preferably diagnosis). Sodium bicarbonate may be necessary to correct life-threatening metabolic acidosis. Hyperammonemia, if

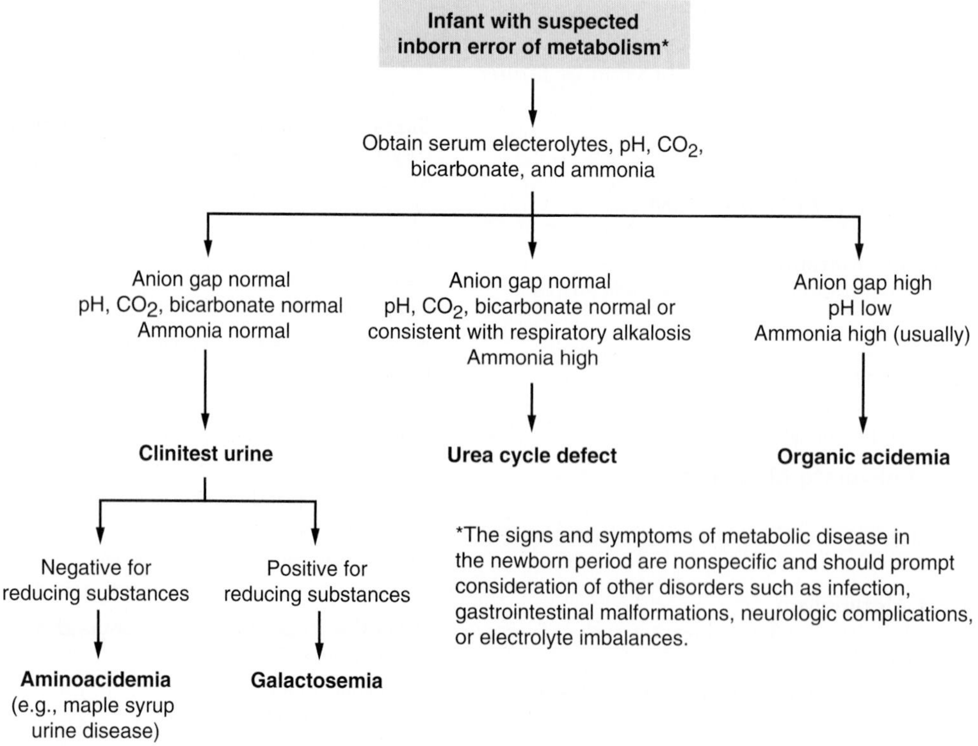

Figure 8-1 Evaluation of an infant with suspected inborn error of metabolism.

TABLE 8-4
REVIEW OF SPECIFIC INBORN ERRORS OF METABOLISM

Disease	Biochemical Disorder	Presentation	Laboratory Evaluation	Treatment	Prognosis
		DISORDERS OF PROTEIN METABOLISM			
Aminoacidopathies: IEMs in which an enzyme defect inhibits the metabolism of specific amino acids, resulting in a buildup of these substances in the plasma					
Phenylketonuria (AR)	Deficiency of phenylalanine hydroxylase, the enzyme that converts phenylalanine to tyrosine (other variants described)	Asymptomatic infant with a positive newborn screen, OR older infant with light hair/skin and unexplained vomiting, irritability, eczematous rash, "musty" odor to urine	Most infants with an elevated phenylalanine level on newborn screen do not have phenylketonuria. Further evaluation (repeat newborn screen, plasma amino acid levels, consultation with a metabolic specialist) is needed.	Life-long dietary intervention (low protein, low phenylalanine diet); tyrosine supplementation	*Treated*: normal growth and development; increased incidence of learning disabilities *Untreated*: severe mental retardation, seizures, behavior problems
Homocystinuria (AR)	Deficiency of cystathionine synthase, the enzyme which converts methionine to cysteine and serine (other variants described)	Asymptomatic infant with a positive newborn screen, OR fair-skinned toddler with developmental delay, OR older child/adolescent with Marfan-like body habitus, ocular lens dislocation, or thromboembolic disease	Elevated plasma or urine homocysteine levels; cultured skin fibroblasts do not demonstrate cystathionine synthase activity	Life-long dietary intervention (low protein, methionine-restricted diet) with cysteine supplementation; some patients respond to pyridoxine	*Treated*: normal growth and development *Untreated*: mild mental retardation, lens dislocation, thromboembolic disease, premature myocardial infarction
Maple syrup urine disease (AR)	Deficiency of branched-chain α-ketoacid dehydrogenase, which is responsible for decarboxylation and metabolism of leucine, isoleucine, and valine	Poor feeding; vomiting within the first week of life; hypertonia, muscle rigidity; progressively depressed sensorium, seizures, coma; "maple syrup" odor to urine and other body fluids	Positive newborn screen; elevated plasma and urine leucine, isoleucine, and valine levels	*Acute:* hemodialysis *Maintenance:* life-long dietary intervention (low branched-chain amino acid diet)	*Treated*: normal growth and development with occasional episodes of acute metabolic decompensation *Untreated*: severe neurologic impairment/death
Organic acidemias (AR)	Deficiency of any of a number of enzymes involved in the catabolism of branched-chain amino acids (leucine, isoleucine, and valine)	Early (within hours to days) onset of poor feeding, vomiting in a previously healthy infant being fed protein; progressively depressed sensorium, seizures, coma; possible	Positive newborn screen; severe metabolic acidosis with elevated anion gap; ketoacidosis; some forms associated with hyperammonemia, abnormal liver function tests,	*Acute*: Hydration, sodium bicarbonate infusion; removal of the excess metabolite; hyperalimentation to prevent ongoing protein catabolism; carnitine	*Treated*: periods of normal function interspersed with episodes of acute metabolic decompensation

(*continued*)

TABLE 8-4
(continued)

Disease	Biochemical Disorder	Presentation	Laboratory Evaluation	Treatment	Prognosis
		identifiable odor to urine and other body fluids	neutropenia; elevated levels of precursors and metabolites in the blood and urine (urine organic acids)	supplementation *Maintenance*: life-long dietary intervention	*Untreated*: severe neurologic impairment/death; milder variants may present during childhood with learning disabilities, unexplained acute metabolic decompensation
Urea cycle defects (AR except for ornithine transcarbamylase deficiency, which is X-L)	Deficiency of any of a number of enzymes involved in the conversion of ammonia to urea	Poor feeding, vomiting, hyperventilation, apnea, hypotonia, lethargy which develops after 24 hours of age in a previously healthy infant being fed protein; progresses to seizures, coma with increased intracranial pressure	Increased plasma ammonia level, decreased blood urea nitrogen; pH, CO_2, serum bicarbonate normal or consistent with respiratory alkalosis; normal anion gap; definitive diagnoses rests on detecting elevated levels of metabolites in the blood or urine	*Acute*: hemodialysis to remove ammonia; hydration; protein-restriction with the balance of calories provided as glucose and lipids *Maintenance*: life-long dietary restriction (low protein diet); supplementation with specific essential amino acids; medical exploitation of alternative pathways	*Treated*: periods of normal function interspersed with episodes of acute metabolic decompensation *Untreated*: death within days of birth
		DISORDERS OF CARBOHYDRATE METABOLISM			
Galactosemia (AR)	Deficiency of galactose-1-phosphate uridyl transferase, which converts galactose-1-phosphate to glucose-1-phosphate;	Poor feeding, vomiting, irritability, jaundice, lethargy, seizures, which develop within days to weeks of birth in a previously normal infant being fed lactose (in	Positive newborn screen; hypoglycemia, direct hyperbilirubinemia, elevated liver function tests, prolonged PT/PTT; urine positive for reducing substances but does not	*Acute*: exclusion of lactose from diet; supportive care *Maintenance*: lactose-free (i.e., soy) formula in place of breastfeeding	*Treated*: normal growth and development with an increased incidence of learning disabilities

(continued)

TABLE 8-4
(continued)

Disease	Biochemical Disorder	Presentation	Laboratory Evaluation	Treatment	Prognosis
	Excess galactose-1-phosphate accumulates in the liver, kidneys, and brain	formula or breast milk). Jaundice, hepatosplenomegaly often present as well. Patient may also present with cataracts or neonatal (*Escherichia coli*) sepsis.	react with glucose oxidase on the test strip (Clinitest); definitive diagnosis by detection of reduced levels of a metabolite in erythrocytes	or cow-milk formula and life-long exclusion of lactose from the diet	*Untreated*: mental retardation, hepatic cirrhosis, death
Glycogen storage disease type I (von Gierke disease) (AR)	Deficiency of glucose-6-phosphatase (all variants of glycogen storage disease involve the deficiency of any of a number of enzymes involved in conversion of glycogen to glucose)	Infants typically present when they begin to sleep through the night (prolonged fasting) with irritability, pallor, insomnia, seizures; hepatomegaly; delays in linear growth; other variants present later in childhood with similar symptoms or with renal stones, short stature, liver disease	Fasting hypoglycemia, lactic acidosis, hyperuricemia, hyperlipidemia, ketonuria; conjugated hyperbilirubinemia; definitive diagnosis by detection of absence of glucose-6-phosphatase in liver tissue	Avoidance of fasting and frequent administration of carbohydrates (including continuous overnight feeds in infants or uncooked corn starch before bed in older patients) Regular monitoring of creatinine kinase, renal and hepatic function	Periods of normal function interspersed with episodes of acute metabolic decompensation; recurrent hyperglycemic seizures may eventually result in irreversible neurologic impairment
DISORDERS OF FAT METABOLISM					
Lysosomal storage diseases					
Tay-Sachs disease (AR, with increased incidence in Ashkenazi Jewish population. Prenatal carrier status testing available)	Deficiency in the enzyme hexosaminidase A, with accumulation of GM-2 gangliosides in neuronal lysosomes; also called GM-2 gangliosiderosis	Initially presents by 3 to 6 months of age with hypotonia, exaggerated startle, motor delay or regression; ophthalmologic examination reveals nystagmus, characteristic cherry-red spots on the retinas	Both genetic and enzymatic tests are available.	Supportive care	Blindness; death by age 2 years

(continued)

TABLE 8-4
(continued)

Disease	Biochemical Disorder	Presentation	Laboratory Evaluation	Treatment	Prognosis
Gaucher disease (AR) Three variants	Deficiency in the enzyme glucosylceramidase, resulting in accumulation of metabolites in the liver, spleen, and bone marrow	May be asymptomatic; otherwise hepatosplenomegaly, bone pain and bony changes (avascular necrosis, osteoporosis, widening of the distal femurs)	Anemia, leukopenia, thrombocytopenia; diagnosis confirmed by detection of low enzyme levels in leukocytes	Recombinant enzyme therapy	Developmental delay, failure to thrive, splenic infarction; death in childhood if severely affected
Niemann-Pick disease	Deficiency in the enzyme sphingomyelinase, resulting in accumulation of sphingomyelin in mononuclear cells and (in some forms) neurons	Several subtypes presenting with variable severity; hepatosplenomegaly is the most consistent finding in children beyond the neonatal period; type A (presenting in early infancy) with failure to thrive, pulmonary disease, and progressive neurodegeneration	Diagnosis confirmed through measurement of sphingomyelinase activity in peripheral white blood cells or presence of "foam cells" (lipid-filled macrophages) on liver or bone-marrow biopsy	Symptomatic treatment; supportive care	Depends on subtype; death in infancy to normal life span
Mucopolysaccharidoses: Disease states caused by defects in any of a number of enzymes involved in the metabolism of glycosaminoglycans, (mucopolysaccharides), resulting in accumulation of these substances in the lysosomes of organs and connective tissues. The specific disorders are distinguished mainly by the enzyme involved and the metabolite that accumulates.					
Hurler syndrome (AR)	Deficiency in the enzyme α-L-iduronidase	Presents in the first 2 years of life with developmental regression, failure to thrive; thickened skin; affected patients develop typical "coarse" facial features including short nose, flat face, and protruding tongue	Diagnosis based on characteristic physical and radiographic signs; quantitative analysis of specific glycosaminoglycans in the urine	Supportive care; research into bone marrow transplantation and gene replacement therapy is ongoing	Joint contractures, kyphosis; deafness; cardiomyopathy; decreased lung function; death before adolescence
Hunter syndrome (X-L)	Deficiency in the enzyme iduronate-2-sulphatase	Developmental delay, hepatosplenomegaly within the first year of life; milder forms may not manifest until adulthood	Diagnosis based on characteristic physical and radiographic signs; quantitative analysis of specific glycosaminoglycans in the urine	Supportive care; research into gene replacement therapy is ongoing	Progressive mental retardation and physical disability; death in adolescence in patients with severe disease

(continued)

TABLE 8-4
(continued)

Disease	Biochemical Disorder	Presentation	Laboratory Evaluation	Treatment	Prognosis
Fatty acid oxidation defects and disorders related to carnitine transport: Disease states caused by defects in any of a number of enzymes involved in the breakdown of stored fat for energy purposes. High levels of fatty acids circulate in the serum, and fasting results in metabolic decompensation.					
Fatty acid oxidation defects (AR)	Multiple variants	Sudden metabolic decompensation (including "near-SIDS") associated with infant sleeping through the night (prolonged fasting) or other metabolic stressor (intercurrent illness); hypotonia on exam; older children complain of muscle pain associated with rhabdomyolysis, or may present with sudden decompensation related to a metabolic stressor (illness, dehydration, fasting)	*Non-ketotic hypoglycemia* is hallmark of defects of fatty acid oxidation; conjugated hyperbilirubinemia may also be present	*Acute*: intravenous 10% dextrose in water to normalize serum glucose (produces rapid, dramatic improvement); maintenance fluids to promote hydration and reduce the risk of renal damage due to rhabdomyolysis; carnitine supplementation *Maintenance*: carnitine supplementation; avoidance of prolonged fasting; fat restricted diet; medium-chain triglyceride oil if indicated	Cardiomyopathy; renal damage
Enzymatic disorders affecting carnitine (AR)	Multiple variants. Carnitine is responsible for the transport of fatty acids into the mitochondria.	Presents in the neonatal period with apnea, seizures, cardiac arrhythmias	Non-ketotic hypoglycemia, elevated plasma ammonia, decreased plasma carnitine	Similar to above	Similar to above

AR, autosomal recessive; X-L, X-linked.

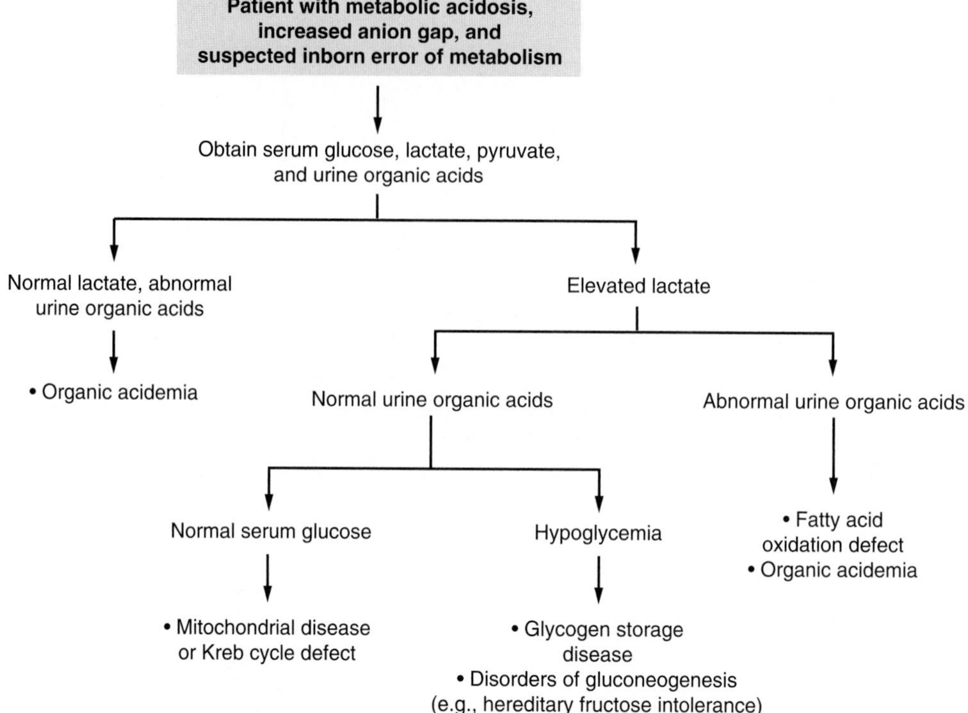

Figure 8-2 Evaluation of a patient with metabolic acidosis and suspected inborn error of metabolism. (Adapted from Cloherty JC. *Manual of Neonatal Care*. 5th ed. Philadelphia: Lippincott Williams & Wilkins; 2003 with permission.)

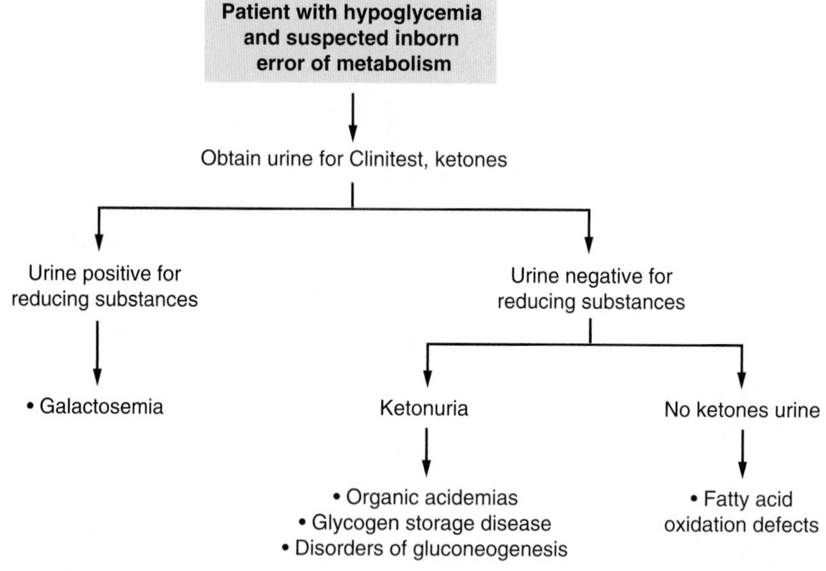

Figure 8-3 Evaluation of a patient with hypoglycemia and suspected inborn error of metabolism. (Adapted from Cloherty JC. *Manual of Neonatal Care*. 5th ed. Philadelphia: Lippincott Williams & Wilkins; 2003 with permission.)

present, is addressed through hemodialysis. The patient's mental status provides important information regarding the success of intervention; progressive neurologic impairment is an ominous development. Maintenance caloric needs must be met to prevent protein breakdown, so energy is provided as parenteral glucose and interlipids. Serum glucose measurements are checked initially and frequently thereafter. Exogenous protein is either completely withheld or administered as essential amino acids at very low concentrations.

SOURCES

Cataltepe SU, Levy HL. Inborn errors of metabolism. In: Cloherty JP, Stark AR, eds. *Manual of Neonatal Care*. 5th ed. Baltimore, MD: Lippincott Williams & Wilkins; 2003:591–606.

Rezvani I. An approach to inborn errors of metabolism. In: Behrman RE, Kliegman RM, Jenson HB, eds. *Nelson Textbook of Pediatrics*. 17th ed. Philadelphia, PA: Saunders; 2004:397–398.

Siegel B, Milunsky J. When should the possibility of a genetic disorder cross your radar screen? *Contemp Pediatr*. 2004;21:30–45.

QUESTIONS

1. The state newborn screen for a 7-day-old in your practice is reportedly positive for phenylketonuria. The baby appears healthy, and the mother reports that he is breastfeeding well. Which of the following is the most appropriate course of action?
A) Send blood for quantitative plasma amino acid levels.
B) Send urine for quantitative urine organic acid levels.
C) Discontinue breastfeeding and substitute phenylalanine-free formula.
D) Continue breast feeding and instruct the parent not to supplement with any commercial formula.
E) Schedule the infant for neurodevelopmental testing.

2. What is the mode of inheritance for the majority of inborn errors of metabolism?
A) Autosomal dominant
B) Autosomal recessive
C) X-linked
D) Mitochondrial
E) Multifactorial

3. Which of the following statements regarding screening tests for inborn errors of metabolism is FALSE?
A) Prenatal testing is available for many inborn errors of metabolism.
B) Genetic screening is offered to people in high-risk populations who wish to determine carrier status.
C) Infants with negative newborn screens do not have the disease.
D) Infants with positive newborn screens may or may not have the disease.
E) Newborn screens may identify affected infants before they become symptomatic.

4. You are called to the newborn nursery to evaluate a 16-hour-old full-term male infant with a normal prenatal course and uneventful delivery who has begun vomiting. He has been offered standard infant formula every 2 to 3 hours since birth and had been feeding well. The patient's physical examination is normal except for irritability and mild hypotonia. You obtain blood and urine for laboratory evaluation. The white blood count is mildly depressed but within normal limits, with a normal differential. Additional results are consistent with metabolic acidosis with an elevated anion gap. Which of the following is the most important additional laboratory value to obtain at this time?
A) Plasma amino acids
B) Urine organic acids
C) Serum pyruvate
D) Serum ammonia
E) Serum lactate

5. You are called to the newborn nursery to evaluate a previously healthy 3-day-old full-term male infant who has begun feeding poorly and vomiting and is now tachypneic. He has been offered standard infant formula every 2 to 4 hours since birth and had been feeding well. The patient's physical examination is normal except for irritability and mild hypotonia. A portable chest radiograph obtained prior to your arrival is negative. You send blood and urine for laboratory assessment and cultures. The white blood count is mildly elevated but within normal limits, with a normal differential. Additional results are consistent with mild respiratory alkalosis. The plasma ammonia level is 840 mcmol per L. In addition to hydration with a glucose-containing intravenous fluid, which of the following is the most appropriate immediate course of action?
A) Make the patient NPO and send cerebrospinal fluid for ammonia level analysis.
B) Make the patient NPO and administer essential amino acids and interlipids through a central line to prevent muscle breakdown.
C) Make the patient NPO and obtain the infant's blood type for potential plasmapheresis.
D) Make the patient NPO and place a Tenckhoff catheter for peritoneal dialysis.
E) Make the patient NPO and administer "ammonia-scavenging" medications while preparing for hemodialysis.

6. You are seeing a new patient who has transferred into your practice. She is a 3-year-old Caucasian female with known classic phenylketonuria. A medical resident asks you about available treatments for this patient's condition. You are correct in telling the resident all of the following EXCEPT:
A) Patients with classic phenylketonuria are managed primarily through the elimination of all phenylalanine from their diets.
B) Patients with classic phenylketonuria usually require tyrosine supplementation.
C) Patients with classic phenylketonuria should be maintained on an appropriate restricted diet for the duration of their lives.
D) Patients with classic phenylketonuria should be maintained on low-protein diets.
E) Patients with classic phenylketonuria should be managed in partnership with a medical professional specifically trained in metabolic disorders.

7. A couple that has attended your prenatal class asks you about genetic screening. They served as missionaries in Laos for three years prior to returning to the United States. While overseas, they had a daughter born at full-term who initially appeared healthy but developed vomiting, irritability, "mousy-smelling" urine, and an eczematous rash. This child died at 18 months of age during a seizure. This clinical history is most consistent with a diagnosis of which of the following?

A) Homocystinuria
B) Phenylketonuria
C) Maple-syrup urine disease
D) Ornithine transcarbamylase deficiency
E) von Gierke disease

8. You are seeing a 13-year-old male in your office for behavior problems at school. The child attends an alternative school for high-functioning children with mild mental retardation. His past medical history is positive for dislocation of the right ocular lens. The physical examination is significant for abnormally long extremities and a heart murmur. Which of the following studies is most likely to be abnormal in this patient?

A) Erythrocyte galactose-1-phosphate uridyl transferase activity
B) Urine leucine, isoleucine, and valine levels
C) Urine homocysteine levels
D) Glucose-6-phosphatase levels in liver tissue
E) Leukocyte β-glucosidase levels

9. An infant presents at 5 days-of-life with poor feeding and vomiting. He is a former full-term neonate with normal prenatal and perinatal histories to date. His mother has noted a "sweet, syrupy" odor to her child's urine. The state newborn screen is consistent with maple syrup urine disease. Following acute management of the patient's disorder, which of the following is the most appropriate dietary intervention?

A) Life-long restriction of phenylalanine in the diet
B) Life-long restriction of methionine in the diet
C) Life-long restriction of branched-chain amino acids in the diet
D) Life-long supplementation with carnitine
E) Life-long supplementation with cysteine

10. Carnitine supplementation is required for which of the following inborn errors of metabolism?

A) Organic acidemias
B) Fatty acid oxidation defects
C) Mucopolysaccharidoses
D) A and B
E) A, B, and C

11. Which of the following is the most appropriate nutritional choice for an infant with galactosemia?

A) Breast or soy milk only
B) Goat milk formula only
C) Breast milk only
D) Cow-milk formula only
E) Soy formula only

12. You are awakened in the middle of an "on-call" night when you are paged by an emergency department physician. She wants to admit one of your patients for observation and evaluation following an ALTE (apparent life-threatening event). The child is a 4-month-old former full-term infant with an unremarkable past medical history who recently began sleeping through the night. The emergency medical technicians in the ambulance were unable to place a line. Upon admission, the infant was responsive to pain with a weak cry. An initial dextrose-stick was 33 g per dL, and there were no ketones in the urine. Hydration and intravenous glucose administration resulted in rapid improvement in the patient's symptoms. This patient will likely require which of the following interventions upon returning home to prevent further episodes of metabolic decompensation?

A) Continuous overnight nasogastric feeds
B) 1 tablespoon baked cornstarch by mouth every evening
C) 1 tablespoon unbaked cornstarch by mouth every evening
D) 1 tablespoon medium-chain triglyceride oil by mouth every evening
E) An apnea monitor

13. You are seeing an 18-month-old male in your office for his regular health maintenance visit. His mother is concerned because he can no longer walk without support. Indeed, the child can pull to a stand, cruise, and walk with his hand held, but cannot walk more than a few steps on his own. The physical examination is significant for hepatosplenomegaly. Which of the following tests is most likely to be diagnostic in this patient?

A) Quantitative analysis of specific glycosaminoglycans in the urine
B) Plasma carnitine
C) Serum lactate/pyruvate ratio
D) Urine reducing substances
E) Radiographic examination of the femur

ANSWERS

1. A
2. B
3. C
4. D
5. E
6. A
7. B
8. C
9. C
10. D
11. E
12. A
13. A

Diseases of Allergy and Immunology

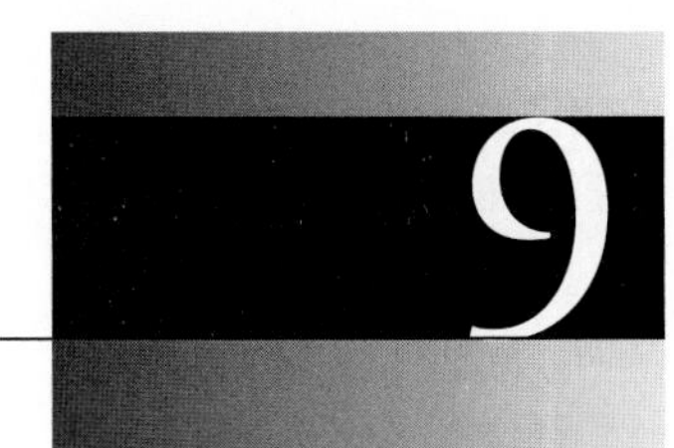

GENERAL FEATURES OF ATOPIC DISEASE

Atopic disorders are characterized by hyperresponsiveness to environmental stimuli, followed by a delayed inflammatory reaction. The response may be generalized (anaphylaxis) or limited to a target organ such as the skin (atopic dermatitis), lungs (asthma), nose (allergic rhinitis), eyes (allergic conjunctivitis), or gastrointestinal tract (food allergies). This chapter is limited primarily to discussion of Type I IgE-mediated allergic disease (Table 9-1). Common environmental allergens include house dust mite, pet, and cockroach allergens; molds and fungi; and seasonal pollinators. Food, drugs, and insect stings may also provoke an allergic response. Chronic allergic inflammation due to persistent exposure or self-perpetuating IgE stimulation results in tissue destruction and irreversible remodeling. A small number of patients with "allergic" symptoms have non-IgE-mediated mast cell degranulation resulting in inflammatory cell infiltration.

TABLE 9-1
CLASSIFICATION OF IMMUNOLOGIC MECHANISMS

Class	Mechanism of Action	Examples
Type I		
Immediate hypersensitivity	IgE-mediated mast cell degranulation	Anaphylaxis
Type II		
Cytotoxic	IgG- or IgM-mediated cytotoxic hypersensitivity	Drug-induced hemolytic anemia
Type III		
Immune complex	IgG or IgM immune-complex deposition with resultant complement-mediated inflammation	Serum sickness; SLE vasculitis
Type IV		
Delayed (cell-mediated) hypersensitivity	T-cells, monocytes, macrophages	Contact dermatitis; PPD skin testing

The worldwide prevalence of atopic disease, specifically asthma, allergic rhinitis, and atopic dermatitis (the *"atopy triad"*), has been increasing over the past 30 years. This phenomenon is exaggerated in developed countries. Factors which influence the risk of developing atopic disease are listed in Table 9-2. Allergic diseases are multifactorial; that is, the interplay of environmental exposures and inherited susceptibility produces signs and symptoms of variable severity within the population. Pediatric patients with one component of the atopy syndrome are three times as likely as their peers to develop a second allergic condition.

TABLE 9-2
FACTORS INFLUENCING THE DEVELOPMENT OF ATOPIC DISEASE

General Risk Factors
A parent with atopic disease (50% of offspring)
Both parents with atopic disease (66% of offspring)
Family history of atopic disease

Allergic Rhinitis
Parent(s) with allergic rhinitis
Family history of allergic rhinitis
Patient history of asthma or eczema
Exposure to house dust mites
Elevated serum IgE levels
Maternal smoking in the first year of life
Mother with asthma

Asthma: Early Wheezing
Maternal smoking (and passive exposure to cigarette smoke)

Asthma: Late-Onset Wheezing
Mother with asthma
Male gender
Elevated serum IgE
Positive allergy skin tests

Asthma: Persistent Wheezing
Patient history of atopic disease
Parental history of atopic disease
Parent(s) with asthma
History of multiple severe episodes of wheezing
History of respiratory syncytial virus necessitating hospitalization
Maternal smoking (and passive exposure to cigarette smoke)

TABLE 9-2
(continued)

Hispanic ethnicity
Male gender
Low birth-weight
Elevated serum IgE
Positive allergy skin tests

Protective Factors
Early day care attendance (all atopic disease)
Early exposure to multiple viral infections (all atopic disease)
Exclusive breastfeeding or use of hypoallergenic formula through age 6 months (delays the onset and decreases the severity of eczema and food allergies during the first 2 years of life)
Delayed introduction of solid foods beyond 4 months of age (impacts eczema risk only)

ALLERGIC RHINITIS

Allergic rhinitis (AR) is the most common chronic disease of childhood, affecting infants, children, and adolescents. AR requires both allergen sensitization and exposure. When the allergen is inhaled, IgE bridging and mast cell degranulation result in an early phase response (within 15 to 30 minutes). The late phase response (LPR) occurs 4 to 8 hours after exposure; infiltration of inflammatory cells leads to tissue damage and the clinical manifestations of AR. Signs, symptoms, and investigative results consistent with AR are listed in Table 9-3 and may be used to differentiate AR from other causes of rhinitis (see Chapter 23). AR may be characterized as intermittent (seasonal) or persistent (perennial) (Table 9-4). Allergic rhinitis in infants is usually perennial in nature; development of seasonal allergies requires repeated exposure and generally does not present prior to age 3 years.

AR is associated with the development of other atopic conditions. Asthma is a frequent comorbid illness, and poor control of AR can exacerbate asthma. Both asthma and AR are exacerbated by respiratory irritants that are not specifically allergens, particularly cigarette smoke.

Management consists of allergen avoidance and pharmacotherapy (Table 9-5). Patients with severe AR unresponsive to the above should be referred to an allergy specialist for possible immunotherapy (discussed later in this chapter). Potential complications of chronic AR are listed in Table 9-6.

TABLE 9-3
ALLERGIC RHINITIS: CLINICAL MANIFESTATIONS AND DIAGNOSIS

Symptoms
Mouth breathing
Snoring
Nasal quality to voice
*Sneezing
*Nasal itching
Sniffing, snorting
Nose blowing
Congestion
Postnasal drainage
Coughing
*Itchy eyes
Watery eyes
Headaches
Fatigue
Disrupted sleep

Signs
Nasal obstruction
*Pale, bluish nasal mucosa
Enlarged, boggy turbinates
Bilateral clear rhinorrhea
Pharyngeal cobblestoning
*Allergic shiners
*Transverse nasal crease due to the "allergic salute"

Diagnostic Studies
Increased eosinophils on nasal smear
*Detection of specific IgE antibodies
*Positive skin prick allergy tests

*specific to AR

ASTHMA

Asthma is a chronic pulmonary condition characterized by variable inflammation of the airways. The inflammation results in bronchial hyperresponsiveness to a variety of "trigger" stimuli, culminating in episodic, reversible airway obstruction. Common precipitants include irritants (cigarette smoke, smog), upper respiratory infections, pet dander, exercise, weather changes, aspirin, and allergen exposure. In fact, almost 90% of children with asthma have demonstrable specific IgE antibodies and/or positive skin prick tests. The extrapyramidal symptoms, consisting of mast cell degranulation, bronchospasm, and airway obstruction, occur within minutes of exposure to the trigger. This "early" bronchospasm either resolves spontaneously or is responsive to β-agonist therapy. The associated release of pro-inflammatory cytokines produces recruitment of neutrophils, lymphocytes, monocytes, and particularly *eosinophils* to the lower airways, leading to a laryngopharyngeal reflux (LPR) (mucous production, delayed bronchospasm) 4 to 8 hours after the initial exposure. This LPR is relatively resistant to β-agonist therapy but can be prevented with systemic glucocorticoid administration. When a sensitized patient develops an exacerbation due to allergen exposure, that patient's disease temporarily

TABLE 9-4
INTERMITTENT VS. PERSISTENT ALLERGIC RHINITIS: MOST LIKELY ALLERGENS

	Strategies to Limit Allergen Exposure
Intermittent	
Pollens	Stay indoors when the pollen count is high
	Keep windows closed and air-conditioning on during pollen seasons
AR due to seasonal allergies occurs cyclically at the same time each year (tree pollen in the spring, grass pollen in the early summer, weed pollen in the late summer). Outdoor molds are present year-round in temperate climates but otherwise disappear with the first frost.	
Persistent	
Dust mites	Seal pillow and mattress in allergen-proof casings
	Use hypoallergenic pillows, sheets, and comforters
	Wash bedding weekly in hot (>130°F) water
	Decrease humidity in the house
Animal dander	Remove the pet from the home
	Less desirable alternative: keep pet out of patient's bedroom
Cockroach allergens	Regular extermination
	Seal cracks and crevices to outside
	Clean up food promptly and store securely
	Fix leaks in faucets or pipes
Indoor molds	Decrease humidity in the home
	Fix leaks in faucets or pipes
	Use HEPA air filters
	Apply bleach solution to obvious areas of mold

TABLE 9-5
MEDICAL MANAGEMENT OF ALLERGIC RHINITIS

Intranasal Steroids

- First-line therapy
- Options include fluticasone, mometasone, budesonide, beclomethasone, triamcinolone, and flunisolide
- Symptom resolution superior to oral antihistamines and leukotriene receptor antagonists
- Can be used in children as young as 2 years of age
- No proven effect on growth
- May be used in conjunction with inhaled steroids for patients with AR and asthma

Second-generation H_1-receptor Antihistamines

- Options include cetirizine (ages 6 months and above), loratadine (ages 2 years and older), and fexofenadine (ages 6 years and older), all oral, and azelastine nasal spray (ages 5 years and above)

Oral Leukotriene Receptor Antagonists

- Montelukast approved for pediatric patients

Decongestants

- Options include oral pseudoephedrine and intranasal ipratropium bromide
- Effective for nasal congestion
- Should be used only intermittently

Intranasal Cromolyn

- Mast cell stabilizer
- Must be dosed every 4 hours
- Delayed onset of action (up to 7 days)

TABLE 9-6
COMPLICATIONS OF CHRONIC ALLERGIC RHINITIS

Physical

Craniofacial abnormalities due to chronic mouth-breathing (palatal arching; elongation of the face; flattening of the midface)

Dental malocclusion due to chronic mouth breathing

Sinusitis due to nasal congestion, increased susceptibility to viral respiratory infections

Otitis media with effusion due to eustachian tube dysfunction, tonsillar/adenoidal hypertrophy

Obstructive sleep apnea due to tonsillar/adenoidal hypertrophy

Social/Academic/Emotional

Impaired **school performance** due to sleep disturbances

Impaired **short term memory** due to sleep disturbances

Frustration over symptoms and appearance

becomes even more reactive to irritant triggers. Chronic airway inflammation leads to tissue remodeling including basement membrane thickening, subepithelial collagen deposition, and smooth muscle and mucous gland hypertrophy and hyperplasia.

The diagnosis of asthma is based on recurrence of symptoms (wheezing, chest tightness, shortness of breath, cough), responsiveness to bronchodilators and/or anti-inflammatory agents, and confirmatory lung function studies (documented reduction in forced expiratory volume in 1 second (FEV_1), with significant improvement follow-ing administration of inhaled β-agonist therapy). Asthma severity is classified according to the frequency and severity of impairment prior to initiation of appropriate therapy. Classification parameters and suggested treatment (based on published National Institutes of Health guidelines) are provided in Table 9-7.

Short-acting inhaled bronchodilators (e.g., albuterol) are added to maintenance therapy during acute exacerbations in all patient groups. Peak effect is reached within 15 minutes and lasts for 4 hours. Side effects include tachycardia, tremor, and nervousness. These are less likely to occur with use of levalbuterol, the active isomer of albuterol. The patient with a moderate-to-severe exacerbation is provided with a 3 to 10 day course of oral steroids (1 to 2 mg/kg/day up to 60 mg of prednisone or methylprednisolone). Doubling the dose of inhaled corticosteroids is a reasonable alternative if symptoms are mild or moderate. A patient with well-controlled asthma who suddenly develops an exacerbation of disease may be exposed to a novel allergen due to a change in location or schedule.

Published management guidelines provided by the National Institutes of Health in 1997 and modified in 2002 include:

- regular monitoring of symptom control and lung function (office visits every 2 weeks until stable, then two to four times a year; annual lung function testing)
- control of factors which contribute to asthma severity (reduced allergen exposure; management of co-morbid conditions, such as AR, sinusitis, and gastroesophageal reflux, which, when active, may contribute to exacerbations)
- appropriate use of medications with emphasis on long-term control and anti-inflammatory pharmacotherapy—Patients may need higher doses of or additional medications to gain control of symptoms initially, with a goal of gradual weaning for optimal control with limited side effects
- patient education regarding daily management and control of acute exacerbations
- referral of all patients with severe asthma, patients with moderate asthma unresponsive to treatment, and patients younger than 3 years of age with moderate-to-severe asthma to a pulmonologist or other asthma specialist

Children who are diagnosed with asthma and their caretakers should be instructed in the correct use of a peak flow meter, with results recorded twice a day initially and at least daily once good control has been achieved. This data allows the physician to provide a written treatment plan for the patient noting recommended medication changes based on readings in the green [peak expiratory flow (PEF) 80% to 100% of personal best], yellow (PEF 50% to 80% of personal best), and red (PEF <50% of personal best) zones of lung function. Families should also be counseled regarding the benefits of limiting allergen exposure.

The patient with an acute exacerbation of his or her underlying pulmonary disease presents with expiratory wheezing, a prolonged expiratory phase, diffuse crackles, rales, rhonchi, nasal flaring, and accessory muscle use. A chest radiograph is generally unnecessary in patients with known asthma unless examination of the chest reveals unequal breath sounds (foreign body, air leak). Hyperinflation, peribronchial thickening, and areas of atelectasis are radiographic findings consistent with obstruction, inflammation, and increased mucous production. Atelectasis associated with an acute asthma exacerbation is due to collapse of airways distal to mucous plugging; it resolves spontaneously and does not require bronchoscopy, antibiotics, or chest physiotherapy.

Severe obstruction is characterized by marked suprasternal and intercostal retractions, the inability to speak more than a few words at a time, cyanosis, quiet breath sounds, and peak expiratory flows <30% predicted. Air leaks (pneumothorax, pneumomediastinum) are more common with this degree of involvement. Severe obstruction is a medical emergency which, if not reversed, may result in hypoxic seizures, respiratory arrest, and death.

Children who present to the emergency department with an acute asthma attack are initially assessed for hypoxemia and degree of airway obstruction. Pulse oximetry measurement is a simple, rapid screen for hypoxemia.

TABLE 9-7
CLASSIFICATION AND MAINTENANCE TREATMENT OF ASTHMA

			Maintenance Medications, Age ≤5 years		Maintenance Medications, Age >5 years	
Severity	**Symptoms**	**Lung Function**	**Preferred**	**Alternative**	**Preferred**	**Alternative**
Mild intermittent	≤2 days/week and/or ≤2 nights /month	PEF or FEV_1≥80% predicted or PEF variability <20%	None	None	None	None
Mild persistent	>2 days/week and/or >2 nights/ month	PEF or FEV_1 ≥80% predicted or PEF variability 20% to 30%	Low-dose inhaled corticosteroid*	Cromolyn or leukotriene receptor antagonist	Low-dose inhaled corticosteroid	Cromolyn, leukotriene receptor antagonist, nedocromil, or sustained-release theophylline
Moderate persistent	Daily and/or >1 night/week	PEF or FEV_1 60% to 80% predicted or PEF variability >30%	Low-to-medium-dose inhaled corticosteroid with or without long-acting β_2-agonist#	Low-to-medium-dose inhaled corticosteroid plus leukotriene receptor antagonist or theophylline	Low-to-medium-dose inhaled corticosteroid with or without long-acting β_2-agonist	High-dose inhaled corticosteroid or low-to-medium-dose inhaled corticosteroid plus leukotriene receptor antagonist or theophylline
Severe persistent	Continual daily and frequent nighttime	PEF or FEV_1 ≤60% predicted or PEF variability >30%	High-dose inhaled corticosteroid plus long-acting β_2-agonist, with systemic corticosteroids	None accepted	High-dose inhaled corticosteroid plus long-acting β_2-agonist, with systemic corticosteroids added if needed	None accepted

PEF, peak expiratory flow; FEV_1, forced expiratory volume in 1 second; PEF, variability comparison of morning PEF level to afternoon or evening PEF level. If the morning level is ≥20% less than the afternoon level, the results are consistent with a diagnosis of asthma.
*Inhaled corticosteroids are recommended as part of maintenance therapy in all patients with persistent asthma. Long-term use of inhaled corticosteroids has been shown to decrease bronchial hyperresponsiveness and inflammation. The most commonly reported side effects are local and include oral candidiasis and hoarseness. Long-term inhaled corticosteroid use has been found to have no significant effect on expected adult height or bone mineral density.
#Long-acting bronchodilators come in inhaled forms (alone or in combination with a corticosteroid) and oral forms. They are dosed twice a day. The side effect profile is similar to that of short-acting bronchodilators.

Arterial blood gas measurements provide information regarding oxygenation, ventilation, and pH in patients with severe distress. Inhaled oxygen therapy is indicated for any patient with arterial hemoglobin saturation <90% to 93%. A rising $PaCO_2$ level signifies impending respiratory failure. A normal $PaCO_2$ in the setting of tachypnea is an equally ominous sign; the $PaCO_2$ should be well below 40 mm Hg when breathing is rapid.

Repetitive nebulized bronchodilators are administered as often as every 15 minutes as needed. Side effects include tachycardia, muscle tremors, and hypokalemia. The addition of inhaled ipratropium bromide, an anticholinergic, may further improve lung function in some patients. Subcutaneous epinephrine or terbutaline rapidly decreases airway reactivity but is reserved for severe obstruction. Oral or intravenous steroids (as previously noted) have a 4 to 6 hour onset of action and are indicated for treatment of inflammation and prevention of the LPR, which is poorly responsive to inhaled bronchodilators. Systemic steroid administration is reserved for hospitalized patients with severe disease (1 mg/kg every 6 hours for 48 hours, followed by a taper). Admission to the hospital is necessary in patients:

- who do not respond with resolution of symptoms following several hours of maximal bronchodilator therapy (*status asthmaticus*)
- who require ongoing oxygen therapy

TABLE 9-8
ASTHMA MORTALITY RISK FACTORS

History of intubation and mechanical ventilation for asthma
History of admission to an intensive care unit for asthma
≥2 hospitalizations or ≥3 emergency room visits for asthma within the past year
Overuse of short-acting bronchodilators (>2 metered dose inhalers per month)
Severe disease requiring chronic systemic steroid use
Poor perception of symptom severity
Non-compliance
Family dysfunction or other significant psychosocial problems
Depression or other psychiatric disease
Atopy

- who cannot tolerate oral medications
- who have an air leak

About 60% of children with asthma will experience resolution by adulthood. Patients with severe asthma and those with atopy are more likely to suffer from persistent disease. The mortality rate of asthma continues to increase in both developing and industrialized areas despite significant advances in management. Table 9-8 lists factors associated with an increased risk of death due to asthma.

Exercise-Induced Asthma

Exercise-induced asthma (EIA) is generally a clinical diagnosis. Characteristics of exercise-induced asthma include the onset of coughing, shortness of breath, and wheezing 5 to 6 minutes after beginning exercise, with gradual improvement over 20 to 30 minutes of rest. Symptoms are not present at other times. EIA may be mistaken for mild persistent asthma if the patient only has symptoms during activity. Symptoms related solely to EIA are responsive to β-agonist therapy. Smog increases the severity of EIA. Prophylactic therapy consists of an inhaled short-acting β_2-agonist 15 to 30 minutes prior to physical activity (second-line therapy: inhaled cromolyn). EIA may be a sign of poorly controlled asthma.

ATOPIC DERMATITIS

Atopic dermatitis (AD, or eczema), the third component of the "atopic triad," is a chronic, relapsing dermatitis that typically begins in infancy or early childhood. The majority of children with AD have elevated serum IgE levels, and 80% go on to develop allergic rhinitis and/or asthma. The strongest risk factor for the development of AD is family history of atopy.

AD is intensely pruritic, leading to frequent scratching with excoriations. Patches of involved skin are erythemic, with scaling and multiple small papular lesions (Fig. 9-1). Infants have primarily scalp, facial, and extensor lesions; in children and adolescents, flexural surfaces are predominately involved. AD is exacerbated when the skin is dry or exposed to temperature extremes (particularly heat), physical trauma (scratching, abrasive or wool clothing), and chemical irritants (strong soaps, detergents). Ingestion of certain foods and exposure to airborne allergens can precipitate or worsen disease in sensitized individuals. Patients with chronic, poorly-controlled eczema develop irreversible lichenification and scarring.

The four elements of AD management consist of:

- skin hydration and lubrication (frequent application of hydrophilic emollients, particularly following bathing)
- elimination or modulation of triggers noted above (wearing loose-fitting cotton garments; limiting exposure to harsh chemicals and perfumes; using only "non-detergent" soaps; skin prick and/or food allergy testing to determine sensitivities)
- topical therapy (glucocorticoid creams and ointments; topical immunomodulators such as tacrolimus and pimecrolimus; tar preparations)
- systemic therapy if necessary for severe or unresponsive disease (antihistamines for itching; systemic glucocorticoids to control inflammation; cyclosporine, interferons in select cases)

Recurrent skin infections are the most frequent complication of AD. Colonization with *Staphylococcus aureus* may progress to frank infection characterized by weeping, honey-crusted lesions and impetigo; local or systemic antistaphylococcal antibiotics are indicated in these cases. Superinfection with herpes simplex virus presents with vesicular and/or crusted erosive lesions, which are Tzanck-stain positive and refractory to antibiotic therapy. The infection may disseminate, resulting in widespread lesions

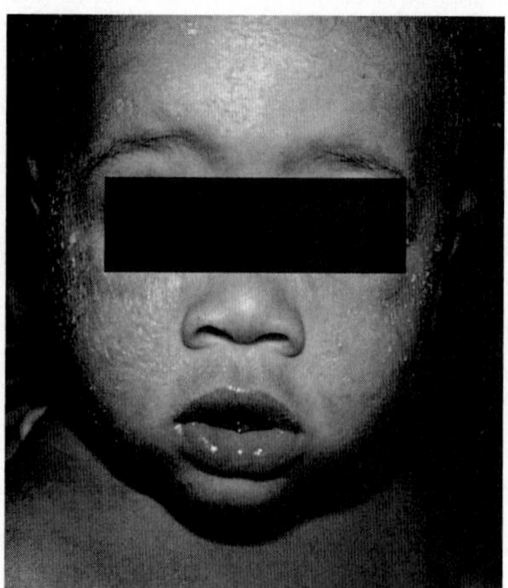

Figure 9.1 Atopic dermatitis in an infant. (From Goodheart HP. *Goodheart's Photoguide of Common Skin Disorders: Diagnosis and Management.* 2nd ed. Philadelphia: Lippincott Williams & Wilkins; 2003 with permission.) *(See Color Insert.)*

(*eczema herpeticum*) and signs of systemic disease. Patients with suspected eczema herpeticum should temporarily stop all immunosuppressive therapy and begin oral antiviral medication. AD also increases susceptibility to other cutaneous viral disease including molluscum contagiosum and warts.

URTICARIA AND ANGIOEDEMA

Urticaria (hives) and angioedema (discreet areas of subcutaneous swelling) may be acute or chronic. Acute forms often result from IgE-mediated responses to allergen (food, drugs), cold, or physical pressure; viral and recent streptococcal infections may also cause urticaria. Hives and/or angioedema that occur only around the inoculation site are localized; those which are widely distributed, occurring in multiple areas distal to the exposure, are systemic.

Cutaneous disease that persists beyond 6 weeks is classified as chronic. Chronic urticaria is often associated with abnormal thyroid function, particularly Hashimoto thyroiditis. Autoimmune disorders, some forms of liver disease, and stress have also been identified as potential causes. Chronic urticaria is not an allergic response, does not involve mast cell degranulation, and does not warrant skin prick allergy testing. Management of chronic urticaria proceeds in a stepwise fashion as outlined in Table 9-9.

Chronic, recurrent angioedema is hereditary in some cases. These patients cannot make a normal inhibitor for complement factor 1. Once C1 is activated (for unknown reasons), the area swells; however, there is no associated pruritis, flushing, or urticaria.

ANAPHYLAXIS

Anaphylaxis is a serious, systemic hypersensitivity reaction precipitated by the sudden release of mast cell mediators following exposure to an allergen. The most common cause of pediatric anaphylaxis in the developed world is food hypersensitivity (see below). Anaphylaxis in hospitalized patients is more often due to drug and latex allergies.

Classic signs and symptoms include any combination of the following:

- Cutaneous—generalized flushing, urticaria, and angioedema
- Respiratory—wheezing, respiratory distress, bronchospasm, laryngeal edema
- Cardiovascular—hypotension, poor perfusion, dizziness
- Gastrointestinal—nausea, vomiting, abdominal pain, diarrhea
- A sense of impending doom

At least 10% of children do not manifest cutaneous signs during anaphylaxis; these patients are at an increased risk of death. Occasionally, this subset of patients will present with a single, nonspecific complaint, such as abdominal pain, which further delays the diagnosis and leads to a poorer outcome.

Emergency therapy consists of administration of epinephrine (intramuscular or intravenous), antihistamines, and corticosteroids. Supplemental oxygen, nebulized albuterol, and airway management are employed as needed. Hypotension is treated with volume expanders and should also respond to epinephrine. Following resolution of the allergic event, the patient and the family are taught to carry and use injectable epinephrine and encouraged to acquire a medical alert bracelet. Allergy testing is indicated if the inciting allergen is not clear from the history. Immunotherapy should be considered if available.

TABLE 9-9
MANAGEMENT OF CHRONIC URTICARIA/ANGIOEDEMA

H_1-receptor antihistamines are the first line of therapy. If the response is sub-optimal, the following agents are added, generally in the order listed:

- Consider the addition of H_2-receptor antihistamines.
- Addition of alternate-day systemic steroids, with a goal of weaning as soon as symptoms are under control
- Addition of leukotriene-receptor antagonists
- In severe refractory cases, intravenous immunoglobulin or plasmapheresis should be considered.

ALLERGIC REACTIONS TO SPECIFIC SUBSTANCES

Food

Food allergy results from sensitization to a specific food protein leading to a hypersensitivity reaction with subsequent exposure. The IgE-mediated (Type I) allergic response produces symptoms within minutes of ingestion and may take the form of urticaria, angioedema, wheezing, shortness of breath, rhinitis, nausea, vomiting, abdominal pain, diarrhea, and/or anaphylaxis (as noted previously). Foods commonly implicated in allergic reactions include milk, soy, eggs, peanuts, seafood, milk, and tree nuts (almonds, cashews, pecans, walnuts). At least 90% of patients with food allergies are allergic to only one or two foods. The vast majority of children with allergies to milk, eggs, soy, and wheat lose sensitivity to the antigen by the age of 5 years. Allergies to peanuts, tree nuts, fish, and shellfish typically persist throughout life. Food allergies can be detected in about 40% of children with AD and about 10% of children with asthma.

Both skin prick and specific IgE antibody testing, together with a positive history, are useful for determining sensitization. Negative tests are conclusive; however patients with positive results may or may not develop clinical symptoms when the food is ingested. Therefore, food elimination and subsequent re-challenge is required to demonstrate that the particular food does indeed result in a systemic allergic or anaphylactic reaction. Obviously, patients with a history of a life-threatening reaction should either be challenged in a hospital setting or diagnosed based on history and skin or blood testing.

Not all food allergies are mediated by IgE. Patients with AD may experience exacerbation of their eczema following ingestion of certain foods. This delayed reaction is thought to be a cell-mediated, Type IV response. Urticaria and wheezing are not present. The most efficacious way to determine if food sensitization is contributing to AD is to institute a restrictive diet that eliminates all foods commonly know to provoke allergic reactions. If the eczema improves within 2 weeks, food allergy is a likely culprit. One food at a time is added back into the diet until the source of the allergy is determined.

Patients who are diagnosed with a food allergy should be educated in how to most effectively avoid the offending protein. If the allergic reaction is IgE-mediated, the patient and family must carry a form of self-injectable epinephrine at all times and be proficient in its administration. Ongoing studies into methods of preventing food allergies in children from atopic families by delaying introduction of specific foods or restricting the maternal diet in cases of breastfeeding may yield additional helpful information.

Food intolerance (e.g., lactase deficiency, irritable bowel syndrome) and food poisoning due to ingestion of organisms or their toxins may be difficult to distinguish from food allergy. Generally, reactions that are accompanied by respiratory symptoms, hives, or other manifestations of atopy are more likely to be due to true food allergies.

Drugs

Adverse reactions to drugs may be allergic or non-allergic. While all four types of immunologic mechanisms are known to occur with use of medication, the immediate (Type 1) hypersensitivity reaction is most closely tied to the term "drug allergy." IgE-mediated drug allergy should be suspected in cases in which:

- the patient has been given the drug before (i.e., has had an opportunity to become *sensitized*)
- the patient develops signs and symptoms within minutes of administration of the drug
- clinical manifestations are consistent with atopic disease (urticaria, wheezing, bronchospasm, laryngospasm, hypotension, anaphylaxis)

Allergy testing is currently available for penicillin; other drug antigens (cephalosporins) are available but not yet clinically useful. A patient who is truly allergic to penicillin has about a 4% to 10% chance of being allergic to cephalosporins as well.

Contrast Media

The risk of anaphylaxis following administration of contrast media is very low. The reaction is not thought to be strictly allergic in nature. Rather, mast cell degranulation appears to result from the hypertonicity of the radiocontrast material. In the patient with a known history of anaphylaxis due to contrast media, this reaction can be prevented in subsequent studies by pretreatment with corticosteroids and antihistamines and use of low-osmolar, nonionic radiocontrast solution.

Hymenoptera

Primary care of Hymenoptera stings is discussed in Chapter 3. Individual reactions are categorized as:

- local—swelling, erythema, itching, and pain limited to the area of the sting; signs and symptoms begin within minutes of being stung and resolve within several hours
- large local—similar signs and symptoms which involve a larger area contiguous to the sting site. The swelling increases over 1 to 2 days and resolves over the next several days
- generalized systemic reactions limited to the skin—involves widespread flushing, urticaria, angioedema, and/or itching which occurs at sites unrelated to the sting
- anaphylaxis—as noted above, presents with wheezing, difficulty breathing due to laryngeal spasm, and hypotension

Diagnosis involves a positive history and demonstration of venom-specific IgE antibodies through skin prick or specific IgE antibody testing. Such studies are only indicated for individuals who have experienced generalized cutaneous or anaphylactic reactions following a sting. Allergic patients should be provided with and instructed in the correct use of self-injectable epinephrine, along with their families, and those with a history of anaphylaxis should wear medical alert bracelets. Hymenoptera insects are attracted to strong perfumes and bright-colored clothing; avoidance of these may decrease the risk of being stung.

True anaphylaxis secondary to Hymenoptera stings is uncommon. Less than 5% of children with a history of non-life-threatening reactions will develop anaphylaxis after subsequent stings. Hymenoptera venom immunotherapy is 98% effective in preventing generalized and anaphylactic reactions in patients who are diagnosed with a venom allergy. Venom immunotherapy is indicated for:

- all patients with histories of anaphylaxis *and* positive skin prick or specific IgE antibody tests
- any patient 17 years of age or older with a history of a systemic cutaneous reaction to a sting *and* a positive skin prick or specific IgE antibody test

Venom immunotherapy is not indicated for patients with negative skin prick or specific IgE antibody tests. In addition, patients ages 16 years and younger with histories of systemic cutaneous reactions, even if positive for venom-specific IgE antibodies, are not appropriate candidates for venom immunotherapy, because studies have demonstrated no increased risk for anaphylaxis in this population.

ALLERGY TESTING

Patients who have symptoms consistent with atopic disease will benefit from specific IgE antibody testing. Allergy testing is not indicated for children who have symptoms or known disorders which are not allergic in origin, such as lactose intolerance or celiac disease. Widespread testing in the absence of atopic symptoms will identify many individuals with antigen-specific IgE, but most will not develop clinical symptoms when exposed to the allergen. Targeted testing is cost-effective; inappropriate testing may provoke needless anxiety if heretofore unknown "allergies" are discovered.

Skin testing is preferable to in vitro testing in most cases. In experienced hands, skin testing is more sensitive than specific IgE antibody immunoassays; in addition, it provides immediate results ("wheal and flare" at the site if positive) and is less costly. False negatives do occur (Table 9-10). Skin testing can be performed in infants but is less sensitive than in older patients. In vitro testing is preferred in patients who cannot discontinue antihistamines, patients with widespread atopic dermatitis, patients with dermographism, and patients with a history of severe, life-threatening anaphylaxis to the allergens being tested. Some allergens, such as latex, are not available for skin prick testing.

IMMUNOTHERAPY

Allergen immunotherapy requires a high degree of patient commitment, because the shots are painful and the duration of treatment can be as long as 5 years. However, immunotherapy is curative in many cases. Possible side effects include pain and swelling at the administration site; adding saline or changing the concentration of the allergen should prevent this. There is also a small but measurable risk of anaphylaxis leading to death, which can be avoided by observing the patient for at least 30 minutes following the injections. If anaphylaxis does occur, distribution of the antigen can be limited by placing a tourniquet proximal to the injection site. Full-dose subcutaneous epinephrine is then administered at both the injection site and in the opposite arm for systemic absorption.

No alternative treatments have been proven to cure allergies, despite claims to the contrary. The use of "fad" therapies (*Candida* immunotherapy, homeopathic desensitization, vitamin replacement) should be discouraged, especially if they cause harm or delay appropriate care.

TABLE 9-10
CAUSES OF FALSE-POSITIVE AND FALSE-NEGATIVE SKIN TEST RESULTS

False Positive
Patient with dermographism

False Negative
Failure to introduce sufficient amount of allergen into the site
Patient use of H_1-receptor antihistamine within a week of testing
Patient use of tricyclic antidepressants, serotonin reuptake inhibitors
Long-term oral or topical steroid use (inhaled steroids do not affect results)

PRIMARY IMMUNE DEFICIENCY DISORDERS

Primary immunodeficiencies are genetic defects which result in abnormalities in the number or function of immune cells or their products. These disorders are typically classified according to which arm of the immune system is predominantly involved (*innate* vs. *adaptive*) and which cells or cellular products are primarily affected. Table 9-11 provides a brief review of some of the more important primary immune deficiency disorders. Secondary immunodeficiencies due to chronic disease, infections, and medications are discussed in respective chapters.

Infections are common in early childhood; immunodeficiency testing is not indicated for most children with recurrent infections. Screening is recommended under the following circumstances:

- Two or more serious bacterial infections including sepsis, meningitis, and osteomyelitis
- Two or more episodes of pneumonia or serious sinus infection within 1 year
- Two or more episodes of cellulitis, lymphadenitis, or draining otitis media
- Any infection with an unusual pathogen or occurring at an unusual site
- Infection with a typical childhood pathogen which results in disease of unusual severity
- Chronic gingivitis or recurrent aphthous ulcers
- Persistence of or appearance of thrush after the ages of 6 to 12 months

Initial screening tests should include a complete blood count with manual differential, erythrocyte sedimentation rate, and more specific screening tests detailed in Table 9-11.

Severe combined immunodeficiency (SCID) is an inherited disorder that affects the functioning of both the adaptive (natural killer) and innate (B and T cells) components of the immune system. There are several genetic variations of the disease, with the common denominator being the absence of functioning T cells. SCID patients present in the first year of life with chronic diarrhea, otitis media, pneumonia, failure to thrive, and recurrent, often severe opportunistic infections. Most patients have low absolute

TABLE 9-11
REVIEW OF PRIMARY IMMUNODEFICIENCIES

Immunodeficiency	Characterization	Typical Presentation	Diagnostic Evaluation	Therapy
Innate immunodeficiencies	**Specific to the disorder**	**Specific to the disorder**	**Specific to the disorder**	**Specific to the disorder**
Chronic granulomatous disease (X-linked or autosomal recessive)	Defect in NAPDH oxidase; inability to produce superoxide anions and destroy catalase-positive organisms	Recurrent bacterial (*Staphylococcus aureus, Burkholderia cepacia, Serratia marscescens, Nocarida* species) and fungal infections (*Candida, Aspergillus* species) involving the skin, lungs, gastrointestinal tract (*Salmonella* species), and lymph nodes; abscess formation	*Screening tests*: complete blood count with manual differential, absolute neutrophil count *Specific confirmatory test*: nitroblue tetrazolium or dihydrorhodamine 123 fluorescence test	Prophylactic therapy: trimethoprim-sulfamethoxazole, itraconazole; subcutaneous interferon-gamma therapy
Complement deficiencies (terminal components)	Recurrent *Neisseria, Gonorrhoeae* infections; increased risk of meningitis	Same	Total hemolytic complement assay (CH_{50})	No specific therapy; aggressive antibiotic therapy for infections
B cell immunodeficiencies	**Recurrent and/or severe infection with encapsulated, extracellular pyogenic organisms**	**Sepsis, pneumonia, sinusitis, meningitis with bacteria such as *Streptococcus pneumoniae, Haemophilus influenzae***	**Screening tests: quantitative immunoglobulins (B cell and subclass numbers); isohemagglutinins (antibody presence and function); antibody titers to tetanus, diphtheria, *Haemophilus influenzae*, and *Streptococcus pneumoniae* vaccination (specific antibody response)**	**Prophylactic therapy: antibody replacement (IVIG therapy)**
X-linked (Bruton) agammaglobulinemia	Above, plus an increased risk of enteroviral meningoencephalitis; lymphoid hypoplasia (small or nonexistent tonsils, lymph nodes) on exam	Typically presents with recurrent infections beginning at 6 to 9 mo of age, when maternal IgG declines	Above; serum immuno-globulin levels of all subclasses are extremely low; absence of circulating B cells on flow cytometry	IVIG therapy
Common variable immunodeficiency	Hypogammaglob-ulinemia with normal levels of circulating B cells; normal or enlarged lymphoid tissue on exam	Typically presents with milder infections involving the above organisms in late childhood or adulthood	Above; serum immunoglobulin levels of all subclasses are low; B cells present on flow cytometry	IVIG or subcutaneous immunoglobulin
Selective IgA deficiency	Near-absent levels of serum IgA	Recurrent bacterial infections of the respiratory, gastrointestinal, and urinary tracts; generally only moderate in severity and responsive to antibiotic therapy	Quantitative serum immunoglobulin levels	Generally none unless other immunoglobulin subclasses are affected as well; **IVIG contraindicated** due to risk of anaphylaxis
T cell immunodeficiencies	**Increased susceptibility to opportunistic infections**	**Severe cytomegalovirus, herpesvirus infections; recurrent infection with *Pneumocystis jiroveci, Candida* species; failure to thrive**	**Screening tests: absolute lymphocyte count (T cell number); *Candida albicans* (or tetanus toxoid, mumps, *Tricophyton*) delayed-type intradermal skin test (T cell function; induration ≥10mm at 48 hours excludes T cell defect)**	**Prophylactic therapy: trimethoprim-sulfamethoxazole**

(continued)

TABLE 9-11 (continued)

Immunodeficiency	Characterization	Typical Presentation	Diagnostic Evaluation	Therapy
DiGeorge syndrome (chromosomal deletion)	Variable degrees of thymic dysplasia; may also include hypocalcemia (absence of parathyroid glands), congenital conotruncal heart and great vessel defects, characteristic facial features (hypertelorism, short philtrum, low-set ears, cleft palate)	Hypocalcemia, congenital heart defects; usually presents in the neonatal period	Absent thymic shadow; abnormal T cell proliferative response to mitogens; possibly low levels of circulating T cells; chromosomal analysis for 22q11.2 microdeletion	Thymic or bone marrow transplantation

neutrophil counts from birth; specialized molecular testing is available for all known variants. Treatment consists of immunologic reconstitution through early bone marrow or stem cell transplantation. All blood products must be negative for cytomegalovirus and irradiated to prevent graft vs. host disease.

Two additional multisystem disorders, Wiskott-Aldrich syndrome (WAS) and ataxia-telangiectasia (AT), involve characteristic immunodeficiencies. WAS consists of eczema, thrombocytopenia, and altered IgM and cellular responses. Patients typically present with prolonged bleeding, petechiae, or excessive bruising in the newborn period. Affected children have an increased susceptibility to infection with encapsulated organisms (e.g., *Streptococcus pneumoniae*) early in life; recurrent opportunistic infections develop later, and most patients do not live to reach adulthood. Reduced IgM levels and impaired T cell mitogenic proliferation are consistent with WAS.

AT, an autosomal recessive disorder, presents in the second year of life with regression of motor milestones and ataxia. Characteristic skin lesions (telangiectasias) develop in early childhood. The clinical picture of immunodeficiency is similar to that of selective IgA deficiency, with recurrent sinopulmonary infections involving encapsulated organisms. Cellular immune deficiencies occur but are less common. Patients are wheelchair-bound by adolescence, with death in early adulthood.

SOURCES

Braganza SF, Ozuah PH. Fad therapies. *Pediatr Rev.* 2005;26:365–370.

Buckley RH. Evaluation of the immune system. In: Behrman RE, Kliegman RM, Jenson HB, eds. *Nelson Textbook of Pediatrics.* 17th ed. Philadelphia: Saunders; 2004:681–683.

El-Gamal YM, Hossny EM. Respiratory food allergy. *Pediatr Ann.* 2006; 35:733–740.

Expert Panel Report 2: Guidelines for the Diagnosis and Management of Asthma. NIH Publication 97-4051. Bethesda, MD; April 1997.

Fasano MB. Dermatologic food allergy. *Pediatr Ann.* 2006;35:727–732.

Fleisher TA. Primary immune deficiencies: Windows into the immune system. *Pediatr Rev.* 2006;27:363–372.

Guill MF. Asthma update: Clinical aspects and management. *Pediatr Rev.* 2004;25:335–344.

Guill MF. Asthma update: Epidemiology and pathophysiology. *Pediatr Rev.* 2004;25:299–305.

Knight AK, Bahna SL. Diagnosis of food allergy. *Pediatr Ann.* 2006;35:709–717.

Kumar S, Mahalingam R. Anaphylactoid reactions to radiocontrast agents. *Pediatr Rev.* 2001;22:356.

Lasley MV. New treatments for asthma. *Pediatr Rev.* 2003;24:222–232.

Mahr TA, Sheth K. Update of allergic rhinitis. *Pediatr Rev.* 2005; 26:278–283.

Phipatanakul W. Environmental factors and childhood asthma. *Pediatr Ann.* 2006;35:646–656.

Wright AL, Holberg CJ, Martinez FD, et al. Epidemiology of physician-diagnosed allergic rhinitis in childhood. *Pediatrics.* 1994;94:895–901.

QUESTIONS

1. You are discussing the epidemiology of asthma with medical students. All of the following statements are correct EXCEPT:

A) The prevalence of asthma is decreasing in developed countries.

B) The prevalence of asthma is increasing in Third World countries.

C) The mortality of asthma is increasing in developed countries.

D) The mortality of asthma is increasing in Third World countries.

E) Children with atopic dermatitis and/or allergic rhinitis are more likely than their unaffected peers to develop asthma.

2. The mother of a newborn asks you if there is anything that she can do to lower the child's risk of developing eczema and food allergies. She reminds you that her other two children had severe eczema as infants and toddlers but responded to limitation of their diet. Which of the following is the most appropriate response to this mother?

A) Excluding milk from the maternal diet will delay the onset of eczema in breastfed infants.

B) Exclusive breastfeeding or hypoallergenic formula feeding in the first 6 months of life has been shown to delay the onset and severity of eczema.

C) Excluding peanuts from the maternal diet during pregnancy and breastfeeding will prevent peanut allergy in the child.

D) Milk allergy generally persists throughout life.

E) Peanut allergy generally persists throughout life.

3. Which of the following is not considered a common environmental allergen?

A) Pet dander

B) Dust mite

C) Tobacco smoke

D) Seasonal pollination

E) Cockroach

4. A mother brings her 13-month-old son to you because "his nose runs a lot of the time," which periodically keeps him out of day care. She wants you to refer him for allergy testing. Which of the following statements concerning this patient's rhinorrhea is TRUE?

A) Her son's rhinorrhea is probably not due to allergies because it is not seasonal.

B) Her son's rhinorrhea cannot be due to allergies because he is too young.

C) The rhinorrhea that she is describing cannot be due to allergies because it is intermittent.

D) The intermittent rhinorrhea that she is describing is more likely to be due to recurrent viral infections associated with day care attendance.

E) Her son is too young to be tested for allergies.

5. A 16-year-old male comes to your office in April complaining of sneezing, nasal pruritis, watery congestion, and itchy eyes. His symptoms started 3 weeks ago. He says he always seems to "get a cold like this in the spring when the weather changes." He has had no fever, cough, or difficulty breathing. On physical examination, you note bilateral clear rhinorrhea and enlarged, boggy turbinates with pale nasal mucosa. This patient's clinical picture is most consistent with which of the following?

A) Viral upper respiratory infection

B) Allergic rhinitis due to food allergies

C) Allergic rhinitis due to grass pollen

D) Allergic rhinitis due to weed pollen

E) Allergic rhinitis due to tree pollen

6. A 5-year-old patient with persistent allergic rhinitis and nasal eosinophilia has a positive skin prick test for cat animal dander. The parent refuses to remove the child's pet cat from the home. In addition to counselling the parent about the natural course of the disease (tissue remodeling) and the importance of allergen avoidance, appropriate management of this patient includes all of the following EXCEPT:

A) Counseling the parent to lower the humidity in the child's room

B) Counseling the parent to keep the child's bedroom door closed so that the cat is excluded from the room

C) Counseling the parent regarding possible complications of chronic allergic rhinitis

D) Counseling the parent regarding the impact of active allergic rhinitis on school performance

E) Counseling the parent regarding the impact of active allergic rhinitis on quality of sleep

7. A 6-year-old female patient with mild persistent asthma is diagnosed with seasonal allergic rhinitis. Her asthma medications include daily-inhaled budesonide and short-acting albuterol for breakthrough symptoms. You counsel the parent regarding allergen avoidance. The most appropriate next step in the management of this patient is the addition of which of the following medications?

A) Oral cetirizine

B) Intranasal fluticasone

C) Oral loratadine

D) Intranasal cromolyn

E) Intranasal azelastine

8. Which of the following patients is least likely to outgrow his asthma?

A) A 3-year-old African-American male whose mother smokes in the home

B) A 3-year-old Hispanic male hospitalized for 2 days as an infant with respiratory syncytial virus

C) A 3-year-old African-American male with atopic dermatitis

D) A 3-year-old Caucasian male born at 32 weeks of gestation

E) A 3-year-old Asian male who lives with his parents and three cats

9. Which of the following statements regarding bronchial hyperresponsiveness in asthma is FALSE?

A) Asthmatic patients have an exaggerated bronchial response to environmental stimuli such as respiratory irritants, changes in weather, and allergens.

B) Asthmatic patients have an exaggerated bronchial response to environmental stimuli which results in obstruction.

C) The early phase bronchial response to environmental stimuli responds to inhaled β-agonist therapy.

D) The late phase bronchial response to environmental stimuli responds to inhaled β-agonist therapy.

E) The late phase bronchial response to environmental stimuli can be prevented by early systemic corticosteroid administration.

10. A 9-year-old female patient with asthma ran out of medication 2 months ago. Her symptoms wake her from sleep about once a week. She wants to try "natural" therapy for her breathing difficulties rather than standard medications. This patient's disease should be classified as which of the following?
A) Nocturnal asthma
B) Severe persistent asthma
C) Moderate persistent asthma
D) Mild intermittent asthma
E) Mild persistent asthma

11. A 4-year-old male is diagnosed with asthma based on history, physical examination, and lung function studies (FEV_1 70% predicted). He has symptoms at least once daily and about 2 nights a month. This patient's clinical severity is most consistent with which of the following?
A) Moderate persistent asthma
B) Severe persistent asthma
C) Mild persistent asthma
D) Mild intermittent asthma
E) Exercise-induced asthma

12. A 6-year-old female with allergic rhinitis is diagnosed with asthma based on history, physical examination, and lung function studies (peak expiratory flow volume variability 40%). She wakes every night with difficulty breathing and has symptoms several times a day. This patient's clinical severity is most consistent with which of the following?
A) Moderate persistent asthma
B) Severe persistent asthma
C) Mild persistent asthma
D) Mild intermittent asthma
E) Exercise-induced asthma

13. A 3-year-old male is diagnosed with asthma based on history and physical examination. His caretaker reports that he has symptoms about 3 days a week and wakes up with nighttime symptoms about twice a month. This child's clinical severity is most consistent with which of the following?
A) Nocturnal asthma
B) Mild intermittent asthma
C) Mild persistent asthma
D) Moderate persistent asthma
E) Severe persistent asthma

14. Which of the following treatments is a reasonable alternative for a 9-year-old patient with mild persistent asthma whose parents are resistant to steroid use?
A) Symptomatic treatment with inhaled β-agonist by metered dose inhaler and spacer
B) Twice daily long-acting β-agonist therapy
C) Symptomatic treatment with inhaled ipratropium bromide
D) Leukotriene-receptor antagonist maintenance therapy
E) Oral theophylline

15. Which of the following is the most appropriate initial medication regimen for a 3-year-old patient with asthma who has symptoms limited to 2 days a week?
A) Symptomatic treatment with inhaled β-agonist by metered dose inhaler and spacer
B) Daily maintenance low-dose inhaled corticosteroid in addition to (A) above
C) Daily maintenance low-dose inhaled corticosteroid plus a long-acting β-agonist in addition to (A) above
D) Daily maintenance medium-dose inhaled corticosteroid plus a long-acting β-agonist in addition to (A) above
E) None of the above

16. Which of the following is the most appropriate initial medication regimen for a 7-year-old patient with asthma who has symptoms 3 days a week and 2 nights a month?
A) Symptomatic treatment with inhaled β-agonist by metered dose inhaler and spacer
B) Daily maintenance low-dose inhaled corticosteroid in addition to (A) above
C) Daily maintenance low-dose inhaled corticosteroid plus a long-acting β-agonist in addition to (A) above
D) Daily maintenance medium-dose inhaled corticosteroid plus a long-acting β-agonist in addition to (A) above
E) None of the above

17. Which of the following is the most appropriate initial medication regimen for a 6-year-old female patient with asthma who has symptoms once or twice a day?
A) Symptomatic treatment with inhaled β-agonist by metered dose inhaler and spacer
B) Daily maintenance low-dose inhaled corticosteroid in addition to (A) above
C) Daily maintenance low-dose inhaled corticosteroid plus oral theophylline in addition to (A) above
D) Daily maintenance medium-dose inhaled corticosteroid plus a long-acting β-agonist in addition to (A) above
E) None of the above

18. A 12-year-old patient with mild persistent asthma comes to your office for her quarterly visit complaining of "symptoms after walking up stairs." At her last visit, her symptoms were reportedly well-controlled on maintenance medications. Her new symptoms started with school this year. She has to walk up two flights of stairs to attend biology class, and her symptoms start within a few minutes of entering the classroom. This patient's

additional symptoms are most likely due to which of the following?
A) Noncompliance with her maintenance medications
B) Exercise-induced asthma
C) Exposure to a new allergen or irritant in biology class
D) Intermittent viral upper respiratory infections
E) Increasing severity of her underlying disease

19. A medical student asks you about the relationship between asthma and "allergies." You are correct in telling her all of the following EXCEPT:
A) Children with a history of atopic disease are more likely than their peers to develop asthma.
B) Children with asthma and a history of at least one additional atopic disease are more likely to see their asthma persist into adulthood than patients who do not have any other atopic condition.
C) Asthma patients with a history of an additional atopic disease are more likely than other asthmatic patients to die from their disease.
D) Early day care attendance and recurrent viral infections are associated with an increased risk for the development of atopic diseases, including asthma.
E) Positive skin prick allergy tests can be found in over half of school-age children with asthma.

20. You are reviewing peak flow meter testing with a nurse practitioner who will be providing ongoing asthma education for your practice. Important teaching points that should be including in presentations to newly-diagnosed asthma patients include each of the following EXCEPT:
A) Peak flow testing should be performed at least twice a day in newly diagnosed patients.
B) Peak flow testing should be performed at least daily in asthma patients who are on established maintenance therapy with good control of their symptoms.
C) Peak flow testing results that are within 80% to 90% of peak values should not provoke any change in maintenance medications.
D) Once good symptom control has been achieved, medication may be weaned under the supervision of a medical professional.
E) Peak flow meter measurements are not reliable in the setting of an acute exacerbation.

21. A 15-year-old patient with asthma arrives at the emergency department in severe respiratory distress. Vitals include a temperature of 37.2°C, respiratory rate of 42 breaths per minute, and heart rate of 160 beats per minute. He has intercostal and suprasternal retractions and can barely speak. His chest examination is significant for full inspiratory and expiratory wheezes, quiet breath sounds over the right anterior chest, and a PMI shifted to the left. Chest radiographs in this patient will most likely reveal which of the following?
A) A right-sided pneumothorax
B) A right-sided foreign body
C) A right-sided pneumonia
D) Right-sided lobar atelectasis
E) Left-sided collapsed lung

22. An 18-month-old male with known asthma arrives at the emergency department in respiratory distress. He has full expiratory wheezing, with a respiratory rate of 60 breaths per minute. The arterial hemoglobin saturation is 87% on pulse oximetry. $PaCO_2$ is 39 mm Hg. Which of the following statements regarding $PaCO_2$ measurement is TRUE?
A) This patient is not significantly distressed because his $PaCO_2$ is in the normal range.
B) A rising $PaCO_2$ level is indicative of impending respiratory failure.
C) A rising $PaCO_2$ can be normalized in the acute setting by metabolic compensatory processes.
D) The $PaCO_2$ measurement is normally elevated in the setting of tachypnea.
E) The $PaCO_2$ measurement is an adequate measure of patient oxygenation status.

23. Which of the following electrolyte abnormalities is most closely associated with repetitive nebulized bronchodilator administration?
A) Hyperkalemia
B) Hypercalcemia
C) Hypokalemia
D) Hypocalcemia
E) Hyponatremia

24. Hospitalization is indicated for which of the following patients in the emergency department with acute exacerbation of asthma?
A) A 12-month-old with his third episode of wheezing who has partial symptom resolution following six hours of intermittent bronchodilator therapy and systemic steroid administration
B) A 15-year-old known asthmatic with a history of intubation and oxygenation of 91% on arterial pulse oximetry
C) A 6-month-old with no prior history of wheezing who continues to vomit his oral steroids
D) A and B above
E) A, B, and C above

25. A 13-year-old male with no history of asthma develops shortness of breath most days during football practice. This is his first foray into organized sports participation. His symptoms of air hunger and coughing begin within 5 to 6 minutes of starting sprints and gradually improve after 20 to 30 minutes of rest. His symptoms are more pronounced when ozone levels are high. The rest of the history and physical examination

are completely normal. Which of the following statements regarding exercise-induced asthma is FALSE?

A) Appropriate first-line prophylactic therapy for this patient consists of an inhaled short-acting bronchodilator 15 to 30 minutes prior to football practice.
B) An appropriate alternative prophylactic therapy for this patient consists of inhaled cromolyn 30 to 45 minutes prior to football practice.
C) Smog increases the severity of exercise-induced asthma.
D) Exercise-induced asthma typically begins 20 to 30 minutes after the initiation of physical activity.
E) Symptoms that are solely due to exercise-induced asthma should respond to β-agonist therapy.

26. A mother brings her 8-month-old infant son for an office visit so you can evaluate his rash. She says that the rash makes him irritable. The physical examination is significant for patches of erythemic skin with multiple small papules and scaling over the scalp, cheeks, and extensor areas. There are no areas of weeping or crusting. The mother has not tried anything for the rash. The child is afebrile, and there are no other significant findings on exam. This patient's rash is most likely due to which of the following?

A) Atopic dermatitis
B) Psoriasis
C) Keratosis follicularis
D) Seborrhea
E) Nummular eczema

27. You are discussing atopic dermatitis with a group of medical students. You are correct in telling them all of the following EXCEPT:

A) Skin hydration and lubrication are important components of atopic dermatitis management.
B) Antihistamines are helpful in reversing the underlying disease process responsible for atopic dermatitis.
C) Hydrophilic emollients should be applied after each episode of bathing.
D) Patients should wear loose-fitting cotton garments rather than wool.
E) Patients should attempt to limit topical exposure to harsh chemicals and perfumes.

28. An 8-year-old female with poorly-controlled atopic dermatitis develops widespread cutaneous vesicular lesions and a fever to 102.5°F. Which of the following is the most appropriate next step in the management of this patient?

A) Give the patient a prescription for topical mupirocin ointment 2%.
B) Admit the patient to the hospital for intravenous oxacillin.
C) Discontinue all immunosuppressive therapy and begin oral acyclovir.
D) Provide a prescription for a more concentrated topical corticosteroid.
E) Provide a prescription for oral glucocorticoid therapy.

29. The parent of a toddler with newly diagnosed atopic dermatitis asks you if there are things that can be done to decrease the frequency of exacerbations. You are correct in telling him all the following EXCEPT:

A) Dry air, heat, and physical trauma are factors that contribute to the severity of atopic dermatitis.
B) The choice of soaps for bathing should be limited to primarily non-detergent cleansers.
C) Hydrophilic emollients should be applied to the skin frequently, and especially after bathing.
D) Atopic dermatitis is associated with type 1 hypersensitivity food allergies in most children.
E) Institution of a restrictive diet for several weeks should result in improvement in children who have atopic cutaneous disease resulting primarily from a food allergy.

30. Which of the following patients is unlikely to obtain clinically relevant information from skin prick allergy testing?

A) A 15-year-old female patient with a history of anaphylaxis during her first visit to an Ethiopian restaurant
B) A 15-year-old female patient with a history of anaphylaxis to an insect sting
C) A 15-year-old female patient with severe persistent asthma
D) A 15-year-old female with persistent allergic rhinitis
E) A 15-year-old female with chronic urticaria

31. An 11-year-old male attending summer camp is brought to you in the camp infirmary after being stung by a wasp. He feels uneasy and nauseous. On physical examination, you note tachypnea, generalized skin flushing, and swelling around his eyes. Which of the following interventions is most appropriate in the immediate management of this patient?

A) Administration of subcutaneous epinephrine
B) Administration of a topical antihistamine
C) Removal of the stinger
D) Administration of an oral antihistamine
E) Administration of oral prednisone

32. You are lecturing to a group of family medicine residents about food allergies in children. Which of the following statements regarding pediatric food allergies is CORRECT?

A) All food allergies in children are mediated by IgE.
B) Positive skin prick allergy testing does not necessarily mean that the patient will have clinical symptoms following ingestion of that particular food.
C) Food elimination and subsequent re-challenge is a less useful form of evaluation than IgE specific antibody testing.
D) Most children with tree nut or fish allergies lose sensitivity to the antigen by the age of 5 years.

E) Wheat sensitivity which is present before the age of 24 months typically persists throughout life.

33. The mother of a child with a severe peanut allergy is considering having another child and asks you what she can do to affect her second child's risk for developing food allergies. Which of the following interventions has been associated with a decrease in severity and delay in the onset of food allergies in children?

A) Exclusive breastfeeding for the first 6 months of life
B) Exclusive hypoallergenic formula feeding for the first 6 months of life
C) Excluding peanuts from the mother's diet during pregnancy and breast feeding
D) A and B
E) A, B, and C

34. Which of the following patients is most likely to be suffering from a food allergy?

A) A 3-month-old former full-term male with persistent vomiting and failure to thrive despite switching to an elemental formula
B) A 4-year-old girl who always develops diarrhea several hours after anything with red food coloring
C) A 14-year-old girl who feels her throat "swelling up" after eating shellfish
D) A 6-year-old male who develops marked swelling of his arm and hand after being stung by a hornet on the wrist.
E) A 3-year-old male who becomes hyperactive after ingesting a lot of sugar

35. A 9-year-old patient with significant impairment due to mental retardation and cerebral palsy had an episode of anaphylaxis following administration of radiocontrast material in the hospital. The child also has an allergy to latex, and the mother wants to know what can be done to make certain that the anaphylaxis was related to the contrast material. Which of the following statements regarding anaphylaxis following administration of contrast material is TRUE?

A) About 5% of patients who receive contrast media develop an allergic reaction.
B) Skin prick testing is the study of choice for evaluating anaphylaxis following contrast media.
C) A patient with a history of anaphylaxis following the administration of contrast media should be pretreated with an inhaled bronchodilator at least 15 minutes prior to any subsequent study.
D) A patient with a history of anaphylaxis following the administration of contrast media should be pretreated with a leukotriene receptor antagonist prior to any subsequent study.
E) A patient with a history of anaphylaxis following the administration of contrast media should be pretreated with corticosteroids and antihistamines prior to any subsequent study.

36. Hymenoptera venom immunotherapy is indicated for which of the following patients?

A) A 17-year-old with a history of generalized urticaria following a yellow jacket sting AND a skin prick allergy test which is reactive to yellow jacket venom
B) A 15-year-old with a history of generalized urticaria following a yellow jacket sting AND a skin prick allergy test which is reactive to yellow jacket venom
C) A 12-year-old with a history of generalized urticaria following a yellow jacket sting AND a skin prick allergy test which is reactive to yellow jacket venom
D) A 15-year-old with a history of generalized urticaria following a yellow jacket sting AND IgE specific antibody to yellow jacket venom
E) A 12-year-old with a history of generalized urticaria following a yellow jacket sting AND IgE specific antibody to yellow jacket venom

37. Which of the following statements regarding in vivo (skin prick) and in vitro (serum for IgE specific antibody) allergy testing is TRUE?

A) In vitro testing is less expensive than in vivo testing.
B) In most cases, in vivo testing is preferable to in vitro testing.
C) In vitro testing is more reliable than in vivo testing.
D) In vivo testing is available for latex allergen.
E) In vitro testing provides more rapid results.

38. An adolescent patient with a history of generalized urticaria following a hornet sting is in your office for the first of his allergy shots. Less than 5 minutes after administration, she develops wheezing, itching, and nausea and begins to panic. Which of the following treatment options is most appropriate for this patient?

A) Place a tourniquet proximal to the administration site and give full-dose subcutaneous epinephrine at the injection site.
B) Inject full-dose subcutaneous epinephrine in the opposite arm.
C) Place a tourniquet proximal to the administration site and give full-dose subcutaneous epinephrine at the injection site and full-dose epinephrine in the opposite arm.
D) Place a tourniquet proximal to the administration site and give half-dose subcutaneous epinephrine at the injection site and half-dose epinephrine in the opposite arm.
E) Place a line with administration of intravenous epinephrine, diphenhydramine, and solumedrol.

39. Immunodeficiency testing should be considered in which of the following patients?

A) A 12-month-old with two documented episodes of *Streptococcus pneumoniae* sepsis
B) A 15-month-old with persistent thrush and normal urinalysis

C) A 24-month-old with four episodes of otitis media in the last 12 months
D) A and B
E) A, B, and C

40. A 14-month-old male is brought to the emergency room with a fever and bloody diarrhea. His history is significant for *Salmonella* gastroenteritis at age 4 months. He has also had intermittent thrush since the age of 3 months, which has been treated several times with oral nystatin. The physical examination is significant for a temperature of 102.5°F and abdominal tenderness. His white blood count is 12.8 X 10^9/L, with 50% neutrophils and 1% bands. The erythrocyte sedimentation rate is slightly elevated. Blood cultures are positive for *Salmonella typhimurium*. In addition to specific and supportive care for his infection, this child should be evaluated for immunodeficiency based on his medical history. Which of the following tests is most likely to be abnormal in this patient?
A) Chromosomal analysis for the 22q11.2 microdeletion
B) T cell proliferative response
C) Quantitative IgM
D) Total hemolytic complement assay
E) Dihydrorhodamine fluorescence test

41. The newborn nursery calls to tell you that one of your patients has been transferred to the neonatal intensive care unit with generalized seizures. The infant is found to be hypocalcemic, and no thymic shadow is visible on chest radiograph. Which of the following tests is the most useful for evaluating the effectiveness of the patient's immune system?
A) T cell proliferation in response to mitogen/antigen stimulation
B) Absolute B cell count
C) Quantitative immunoglobulins
D) Absolute lymphocyte count
E) Absolute neutrophil count

42. Which of the following pairings contains both an immunodeficiency and an organism more likely to infect patients with the defect?
A) Chronic granulomatous disease—*Pseudomonas aeruginosa*
B) Terminal complement deficiency—*Neisseria meningitides*
C) Selective IgA deficiency—*Pneumocystis jiroveci*
D) Common variable immunodeficiency—*Burkholderia cepacia*
E) X-linked agammaglobulinemia—*Candida albicans*

43. A 7-year-old male presents to your office in midsummer with a 3-week history of sneezing, nasal itching, and clear rhinorrhea. His mother states that he has had similar symptoms each of the past 2 years around this same time. The patient's history and physical examination are consistent with seasonal allergic rhinitis. Which of the following medications would you prescribe as first-line therapy to address his nasal symptoms?
A) Oral H_1-receptor antihistamine
B) Oral H_2-receptor antihistamine
C) Intranasal corticosteroid
D) Intranasal ipratropium bromide
E) Oral leukotriene-receptor antagonist

44. Which of the following symptoms is MOST specific for allergic rhinitis?
A) Impaired sleep
B) Headache
C) Postnasal drainage
D) Jasal itching
E) Coughing

45. Which of the following statements regarding corticosteroid use in asthma therapy is TRUE?
A) Inhaled corticosteroid use prevents early stage bronchospasm.
B) Oral corticosteroid use prevents early stage bronchospasm.
C) Use of newer inhaled corticosteroids for >2 years has been associated with a 2-cm deficit in adult height.
D) Asthma patients who are subsequently diagnosed with allergic rhinitis must not use intranasal corticosteroids if they are already on inhaled corticosteroids.
E) Systemic corticosteroid use prevents late stage bronchospasm.

ANSWERS

1. A	16. B	31. A
2. B	17. D	32. B
3. C	18. C	33. D
4. D	19. D	34. C
5. E	20. E	35. E
6. A	21. A	36. A
7. B	22. B	37. B
8. C	23. C	38. C
9. D	24. E	39. D
10. E	25. D	40. E
11. A	26. A	41. A
12. B	27. B	42. B
13. C	28. C	43. C
14. D	29. D	44. D
15. A	30. E	45. E

Infectious Disease

10

IMMUNIZATION

Active Immunization

Active immunization consists of administration of antigens to a host in order to prime an immune response against a specific pathogen upon subsequent exposure. Polysaccharide antigens stimulate T cell-independent B cell proliferation and antibody production. The 23-valent pneumococcal vaccine and the quadrivalent meningococcal vaccine are examples of *polysaccharide vaccines*. In contrast, vaccines which contain protein antigens or are conjugated with proteins stimulate both T cell and B cell responses, resulting in improved immunity against a pathogen. T cells secrete cytokines (e.g., IL-4) which result in the production of memory B cells. All childhood vaccinations stimulate T cell-dependent immune responses. Recommended childhood and adolescent vaccinations are discussed in detail in Chapter 3.

Passive Immunization

Passive immunization involves administration of immune globulin (IG), the product of B cells, to patients who are immunodeficient or have been exposed to an illness which places them at risk for severe disease. Antibodies in IG bind antigens and facilitate their clearance from the body. The proteins in IG are antigenic, and therefore can trigger anaphylaxis in some individuals. IG is contraindicated in patients with selective IgA deficiency; IgA contained in IG produces a type 1 hypersensitivity reaction (anaphylaxis) in these patients. *Intravenous IG* (IVIG) is primarily made up of IgG, although IgA is also present. *Intramuscular IG*, while similar in composition, is less expensive, easier to administer, and more readily available than IVIG.

HOST RESPONSE TO INFECTIOUS DISEASE

Cytokines are inter-cell signaling proteins which regulate immune responses, fuel inflammation, and stimulate cell production in the marrow. Examples include:

- *interleukin-1*: secreted by macrophages; induces acute phase inflammatory reaction
- *interleukin-6*: secreted by macrophages; induces acute phase inflammatory reaction
- *interleukin-8*: a major chemotactic cytokine; attracts neutrophils to pathogenic organisms
- *interferon-alpha*: secreted by leukocytes and tissue cells; a potent pyrogen; involved in antiviral, anti-tumor responses
- *interferon-gamma*: secreted by T cells, natural killer cells; induces macrophage killing of intracellular bacteria
- *tumor necrosis factor*: pyrogen secreted by white blood cells and other tissues; induces systemic inflammatory response; activates *mononuclear phagocytes*, antigen-presenting cells that are instrumental in the defense against intracellular pathogens

Fever is an adaptive response to endogenous (cytokines) or exogenous (pathogens, toxin) pyrogens. Fever promotes leukocyte mobility/function and interferon production. Pyrogens also directly stimulate neutrophils, leukocytes, monocytes, and macrophages.

INFECTION IN THE IMMUNOCOMPROMISED HOST

Organisms which do not normally inflict disease in immunocompetent individuals can cause severe opportunistic infections in the compromised host (with leukemia, lymphoma, cancer treatment, AIDS, nephrotic syndrome, asplenia, or sickle cell disease). When a child with chronic disease presents with fever and neutropenia, empiric therapy includes coverage for gram-positive (*Staphylococcus aureus, Staphylococcus epidermis*) and gram-negative (*Escherichia coli, Pseudomonas aeruginosa*) bacteria. Depending on disease severity, probable pathogens, and susceptibility patterns, three acceptable regimens include:

- a first-generation cephalosporin plus an aminoglycoside plus an extended-spectrum antipseudomonal penicillin
- an aminoglycoside plus an extended-spectrum antipseudomonal penicillin
- a single extended-spectrum agent which includes antipseudomonal coverage (ceftazidime, imipenem)

PREVENTION OF INFECTIOUS DISEASE IN THE HOSPITAL SETTING

Disease Spread and Isolation Precautions

Strict adherence to correct hand washing remains the most important and effective preventive measure against hospital-acquired infectious illness. Table 10-1 details the categories of isolation precaution recommended by the Hospital Infection Control Practices Advisory Committee (1996; revised 2002).

Infectious Disease in Hospital Personnel

The following should be obtained from all health care workers at the outset of hospital employment:

- Documentation of varicella vaccination, a reliable history of varicella infection, or positive serologic studies; Individuals who are non-immune should receive the varicella vaccine unless contraindicated.
- Documentation of primary vaccination against tetanus and diphtheria; Individuals should also have received a booster within 10 years of their original vaccination.
- Documentation of vaccination against hepatitis B; Individuals who are non-immune should undergo vaccination.
- Documentation of primary vaccination against polio, measles, mumps, and rubella

Health care workers should be offered yearly vaccination against influenza. Although vaccination against hepatitis A and pneumococcus are not universally required for medical personnel, counseling should identify individuals for whom these inoculations are indicated.

NEEDLE-STICK INJURY AND PROPHYLAXIS

Despite numerous precautions, needle-stick injuries are not rare in hospitals, clinics, and laboratories. When a needle-stick injury occurs:

- the wound should be rigorously cleaned and irrigated
- the patient should be tested for HIV and hepatitis B and C
- the affected health care worker should be tested for HIV and hepatitis B and C

TABLE 10-1
ISOLATION PRECAUTIONS

Standard Precautions (used with all patients and for all contact with body fluids, secretions, and excretions)

- *Appropriate hand hygiene*—washing with soap and water or an approved waterless antiseptic agent after removing gloves and before and between all patient contacts
- *Gloves* as barrier protection when handling any of the above, which should be removed promptly after use and changed between tasks
- *Masks* and *eye and face shields* when there is a risk of mucous membrane contact with any of the above
- *Gowns* when there is risk of skin or clothing contact with any of the above
- Strict adherence to established protocols when handling or cleaning *sharp contaminated objects*
- Widespread availability of *ventilation equipment* to avoid the need for direct mouth-to-mouth resuscitation

Airborne Precautions (prevent disease transmission through dissemination of contaminated airborne droplets, dust particles, or fungal spores)

- *Isolating* the infected patient within a private room or cohorting patients with the same disease
- Negative air-pressure *ventilation* through a HEPA filter or external exhaust system
- *Exclusion of susceptible individuals* from rooms of patients with measles or varicella (unless wearing a mask)

Examples: measles, varicella-zoster, Mycobacterium tuberculosis, Aspergillus fungal spores

Droplet Precautions (prevent disease transmission through large droplets propelled only a short distance)

- Special air-handling and ventilation not required
- *Isolating* the infected patient within a private room or cohorting patients with the same disease
- Wearing a *mask* if within 3 feet of an infected patient

Examples: adenovirus, invasive Haemophilus influenzae, influenza, mumps, invasive Neisseria meningitidis, parvovirus B19, pertussis, rubella

Contact Precautions (prevent disease transmission through direct contact with the infected patient or contact with a contaminated object)

- *Isolating* the infected patient within a private room or cohorting patients with the same disease
- Wearing *gloves and gowns*, which should be removed and discarded before leaving the room

Examples: any multi-drug resistant pathogens; Clostridium difficile, conjunctivitis, enteroviruses, E. coli O157, hepatitis A virus, herpes simplex virus, herpes zoster, respiratory syncytial virus, rotavirus, Shigella

- screening questions, test results, and characteristics of the injury result in relative risk assessment
- HIV prophylaxis (if indicated) is administered (zidovudine and lamivudine for 4 weeks; indinavir or nelfinavir added if extensive exposure)
- vaccination against hepatitis B and hepatitis B immune globulin are administered if the health care worker is non-immune
- vaccination against diphtheria and tetanus are completed if the health care worker has not been inoculated within the past 5 years

PREPARATION FOR FOREIGN TRAVEL

With regard to infectious disease, preventive counseling prior to foreign travel should include information regarding:

- *recommended vaccinations* (This includes being up-to-date on routine vaccinations and need for any specialized vaccinations depending on travel destination and anticipated access to health care. Non-routine inoculations which may be required include quadrivalent meningococcal, typhoid, rabies, and Japanese encephalitis vaccines.)
- *malaria prophylaxis* (Travelers to endemic areas should begin prophylaxis 1 to 2 weeks prior to travel and continue for 4 weeks after returning home. Choice of prophylactic medication is dictated by malaria species present and susceptibility patterns in the destination area. Other preventive measures include wearing long sleeves and long pants, avoiding being outside at dusk and dawn, bed nets, and using insect repellent.)
- *prevention of food- and waterborne illnesses* (This includes using bottled water for drinking and brushing teeth if a reliable source of uncontaminated water is not available; eating fully cooked meat; eating only raw fruit and vegetables that can be peeled.)

Specifics regarding the above can be found at the Centers for Disease Control and Prevention's (CDC) travel health Web site, a good resource for both travelers and physicians.

INFECTIOUS DISEASE IN IMMIGRANT CHILDREN

Children who have recently emigrated from developing foreign countries should be tested for hepatitis B, human immunodeficiency virus, and tuberculosis.

SPECIFIC VIRAL PATHOGENS

Cytomegalovirus

Primary cytomegalovirus (CMV) infection in immunocompetent children and adolescents is generally asymptomatic or produces only a mild, nonspecific illness. Under these circumstances, active infections and viral shedding may persist for months to years. The virus is present in saliva, tears, blood, urine, semen, cervical secretions, and breast milk. CMV is transmitted through direct contact with infected bodily fluids (e.g., close personal and sexual contact; breastfeeding; care of young children; blood transfusion; organ transplantation). The incubation period ranges from 3 to 12 weeks in the normal host.

CMV may also be acquired during gestation (see Chapter 5) or in the perinatal period (through contact with cervical secretions during birth or ingestion of infected breast milk). CMV is the most common congenital infection in the United States and is associated with severe long-term sequelae such as hearing loss, developmental delay, mental retardation, and cerebral palsy. These complications are not thought to occur following infections acquired in the perinatal period or thereafter. CMV is part of the differential diagnosis of fever of unknown origin (FUO) in the pediatric population. Although uncommon, older children and adolescents who become infected may develop a mononucleosis-type syndrome.

Traditional (2 weeks) and rapid (~24 hours) viral culture studies detect CMV in urine or saliva samples. Antigen detection can be performed on bronchoalveolar lavage and blood specimens, and molecular probes are available for serum specimens as well. If CMV is detected prior to 3 weeks of age, the patient was infected in utero. Differentiating congenital CMV from perinatally-acquired CMV is difficult but should be attempted due to divergent prognoses and follow-up needs.

Infection in the immunocompromised host may follow reactivation or may be primary through exposure to infected individuals, transfusion with CMV-positive blood products, or transplantation of an organ from a CMV-positive donor. Patients with impaired T-cell function (HIV infection, bone marrow transplantation, post-transplantation suppression therapy) are particularly at risk for severe, life-threatening disease; in these individuals, the incubation period is hours to days. Transplant patients present with fever and leukopenia, followed by rash and myalgia; multi-organ dysfunction and failure may ensue. Patients with HIV often develop CMV retinitis or gastrointestinal disease (esophagitis, colitis). Detection and quantification of the virus in the blood through immunofluorescence or PCR is the most useful laboratory test in immunocompromised patients. Ganciclovir, foscarnet, or cidofovir is indicated for treatment of CMV in the immunocompromised host. CMV-infected HIV patients are indefinitely maintained on ganciclovir to prevent retinitis and blindness, among other complications. Prophylactic antiviral therapy, the use of seronegative blood products, and CMV immune globulin have been instrumental in preventing CMV infection in transplant patients.

Epstein-Barr Virus

Epstein-Barr virus (EBV) infects virtually the entire world population. The organism is transmitted through infected saliva, blood transfusions, or transplantation of EBV-positive organs or marrow. Primary infection in early childhood is usually asymptomatic or causes only a mild upper respiratory illness. However, some children and many adolescents who contract EBV present with infectious mononucleosis. Older children and adolescents with primary EBV who are inadvertently treated with ampicillin develop a morbilliform rash after 3 to 6 days of antibiotic therapy which is highly suggestive of EBV infection. Following primary infection, EBV establishes latent infection in B-cells of the immunocompetent individual, resulting in intermittent or nearly continuous asymptomatic viral shedding. However, in patients with T-cell immunodeficiencies, EBV induces ongoing B-cell proliferation, which is related to the increased incidence of lymphoproliferative disorders and malignancies (Burkitt lymphoma, Hodgkin disease) in this population.

Other pathogens that can cause symptoms consistent with infectious mononucleosis (IM) include CMV, *Toxoplasma gondii,* adenovirus, human herpesvirus 6, and HIV. In most cases, the diagnosis of IM is made based on a constellation of clinical findings (fever, tonsillopharyngitis with or without exudate, cervical or generalized lymphadenopathy, hepatosplenomegaly, and profound malaise) in conjunction with characteristic laboratory results (moderately elevated white blood count with a predominance of lymphocytes and >10% atypical lymphocytes). The majority of patients ≥4 years old have detectable heterophile antibodies on rapid testing. Serologic testing can differentiate between acute and latent infection and should be considered in heterophile-negative patients (Fig. 10-1). Detection of viral capsid antigen-specific IgM is diagnostic of acute infection. Additional testing for other pathogens listed above may be beneficial in patients with classic IM who do not have serologic evidence of EBV.

Symptomatic treatment alone is sufficient in the majority of patients with primary EBV infection, as the disease is self-limited. Patients with infectious mononucleosis and splenomegaly should avoid contact sports until physical examination confirms normal size of the organ. Systemic steroids are given to patients with impending airway obstruction due to markedly enlarged tonsils, adenoids, and/or cervical lymph nodes. Neither steroids nor antiviral medications shorten the duration of symptoms or shedding; thus, they are not indicated for the treatment of uncomplicated EBV.

Herpes Simplex Virus

There are two serotypes of herpes simplex virus (HSV), a double-stranded DNA virus:

- HSV-1 is typically implicated in infections of the face, skin, and extremities, but also causes about a quarter of genital infections. The virus is transmitted through direct contact with infected oral secretions or lesions.
- HSV-2 typically infects the genitalia, although oral lesions may develop following direct contact with genital lesions. Transmission takes place through direct exposure to infected genital secretions or lesions as a result of sexual contact or vaginal delivery. Any genital HSV-2 infection diagnosed in a prepubertal child strongly suggests sexual abuse.

The incubation period of HSV in the immunocompetent individual is 2 to 14 days. Characteristic herpetic lesions consist of clustered 1 to 2 mm papules which quickly

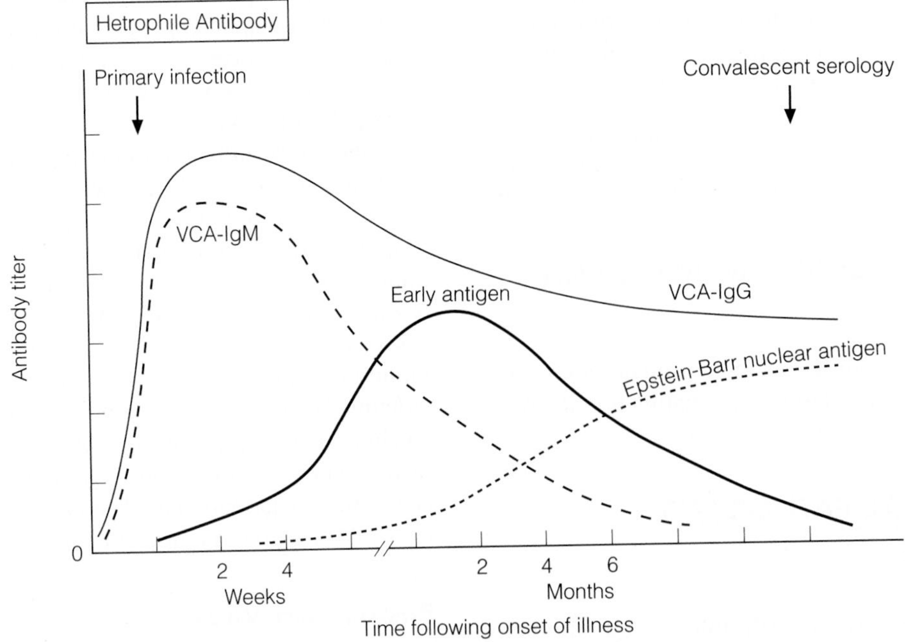

Figure 10-1 Antigen detection and serologies during EBV infection. VCA, viral capsid antigen. (From Marino BS and Fine KS. *Blueprints Pediatrics.* 4th ed. Philadelphia: Lippincott Williams & Wilkins; 2006 with permission.)

evolve into vesicles. These vesicles are unroofed within 3 to 4 days to reveal pustular, hemorrhagic bases which then resolve. Once infected, individuals harbor latent virus and may experience disease recurrences. They are capable of transmitting the virus to others during primary infection, recurrences, and frequent periods of asymptomatic shedding. Primary HSV infection produces viral shedding for a week or more, whereas shedding with recurrences is more limited; however, most infected individuals acquire HSV from someone with asymptomatic shedding.

Neonatal HSV disease is discussed in Chapter 5. Chapter 24 contains information regarding genital herpes infections. Most infants and older children who contract HSV beyond the neonatal period are asymptomatic during primary infection. Several distinct clinical scenarios associated with mucocutaneous HSV (generally HSV-1) are listed as follows:

- *Gingivostomatitis*: painful ulceration of the gingiva and oral mucous membranes accompanied by fever and local adenopathy. The pain is usually marked and may preclude eating and drinking in young children, resulting in dehydration.
- *Herpes labialis*: typical "cold sores" or "fever blisters." Lesions appear at the vermillion border and are preceded by a "tingling" sensation.
- *Herpetic whitlow*: multiple herpetic lesions localized to a single finger
- *Herpetic gladiatorum*: multiple herpetic lesions clustered on the face, head, torso, and/or upper extremities of wrestlers
- *Eczema herpeticum* (see Chapter 9): widespread cutaneous lesions occurring in patients with atopic dermatitis; dissemination and systemic disease may follow

Most cases of mucocutaneous HSV are benign and self-limited; no specific therapy is required (exception: eczema herpeticum). Topical acyclovir is ineffective. Systemic acyclovir (intravenous or oral) is reserved for patients at high risk for disseminated disease. Unfortunately, acyclovir requires frequent dosing (i.e., three times a day intravenous or five times a day oral). The most common adverse effects attributed to acyclovir are abdominal pain, nausea, vomiting, and diarrhea. Acyclovir should be used with caution in patients with impaired renal function.

HSV conjunctivitis generally results from autoinoculation and can occur with both primary and recurrent infections. Conjunctival HSV must be managed in consultation with an ophthalmologist because of the risk of progression to keratitis (corneal inflammation) and scarring. Eye drops are effective in uncomplicated cases. Topical corticosteroids are contraindicated in cases of suspected HSV conjunctivitis.

HSV encephalitis is uncommon beyond the neonatal period but does occur. Most cases are due to HSV-1, and both primary and recurrent infections can result in encephalitis. Clinical manifestations include fever, altered sensorium, focal neurologic signs, and seizures. Analysis of cerebrospinal fluid (CSF) demonstrates an elevated white blood cell count with lymphocytic predominance. In about one half of patients, the CSF also contains red blood cells which do not clear from the first tube to the last. An electroencephalogram showing periodic lateralizing epileptiform discharges emanating from the temporal lobe is highly suggestive of HSV encephalitis. Long-term complications (persistent seizures) and significant cognitive impairment are common, even with timely, appropriate therapy.

In patients with immunodeficiency, local HSV disease can rapidly disseminate and infect multiple organs. Early, aggressive antiviral therapy may prevent this. Immunodeficient patients with local HSV must be started on systemic antiviral therapy (i.e., acyclovir) as soon as possible.

When characteristic lesions are present and the clinical course matches a typical HSV disease state (e.g., genital herpes), laboratory confirmation is generally unnecessary. Tests that detect the virus (Table 10-2) should be considered in atypical cases, neonatal HSV, encephalitis, and infections in the immunocompromised host. A Tzanck smear with multinucleated giant cells confirms the presence of a herpesvirus but is not specific for HSV.

Varicella-Zoster Virus

Primary infection with varicella-zoster virus (VZV), a herpesvirus, causes chickenpox. Herpes zoster ("shingles") results from reactivation of the virus, which lies dormant in various sensory ganglia. VZV is transmitted via direct

TABLE 10-2
HSV: LABORATORY EVALUATION

Viral Culture

- Best if specimen obtained from unroofed vesicle
- Specimen may also be obtained from conjunctivae, nasopharynx, or blood
- Most patients with HSV encephalitis have negative CSF cultures
- Positive results usually available within 72 hours; read as negative after 2 weeks

Direct Fluorescent Antibody Staining (DFA; antigen detection)

- Best if specimen obtained from unroofed vesicle
- Specimen may also be obtained from conjunctivae, nasopharynx, and blood
- Less sensitive than culture, so better used to differentiate serotypes once culture becomes positive

Enzyme Immunoassay of HSV Antigens (ELISA; antigen detection)

- Best if specimen obtained from unroofed vesicle
- Specimen may also be obtained from conjunctivae, nasopharynx, and blood
- Less sensitive than culture, so better used to differentiate serotypes once culture becomes positive

Polymerase Chain Reaction (PCR); Molecular Probes

- Highly sensitive for detecting HSV DNA in the CSF

contact with infected mucosa, respiratory secretions, or vesicle fluid; in patients with herpes zoster, only the lesions contain infectious material. The incubation period is 10 to 21 days. Individuals are most infectious during the 4-day period surrounding the appearance of the rash. About 90% of susceptible contacts will contract the disease when exposed. Primary infection during pregnancy may result in *congenital varicella* (see Chapter 5).

Chickenpox presents as 1 to 2 days of fever and malaise followed by the appearance of characteristic lesions. The rash begins on the face or upper body as intensely pruritic erythematous papules that evolve into vesicles, which then rupture, crust, and scar. Lesions in all stages of development are present simultaneously; in fact, unlike smallpox, lesions located on any single body area represent different stages of evolution. Patients are infectious until all sores are crusted over, which usually occurs about 5 days after the appearance of initial lesions. Secondary bacterial infections are the most common serious complication. Group A Streptococcus in particular is capable of causing severe invasive disease in patients with chickenpox; the risk may be even greater in patients treated with nonsteroidal anti-inflammatory medications.

Management is largely supportive. Nonsteroidal anti-inflammatory agents and aspirin should be avoided in children with VZV. Oral acyclovir is reserved for patients older than 12 years of age and those at increased risk for severe disease (patients who are immunocompromised, receiving long-term salicylate therapy, or have chronic lung or skin disease). The medication must be initiated within 72 hours of symptom onset to affect the course of illness. Recommendations regarding post-exposure prophylaxis are detailed in Table 10-3.

TABLE 10-3
VARICELLA-ZOSTER VIRUS: POST-EXPOSURE PROPHYLAXIS

Varicella Vaccination

- Indicated for prevention of disease in susceptible individuals
- Prevents disease if administered within 3 days of exposure
- Safe for use in patients with no history of clinical disease who are antibody-positive
- IVIG should not be given within 2 weeks of vaccination.

Varicella-Zoster Immune Globulin (VZIG)

- Prevents or lessens the severity of disease if administered within 4 days of exposure
- Indicated for the prevention of disease in susceptible pregnant women
- Indicated for prevention of infection in individuals at risk for severe disease (including infants born to mothers who develop lesions 5 days before to 2 days after delivery)
- Monthly injections recommended for some immunocompromised patients to protect them from infection
- Varicella vaccination should be delayed for at least 3 months, preferably up to 1 year.

Post-exposure prophylaxis is not indicated following exposure to vaccine-associated virus.

Herpes zoster presents as localized pain and pruritis, followed by the characteristic vesicles clustered within a sensory dermatome. Herpes zoster is uncommon in the pediatric population; however, its appearance in a child is not necessarily indicative of immunodeficiency.

The diagnoses of both chickenpox and herpes zoster are usually evident on physical examination; laboratory confirmation is rarely indicated. A Tzanck smear of vesicle scrapings demonstrates multinucleated giant cells identical to those identified in HSV infections. Antigen detection (DFA, ELISA) is available for VZV diagnosis in questionable cases and provides rapid, sensitive, specific results.

The varicella vaccine is a live-attenuated preparation approved for use in children older than 12 months of age. Two doses are recommended. Recipients may break out in a mild vesicular rash within a week of vaccination. Transmission of vaccine-associated VZV is extraordinarily rare; however, many school districts do not allow children with vaccine-associated lesions to attend school until the sores are crusted over.

Patients who are immunocompromised, especially those with congenital or acquired T cell defects, leukemia, or lymphoma, are at risk for severe, disseminated varicella. Pneumonitis, meningoencephalitis, hepatitis, and hemorrhagic varicella can occur in immunocompetent hosts but are far more common in patients with immune deficiencies. Herpes zoster often has a more protracted course in immunocompromised individuals; systemic disease with or without the aforementioned complications may be associated with zoster in these patients. Intravenous acyclovir should be started within 24 hours of the appearance of rash. Infected family members and close contacts of immunocompromised individuals should maintain airborne and contact precautions for 21 days after the onset of the rash.

Measles Virus

Measles virus is an RNA paramyxovirus which causes a distinct clinical syndrome in infected individuals. The virus is transmitted through contact with contaminated respiratory droplets. Infected individuals are contagious for several days prior to until 4 days after the appearance of the rash, and 90% of exposed susceptible contacts acquire the disease. A prodromal stage follows a 10 to 12 day asymptomatic incubation period. Koplik spots, consisting of small, discrete, grayish-white lesions with red centers that appear on the buccal mucosa, are pathognomonic for measles. Other prodromal symptoms include low-grade fever and the three C's (cough, coryza, conjunctivitis). Within 3 to 5 days, the patient develops a high fever accompanied by marked lymphadenopathy and an erythematous maculopapular rash that spreads in a cephalocaudal direction. The virus can be cultured from nasopharyngeal or conjunctival specimens, blood, or urine. IgM specific for measles is present within 3 days of the onset of the rash and remains elevated for about a month. Uncomplicated cases resolve within 5 to 7 days. The most significant complications of measles infection are pneumonia (measles or secondary bacterial) and acute encephalitis, which carries a high mortality rate. Measles suppresses T-cell function; in chronically malnourished patients, particularly those with vitamin A deficiency, serious secondary bacterial infections may occur. The American Academy of Pediatrics recommends vitamin A supplementation for all children ages 6 months to 2 years who are hospitalized for measles and for any child with measles who is also malnourished.

A combination live-attenuated vaccine for measles, mumps, and rubella is available; two doses provide complete protection in >99% of recipients. The vaccine will also prevent disease in susceptible contacts if administered within 72 hours of exposure, and is approved for this indication in infants as young as age 6 months. Any measles inoculation given prior to 12 months of age does not count toward completion of the two-dose series. Intramuscular measles immunoglobulin should be administered within 6 days to *all* susceptible household contacts who do not receive the vaccine in a timely manner; susceptible subjects may be vaccinated 6 months thereafter.

Mumps Virus

Mumps is a paramyxovirus which causes systemic disease through direct infection of multiple organs. The organism is spread via respiratory droplets. Following an incubation period of 14 to 18 days, affected patients develop nonspecific prodromal symptoms including low-grade fever, malaise, myalgia, and headache. The virus infects the salivary glands, resulting in uni- or bilateral parotitis which presents early in the illness as earache and tenderness at the angle of the jaw. Up to 50% of post-pubertal males develop orchitis. The virus also infects the meninges, leading to symptomatic aspetic meningitis in a significant minority of patients. Pancreatitis is uncommon but does occur. Children are less likely than adults to manifest symptomatic organ involvement. Mumps is sub-clinical or mild and nonspecific in at least half of those infected. The virus can be cultured from the nasopharynx, urine, and buccal cavity, but serology (IgM titers) is the preferred method of diagnosis. The mumps vaccine induces seroconversion in 97% of individuals.

Rubella Virus

Rubella is an RNA virus spread through respiratory droplets. At least half of acquired cases are asymptomatic. Following an incubation period of about 14 days, affected children develop a low-grade fever and a pale, erythematous maculopapular rash which begins on the head and progresses caudally, fading within 3 to 4 days. Unlike measles, the rubella exanthem never coalesces. Patients are most contagious during eruption of the rash. Lyphadenopathy (particularly occipital) is a common associated feature. Infected adults are more likely to experience a prodromal phase of fever and malaise; many also develop myalgia and arthralgia. Congenital rubella syndrome is discussed in Chapter 5. The virus can be cultured from multiple sites, but serology (rubella IgM) is the simplest method of diagnosis. The presence of rheumatoid factor, heterophile antibody, and parvovirus may result in false positive results under certain circumstances. The vaccine confers immunity in about 97% of individuals inoculated with two doses; however, immunity may wane, and there are rare reports of infants with congenital rubella born to documented rubella-immune mothers. Post-exposure vaccination and immune globulin are not effective for prevention of disease.

Roseola and Erythema Infectiosum

Roseola and erythema infectiosum are two benign, self-limited viral infections of early childhood (generally prior to age 3 years) that have distinct clinical presentations. Roseola, caused by human herpes virus type 6 (HHV-6), begins with the sudden onset of a high fever which lasts for about 3 days and may provoke febrile seizures. The characteristic widespread pink maculopapular rash appears as the fever resolves. In both roseola and erythema infectiosum, the child is most contagious during the period of viremia, which concludes with the onset of the rash. Erythema infectiosum, also called fifth disease, results from infection with parvovirus B19, the same virus capable of causing bone marrow suppression and aplastic crisis in patients with hemolytic anemia. An infected child often comes to medical attention due to the characteristic "slapped-cheek" facial appearance and the lacy, faintly erythematous rash on the trunk and extremities. The illness may or may not be preceded by mild fever and fussiness. Infection with parvovirus B19 can cause arthralgia and arthritis in the older child and adult. Hydrops fetalis, a form of fetal demise associated with maternal B19 infection, is mentioned in Chapter 5.

Enteroviruses

Enterovirus is a family of RNA viruses that includes coxsackieviruses (groups A and B), echoviruses, and polioviruses. In temperate climates, infections are more common in the summer and fall. Enteroviruses are transmitted primarily via the fecal-oral route, although respiratory and fomite transfer do occur. Attack rates are highest in infants and children ≤3 years of age. Affected individuals are contagious during the course of their symptoms and continue to shed the virus in their stool for several weeks. Symptoms vary depending on the specific causative organism (Table 10-4). Most children develop a nonspecific, self-limited febrile

TABLE 10-4
CLINICAL SYNDROMES ASSOCIATED WITH SPECIFIC ENTEROVIRUSES

Group A coxsackieviruses: encephalitis, hand-foot-mouth disease, acute hemorrhagic conjunctivitis

Group B coxsackieviruses: myocarditis, pleurodynia, herpangina, meningitis

Echoviruses: meningitis, neonatal hepatitis

illness, which may consist of upper respiratory (pharyngitis, nasal congestion) and/or gastrointestinal (vomiting, diarrhea) symptoms. Herpangina and hand-foot-mouth disease are also caused by enteroviruses. These organisms can infect a variety of organs and tissues, sometimes resulting in significant symptoms or serious illness (acute hemorrhagic conjunctivitis; pneumonia with or without pleurodynia; myocarditis, pericarditis; hepatitis; aseptic meningitis, encephalitis). Neonates in particular may develop severe disease, including myocardial dysfunction and hepatitis. Although laboratory confirmation is unnecessary in most cases, the virus may be identified in CSF, stool, rectal or nasopharyngeal swabs, and urine samples through PCR or culture. Treatment consists of symptom reduction, supportive care, and management of serious complications.

Wild poliovirus was eliminated from the western hemisphere in 1994; the World Health Organization has a goal of worldwide eradication in the near future.

Influenza Virus

"The flu" represents infection with influenza A or B, members of the orthomyxovirus family of RNA viruses. Influenza virus is transmitted via respiratory droplets and causes an acute upper respiratory illness during the mid-winter months. Symptoms include moderate-to-high fever, headache, sore throat, malaise, myalgia, and cough. Abdominal pain may occur in younger children. Viral pneumonia or croup may complicate the disease course. During peak flu season, clinical presentation alone is usually sufficient for diagnosis. Confirmatory studies are indicated for young infants, patients with severe disease or focal lung findings, and patients who do not improve over several days. Rapid antigen (ELISA) testing of nasopharyngeal swab specimens yields results in minutes. Viral culture is available but less useful. Most patients require only supportive care. However, antiviral therapy is available for patients at high risk for complications and those with severe disease (Table 10-5). The live-attenuated influenza vaccine is reformulated yearly to reflect specific anticipated antigenic strains. Annual vaccination is recommended for all children ages 6 to 59 months of age, any patient at risk for severe disease (e.g., those with congenital heart defects, cystic fibrosis, asthma, or other chronic illnesses), household contacts of the above and infants younger than 6 months of age, pregnant women, and medical personnel. An intranasal vaccine is approved for use in healthy patients ≥5 years of age; a recent study suggests similar safety and efficacy in children as young as 12 months of age.

TABLE 10-5
APPROACHES TO THE TREATMENT AND PREVENTION OF INFLUENZA

Amantadine
- Licensed for use in children ≥12 months of age
- Effective against influenza A only
- Approved for prophylactic use

Rimantadine
- Licensed for use in children ≥12 months of age
- Effective against influenza A only
- Approved for prophylactic use

Oseltamivir*
- Licensed for use in children ≥13 years of age
- Effective against influenza A and B
- Approved for prophylactic use

Zanamivir*
- Licensed for use in children ≥7 years of age
- Effective against influenza A and B
- NOT approved for prophylaxis

*Reports of mental status changes in a small minority of children treated with these medications may limit their widespread use in pediatrics.

Amantadine and rimantadine are tricyclic amines which inhibit replication of influenza A. Oseltamivir and zanamivir are neuraminidase inhibitors effective against both influenza A and B. If administered within 48 hours of development of symptoms, all four can reduce severity of illness and shorten duration by about a day. Post-exposure prophylaxis (PEP) consists of administration of the influenza vaccine and chemoprophylaxis with an appropriate agent for 2 weeks following injection.

Prophylactic antiviral medication is indicated for individuals who are:

- at risk for severe disease during the 2-week interval between vaccination and full protection if influenza is already present in the community
- at risk for severe disease for whom the flu vaccine is contraindicated
- at risk for severe disease if the vaccine is not protective against the strains circulating in the community
- nonimmunized close contacts of patients at risk for severe disease
- immunocompromised children regardless of vaccination status
- nonimmunized residents of any group home in which an outbreak occurs

Respiratory Syncytial Virus

Respiratory syncytial virus (RSV) causes minor upper respiratory illness in most immunocompetent children and adults. However, it is the most significant cause of seasonal (late fall to early spring) lower respiratory disease, most notably *bronchiolitis* and pneumonia, in infants. Virtually all children become infected with RSV within the first 2 years of life. Transmission takes place when infected respiratory secretions come in contact with host ocular or nasal tissue. Patients with RSV shed the virus for a week or more. RSV can survive on surfaces for several hours, making it an ideal nosocomial pathogen. Following 2 to 8 days of incubation, the affected patient develops clear rhinorrhea and persistent coughing. Infants are likely to be febrile during an initial RSV episode and may develop otitis media as well. In about one half of these infants, the disease progresses to bronchiolitis or pneumonia, suggested clinically by tachypnea, retractions, wheezing, and rales/rhonchi. Hypoxemia is not uncommon. A chest radiograph demonstrating hyperaeration and peribronchial cuffing is consistent with RSV bronchiolitis. Premature, very-low–birth weight infants occasionally present with apnea in the absence of respiratory symptoms.

Once RSV infection has been documented within a community, most cases are diagnosed clinically. However, RSV should be confirmed in patients with severe disease and those requiring hospitalization (due to isolation requirements). ELISA or DFA testing of nasal wash specimens allows rapid diagnosis of RSV. If appropriate, viral culture confirms the diagnosis. Hospitals should make sure that medical personnel maintain good hand washing procedures and understand the protocols of contact isolation.

Neither systemic corticosteroids nor bronchodilator therapy has been shown to be of any benefit for patients with RSV. Ribavirin is an antiviral aerosol which results in clinical improvement in some patients but does not affect length of hospital stay.

Former premature and/or very-low–birth weight infants, infants with congenital heart disease or bronchopulmonary dysplasia, and immunocompromised children are at increased risk for severe RSV disease, and mortality associated with the virus is higher in these patient populations. Two RSV antibody products are currently approved for prophylactic use in high-risk patients (Table 10-6). Children with a history of hospitalization due to RSV are more likely than their peers to develop asthma later in life; however, current theory suggests that underlying airway hyperresponsiveness predisposes to severe RSV, rather than early RSV increasing future likelihood of wheezing.

Parainfluenza Virus

Parainfluenza virus is the predominant cause of acute laryngotracheobronchitis (croup) in children, although infection with influenza A and B, adenovirus, and RSV may also result in croup. More cases occur during spring and fall months. The virus is transmitted through contact with infected respiratory secretions. Parainfluenza is also implicated in cases of bronchiolitis and pneumonia, but usually causes only mild-to-moderate upper respiratory symptoms in older children and adults. Croup presents with partial upper airway obstruction, stridor, and a "barky" cough. Symptoms generally respond to cool mist or humidified air. Nebulized racemic epinephrine and systemic corticosteroids are reserved for patients in respiratory distress. Rapid antigen studies are available for diagnosis using respiratory fluid specimens.

TABLE 10-6
COMMERCIAL ANTIBODY PREPARATIONS FOR PREVENTION OF RSV DISEASE

Palivizumab

- Monthly intramuscular injection associated with decreased incidence of hospitalization and less severe disease
- Contraindicated in infants with congenital heart disease

RSV immune globulin

- Monthly intravenous infusion associated with decreased incidence of hospitalization and less severe disease
- Blood product
- Interferes with the use of live vaccines
- Contraindicated in infants with congenital heart disease

The American Academy of Pediatrics recommends prophylaxis with one of the above products during RSV season in children younger than 24 months of age who:

- Have chronic lung disease requiring ongoing medical therapy
- Were born at ≤32 weeks' gestation

Prophylaxis should also be considered for patients who:

- Are <24 months of age and were born between 32 and 35 weeks' gestation
- Are immunocompromised

Adenovirus

Adenovirus is a family of DNA viruses implicated in respiratory and gastrointestinal illnesses. Cases peak in winter and spring but occur year-round, even in temperate climates. The virus is transmitted through contact with infected respiratory droplets, conjunctival fluids, or stool, with symptoms developing after a 5 to 10 day incubation period. Asymptomatic shedding persists for months to years. Clinical manifestations include fever, headache, rhinorrhea, cough, conjunctivitis (Table 10-7), pharyngitis (with or without exudate), or, in the case of enteric pathogens, vomiting and diarrhea. In fact, adenovirus is second only to rotavirus as a causative organism of acute diarrhea. Severe lower respiratory disease due to adenovirus may occur in neonates and immunocompromised patients. Bronchiolitis obliterans is a rare but important complication of adenovirus

TABLE 10-7
OPHTHALMOLOGIC SYNDROMES ASSOCIATED WITH ADENOVIRUS INFECTION

Conjunctivitis associated with viral upper respiratory illness
Acute follicular conjunctivitis (isolated conjunctivitis or "pinkeye")
Pharyngoconjunctival fever (conjunctivitis accompanied by fever and sore throat)
Epidemic keratoconjunctivitis (acute follicular conjunctivitis which progresses to diffuse corneal inflammation, photophobia, lid swelling, and discharge)

pneumonia; the terminal bronchioles become irreversibly obstructed with granulation tissue, resulting in chronic obstruction and shortness of breath. Infection with adenovirus has also been associated with intussusception, myocarditis, and hemorrhagic cystitis. Rapid antigen detection is available in cases of serious disease when the diagnosis is in doubt. In most patients, adenovirus illness is mild and self-limited. Treatment is supportive.

Rotavirus

Rotavirus is an RNA virus that causes gastrointestinal illness during the winter months. The pathogen is spread by fecal-oral route and can live for a variable amount of time on surfaces; not surprisingly, it is frequently associated with diarrheal outbreaks in child care centers. Rotavirus is present in stool prior to the onset of symptoms, and shedding persists for up to two weeks. Following a 1 to 3 day incubation period, the affected individual develops greenish, watery diarrhea which lasts up to a week. The stool may rarely be streaked with blood, especially in younger patients. Vomiting often occurs early in the disease course, but fever is generally absent. Severe disease, characterized by profuse diarrhea, dehydration, electrolyte imbalances, and hypovolemic shock, is rather rare and occurs more frequently in patients younger than 12 months of age; hospitalization for intravenous rehydration is not uncommon in this age group. Rapid antigen testing of stool samples is both sensitive and specific. A previous vaccine was associated with an increased incidence of intussusception and was pulled from the market. A newer vaccine is available and recommended by the ACIP for use in infants younger than 12 weeks of age.

Norwalk Virus

Norwalk virus and Norwalk-like viruses cause acute diarrheal illnesses lasting <72 hours in most infected individuals. The pathogen is spread through the fecal-oral route and by ingestion of contaminated food (raw seafood) and water. Norwalk virus has frequently been identified in outbreaks of gastrointestinal illness in childcare centers, nursing homes, and cruise ships.

TABLE 10-8
EXAMPLES OF ENCEPHALITIS RESULTING FROM ARBOVIRUS INFECTION

Eastern equine encephalitis
Western equine encephalitis
West Nile encephalitis
Colorado tick fever

Arboviruses

Arboviruses are a significant cause of viral encephalitis (Table 10-8) and aseptic meningitis. The pathogen is transmitted through the bites of mosquitoes and ticks. Individuals who develop arbovirus encephalitis typically present with high fever, disorientation, and failure to recognize familiar people. Specific arboviruses are associated with polyarthropathy (chronic, destructive arthritis) and acute hemorrhagic fever (e.g., dengue fever). Serology is the preferred method of diagnosis. Treatment is supportive.

Hepatitis A

Hepatitis A (HAV) is responsible for about one third of cases of viral hepatitis in the United States. The virus is highly contagious and is spread through ingestion of contaminated food or water products, contact with an infected individual, in day care settings with young children still in diapers, through anal sexual activity, and by intravenous drug use. Infections in young children are generally asymptomatic or very mild; hence, they serve as an important infectious reservoir. The average incubation period is about three weeks, and infected individuals are most contagious in the two-week period surrounding the onset of symptoms. In older children and adults, hepatitis A presents with fever, malaise, headache, nausea, vomiting, and diarrhea lasting up to a week. Jaundice develops as symptoms resolve and is often accompanied by pruritus, dark-colored urine, clay-colored stools, and right upper quadrant pain. HAV does not cause chronic hepatitis but can progress to fulminant hepatitis in rare cases. Diagnosis rests on detection of serum anti-HAV IgM antibodies during acute infection (Fig. 10-2). Associated laboratory findings in acute disease include elevated levels of serum aminotransferases (AST, ALT), total and direct bilirubin, and alkaline phosphatase. Measurable serum HAV IgG indicates immunity. Intramuscular immune globulin is recommended for unvaccinated household contacts, day care attendees, food handlers, and restaurant patrons within 14 days of exposure to hepatitis A.

Hepatitis B

Hepatitis B (HBV) is transmitted through percutaneous or mucosal exposure to infectious body fluids. Intravenous drug users, those who have unprotected sex with multiple

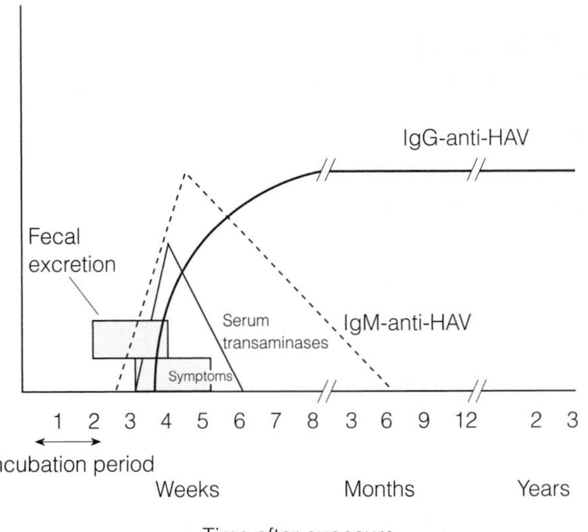

Figure 10-2 Typical course of acute hepatitis A. (From Marino BS and Fine KS. *Blueprints Pediatrics*. 4th ed. Philadelphia: Lippincott Williams & Wilkins; 2006 with permission.)

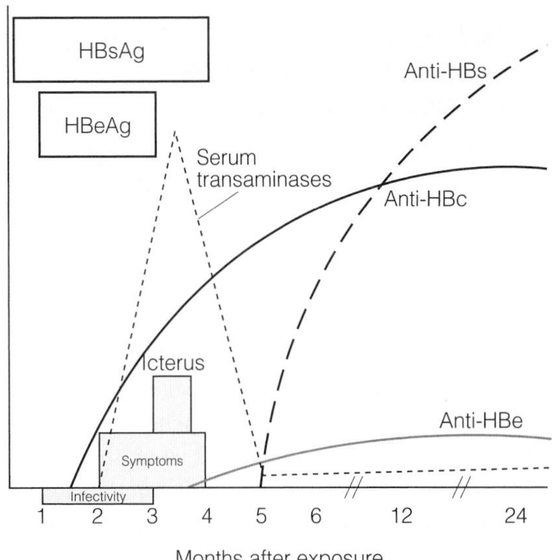

Figure 10-3 Typical course of acute hepatitis B. (From Marino BS and Fine KS. *Blueprints Pediatrics*. 4th ed. Philadelphia: Lippincott Williams & Wilkins; 2006 with permission.)

partners, medical personnel, and those who require regular blood transfusions are at increased risk for exposure to the virus. HBV is also capable of infecting the fetus of an infected mother. The average incubation period is about 8 to 12 weeks, and infected individuals are most contagious in the weeks just before and after symptoms develop. The presentation is similar to that of hepatitis A, except that symptoms generally persist for 4 to 6 weeks. Hepatitis B surface antigen (HBsAg) is the serologic hallmark of active infection with HBV; it is detectable prior to the onset of symptoms and persists for 4 to 6 months. The appearance of anti-HBs (HBV surface antigen antibody) heralds resolution of the illness and confers life-long immunity (Table 10-9, Fig. 10-3).

Perinatally-acquired HBV is usually asymptomatic; however, affected infants are at high risk for chronic disease. Detection of serum HBsAg for >6 months indicates chronic infection. Chronic persistent HBV causes minimal cellular inflammation and usually resolves within a year.

TABLE 10-9
DISEASE STATES ASSOCIATED WITH HEPATITIS B INFECTION

Test	Acute HBV	Resolved HBV	Chronic HBV
HBsAg	+	−	+
Anti-HBs	−	+	−
Anti-HBc	+	+	+
HBeAg	±	−	±
Anti-HBe	−	+	±

Anti-HBc, total antibody to hepatitis B core antigen; anti-HBe, total antibody to hepatitis B e antigen; anti-HBs, total antibody to hepatitis B surface antigen; HBeAg, hepatitis B e antigen; HBsAg, hepatitis B surface antigen; HBV, hepatitis B virus.

These individuals are asymptomatic carriers and can transmit HBV to others. Chronic active hepatitis is more aggressive, with progression to cirrhosis and, eventually, hepatocellular carcinoma. Pediatric patients with chronic HBV infection are treated with alpha-interferon and lamivudine. Universal vaccination against HBV is recommended for disease prevention.

Hepatitis C

Patients who acquire hepatitis C have an 80% chance of developing chronic hepatitis and a 15% likelihood of subsequent liver cirrhosis. Risk factors for acquiring hepatitis C include blood transfusion, intravenous drug use, multiple sexual partners, anal intercourse, and (in the neonate) maternal hepatitis C. Molecular probes are available for the diagnosis of hepatitis C. Interferon therapy is not approved for pediatric use in the United States but has been associated with improvement in the majority of treated children.

Human Immunodeficiency Virus

Human immunodeficiency virus (HIV) is an RNA virus that infects CD4+ lymphocytes, monocytes, and macrophages. The virus remains dormant until the host immune cell undergoes antigenic stimulation, whereupon it replicates, bursts from the cell, and infects other CD4+ cells. HIV is transmitted through contact with genital secretions (e.g., semen) or infected blood or blood products. The incubation period ranges from a few weeks to months or even years, allowing asymptomatic individuals who do not know that they have the disease to continue to spread the illness to others long after they become infected. The highest

TABLE 10-10
SEVERE IMMUNOSUPPRESSION AS CLASSIFIED BY THE CDC

Birth to age 12 months: CD4+ lymphocyte count <**750**/mm^3
Ages 1 to 5 years: CD4+ lymphocyte count <**500**/mm^3
≥age 6 years: CD4+ lymphocyte count <**200**/mm^3

transmission rates occur in those with high viral loads, usually found in new-onset or untreated infections.

HIV-positive patients are considered to have acquired immune deficiency syndrome (AIDS) when they have contracted an opportunistic infection OR when they reach the CD4+ criteria defined by the CDC as "severe immunosuppression" (Table 10-10). Low CD4+ counts are associated with a poorer prognosis.

Perinatal transmission is by far the most common source of pediatric HIV. The rate of newly diagnosed pediatric HIV infections has declined during the most recent decade, primarily due to widespread maternal/neonatal antiretroviral therapy (see Chapter 5), which lowers the risk of perinatal transmission from 25% to <2%. Infants of women who engage in or partner with men who engage in certain high-risk behaviors (e.g., intravenous drug use) are more likely to be infected with HIV. Currently, however, more infected infants overall are born to mothers who have acquired the disease through heterosexual contact.

At present, the rate of adolescent HIV cases is increasing in the United States. Intravenous drug use and unprotected sexual intercourse are the primary modes of transmission in adolescence and beyond. Abstinence and consistent use of barrier contraceptives (condoms) are the best methods of protection against sexual transmission of HIV. Adolescents who become infected with HIV often present within six weeks with symptoms suggestive of infectious mononucleosis; persistent systemic lymphadenopathy may be noted in others.

Overall, HIV and AIDS can present in a number of different ways, depending on the patient's age and degree of immunosuppression (Table 10-11). Children with perinatally-acquired HIV typically present between 5 and 12 months of age with pneumonia (accompanied by respiratory distress and hypoxia) which does not improve with antibiotic therapy. *Pneumocystis jiroveci*, an opportunistic pathogen, is recoverable by bronchial lavage. Treatment consists of corticosteroids and trimethoprim/sulfamethoxazole, which is then continued indefinitely as prophylaxis. Other pathogens which may present with similar radiographic and clinical features in patients with HIV include *Streptococcus pneumoniae*, *Mycoplasma* sp., *Legionella* sp., *Chlamydia*, and respiratory viruses. Identification of the causative organism is paramount and may require aggressive investigative procedures such as bronchoalveolar lavage or bronchoscopy with lung biopsy.

TABLE 10-11
TYPICAL PRESENTATIONS OF HIV BY AGE

Congenital
- Chapter 5

Perinatal (age 2 months to 2 years)
- *Pneumocystis jiroveci* pneumonia
- Lymphoid interstitial pneumonitis
- Recurrent bacterial infections (otitis media, sinusitis, pneumonia, bacteremia)
- Failure to thrive
- Refractory thrush/*Candida* diaper rash
- Petechiae, splenomegaly, thrombocytopenia, and/or systemic adenopathy

Early Childhood (ages 2 to 6 years)
- Recurrent bacterial infections (otitis media, sinusitis, pneumonia)
- Persistent, generalized lymphadenopathy

Late Childhood/Adolescence
- Candidal disease (pneumonia, esophagitis, vaginitis)
- Herpes zoster
- Cytomegalovirus retinitis
- Infection with *Mycobacterium avium-intracellulare* or *Cryptosporidium* sp.
- Severe/protracted recurrent HSV episodes
- Parotitis

Lymphoid interstitial pneumonitis (LIP) is a respiratory illness that results when an HIV-positive child becomes infected with EBV. A characteristic "honeycomb" pattern is noted on chest radiograph. The condition responds to systemic corticosteroids and oxygen therapy.

Whenever HIV is considered in a child's differential diagnosis, the history should include questions regarding:

- perinatal course and parental risk behaviors prior to and during pregnancy
- recurrent bacterial infections such as otitis media, sinusitis, bacteremia, and pneumonia
- persistent or unusual infections such as thrush or herpes zoster
- poor growth
- developmental delay or regression

Adolescents should be questioned about their sexual history, number of partners, contraceptive choices, and drug use.

HIV diagnostic studies can be divided into those which detect antibodies to the virus and those which detect the virus itself (Table 10-12). Appropriate screening tests include the OraQuick HIV rapid test and the HIV ELISA. Positive results on either test require confirmation with Western blot. Individuals who have been infected for <6 months may have negative HIV antibody tests. Patients with suspected disease who are antibody negative should be offered virus-specific testing (HIV DNA or RNA PCR) to determine if they have the disease. Individuals found to be infected with HIV are encouraged to undergo evaluation for other sexually transmitted diseases, particularly syphilis.

TABLE 10-12
USE OF DIAGNOSTIC TESTING IN THE DIAGNOSIS OF HIV/AIDS

Antibody Tests (may not be positive for up to 6 months after infection)
OraQuick HIV rapid test

HIV ELISA (enzyme-linked immunosorbent assay)

- Performed on serum samples
- Must be confirmed by Western blot (a positive HIV ELISA is not diagnostic)

Western blot

- Identifies individual antibodies to HIV antigens
- Patient with a negative Western blot does not have HIV, even if ELISA positive (unless the infection was recently acquired).
- Any patient older than 18 months of age with positive ELISA and Western blot is infected with HIV.

Viral-Specific Tests (if positive, these tests are diagnostic of HIV infection)
HIV RNA PCR (polymerase chain reaction which quantitates plasma **viral load**)

- Considered positive if viral load exceeds 10,000 copies/mL
- Considered high if viral load exceeds 100,000 copies/mL
- High viral load is associated with increased infectivity and poor prognosis.
- Used to follow the efficacy of treatment (viral load should approach zero with optimal therapy)

HIV DNA PCR

- Detects DNA in the host cell genome that has been reverse transcribed from HIV RNA
- Remains positive, even in optimally treated patients

Additional Laboratory Abnormalities Which May Be Present
Anemia, neutropenia, thrombocytopenia (bone marrow suppression)

CD4/CD8 ratio <1

Elevated immunoglobulin levels

Elevated liver enzymes

TABLE 10-13
ANTIRETROVIRAL THERAPY: CLASSIFICATIONS

Nucleoside analogue reverse transcriptase inhibitors (NRTIs) (AZT, didanosine (ddI), stavudine (d4T), lamivudine (3TC), zalcitabine (ddC), abacavir (ABV), tenofovir)

Nonnucleoside analogue reverse transcriptase inhibitors (NNRTIs) (nevirapine, efavirenz, delavirdine)

Protease inhibitors (nelfinavir, ritonavir, indinavir, saquinavir, amprenavir, lopinavir)

The CDC has recently recommended universal screening of adolescent and adult patients in the medical setting. In particular, all women who are pregnant or considering pregnancy should be tested. Any infant born to an HIV-positive woman will have a positive HIV ELISA and Western blot at birth due to passive transplacental transfer of maternal IgG. Therefore, positive HIV antibody tests are not diagnostic in any child younger than 18 months of age, and viral-specific testing is required (HIV culture, DNA or RNA PCR).

The earlier treatment is initiated, the better the outcome. Ideally, therapy is started before the patient becomes symptomatic, increasing the likelihood of maintaining a functional immune system. Three classes of antiretroviral medication are listed in Table 10-13. Initial therapy usually consists of two NRTIs and one additional medication. Regimens are changed periodically to prevent emergence of resistance. Prophylaxis against opportunistic infections should be started when the patient becomes severely immunosuppressed based on CD4+ lymphocyte count or sooner if the patient becomes infected. Live vaccines are withheld in HIV-positive patients with abnormal CD4+ counts.

In general, HIV-positive children should not be excluded from day care or school; the virus is not transmitted through saliva, tears, urine, or feces. Moreover, parental disclosure of a child's HIV status is not required by law for school attendance. All establishments attended by children should follow standard precautions to avoid contact with blood or other bodily fluids, including using gloves to clean up contaminated areas with an appropriate cleaning solution.

Rabies Virus

Rabies is an RNA virus which primarily infects the peripheral and central nervous systems. It is a zoonotic disease, passed from animal to human through infected saliva. Human-to-human transmission does not occur. In countries with strict animal immunization programs, wild animal species such as skunk, racoon, fox, wolf, and bat are the primary reservoirs of the virus. Small rodents are not a significant source of human disease because of their rapid demise following infection. In countries with little or no rabies prevention standards, humans are more likely to become infected by domestic animals such as dogs and cats. People whose occupations or travel plans place them at significant risk of rabies exposure (veterinarians, animal control workers) should receive the three-dose primary (killed virus) series, with boosters every 2 to 3 years.

The typical human case involves an extended period of incubation (1 to 3 months, but may be as long as a few years), followed by nonspecific prodromal signs and symptoms (fever, headache, malaise, vomiting, diarrhea) and possibly itching or paresthesia at the site of the bite. Over 7 to 10 days, the patient develops anxiety, personality changes, and photophobia. Neurologic signs include nuchal rigidity, seizures, paralysis, irregular breathing, and coma. Death is the near-universal outcome.

Post-exposure prophylaxis (rabies immune globulin, vaccine) should be considered for all patients who have been bitten by an animal:

- which has not been sufficiently vaccinated
- which is of unknown or undocumented vaccination status
- which is not available for evaluation (euthanasia and examination of the brain) or monitoring

Post-exposure prophylaxis should also be provided to any individual sleeping in a room found to be infested with bats, because humans have been known to acquire infection from bats without history of a known bite.

Animal wounds should be thoroughly washed and debrided. When indicated, rabies immune globulin is administered at the site of the bite and at an additional intramuscular site away from the wound. The patient is then inoculated with the rabies vaccine at the initial visit and on days 3, 7, 14, and 28 following exposure.

Antiviral Medications

Acyclovir, ganciclovir and antiviral therapy for influenza are discussed previously in specific sections.

Foscarnet is an antiviral drug which is effective against cytomegalovirus, herpes simplex virus, and varicella zoster virus. It is reserved for the treatment of acyclovir- or ganciclovir-resistant strains of these pathogens, which occur more frequently in HIV/AIDS patients (e.g., CMV retinitis). Serious adverse effects have been associated with foscarnet use, most commonly nephrotoxicity and electrolyte imbalances; serum creatinine and electrolyte levels must be monitored routinely in patients treated with foscarnet.

SPECIFIC BACTERIAL PATHOGENS

Clostridium Botulinum

C. botulinum is an anaerobic spore-forming gram-positive bacterium. It is acquired through either ingestion of spores in contaminated food/water or spore deposition in an open wound. Botulism is uncommon in the developed world; most reported cases involve infants. Risk factors for infant botulism include age ≤6 months, ingestion of honey, living in areas with extensive soil disruption and/or a high concentration of *C. botulinum* spores, and constipation. Following ingestion, the spores germinate, resulting in bacterial colonization and the release of a toxin which inhibits motor nerve acetylcholine release, effectively preventing muscle contraction. Botulism should be suspected in any infant aged 6 months or younger who presents with constipation, poor feeding, listlessness, decreased head control, a weak cry, drooling, facial asymmetry suggesting cranial nerve paralysis, and hypotonia. The physical examination may also reveal a decreased gag reflex and the loss of deep tendon reflexes. When respiratory muscles become affected, the infant develops irregular breathing followed by apnea. The symptoms progressively worsen over 1 to 2 weeks, with gradual resolution over the next month. Diagnosis rests on detection of botulinum toxin in the stool/serum or isolation of toxin-producing *C. botulinum* from the stool. As is true whenever anaerobic bacteria are suspected, special specimen collection parameters must be met to achieve successful culture. Infected infants who receive early intravenous botulinum immunoglobulin have an excellent prognosis for return to full health.

Clostridium difficile

C. difficile is a gram-positive, spore-forming anaerobic bacterium associated with nosocomial and post-antibiotic diarrheal illness. The spores are virtually ubiquitous in hospital and residential care settings. When normal colonization of the gut is compromised by antibiotic therapy, organisms from ingested spores are able to persist and elaborate toxins which cause colitis. Typical symptoms include cramping abdominal pain and watery diarrhea. Severe disease is characterized by high fever, diarrhea mixed with blood and mucous (due to pseudomembranous colitis), and significant abdominal pain and tenderness. Many patients remain asymptomatic and become infectious carriers; carriage rates in infants run as high as 25%. Diagnosis rests on detection of toxins in the stool by ELISA. Symptomatic patients are treated with metronidazole. Treatment is not indicated for infants with diarrhea who test positive for *C. difficile* toxin unless the gastrointestinal symptoms are conclusively related to the presence of the organism.

Diphtheria and Tetanus

Diphtheria is a toxin-mediated disease resulting from infection with a toxigenic strain of *Corynebacterium diphtheriae*. The current pediatric diphtheria-tetanus-pertussis vaccine contains a toxoid that produces immunity to the *C. diphtheriae* toxin. Infection with the organism can still cause mild upper respiratory or cutaneous disease. Erythromycin and penicillin are both appropriate choices for antibiotic therapy.

Tetanus (lockjaw) results from infection with the exotoxin-producing bacterium *Clostridium tetani*. The organism usually enters the body through a wound. Toxins interfere with release of neurotransmitters, leading to sustained skeletal muscle contraction and spasm of the neck and jaw muscles and vocal cords. Neonatal tetanus can occur when the mother is not immune and the umbilical cord is cut under nonsterile conditions. The aforementioned vaccine confers immunity to the toxin and severe disease; a booster should be administered every decade, or sooner if a patient presents with an open wound and no history of vaccination within the past 5 years. Nonimmune individuals who develop tetanus and are treated with antitoxin immune globulin do not develop immunity and should be vaccinated upon resolution of their illness.

Bordetella Pertussis

B. pertussis infects the ciliated respiratory epithelium and causes whooping cough in infants and young children. Infected older children and adults present with prolonged, persistent coughing in absence of other respiratory symptoms. The organism is spread through aerosolized droplets, and undiagnosed adults constitute the major reservoir. Symptoms begin 7 to 10 days after infection. The three clinical stages of pertussis include:

- the catarrhal state, characterized by nonspecific upper respiratory symptoms, during which the patient is most contagious
- the paroxysmal stage, so named because of the paroxysms of coughing which may or may not be followed by a loud "whoop" suggesting the diagnosis (note: infants younger than 6 months of age do not produce the whoop; pertussis may present with isolated apneic episodes in this population)
- the convalescent stage, lasting from when the cough begins to improve until resolution of symptoms several weeks later

The virus can be cultured from nasopharyngeal specimens but is fastidious and requires specific specimen collection and growth conditions. Direct fluorescent antibody testing is rapid but less sensitive and specific. Most but not all patients with pertussis have elevated white blood counts and lymphocytosis.

Infants with pertussis who are less than 6 months of age should be admitted to the hospital on respiratory isolation for observation and supportive care. Pertussis is treated with erythromycin estolate for 14 days (alternative therapy: trimethoprim-sulfamethoxazole). Treatment eliminates the organism (thereby interrupting infectivity) but does not affect the course of the disease unless administered during the catarrhal stage. Individuals with pertussis should be isolated or excluded from school or day care until they have completed 5 days of erythromycin. Household and close contacts, including school or day care contacts, should receive erythromycin (or azithromycin if younger than 6 weeks of age) prophylaxis, and those younger than 7 years who have not received a dose of vaccine within the past 3 years should do so. Vaccine efficacy ranges from 80% to 85%, so a significant proportion of individuals who are adequately immunized are not immune to the disease. Bronchiectasis is a rare but measurable long-term complication of pertussis pneumonia.

Listeria Monocytogenes

L. monocytogenes is an anaerobic gram-positive rod which rarely results in disease in healthy subjects but is an important cause of neonatal sepsis. *L. monocytogenes* bacteremia occurs in immunocompromised patients, who may present with bacterial meningitis. Listeriosis is usually a food-borne illness in humans; raw vegetables, unpasteurized milk, fish, poultry, beef, and particularly hot dogs and deli meats may be contaminated. Both vertical and perinatally-acquired transmission are possible in infants. The mother may experience gastrointestinal symptoms (cramping and diarrhea) or a mild flu-like illness with infection, which results in fetal demise in about 20% of cases and preterm birth in some others. Infants who survive present with early- or late-onset disease (Table 10-13). Listeriosis is diagnosed when the pathogen is cultured from a normally sterile site (blood, CSF, urine) (Table 10-14). Management consists of antibiotic therapy with ampicillin and gentamicin for 10 to 14 days (14 to 21 days for meningitis). Pregnant women should avoid soft cheeses and deli meats.

The CDC recommends the following precautions to prevent transmission of *L. monocytogenes:*

- Thoroughly wash all raw vegetables.
- Thoroughly cook all meats.
- Avoid unpasteurized dairy products.
- Keep uncooked meats separated and thoroughly clean all surfaces, knives, and cutting boards.

Haemophilus Influenzae Type B

Haemophilus influenzae type b (Hib) is an encapsulated gram-negative coccobacillus which causes invasive bacterial disease in infants and young children. The organism is spread through inhalation of or direct contact with infected respiratory secretions. Prior to the development of effective vaccines, Hib was the leading cause of bacterial meningitis and epiglottitis in children younger than 5 years of age. The attack rate was particularly high in patients younger than 18 months. Other presentations of Hib disease in this age group include pneumonia, septic arthritis, cellulitis,

TABLE 10-14
COMPARISON OF EARLY- AND LATE-ONSET PERINATAL LISTERIOSIS

Early-Onset Neonatal Listeriosis

- Mother becomes symptomatic a few days prior to delivery, which may be preterm
- Most common presentation is sepsis in an infant 1 to 3 days old
- May also present as respiratory distress syndrome/pneumonia, widespread cutaneous and internal granulomas, meningitis, or chorioamnionitis

Late-Onset Neonatal Listeriosis

- Less common than early-onset disease
- Usually no history of illness in the mother
- Most common presentation is meningitis which presents about 14 days after birth in a previously healthy full-term infant

and otitis media. Hib can be recovered and cultured from multiple sites; an initial gram-stain may suggest the diagnosis. Serotyping is necessary to confirm that the infection is caused by type b *H. influenzae*. All Hib isolates should be tested for beta-lactamase production; those which inactivate the lactam-ring require treatment with a beta-lactamase-resistant antibiotic (see "Antibiotic Therapy" later in the chapter). Latex agglutination antigen testing is used to detect Hib in the CSF but is not specific enough to exclude the possibility of infection. Invasive Hib infections require treatment for 10 to 14 days with a third-generation cephalosporin (either cefotaxime or ceftriaxone) or ampicillin and chloramphenicol. Once sensitivities are know, ampicillin alone may be sufficient. Household contacts should receive rifampin prophylaxis post-exposure if there is any infant, inadequately-immunized, or immunodeficient individual in the home. If more than two cases of Hib infection occur during a 60-day period in a child- or day care center, all attendees and employees should be given rifampin for prophylaxis, and children who are inadequately vaccinated should be identified and inoculated as well. Details regarding use of the available Hib vaccines are provided in Chapter 3. Development and routine administration of highly antigenic Hib conjugate vaccines has led to a striking decrease in the incidence of invasive Hib disease.

Streptococcus Pneumoniae

S. pneumoniae is a gram-positive encapsulated coccus with multiple serotypes. The organism is spread person-to-person by large respiratory droplets. A significant minority of young children are colonized with pneumococci at any one time, resulting in asymptomatic nasopharyngeal carriage. Carriage rates are highest in infants and children who attend day care. Pneumococcal antibiotic resistance due to altered penicillin binding sites is growing, necessitating specialized knowledge about local and individual patient resistance patterns for effective treatment. Strains which are resistant to beta-lactam antibiotics can be eradicated by those medications at higher doses in many instances.

The most common presentation of *S. pneumoniae* disease in children is otitis media. The pathogen causes up to 40% of bacterial ear infections and rarely resolves without antibiotics. *S. pneumoniae* is also responsible for a significant proportion of pediatric sinusitis and pneumonia. Patients with pneumococcal pneumonia typically appear very ill, with high fevers, tachypnea, and focal findings on chest auscultation. Consolidation is often noted on chest radiographs. Empyema is an uncommon complication but occurs more frequently with *S. pneumoniae* than other organisms. Pneumococci are known to cause several invasive disease states including:

- occult bacteremia and sepsis
- meningitis, which may be sudden or gradual in onset and has a high rate of residual neurologic complications, including sensorineural hearing loss
- septic arthritis, most commonly involving the hip or knee joint
- osteomyelitis, most commonly involving the femur or humerus

The diagnosis of pneumococcal infection is strongly suggested by Gram stain and confirmed by culture. The organism can be recovered from virtually any infected site. Positive nasopharyngeal specimens are not diagnostic of pneumococcal disease due to carriage patterns. Given the high rate of antibiotic resistance, susceptibility testing is routinely carried out on all isolates. Susceptibility reports include minimum inhibitory concentrations (MIC, the minimum concentration of a particular antibiotic that prohibits growth and reproduction of the organism) and minimum bactericidal concentrations (MBC, the minimum concentration needed to kill the pathogen). These tests do not take into account the site of infection or whether an MIC or MBC can be achieved there without substantial toxicity to the rest of the body.

Empiric treatment is based on susceptibility patterns:

- Meningitis and other invasive disease, serious pneumonia: vancomycin plus cefotaxime or ceftriaxone (vancomycin plus rifampin for allergic patients)
- Sinusitis and otitis media: high-dose amoxicillin (active against resistant strains as well at the increased dosage)

Chapter 3 provides a discussion of the heptavalent pneumococcal conjugate vaccine (PCV7) and the 23-valent pneumococcal polysaccharide vaccine (PPV23) and their proper usages. Routine vaccination of children under 24 months of age with the PCV7 vaccine (protective against serotypes 4, 6B, 9V, 14, 18C, 19F, and 23F) has resulted in a significant decrease in invasive pneumococcal disease (including meningitis) and pneumonia with these serotypes, without an corresponding increase in disease due to non-vaccine serotypes. Although there has also been a decline in vaccine serotype pneumococcal otitis media, this has been paralleled by a recognizable increase in otitis media due to other pathogens. As a group, however, children who received the PCV7 series saw a significant reduction in tympanostomy tube placement.

Neisseria Meningitidis

N. meningitidis, an aerobic gram-negative diplococcus, is an important cause of meningitis, meningococcemia, and less commonly focal infections. Five specific serotypes are responsible for the majority of invasive disease (A, B, C, Y, and W-135). The organism is transmitted through aerosolized respiratory droplets or contact with nasopharyngeal secretions from a diseased or carrier individual. The incubation period is about 3 to 5 days. Characteristic disease presentations include:

- meningitis—Almost half of patients with meningococcal bacteremia develop purulent meningitis. Signs and symptoms include the sudden onset of a high fever, headache, stiff neck, nausea/vomiting, photophobia, and mental status changes. Meningococcal meningitis has a high mortality rate, and about one in five survivors suffers serious and irreversible complications (e.g., hearing loss).

- meningococcemia—Presents with the sudden onset of high fever, petechial or purpuric rash, and systemic shock with hypotension which may progress to multiorgan failure. Acute adrenal hemorrhage is not uncommon. Meningococcemia has a high mortality rate.
- pneumonia
- septic arthritis

A Gram stain demonstrating gram-negative diplococci is highly suggestive of meningococcal disease, particularly in CSF specimens. The Gram stain is extremely useful early in the disease and/or when the patient has already been given antibiotics which may interfere with culture results. Diagnosis rests of the isolation of *N. meningitidis* from a normally sterile site. Susceptibility testing must be performed on all isolates. Antigen detection testing is variably reliable. Once the organism has been identified, penicillin is adequate for treatment in the majority of cases. However, penicillin does not reliably eradicate *N. meningitidis* from the nasopharynx, so additional therapy may be needed once the patient is in recovery.

Chemoprophylaxis is recommended for all close contacts of infected individuals, including household members, child care/nursery school contacts, and medical personnel exposed to the patient's oral secretions. Options include rifampin, ciprofloxacin, and ceftriaxone, all of which prevent or eradicate carriage.

Staphylococcus Aureus

S. aureus is a gram-positive, catalase-positive cocci transmitted person-to-person through direct contact. Hand washing is the most effective means of preventing spread. The bacteria are coagulase-positive, as opposed to *Staphylococcus epidermidis* and other coagulase-negative species. *S. aureus* frequently colonizes the skin and nasopharynx. The many clinical presentations of *S. aureus* infection include:

- skin infections—impetigo (crusted or bullous), folliculitis/furuncles/carbuncles, wound infections, cellulitis
- pneumonia, which may be complicated by empyema, pneumatoceles, and/or pyopneumothorax
- localized soft tissue (skin, muscle) or organ (renal, perinephric) abscesses, which must be drained in order for antibiotic therapy to be effective
- bacteremia and septicemia, which is associated with a high mortality rate
- endocarditis—follows *S. aureus* bacteremia; requires treatment with vancomycin or nafcillin plus gentamicin and rifampin
- Toxic shock syndrome (TSS)—a toxin-mediated infection characterized by the acute onset of high fever, vomiting, diarrhea, and myalgias. Signs on physical exam include hyperemia of the conjunctival, oral, and vaginal mucosa, strawberry tongue, and an erythematous rash; desquamation of the hands and feet occurs during recovery. Hypotension is a consistent finding, and patients may develop severe multisystem disease. As a population, menstruating women who use tampons are disproportionately affected, but TSS occurs in both genders and all age groups and can be associated with virtually any clinical presentation. Management consists of recovery of the organism for sensitivity testing, antibiotics as discussed below, drainage of any collected pus or foreign body (including a tampon), and fluids and inotropic support for hypotension.
- Staphylococcal scalded skin syndrome—dissemination of toxin-producing *S. aureus* presents as generalized painful erythroderma associated with a Nikolsky sign (blister formation or sloughing of the skin following rubbing). Mainly a disease of infants and toddlers.
- staphylococcal scarlet fever
- *Food poisoning* results from ingestion of *S. aureus* enterotoxins. Vomiting begins 2 to 6 hours after ingestion of the toxin, lasts for up to 24 hours, and may be accompanied by watery diarrhea.

Diagnosis is suggested by signs and symptoms consistent with any of the above staphylococcal diseases and recovery of gram-positive, catalase-positive, coagulase-positive organisms in clumps from a site not normally colonized with *S. aureus.* Antibiotic sensitivity testing should be performed in cases of severe or invasive disease due to emergence of resistance to beta-lactam antibiotics (i.e., MRSA). Vancomycin is appropriate empiric therapy until sensitivities are known, with clindamycin added for suspected toxin-mediated disease. If the causative organism is sensitive to beta-lactam antibiotics, nafcillin, oxacillin, or a first- or second-generation cephalosporin provides adequate coverage. MRSA infection requires a complete course of vancomycin and MRSA isolation.

Treatment of patients with mild infection or those who are ready to be switched to oral antibiotics should be guided by sensitivities. Options include first-generation cephalosporins, amoxicillin-clavulanic acid, dicloxacillin, clindamycin, or trimethoprim-sulfamethoxazole.

Staphylococcus Epidermidis

S. epidermidis is one of several species of gram-positive, catalase-positive, coagulase-negative bacteria. *S. epidermidis* is normally found on human skin. Most infections with this organism occur in relation to indwelling foreign bodies such as catheters (peripheral and central), shunts, sutures, and grafts. Other patients subject to invasive disease include immunocompromised individuals and neonatal intensive care unit patients, which may acquire nosocomial infections and present with late-onset neonatal sepsis.

Vancomycin is administered until sensitivities are known. Infections associated with implanted devices usually necessitate removal. The vast majority of blood cultures reported as positive for coagulase-negative *Staphylococcus* are contaminated at collection. However, cultures which turn positive within 24 hours, repeat cultures which grow *S. epidermidis,* and cultures drawn through an indwelling line are more likely to represent true infection.

Group A *Streptococcus*

Group A *Streptococcus* (GAS) is a gram-positive cocci which causes a myriad of infectious diseases in humans (Table 10-15). The organism is transmitted person-to-person by direct contact. The clinical presentations of two post-streptococcal illnesses, acute rheumatic fever (ARF) and postinfectious glomerulonephritis (PSGN), are provided in Table 10-16.

Treatment options are included in Table 10-17. GAS is universally sensitive to penicillin. Infected individuals remain contagious for 24 hours following initiation of therapy. Documentation of a negative throat culture is not indicated in patients who are asymptomatic following an appropriate course of antibiotics. Patients with persistent symptoms may be re-infected with a different strain of GAS, chronic carriers with intercurrent viral pharyngitis, or noncompliant with medication; these individuals should be re-cultured and treated if symptomatic and GAS-positive.

Group B *Streptococcus*

Group B *Streptococcus* (GBS), an encapsulated gram-positive diplococcus, is a significant cause of maternal and perinatal disease. The infection may be acquired in utero or during passage through the birth canal. Affected neonates present with early- or late-onset disease (Table 10-18). Blood and CSF cultures should be gathered from neonates with suspected sepsis. Diagnosis rests on culture of the pathogen from a normally sterile site. A Gram stain demonstrating gram-positive cocci suggests GBS infection. Antigen detection may be helpful in patients treated with antibiotics prior to diagnosis.

Colonization of the maternal genital tract may be chronic or intermittent. Vaginal and rectal cultures are obtained in all pregnant women between 35 and 37 weeks of gestation. Women who have had positive cultures in a

TABLE 10-15
CLINICAL PRESENTATIONS OF GROUP A *STREPTOCOCCUS*

Pharyngitis

Epidemiology: Up to one third of cases of acute pharyngitis in children are due to GAS; highest incidence in children ages 5 to 11 years

Disease course: Self-limited illness lasting 3 to 5 days even without treatment

Typical presentation: Sudden onset of fever, throat pain, headache, dysphagia, and possibly abdominal pain. Suggestive physical findings include exudative pharyngitis, palatal petechiae, inflammation of the uvula, and tender anterior cervical lymphadenopathy. May be accompanied by *scarlet fever*, a fine, red, papular sandpaper-like rash which begins on the face and neck and spreads caudally over 24 to 48 hours. The rash blanches with pressure, spares the circumoral area, and is usually more concentrated in flexor skin creases. Symptoms which are *inconsistent* with GAS pharyngitis: rhinorrhea, conjunctivitis, cough, hoarseness.

Diagnosis: Rapid antigen testing should be considered in all patients with signs and symptoms consistent with GAS pharyngitis. Negative tests require confirmation by culture. Testing is unnecessary in patients younger than 3 years of age [low incidence of acute rheumatic fever (ARF) and rheumatic heart disease (RHD)] and is discouraged for patients without classic symptoms. Individuals who are asymptomatic carriers will have positive rapid antigen and culture results but are not at risk for invasive disease or ARF and do not require treatment.

Treatment: Primary goals of treatment are reduction of suppurative complications and prevention of ARF and RHD, which is achieved when antistreptococcal medication is initiated within nine days of the start of symptoms. Antibiotic therapy also hastens resolution of symptoms and limits transmission. Treatment should be preceded by positive studies because GAS pharyngitis is over-diagnosed in the absence of testing.

Complications:

Peritonsillar abscess—more common in adolescents; presents with sore throat, muffled voice, deviation of the uvula, and bulging of the peritonsillar area on the affected side

Retropharyngeal abscess—more common in younger children, who present with classic GAS pharyngitis and hyperextension of or reluctance to move the neck. Diagnosed on radiograph or computed tomography.

Streptococcal Toxic Shock Syndrome: Typically associated with localized soft tissue infection (e.g., cellulitis). Presentation is similar to that of staphylococcal TSS: hypotension, multi-organ system disease, and, in TSS caused by GAS, a scarlatiniform rash (described above).

Other Presentations: impetigo, cellulitis, osteomyelitis, necrotizing fasciitis

Diagnosis of Invasive Disease: Gram stain from infected site or blood demonstrating gram-positive cocci in clusters and chains. Culture of an infected specimen on blood agar plate demonstrates small gray-white colonies with zones of beta-hemolysis. Beta-hemolytic organisms can be confirmed by latex agglutination or inhibition of growth around a bacitracin disc placed on the plate.

TABLE 10-16
POST-STREPTOCOCCAL SYNDROMES

Acute rheumatic fever (ARF) due to GAS pharyngitis follows a 2 to 4 week asymptomatic period. It does not occur in patients who are adequately treated. The diagnosis is made by documenting a preceding GAS infection (rising streptococcal antibody titers (antistreptolysin or antiDNAse B titers) or positive rapid antigen or culture results) in a patient who meets the revised Jones criteria:

- Patient must have one *major* and two *minor* OR two *major* criteria:
  Major: carditis, polyarthritis, chorea, erythema marginatum, subcutaneous nodules
  Minor: arthralgia, fever, elevated acute-phase reactants (ESR, CRP), prolonged PR interval

Patients with ARF are initially treated with anti-inflammatory medications (salicylates, corticosteroids) and antibiotics, then maintained on anti-GAS prophylaxis.

Postinfectious (poststreptococcal) glomerulonephritis follows GAS pharyngitis (by 3 to 4 weeks) or cellulitis (by 7 to 14 days) and results from deposition of immune complexes in the glomerulus. It can occur regardless of adequate treatment. Patients present with hematuria, hypertension, oliguria (markedly decreased urine output), and edema. Treatment is supportive. For further discussion, see Chapter 16.

previous pregnancy are presumed to be positive without additional testing. Intrapartum antibiotic prophylaxis (IAP) is indicated for women who:

- are GBS culture-positive on universal screening described above, unless the baby is born via C-section without labor or rupture of membranes
- are of unknown GBS status and have risk factors noted in Table 10-18
- had a positive GBS culture during a previous pregnancy or had a previous child infected with GBS

Ampicillin, penicillin, and cefazolin are all appropriate medications for IAP when administered ≥4 hours prior to delivery. Vancomycin is an alternative in penicillin-allergic women. The institution of routine IAP has decreased the incidence of neonatal GBS by >50%.

Enterococcus

Enterococcus is a family of gram-positive cocci which causes urinary tract infections, neonatal meningitis, peritonitis, and bacteremia-associated endocarditis. The organism is transmitted through direct fecal contamination. Most enterococci, even some resistant to vancomycin, are sensitive to ampicillin. Vancomycin resistance remains a growing problem, however; currently, no drugs capable of eradicating ampicillin/vancomycin resistant pathogens are approved for use in children. Enterococci are generally resistant to cephalosporins, aminoglycosides, ciprofloxacin, and trimethoprim-sulfamethoxazole.

Neisseria Gonorrhoeae

N. gonorrhoeae is a species of gram-negative cocci which primarily causes sexually transmitted disease. It is discussed in detail in Chapter 24.

TABLE 10-18
GBS IN THE NEONATE: EARLY- AND LATE-ONSET DISEASE

Early-Onset Disease (probably acquired in utero)
Risk Factors: maternal colonization, history of GBS urinary tract infection during pregnancy, history of previous infant with GBS, delivery prior to 37-weeks gestation, maternal intrapartum temperature >38°C, prolonged rupture of membranes (>18 hours)
Presentation: presents at birth or within the first week of life (usually before 72 hours of age) as asymptomatic bacteremia, sepsis (shock, disseminated intravascular coagulation, multiorgan system disease/failure), pneumonia (tachypnea, respiratory distress, apnea, cyanosis), empyema, or meningitis (bulging fontanelle, seizures, lethargy)
Treatment: intravenous ampicillin (plus an aminoglycoside until GBS is confirmed as the pathogen); supportive care

Late-Onset Disease (probably acquired during delivery)
Presentation: presents at 1 to 4 weeks of age with bacteremia, sepsis, meningitis, pneumonia, osteoarthritis, or soft-tissue infection
Treatment: intravenous ampicillin or high-dose penicillin (plus a third-generation cephalosporin until GBS is confirmed); supportive care

TABLE 10-17
TREATMENT OPTIONS FOR GAS

GAS Pharyngitis
Preferred: oral penicillin (250 to 500 mg b.i.d. for 10 days) or single dose of intramuscular benzathine penicillin G
Alternate: amoxicillin, erythromycin, clarithromycin, azithromycin

GAS Peritonsillar or Retropharyngeal Abscess
Preferred: incision and drainage by otolaryngologist, followed by ampicillin-sulbactam (with or without clindamycin)

Streptococcal TSS
Preferred: penicillin plus clindamycin (which has an antitoxin effect); supportive care; surgical management and debridement of infected areas

Pasturella Multocida

P. multocida is a gram-negative coccobacillus implicated in the majority of animal (particularly cat) bite wound infections in humans. Patients typically present within 24 to 48 hours of the bite with the rapid development of marked erythema, pain, swelling, and purulent discharge from the wound. Fever and regional lymphadenopathy may also be present. Complications of local cellulitic *P. multocida* infection include abscess formation, sepsis, meningitis, endocarditis, pneumonia, and (when the wound is near a joint or bone) septic arthritis and osteomyelitis. The organism is recoverable from infected sites and is diagnosed by culture. *P. multocida* is sensitive to penicillin, although patients with infected wounds are often placed on amoxicillin-clavulanic acid to provide additional coverage against anaerobic and staphylococcal organisms. Ampicillin, cefuroxime, trimethoprim-sulfamethoxazole, and doxycyline are also effective.

Borrelia Burgdorferi

B. burgdorferi is a spirochete transmitted by ticks (*Ixodes scapularis* (deer ticks) on the East Coast and in the Midwest; *Ixodes pacificus* on the West Coast). The tick must be attached to a person for at least 48 hours in order to transmit the organism. Some individuals clear the infection with no overt evidence of disease. Lyme disease presents in three clinical stages:

- Localized—*erythema migrans*, which begins as a red papule at the site of the tick bite and expands to a "bull's-eye" lesion several centimeters in diameter with clearing around a red center; Similar lesions may be seen on nearby areas of the skin. Many patients also experience nonspecific flu-like symptoms during this period, including fever, myalgias, and lymphadenopathy.
- Disseminated—intermittent arthritis, malaise, cranial nerve palsies, and atrioventricular block; The joint swelling generally affects large joints, does not restrict motion, and is not associated with fever.
- Persistent—prolonged arthritis, encephalitis, myelitis, and partial paralysis of the lower limbs; Patients with prolonged arthritis may be misdiagnosed with juvenile idiopathic arthritis.

Antibody titers (IgM and IgG) should be obtained in patients with symptoms of Lyme disease; however, these are not elevated during stage 1 disease. Positive titers require Western blot confirmation. Antibody titers are also elevated in CSF samples of patients with neurologic symptoms; pleocytosis with mononuclear cell predominance is present as well. Synovial fluid taken from patients with arthritis shows highly elevated white blood cell counts. Antibody studies indicate exposure to *B. burgdorferi*, not necessarily infection; however, as culture is only available in research laboratories, symptoms consistent with Lyme disease in a patient with elevated titers are sufficient for diagnosis. Titers should not be drawn in individuals who do not have classic symptoms of Lyme disease because of the high rate of false positives resulting from cross-reactivity with other antigens.

Patients diagnosed with Lyme disease are treated for 30 to 60 days with doxycycline if ≥8 years of age or amoxicillin if younger. Patients ≤8 years of age who are allergic to penicillin can take erythromycin. Cefuroxime or ceftriaxone is indicated for hospitalized patients requiring intravenous therapy and patients with Lyme meningitis.

Salmonella Species

Salmonella are gram-negative rods which primarily cause self-limited gastrointestinal disease. These organisms are spread through fecal-oral transmission or the ingestion of contaminated water or food. Undercooked eggs and poultry products and unpasteurized milk constitute the main sources of food-borne infection. Many "domesticated" reptiles (snakes, iguanas) and amphibians (turtles) are colonized with *Salmonella*. Following an incubation period of 1 to 3 days, most individuals develop low-grade fever, nausea, diarrhea, and cramping abdominal pain with diffuse diarrhea which may be mucoid and/or bloody. Children with severe disease present with high fever, altered sensorium, seizures, and abdominal tenderness. Neonates and immunocompromised patients are at risk for widespread dissemination, multiorgan system failure, and death. *Salmonella* species can also cause focal infections such as meningitis (more common in AIDS patients) and osteomyelitis (increased incidence in patients with sickle cell disease).

Patients with *Salmonella* gastroenteritis have blood and polymorphonuclear cells in their stool and may also have a mildly elevated white blood count. However, definitive diagnosis rests on culture results of the stool or, in cases of invasive disease, the CSF, joint fluid, or blood. Once the organism has been isolated, serotype is determined by rapid latex agglutination.

Antimicrobial therapy is not indicated for patients with isolated *Salmonella* gastroenteritis, because antibiotics do not shorten the duration of illness or prevent shedding. In contrast, antimicrobial therapy may suppress normal gut flora and prolong fecal excretion. However, infants younger than 3 months of age, those at increased risk for severe disease, and children with demonstrated *Salmonella* invasive or focal disease should be treated with ampicillin, trimethoprim-sulfamethoxazole, or chloramphenicol. Susceptibility testing is routinely performed on all isolates due to emerging resistance to the above antibiotics as well as third-generation cephalosporins.

Shigella Species

Shigella is a gram-negative bacillus that causes gastrointestinal disease in humans at a fairly low inoculum dose. The organisms are spread person-to-person, through fecal-oral transmission, and via contact with infected fomites. The attack rate is highest in young children; *Shigella* is frequently associated with outbreaks of diarrheal disease in child care centers. Following an incubation period of several days, the patient develops fever, abdominal cramping, and watery diarrhea (with or without vomiting), which progresses over the next 24 to 48 hours to symptoms of colitis. This is the classic presentation; however, disease severity ranges from mild diarrhea to severe invasive illness. Complications include seizures (presumably due to elaboration of a neurotoxin), bacteremia, and *hemolytic-uremic syndrome*.

Shigella can be isolated from stool samples; stool microscopy demonstrating large numbers of neutrophils is consistent with bacterial gastroenteritis and may be informative early in the course of illness. Isolates should undergo sensitivity testing, because antimicrobial resistance complicates treatment. Most species are susceptible to third-generation cephalosporins; once sensitivities are known, the patient may be switched to ampicillin or trimethoprim-sulfamethoxazole. Amoxicillin is not effective against *Shigella* organisms. As opposed to *Salmonella* cases, all patients diagnosed with *Shigella* infection should be treated with antibiotics; such therapy shortens the duration of symptoms and transmissibility. Children who attend preschool or child care centers should not be allowed to return until stool cultures are negative.

Yersinia Enterocolitica

Y. enterocolitica is a gram-negative bacillus frequently found in pigs and other animals. The organism is transmitted through ingestion of contaminated food (undercooked pork, unpasteurized milk) or ground water, through direct contact with an infected animal, and possibly person-to-person. Young children typically present with fever and diarrheal stools containing blood, mucous, and fecal leukocytes. A "pseudoappendicitis" syndrome consisting of fever, right lower quadrant tenderness, and leukocytosis, probably related to mesenteric adenitis, is occasionally seen in older children and adolescents. Infection with *Y. enterocolitica* has been associated with Reiter syndrome in adolescents and with the development of reactive arthritis in patients with HLA-B27 haplotype.

Y. enterocolitica can be cultured from the stool in patients with or without diarrhea. Specific culture conditions are required, so the laboratory should be notified that the organism is a possibility. Antibiotic therapy is recommended for patients with invasive disease or incompetent immune systems. When the disease is limited to enterocolitis, pseudoappendicitis, or mesenteric adenitis, antibiotics do not affect disease course or outcome but do limit transmission by shortening the duration that the organism is present in the stool. Their use in this setting is controversial. *Y. enterocolitica* is susceptible to trimethoprim-sulfamethoxazole, cefotaxime, aminoglycosides, and tetracycline but is resistant to first-generation cephalosporins and most penicillins.

Yersinia Pestis

Y. pestis is found in rodents and their fleas and usually is transmitted to humans through the bite of an infected flea. This organism causes bubonic plague and has the potential to be used as a biologic weapon. Eradication of vermin is an effective prevention strategy.

Camphylobacter Species

C. jejuni and *C. fetus* are responsible for the majority of human *Camphylobacter* disease. Patients with *Camphylobacter* gastroenteritis usually develop symptoms within 1 to 5 days of exposure to the pathogen, either through ingestion of contaminated water or food (undercooked poultry, unpasteurized milk) or via fecal-oral transmission. The inoculum dose required to produce disease is very low. *Camphylobacter* requires a specific specimen collection regimen to assure growth in culture. Treatment with erythromycin, azithromycin, or ciprofloxacin early in the course of disease is thought to decrease the duration of symptoms.

C. fetus is capable of causing severe systemic disease, including sepsis and meningitis, in the neonate. Perinatal transmission occurs during passage through an infected birth canal. Invasive disease is treated with intravenous aminoglycosides or chloramphenicol.

Helicobacter Pylori

H. pylori is a gram-negative spiral-shaped bacterium which infects the glands lining the stomach. While many affected patients remain asymptomatic, others develop peptic ulcer disease (PUD), which is uncommon in children. PUD (antral gastritis, duodenal ulcers) can present as epigastric pain, which is often worse at night; nausea and recurrent vomiting; upper gastrointestinal bleeding or melena; or anemia. Risk factors for *H. pylori* infection include living in overcrowded conditions, being of low socioeconomic status, residing in a long-term care facility or institution, and living in an underdeveloped country. The gold standard for diagnosis is recovery of the organism from endoscopic biopsy of ulcerative lesions. Rapid antigen testing is available but less sensitive and specific. The urea breath test is a less invasive method of detecting the presence of *H. pylori* but is not yet widely available and cannot be used to ascertain whether the organism is causing disease. Antibody titers are not generally very helpful in children; *H. pylori*–specific IgG is elevated in both patients who are currently infected and those who have been infected in the past but no longer harbor the organism. Eradication of the organism in a treated individual is documented by a negative *H. pylori* fecal antigen test, which should be performed on all patients 30 days after medical therapy is completed. Treatment is indicated for infected patients who also have gastritis or duodenal ulcers, but not for those with vague, unrelated gastrointestinal complaints (e.g., irritable bowel syndrome). Management consists of 14 days of any of the following regimens:

- Amoxicillin plus clarithromycin plus omeprazole
- Amoxicillin plus metronidazole plus omeprazole
- Clarithromycin plus metronidazole plus omeprazole
- Lansoprazole or another proton pump inhibitor may be substituted for omeprazole
- Note: ciprofloxacin is not an effective treatment for *H. pylori*-associated PUD.

H. pylori infection is a risk factor for the development of gastric lymphoma in adults. It is unclear whether eradication of the organism reduces that risk.

Escherichia Coli

E. coli are gram-negative bacilli. Many species of *E. coli* are part of the normal colonization of the gastrointestinal tract. Infection with enterotoxigenic *E. coli* (ETEC) follows ingestion of contaminated food or water, causing a moderate self-limited illness ("traveler's diarrhea") characterized by abdominal cramping and watery, nonbloody diarrhea. ETEC disease is rarely severe enough to require medical attention. Enteropathogenic *E. coli* (EPEC) is a toxin-producing, noninvasive strain which is associated with outbreaks of nonbloody watery diarrhea in nurseries. EPEC is also a frequent cause of diarrhea in children under the age of 12 months. The most important pathogenic strain of *E. coli* is the enterohemorrhagic 0157:H7 (Table 10-19), which is associated with *hemolytic-uremic syndrome* (HUS) in children and *thrombotic thrombocytopenic purpura* (TTP) in adolescents and adults. Infected individuals develop watery diarrhea which becomes frankly bloody over 24 to 48 hours. Nausea, vomiting, and painful abdominal cramping are present and may be accompanied by fever.

TABLE 10-19
CHARACTERISTICS OF *E. COLI* 0157:H7 (ENTEROHEMORRHAGIC *E. COLI*)

Seasonal Variance
- More common in the summer months
- Often occurs in outbreaks

Transmission
- Ingestion of food or fluids contaminated with fecal material (including poorly cooked ground beef, unpasteurized dairy products or juices, and leafy greens)
- Swimming in water contaminated with fecal material
- Direct contact with farm animals who shed the organism in their stool
- Person-to-person transmission and transmission via fecal-oral route

Incubation
- 2 to 7 days

Pathogenesis of Disease
- Localized intestinal infection with elaboration of *Shigella*-like verotoxin, which is systemically absorbed and results in widespread thrombus formation
- Associated with HUS (thrombocytopenia, hemolytic anemia, hematuria, and oliguria) and TTP, which occur within 2 to 4 weeks of the onset of symptoms

Clinical Manifestations/Severity
- Mild, watery diarrhea
- Bloody diarrhea
- Colitis (stool mixed with blood and mucous)
- Toxic megacolon (abdominal pain, distension, diffuse tenderness; fever; dehydration; may progress to septic shock)
- HUS
- TTP

Diagnosis
- Since *E. coli* species are normally present in the bowel, isolation of *E. coli* 0157:H7 requires specific testing (this species cannot ferment sorbitol, unlike other *E. coli* species)

Treatment
- Supportive care only
- Antimicrobial therapy increases the risk of HUS

Pseudomonas Aeruginosa

P. aeruginosa is a gram-negative rod associated primarily with opportunistic infections in humans. Individuals who are immunocompromised or have chronic illness, particularly patients with cystic fibrosis, can develop severe, life-threatening illness. In fact, the vast majority of cystic fibrosis patients become colonized with multiple strains of *Pseudomonas*. This organism is also an important nosocomial pathogen, frequently colonizing tracheostomy tubes and other indwelling devices in intensive care units. When the organism is recovered under these circumstances and the patient's clinical status is unchanged, colonization is more likely than infection. *Pseudomonas* can cause invasive disease in neonates, particularly those who are hospitalized. The pathogen is sensitive to oral ciprofloxacin and intravenous piperacillin-tazobactam, imipenem, ceftazidime, and the aminoglycosides.

Pseudomonas infection is uncommon in non-hospitalized, immunocompetent individuals. The organism does cause a fair amount of otitis externa, "hot tub" folliculitis, and skin and/or bone infection following a puncture wound to the foot. *P. aeruginosa* may also present as an enlarging necrotic skin lesion termed ecthyma gangrenosum.

Treponema Pallidum

Infection with *Treponema pallidum*, a spirochete, results in syphilis. The organism is transmitted through intimate sexual contact and can also cross the placental barrier to infect the fetus. Congenital syphilis is discussed in detail in Chapter 5. Acquired syphilis in the pediatric population is primarily seen in adolescents.

- Primary syphilis presents with a papule on the genitals which evolves into a painless ulcer (chancre). Chancres are highly infectious and may be associated with regional lymphadenopathy; they resolve within 4 to 6 weeks without treatment.
- Secondary syphilis is a systemic illness consisting of fever, malaise, headache, and sore throat accompanied by a characteristic nonpruritic full-body maculopapular rash which includes the palms and soles. The organism may infect the CSF (neurosyphilis) with or without symptomatology. Following clinical resolution, the virus becomes dormant; recurrences are not uncommon.
- Tertiary syphilis and its associated cutaneous, cardiovascular, and neurologic manifestations are rare in the pediatric population.
- The late manifestations of untreated congenital syphilis include the gradual onset of any of the following before the age of 20 years: bony abnormalities (forehead prominence, anterior tibial bowing, scaphoid scapula, saddle nose deformity); dental problems (including Hutchinson teeth); partial paralysis; blindness; deafness.

Testing for syphilis is either non-treponemal or treponemal (Table 10-20). *T. pallidum* is universally sensitive to penicillin, which is the treatment of choice. Patients who are allergic to penicillin should be desensitized and treated with penicillin if at all possible. Doxycycline is a less desirable alternative. Condoms reduce transmission of the disease when used as directed. Testing should be offered to and encouraged for all sexually active patients; those who test positive should also be tested for other sexually transmitted diseases, including HIV.

TABLE 10-20

SEROLOGIC TESTING FOR SYPHILIS: NON-TREPONEMAL AND TREPONEMAL STUDIES

Non-Treponemal Tests

- Include Venereal Disease Research Laboratory (VDRL) and rapid plasma reagin (RPR)
- More sensitive, less specific than treponemal tests
- Good for screening, but not specific for syphilis
- Quantitative results correlate with disease activity, so they can be used to monitor response to treatment.
- Can detect re-infection
- Positive non-treponemal test on CSF is diagnostic of neurosyphilis.
- False-positive results may occur in patients with certain autoimmune diseases.

Treponemal Tests

- Include fluorescent treponemal antibody absorption test (FTA-ABS) and microhemagglutination assay for *T.pallidum* antibodies (MHA-TP)
- Detect specific antibodies to *T. pallidum*; used to confirm results of a non-treponemal test
- Titers become positive early in infection and remain so throughout life.
- Cannot be used to monitor response to treatment

Mycobacterium Tuberculosis

M. tuberculosis, the organism which causes tuberculosis (TB), is transmitted person-to person via airborne droplets. Children with active TB are less infectious than adults. The primary site of infection is usually the lungs. Macrophages ingest the rod-shaped bacilli and transport them to regional lymph nodes, resulting in lymphadenitis. *M. tuberculosis* can spread through the bloodstream to numerous sites, resulting in a range of presentations including:

- lymphadenitis (most commonly cervical and supraclavicular nodes)
- pneumonia
- arthritis
- meningitis
- renal TB
- osteomyelitis

Pulmonary TB results from infection of the lungs and regional lymph nodes. Symptoms include a non-productive cough and occasionally constitutional complaints such as fever, chills, night sweats, and weight loss. Hilar lymphadenopathy may be impressive on chest radiograph. Focal hyperinflation, segmental atelectasis, and pleural effusions are seen later in disease. Miliary TB is a variation of pulmonary disease manifested by multiple small nodules scattered over both lung fields.

Latent TB is defined as a reactive tuberculin (Mantoux) skin test (Table 10-21) with no clinical or radiologic manifestations of the disease.

TABLE 10-21

INDURATION* CRITERIA DEFINING POSITIVE MANTOUX SKIN TESTING FOR TB*

Induration ≥5 mm is positive in:

- known close contacts of an index case
- patients with clinical (cough) or radiographic (pulmonary) evidence of disease
- patients with T cell immunodeficiencies and patients on immunosuppression therapy

Induration ≥10 mm is positive in:

- patients ≤4 years of age
- patients with chronic disease
- patients with known exposure to TB
- patients born in or recently immigrated from a country with endemic TB
- patients with recent travel to a country with endemic TB

Induration ≥15 mm is positive in:

- children >4 years of age with no known TB contacts or risk factors for disease

*Induration should be measured 48 to 72 hours after placement.

Patients with HIV/AIDS are at particular risk for the development of pulmonary and/or invasive TB, and mortality rates are substantially higher in this population. Isolates recovered from patients with depressed CD4+ cell counts have higher rates of drug resistance and are more difficult to eradicate. HIV testing should be considered for any pediatric patient who presents with TB.

Definitive diagnosis is achieved by isolation of the acid-fast bacilli from sputum or early morning gastric fluid samples. The organism can be difficult to recover, however, so in practice TB is diagnosed when a patient has a positive skin test, clinical or radiographic evidence of disease, and known TB exposure. Lowenstein-Jensen media is required for successful culture of the organism. All recovered isolates require sensitivity testing.

Management is based on sensitivity testing and sites of involvement. Immunocompetent patients with pulmonary disease should be treated with isoniazid and rifampin for 6 months plus pyrazinamide for the first 2 months. Streptomycin or ethambutol is added in patients with compromised T cell function due to the increased incidence of resistance. Patients with latent TB must complete a 9-month course of isoniazid. Individuals who are family members or close contacts of an index case should be evaluated for TB. If the initial skin test is negative, the contact individual is treated with isoniazid for 12 weeks, followed by repeat Mantoux testing; isoniazid is discontinued if the second test is also negative. Success rates are significantly higher when patients are required to take their medications in the presence of a health worker.

Airborne isolation with use of approved personal sealed respiratory devices for medical personnel is indicated for patients who require hospitalization. Children with TB who are not coughing do not produce sputum and are therefore not contagious unless cavitary lesions are noted on chest radiograph.

Medical personnel who are diagnosed with tuberculosis should be restricted based on the type of disease they have. Those who have a positive PPD but a negative chest radiograph have latent TB and do not pose a threat to other individuals; that is, they are not contagious. An individual with a positive PPD and an abnormal chest radiograph has active pulmonary tuberculosis and is highly infectious. He or she should not work until adequately treated (cough has resolved and negative sputum results on three consecutive days). All office contacts of this individual should have skin testing and chest radiographs.

Management of a newborn infant born to a woman infected with TB is detailed in Table 10-22.

TABLE 10-22
TREATMENT OF INFANTS BORN TO WOMEN WITH TUBERCULOSIS

Positive PPD, normal chest radiograph, asymptomatic	No special evaluation or therapy
Positive PPD, abnormal chest radiograph, asymptomatic	Isolation from the mother until she is placed on antituberculosis therapy
Positive PPD, abnormal chest radiograph, symptomatic	Isoniazid, rifampin, pyrazinamide, and streptomycin or kanamycin until exclusion of congenital tuberculosis and tuberculosis meningitis, then continued treatment with isoniazid
Mother infected with multi-drug resistant TB	Isolation from the mother Consider prophylactic bacillus Calmette-Guérin immunization (BCG)

Nontuberculous Mycobacteria

Nontuberculous Mycobacteria (NTB) cause a variety of diseases in immunocompetent children, including lymphadenitis, mastoiditis, cutaneous and soft tissue infections, catheter-related infections, pneumonia, and disseminated disease. *Mycobacteria avium complex* (MAC) is the most common isolate in nontuberculous infections; AIDS patients have a particularly high incidence of disseminated MAC disease. Lymphadenitis, the most common presentation of NTB infection in children, is detailed in Table 10-23. Cases of NTB lymphadenitis involving the facial nerve or parotid gland may respond to antimicrobial therapy (clarithromycin, doxycyline, trimethoprim-sulfamethoxazole, among others). Patients with invasive disease require intravenous therapy with tobramycin or amikacin. Antibiotics need to be given for long periods of time (3 to 6 months) and in combination to combat the development of resistance.

TABLE 10-23
NTB LYMPHADENITIS: PRESENTATION AND TREATMENT

Lymphadenitis

- The most common presentation of NTB infection in children
- Typically involves unilateral cervical lymph node(s)
- Needs to be distinguished from TB adenitis because the latter requires antimicrobial therapy and NTB adenitis often does not
- Child is asymptomatic; chest radiograph is normal; purified protein derivative skin test results variable due to cross-reactivity
- Treatment is complete surgical excision of the node; diagnosis confirmed through biopsy specimens; susceptibility testing of identified isolates
- Antimicrobial therapy indicated for patients with sinus tract formation; cases in which excision of the node has a high risk of damage to the facial nerve; and patients with intraparotid adenitis (in an attempt to avoid resection)
- When antimicrobial therapy is recommended, clarithromycin, in combination with rifabutin and/or ethambutol, should be continued for 3 to 6 months.
- Complications: chronic sinus tract formation; damage to facial nerve

Patients with AIDS require MAC prophylaxis (clarithromycin) once the initial infection has been treated. The preferred treatment of NTB lymphadenitis is surgical excision of the node.

Antibiotic Therapy

Resistance to first- and second-line antibiotic therapy continues to emerge. Excessive and inappropriate antibiotic use has contributed to the development of bacterial resistance in certain communities and across the country. For example, extensive use of cephalosporins as first-line therapy for uncomplicated sinusitis, pharyngitis, and otitis media has contributed to broad-spectrum antibiotic resistance.

Antibiotics effective against specific infections are previously noted.

Penicillins

Penicillins (Table 10-24) are relatively inexpensive and well-tolerated, with a low incidence of side effects. The most common complaints reported during therapy are nausea and diarrhea. Allergy to penicillins is not rare; a small percentage (≤10%) of penicillin-allergic patients are allergic to cephalosporins as well.

TABLE 10-24
PENICILLINS COMMONLY USED IN PEDIATRIC PRACTICE

	Formulations	Indications	Key Points
Natural (narrow-spectrum) Penicillins			
Penicillin V	oral	Antibiotic of choice for ■ group A *Streptococcus* pharyngitis ■ prophylaxis against acute rheumatic fever recurrences ■ treatment of syphilis in children Also used to treat ■ oral, dental infections ■ group B *Streptococcus* infections	Better gastrointestinal absorption than oral penicillin G
Penicillin G	aqueous crystalline salts (potassium, sodium)—IV or IM; require frequent dosing IM procaine penicillin G—results in low serum concentration for 12 hours IM benzathine penicillin G—results in low serum concentration for up to 4 weeks; painful injection	Indications (intravenous penicillin G salts) ■ Treatment of susceptible infections in hospitalized patients (including meningitis) ■ Aspiration pneumonia Indications (procaine penicillin G) ■ Neonatal congenital syphilis ■ Patients who need to begin a course of penicillin but cannot yet tolerate oral medications Indications (benzathine penicillin G) ■ Asymptomatic neonatal syphilis ■ Treatment of syphilis in children ■ Group A *Streptococcus* pharyngitis ■ Prophylaxis against acute rheumatic fever recurrences	Coverage identical to penicillin V

(continued)

TABLE 10-24
(continued)

	Formulations	Indications	Key Points
Narrow-Spectrum Penicillinase-Resistant* (anti-staphylococcal) Penicillins			
	intravenous dicloxacillin, oxacillin, and nafcillin (methicillin no longer used but part of this class)	Effective against pathogens listed above, as well as methicillin-sensitive *Staphylococcus aureus* (MSSA) and *Staphylococcus epidermidis*	Methicillin-resistant *Staphylococcus aureus* (MRSA) is resistant to all penicillins. Nafcillin dosing does not need to be adjusted in patients with renal failure.
AminopEnicillins (moderate-spectrum penicillins)			
Amoxicillin	oral	Spectrum of activity identical to ampicillin	Excellent gastrointestinal absorption In combination with clavulanic acid, increased activity against *Klebsiella* and *Proteus* species, *Staphylococcus aureus*, and *Haemophilus influenzae*
Ampicillin	intravenous	Effective against most streptococci, enterococci, non-β-lactamase-producing *Haemophilus influenzae*, and gram-negative enteric pathogens (e.g., *Escherichia coli*)	In combination with sulbactam, increased activity against *Klebsiella* and *Proteus* species, *Staphylococcus aureus*, and *Haemophilus influenzae*
Extended-Spectrum (antipseudomonal) Penicillins			
Piperacillin	intravenous	Effective against organisms listed for ampicillin, plus extended activity against many gram-negative organisms (*Proteus*, *Enterobacter*, and *Pseudomonas* species)	In combination with tazobactam, increased activity against *Klebsiella* species, *Staphylococcus aureus*, and *Haemophilus influenzae*
Ticarcillin	intravenous	Same as piperacillin	In combination with clavulanic acid, increased activity against *Klebsiella* species, *Staphylococcus aureus*, and *Haemophilus influenzae*

*Group of semi-synthetic penicillins effective against β-lactamases, enzymes elaborated by certain types of bacteria which inactivate the antibiotic by breaking down the β-lactam ring (common feature of all β-lactam antibiotics).

Cephalosporins

Cephalosporins come in a wide variety of oral and parenteral preparations, and the classes vary with regard to spectra of activity (Table 10-25). The most common side effects are gastrointestinal (diarrhea). Nephrotoxicity is rare; however, cephalosporin dosing must be adjusted in patients with renal insufficiency. Cefepime, a fourth generation cephalosporin with coverage similar to cefotaxime, shows promise in the treatment of pneumonia, urinary tract infections, and skin and soft tissue infections. It is also approved for use as empiric therapy in patients as young as 2 months of age with febrile neutropenia.

TABLE 10-25
CEPHALOSPORINS COMMONLY USED IN PEDIATRIC PRACTICE

	Formulations	Indications	Key Points
First-generation cephalosporins	cephalexin (oral) cefazolin (intravenous) cephalothin (intravenous)	Effective against gram-positive cocci (including methicillin-sensitive *S. aureus*, *Streptococcus pyogenes*, penicillin-susceptible *S. pneumoniae* Effective against susceptible strains of *E. coli* and *Klebsiella*, *Proteus* species Primary indication—skin and soft tissue infections, including infected wounds, cellulitis, and abscesses	Does not reach high concentrations in the CSF, so ineffective in treating meningitis
Second-generation cephalosporins	cefuxoxime axetil (oral) and cefuroxime (intravenous) cefprozil (oral) cefaclor (oral) loracarbef (oral) cefoxitin (oral)	Enhanced activity against gram-positive organisms, including some penicillin-resistant *S. pneumoniae*; however, decreased activity against *S. aureus* Effective against *H. influenzae* and *M. catarrhalis* (even when β-lactamase-producing) as well as *E. coli*, *Proteus*, *Klebsiella*, and *Citrobacter* species Indications include community-acquired pneumonia, otitis media which has failed high-dose amoxicillin therapy, and sinusitis	Cefaclor should not be used to treat otitis media, as it is relatively susceptible to inactivation by β-lactamase. Cefaclor is associated with a relatively high incidence of *serum sickness*, in which fever, rash, lymphadenopathy, and joint pain present within 7 days of completion of the medication. Serum sickness is occassionaly mistaken for a drug allergy.
Third-generation cephalosporins	cefpodoxime proxetil (oral) cefdinir (oral) ceftibutin (oral) cefotaxime (intravenous) ceftriaxone (intravenous, intramuscular) ceftazidime (intravenous)	Effective against most aerobic gram-negative bacilli (*H. influenzae*, *M. catarrhalis*, *N. meningitidis*, enteric bacilli) and *Streptococcus pneumoniae* Indications include presumed meningitis or other serious infection, persistent otitis media/sinusitis despite first- and second-line options, urinary tract infections, and Lyme disease	Third-generation cephalosporins are broad-spectrum antibiotics. Third-generation cephalosporins have excellent penetration into the CSF. Third-generation cephalosporins are less toxic than aminoglycosides, require no monitoring of levels or renal studies, and are more effective in treating deep tissue infections. Ceftazidime is effective against *Pseudomonas aeruginosa* and is frequently used in combination with an aminoglycoside to treat this pathogen in patients with cystic fibrosis Ceftriaxone should not given to infants during the first several weeks after birth due to displacement of albumin-bound bilirubin and increased risk of kernicterus

Macrolide Antibiotics

Macrolides are active against many gram-positive cocci and are the antibiotics of choice for treating *Mycoplasma pneumoniae, Chlamydia pneumoniae, and Legionella pneumoniae* in children and adolescents. The proper usage of the various forms of erythromycin and other macrolides, as well as major adverse effects and reactions, are noted in Table 10-26.

Aminoglycosides

Aminoglycosides are parenteral antibiotics effective against (mostly aerobic) gram-negative organisms such as *M. catarrhalis, H. influenzae, E, coli, Klebsiella, Proteus,* and *Enterobacter* species, and *Pseudomonas,* as well as non-tuberculosis *Mycobacterium.* Aminoglycosides are often administered in conjunction with β-lactam antibiotics to improve coverage and provide synergy. The most serious adverse effects are renal and ototoxicity. Drug levels must be maintained within a narrow therapeutic range by frequent monitoring of serum drug levels and renal function. Because some cephalosporins can displace albumin-bound bilirubin, aminoglycosides are frequently used in the neonate to avoid increasing the risk of kernicterus. Drugs in this family include gentamycin, tobramycin, and amikacin.

Tetracyclines

Pertinent facts regarding the use of tetracyclines are noted in Table 10-27.

Carbapenems

Meropenem and imipenem are broad-spectrum antibiotics, active against gram-positive, gram-negative, and anaerobic organisms. Their use should be restricted to treatment of nosocomial infections with multi-drug resistant organisms. Unfortunately, these medications (more so imipenem) appear to lower the seizure threshold, especially in patients with CSF infections.

Quinolones

Fluoroquinolones (ciprofloxacin, levofloxacin) are broad-spectrum antibiotics which are active against most gram-negative organisms. Their use is limited in children younger than 18 years of age due to the potential for damage to immature cartilage. Fluoroquinolones are primarily indicated for patients older than 18 years of age, and those younger than 18 years of age who:

- have cystic fibrosis and require oral antipseudomonal coverage
- have *Pseudomonas* urinary tract or other serious infection when no other oral antibiotic is effective
- have life-threatening infection, including meningitis, caused by multidrug-resistant gram-negative organisms

Dosing may need to be adjusted in patients receiving phenytoin, diazepam, cyclosporine, or warfarin; blood levels of these medications rise and may become toxic during treatment with a fluoroquinolone.

Vancomycin

Vancomycin is a glycopeptide antibiotic developed for the treatment of infections with gram-positive cocci (staphylococci, streptococci, enterococci). Its use has traditionally been limited to pathogens which are resistant to other

TABLE 10-26
MACROLIDES COMMONLY USED IN PEDIATRIC PRACTICE

	Indications	Adverse Effects
Erythromycin (oral and intravenous)	■ Treatment of respiratory illness resulting from susceptible strains of *Haemophilus influenzae, Moraxella catarrhalis, Streptococcus pyogenes, Chlamydia* sp., pertussis, *Legionella*, and non-tuberculosis *Mycobacterium* (MAC) ■ Alternative to penicillin; no risk of anaphylaxis in patients with penicillin allergy	Associated with the development of hypertrophic pyloric stenosis in infants Most common adverse effects: (gastrointestinal) nausea, vomiting, diarrhea, abdominal cramps Avoid in patients with pre-existing prolonged QT interval
Clarithromycin (oral)	Same as above; longer half-life, less frequent dosing (b.i.d.), fewer gastrointestinal side effects, greater bioavailability than erythromycin	
Azithromycin (oral and intravenous)	Same as above; longer half-life, less frequent dosing (qD), fewer gastrointestinal side effects, greater bioavailability than erythromycin; fewer drug interactions than erythromycin and clarithromycin	

TABLE 10-27
USE OF TETRACYCLINES IN PEDIATRIC PRACTICE

	Activity Against:	Indications	Key Points
Tetracycline	*Borrelia burgdorferi* *Rickettsia rickettsii* *Ehrlichia* species *Chlamydia trachomatis*	■ Primarily used for treatment of acne ■ Role has been largely supplanted by doxycycline	Use of tetracyclines may cause permanent discoloration of tooth enamel; important factor is total dose prior to 8 years of age. Must be taken on an empty stomach
Doxycycline	same as above	■ Uncomplicated Lyme disease ■ Pelvic inflammatory diseased, other sexually transmitted diseases (in combination with other medications) ■ Used to treat Rocky Mountain spotted fever and ehrlichiosis in patients of any age	Used more frequently than tetracycline Dosed twice a day; can be taken on an empty or full stomach Risk of dental staining is slightly less than with tetracycline, but still should be avoided if possible in children younger than 8 years of age.

antibiotics. However, vancomycin-resistant enterococci and staphylococci now exist. According to posted CDC guidelines, vancomycin should be reserved for the following:

- Serious disease caused by β-lactamase-producing gram-positive organisms
- Serious disease caused by gram-positive organisms in patients who are allergic to β-lactam antibiotics
- *Clostridium difficile* colitis unresponsive to metronidazole
- Endocarditis prophylaxis
- Prophylaxis in patients undergoing surgical insertion of a prosthetic device if the hospital has a significant rate of methicillin-resistant gram-positive infections

Other Antibiotics Commonly Used in Pediatric Practice

Table 10-28 discusses the indications for and adverse effects associated with several other antibiotics prescribed in children.

Rickettsial Disease

Rickettsia rickettsii is the gram-negative obligate intracellular organism responsible for Rocky Mountain spotted fever (RMSF). Over half of reported cases occur in North Carolina, South Carolina, Tennessee, Oklahoma, and Arkansas, mostly between April and October. The wood tick, dog tick, and Lone Star tick all serve as disease vectors. *R. rickettsii* is typically transmitted to humans through the saliva of an infected tick that has been attached for at least 12 to 24 hours.

Fever, headache, and rash are the classic signs and symptoms of RMSF. Following an incubation period of several days, the patient develops vague nonspecific constitutional signs and symptoms (fever, nausea, vomiting, malaise, myalgia, headache). The characteristic rash appears 2 to 5 days after the onset of symptoms, consisting of blanching erythematous macules which begin on the wrists and ankles and spread to the feet, soles, hands, palms, and finally the trunk within several hours. Petechiae begin to appear several days into the rash. A small proportion of infected patients do not develop a rash. The headache associated with RMSF is severe and may be accompanied by mental status changes and other signs of central nervous system or meningeal irritation. Complications include shock, disseminated intravascular coagulation, and gangrenous digits. Meningococcemia and ehrlichiosis have very similar clinical and laboratory presentations and may be confused with RMSF. Laboratory studies consistent with RMSF include hyponatremia and thrombocytopenia; the white blood count is generally normal or depressed. Specific serologic testing is helpful for diagnosis.

When RMSF is suspected, antimicrobial therapy should be initiated immediately; delay in treatment is associated with increased morbidity and mortality. The decision to treat should be based on clinical manifestations and epidemiological patterns. Doxycycline is first-line therapy in all age groups, in part because it provides coverage against both *R. rickettsii* and *Ehrlichia* organisms, and should be continued until three days after the patients becomes afebrile and substantially improved.

TABLE 10-28
OTHER ANTIBIOTICS COMMONLY USED IN PEDIATRICS

	Activity Against:	Indications	Key Points
Clindamycin (oral, intravenous)	■ Most gram-positive cocci (aerobic and anaerobic) ■ Most anaerobes ■ Certain protozoa in conjunction with other agents	■ Inhibits production of staphylococcal exotoxin (TSS) ■ Treatment of severe staphylococcal or streptococcal infections in patients allergic to penicillin ■ Treatment of presumed anaerobic infections of the lower respiratory tract, abdomen, pelvis, mouth, and teeth ■ Deep tissue infections thought to be caused by gram-positive organisms ■ Invasive group A streptococcal infections (retropharyngeal abscess; necrotizing fasciitis)	Reaches therapeutic concentrations in virtually all body fluids and tissues except CSF and bile Most common adverse side effect is diarrhea. Treatment with clindamycin can permit overgrowth of *C. difficile* in the intestines, leading to toxin production and pseudomembranous colitis.
Sulfonamides	Limited alone; synergistic when used in combination	■ Inflammatory bowel disease ■ Burn therapy ■ Umbilical cord therapy ■ Bacterial conjunctivitis	Most common adverse reaction is allergic (rash, pruritus). Use results in acute hemolysis in patients with G-6-PD deficiency (including neonates) Sulfonamide use is also associated with development of various febrile mucocutaneous syndromes (erythema multiforme; Stevens-Johnson syndrome; toxic epidermal necrolysis).
Trimethoprim-sulfamethoxazole (oral, intravenous)	■ Susceptible strains of *Streptococcus pneumoniae, Moraxella catarrhalis, Escherichia coli*, and *Klebsiella* species ■ *Pneumocystis jiroveci* ■ *Susceptible Shigella, Salmonella species*	■ Treatment of susceptible isolates in urinary tract infections; prophylaxis in children with reflux ■ Prevention and treatment of *Pneumocystis jiroveci* (PCP) in HIV/AIDS patients ■ *Shigella* gastroenteritis, as well as *Salmonella* gastroenteritis when treatment is indicated ■ Infection with methicillin-resistant *Staphylococcus aureus*	
Chloramphenicol (capsules, oral suspension, parenteral)	■ *Haemophilus influenzae* ■ *Streptococcus pneumoniae* ■ *Neisseria meningitidis*	■ Not indicated as first-line treatment for any pediatric infection ■ Used to treat pathogens at left under certain circumstances (allergic patients) ■ Typhoid fever in countries with low levels of resistance	High rate of adverse effects (dose-related bone-marrow suppression, irreversible aplastic anemia) limits use Serum concentrations are erratic and must be monitored weekly. Serum concentrations increased by concomitant use of phenytoin; decreased by phenobarbital, rifampin Acheives high concentrations in the CSF Use should be avoided in neonates (gray baby syndrome)

(*continued*)

TABLE 10-28 (continued)

	Activity Against:	Indications	Key Points
Rifampin (oral, intravenous)	■ Coagulase-positive and negative staphylococci ■ Other gram-positive cocci (*Streptococcus pyogenes*, penicillin-sensitive *Streptococcus pneumoniae*, enterococci ■ Gram-negative organisms such as *Neisseria meningitidis, Neisseria gonorrhoeae, Haemophilus influenzae* ■ *Chlamydia* species ■ *Mycobacterium tuberculosis*	■ Tuberculosis (as part of combination regimen) ■ Prophylaxis when isoniazid is contraindicated or when the organism is resistant ■ Eradication of the carrier state in close contacts of patients with invasive *Neisseria meningitidis* or *Haemophilus influenzae*	Adverse effects: stains contact lenses, turns saliva reddish-orange; hepatitis Affects blood levels of warfarin, digoxin, thyroxine, oral contraceptives, and chloramphenicol Should not be used during pregnancy

FUNGAL PATHOGENS

Candida Species

Candida albicans is normally present on the skin and in the mouth, gastrointestinal tract, and vagina of the immunocompetent individual. Factors which predispose a patient to the development of superficial (thrush, vaginitis) and systemic candidiasis include broad-spectrum antibiotic use, presence of an indwelling catheter, total parenteral nutrition, and immunodeficiency (HIV, neutropenia, diabetes) or suppression (corticosteroid use).

The treatment of candidal vulvovaginitis is discussed in Chapter 24. The agent of choice for treatment of oral or esophageal candidiasis is fluconazole. Patients with recurrent non-systemic *Candida* infections should be screened for diabetes and specific immunodeficiencies as outlined in Chapter 9.

Other Fungal Pathogens

Pertinent information regarding four additional fungal infections which may be encountered in the pediatric population (coccidiosis, aspergillosis, histoplasmosis, and sporotrichosis) is provided in Table 10-29.

ANTIFUNGAL MEDICATIONS

Amphotericin B and Flucytosine (5-FC)

Amphotericin B is a broad-spectrum antifungal agent effective against most fungal pathogens. It is the preferred initial treatment for serious Histoplasma, Coccidioides, and Aspergillus infections. The most common electrolyte abnormality associated with amphotericin B use is refractory hypokalemia, which usually occurs between 2 to 7 days of initiating therapy. Fever and chills/rigors are not uncommon during amphotericin B infusion; pretreatment with antipyretics may prevent these in susceptible patients. Nephrotoxicity is an uncommon but serious side effect. The liposomal formulation of amphotericin B must be used in patients with renal insufficiency.

Flucytosine is an antimetabolite which has antifungal activity against *Candida* species and *Cryptococcus* when used in conjunction with amphotericin B and fluconazole, respectively. Flucytosine should not be used in isolation. It is only available in an oral form, cannot be administered to patients with renal insufficiency, and requires serum level monitoring.

Azole Antifungal Agents

Azole antifungal medications are divided into imidazoles and triazoles. Ketoconazole, clotrimazole, and miconazole are imidazoles. Oral ketoconazole was used extensively for systemic fungal infections in the past but is now viewed as more of a "second-line" agent due to erratic absorption and the incidence of adverse side effects (nausea, vomiting, diarrhea, rash; hepatotoxicity). Ketoconazole also interferes with internal steroid synthesis. Fluconazole and itraconazole, two triazole agents, are now preferred for the treatment of most non-cutaneous fungal infections. Unlike ketoconazole, fluconazole has excellent CSF penetration and can be used to treat fungal meningitis. Fluconazole is effective against *Candida albicans, Histoplasma capsulatum*, and *Sporothrix schenckii*. It is the agent of choice for uncomplicated invasive fungal disease in patients who are clinically stable. The most common adverse effects are nausea, abdominal pain, vomiting, and diarrhea. Co-treatment with rifampin decreases serum levels of fluconazole. Fluconazole use increases

TABLE 10-29
ADDITIONAL PEDIATRIC FUNGAL DISEASES OF IMPORTANCE

Aspergillosis
Causative Organism: *Aspergillus* species (fungi), which is ubiquitous in the environment
Transmission: inhalation of the organism in outdoor or indoor air
Clinical Presentations
Local: *Isolated sinusitis*
Isolated pneumonia
Allergic pulmonary aspergillosis (occurs in asthmatic patients who have hypersensitivity reaction to the organism; presents as fever, wheezing, dyspnea, and productive cough)
Systemic: *Invasive pulmonary aspergillosis* (presents with fever, cough, hemoptysis, respiratory distress) *with hematogenous spread* in patients with neutropenia or immunosuppressive therapy. Infection may seed the brain, gastrointestinal tract, heart, liver, or kidneys.
Treatment: amphotericin B or azoles

Histoplasmosis
Causative Organism: *Histoplasma capsulatum*
Transmission: inhalation of spores due to disruption of soil contaminated with animal (bird or bat) droppings
Clinical Presentations
Asymptomatic infection (50%)
Local: *acute pulmonary histoplasmosis*—symptoms include abrupt onset of fever, nonproductive cough, headache, malaise, and myalgias. Patchy infiltrates and hilar adenopathy are present on chest radiograph.
Systemic: disseminated disease in immunocompromised individuals
Treatment: amphotericin B; certain azoles

Sporotrichosis
Causative Organism: *Sporothrix schenckii*
Transmission: intradermal introduction of spores from contaminated thorns or other spiky plant materials. Nursery workers are at particular risk.
Clinical Presentations
Local: lymphocutaneous sporotrichosis (initially small painless subcutaneous nodule which enlarges, becomes fluctuant, and eventually ulcerates as other subcutaneous nodules appear along tracts of lymphatic drainage)
Systemic: hematogenous dissemination leads to infection of bone (multiple lytic lesions, most commonly tibial) and/or joint (cartilage degeneration, usually involving the knee)
Treatment: guided by susceptibility studies

Coccidioidomycosis
Causative Organism: *Coccidioides* species (fungi)
Transmission: inhalation of spores due to soil disruption; generally limited to the Southwestern United States, Mexico, and Central America
Clinical Presentations
Local: acute, self-limited respiratory infection
Systemic: dissemination is uncommon in immunocompetent individuals; hematogenous seeding of skin, bone, joints, lymph nodes, adrenal glands, and/or central nervous system
Treatment: none required for local disease; amphotericin B or azoles for disseminated disease

serum levels of phenytoin, cyclosporine, and tacrolimus. Itraconazole has a broader spectrum of activity than fluconazole but penetrates poorly into the CSF.

PARASITIC INFECTIONS

Giardia lamblia

Giardiasis is a diarrheal illness that results from infection with *G. lamblia*. Cysts may be passed from person-to-person through fecal-oral transmission or fomite contact and ingested with contaminated water. A relatively low inoculum dose is required to produce symptomatic infection. Child care centers have relatively high rates of infection which may be lowered with rigorous attention to proper hand washing. Symptoms develop following a 1 to 4 week incubation period and include watery diarrhea, abdominal cramping, anorexia, and weight loss or failure to thrive. Infected individuals with asymptomatic shedding may be contagious for months. Detection of *G. lamblia* trophozoites, cysts, or antigens in the stool is diagnostic. A 5-day course of metronidazole is generally effective.

Cryptosporidium Parvum

C. parvum is spread through ingestion of contaminated water or food and fecal-oral transmission. Cryptosporidiosis is usually asymptomatic in immunocompetent children; however, some immunocompetent individuals develop diffuse watery diarrhea, abdominal cramping, and upper respiratory symptoms. The gastrointestinal symptoms may last up to 1 month. In children who are malnourished or immunodeficient, infection with *C. parvum* can result in severe diarrhea and marked dehydration requiring hospitalization or persistent diarrhea leading to malnutrition and poor growth.

Trichomonas

Trichomonas causes sexually-transmitted disease and is discussed in detail in Chapter 24.

Toxocara Infections

Species of *Toxocara* include both dog and cat roundworms. Humans become infected when they ingest contaminated soil containing roundworm eggs. Although roundworm infection can also result in asymptomatic disease, the classic presentation is visceral larva migrans (VLM), which presents with fever, hepatomegaly, and wheezing. Impressive eosinophilia and hypergammaglobulinemia are supportive evidence of disease. Diagnosis rests on serology testing. VLM is treated with anti-helminthic medication and oral steroids.

Pneumocystis Jiroveci (Carinii)

Pneumocystis jiroveci is an opportunistic pathogen which causes what is still termed PCP (pneumonia) in patients who are immunocompromised, particularly patients with leukemia, severe-combined immunodeficiency disease, or HIV/AIDS. In fact, these conditions may initially present with PCP. The diagnosis should be suspected in any patient who presents with fever and respiratory signs (tachypnea, retractions, and hypoxia) in the absence of wheezing or focal auscultory findings, especially when that patient does not improve with antibiotic therapy. Common radiographic results include hyperinflation and diffuse interstitial perihilar infiltrates. PCP is diagnosed through identification of the organism in sputum, bronchoscopy lavage washings, or bronchoalveolar biopsy samples. Most physicians treat symptoms consistent with PCP in high-risk patients without waiting for confirmatory results. Appropriate treatment regimens include systemic corticosteroids in conjunction with any of the following:

- Trimethoprim-sulfamethoxazole
- Dapsone
- Intravenous pentamidine
- Clindamycin/primaquine

Prophylactic trimethoprim-sulfamethoxazole (or dapsone) is indicated for any HIV patient with a low CD4+ cell count or prior episode of *P. jiroveci*.

Enterobius Vermicularis

E. vermicularis causes pinworms, the most common intestinal nemotode infection in the United States. Symptomatic infection is most common during young and middle childhood. Significant perianal pruritis is the predominant symptom, leading to scratching, retention of infectious eggs under the nails, and subsequent fecal-oral transmission. The eggs are not excreted in stool but are deposited on perianal tissue during the night and can be collected with adhesive tape for microscopic diagnosis. Mebendazole is usually prescribed for all family members, with another dose repeated two weeks later. Nails should be cut short, and the primary source should be bathed upon wakening to remove eggs deposited overnight.

Plasmodium (Malaria) Parasites

Infection with the protozoan parasites *P. falciparum, P. vivax, P. ovale*, or *P. malariae* causes malaria, one of the world's most common infectious diseases. The illness is most prevalent in Africa, South and Southeast Asia, northern South America, and other countries around the equator. Individuals traveling to endemic areas should refer to the CDC's Web site for information regarding which prophylactic medication is most appropriate to prevent infection with specific strains found in each geographic area and the prevalence of resistance.

Malarial organisms are transmitted through the bites of female mosquitoes. Symptoms include cyclic (every 2 to 3 days) high fevers, chills, malaise, myalgia, and arthralgia. Malaria parasites replicate within and destroy red blood cells, so hemolytic anemia and hemoglobinuria are common. Death rates are elevated in children younger than 5 years of age and pregnant women. Identification of the organism through microscopic examination of red blood cells is the gold standard; antigen testing is also available. The choice of antimalarial medication is based on the species identified and susceptibility testing (Table 10-30). Malarial organisms present in the blood more than 5 days after initiation of therapy indicate resistance to the medication chosen for treatment.

Trichinella Spiralis

Trichinosis is relatively uncommon in the United States. *Trichinella* larvae present in undercooked pork infect the lining of the small intestine. There they mature, mate, and produce additional larvae which undergo hematogenous dissemination, resulting in widespread cardiac, CNS, and muscle involvement. Following an initial period of nausea, vomiting, and diarrhea, infected individuals develop fever, muscle tenderness, and symptoms of multisystem

TABLE 10-30
ANTIMALARIAL MEDICATIONS

Chloroquine

- Inexpensive
- Well-tolerated
- Requires only a short course for treatment
- Oral and parenteral formulations available
- *P. ovale* and *P. malariae* are generally chloroquine-sensitive; however, the majority of malaria is caused by infection with *P. falciparum, P. vivax.*

Quinine

- First-line agent in children with severe disease infected with susceptible strains
- Intravenous and oral preparations; oral quinidine may be substituted if quinine not available
- Adverse effects include tinnitus, irreversible high-tone hearing loss, prolongation of the QT interval

Sulfadoxone-Pyrimethamine

- Relatively inexpensive
- Single dose treatment for some strains
- Treatment medication of choice in areas with high levels of resistance
- Not indicated for prophylaxis

Mefloquine

- Expensive
- Used in areas with high levels of resistance
- Oral formulation only
- Causes severe gastrointestinal upset, so cannot be used in patients with nausea and vomiting.

involvement. Management consists of symptomatic and supportive care and systemic corticosteroids to reduce the host inflammatory response to mass larval death.

Ascaris Lumbricoides

A. lumbricoides causes ascariasis, a common helminthic infestation. Infection follows ingestion of eggs in soil contaminated with human feces. The worms mature in the small intestine, but subsequent crops of larvae migrate to the lungs and other organs. Most infected individuals remain asymptomatic. Children are more likely to experience symptoms of infection, including colicky abdominal discomfort, abdominal distention, nausea, and occasionally vomiting. An extremely heavy worm burden may result in intestinal obstruction. Demonstration of eggs via microscopy or identification of an adult worm which has exited the nose, mouth, or anus makes the diagnosis. Treatment consists of pyrantel pamoate, mebendazole, or albendazole. The stool of household contacts should be examined for eggs as well.

Entamoeba Histolytica

E. histolytica infection causes primarily gastrointestinal amebiasis, characterized by colicky abdominal pain, tenesmus, and diarrhea which becomes mixed with blood and mucous. In young children, the disease can progress to fulminant colitis, toxic megacolon, or ulceration with frank perforation of the bowel. Dissemination of the organism is not rare; liver abscesses are the most frequent complication and should be suspected in the systemically ill patient. Liver function tests remain normal in these patients; abdominal ultrasonography is the study of choice for detecting hepatic disease. Chronic amebiasis results in clinical disease and bowel lesions which may be mistaken for inflammatory bowel syndrome. Some infected individuals remain asymptomatic but shed infectious cysts in their stool. Diagnosis relies on detection of trophozoites (spore-forming protozoans) or cysts in the stool. Symptomatic patients are treated with metronidazole followed by iodoquinol or paromomycin; either of the latter two agents is sufficient for the asymptomatic shedder.

OTHER INFECTIOUS PATHOGENS

Chlamydia Trachomatis and *Chlamydophila* Pneumoniae

Chlamydia species are obligate intracellular pathogens. *C. trachomatis* is transmitted through sexual contact and to neonates during passage through an infected birth canal. Sexually transmitted disease associated with *C. trachomatis* is discussed in detail in Chapter 24. Neonatal conjunctivitis is covered in Chapter 22. It is important to note that infants who are diagnosed with chlamydial conjunctivitis should receive systemic antibiotic therapy with oral erythromycin to avert development of pneumonia. Chlamydial pneumonia presents at 4 to 12 weeks of age with cough, congestion, tachypnea, and rales on auscultation. Fever and wheezing are typically absent. The chest radiograph may show hyperinflation. Peripheral eosinophilia is consistent with chlamydial pulmonary disease. *C. trachomatis* may also infect the vagina and rectum of the perinatally-exposed neonate; such infections are usually asymptomatic but persistent (up to 3 years) and may be mistaken for sexual abuse. Sexually-acquired chlamydial infections are generally asymptomatic in pre-adolescent children as well.

The diagnosis of chlamydial infection in infants and children rests on culture of the organism from an infected site or demonstration of inclusions by fluorescent antibody staining. Other methods are available but are either less sensitive and specific or unstudied in pediatric disease (e.g., nucleic acid amplification tests). Culture is the only appropriate method of detection for specimens gathered as forensic evidence. *C. trachomatis* is susceptible to erythromycin, tetracycline, azithromycin, doxycycline, ofloxacin, and levofloxacin.

C. pneumoniae causes atypical pneumonia which is clinically indistinguishable from Mycoplasma pneumonia, although pharyngitis may be more prominent when this pathogen is the causative agent.

Mycoplasma Pneumoniae

M. pneumoniae causes pneumonia and upper respiratory infections in children and adolescents but is an uncommon source of disease in children younger than 2 years of age. The organism is spread person-to-person through contact with infected respiratory secretions, with an incubation period of 1 to 4 weeks. Often the illness begins with low-grade fever, malaise, headache, and/or vague gastrointestinal symptoms. Cough is the most prominent symptom; it is typically non-productive and may last for several weeks. Rhinorrhea and pharyngitis are uncommon. Auscultation of the lungs may reveal wheezing and/or diffuse crackles. Extrapulmonary disease manifestations (erythematous macular skin rashes, urticaria, arthritis) occur in up to 10% of patients.

Cold agglutinin titers have been used in the past as supportive evidence of infection with Mycoplasma; however, they are no longer considered sensitive or specific enough for this purpose. Two to 3 weeks are required for culture results. Elevated serum IgM specific Mycoplasma titers (via ELISA or complement fixation) in the presence of lower respiratory disease are generally considered diagnostic. An increase in IgG titers over several weeks indicates recent infection.

The older child or adolescent with suspected *Mycoplasma* pneumonia is typically treated with a 5-day course of azithromycin; longer courses of erythromycin, clarithromycin, and tetracycline are also effective.

Bartonella Henselae

B. henselae is a gram-negative bacillus which infects cats when they are bitten by infested fleas. Higher rates of infection are found among kittens and strays. When an individual is exposed to the pathogen, often but not always through a scratch or bite, a characteristic brownish-red skin papule develops at the site of inoculation within 2 weeks, followed by regional lymphadenopathy. In fact, cat-scratch disease (CSD) is one of the most common causes of chronic lymphadenitis in children. Cervical and axillary nodes are most commonly involved, but virtually any superficial nodes may be affected. Infected individuals may have very high fevers and other non-specific symptoms such as malaise. Affected lymph nodes are typically enlarged, erythematous, and tender to palpation. The differential diagnosis of chronic lymphadenitis includes other infectious etiologies (nontuberculous *Mycobacteria*, tuberculosis, tularemia, toxoplasmosis, brucellosis), neoplasms (leukemia, lymphoma), and sarcoidosis. Immunocompetent individuals who become infected with *Bartonella* may also present with *oculoglandular syndrome* (painless conjunctival injection with preauricular lymphadenitis), hepatic microabscesses, lytic bone lesions, or encephalitis.

Immunocompromised patients are at risk for life-threatening disease due to infection with *Bartonella* organisms. In particular, individuals with HIV/AIDS can develop *bacillary angiomatosis*, an AIDS-defining illness consisting of widespread nontender, firm, red or purplish papules or flesh-colored nodules ranging from 3 to 20 mm in size. Dissemination to multiple organs is suggested by constitutional symptoms such as fever and weight loss. Timely antimicrobial treatment may prevent invasive disease in these patients.

Biopsies of skin lesions and affected lymph nodes reveal granulomas and microabscesses. The bacilli can also be detected in blood vessel walls and red blood cells, and usually stain with Warthin-Starry silver. However, the preferred method of diagnosis is demonstration of specific IgM and IgG antibodies to *B. henselae* using enzyme immunoassay or immunofluorescent antibody testing. The pathogen is fastidious and difficult to culture. Antibiotics are of no proven benefit in non-invasive, uncomplicated disease. Needle aspiration of suppurative lymph nodes may provide symptomatic relief. Most cases resolve within 4 months, but enlarged nodes may persist for years. Patients with invasive disease or bacillary angiomatosis should be treated with erythromycin or doxycycline, with or without gentamycin or rifampin. Elimination of fleas is the most effective preventive measure.

SOURCES

Adderson E. Histoplasmosis. *Pediatr Infect Dis J*. 2006;25:73–74.

Adler SP, Marshall B. Cytomegalovirus infections. *Pediatr Rev*. 2007; 28:92–100.

American Academy of Pediatrics, Committee on Infectious Diseases. *Red Book: 2006 Report of the Committee on Infectious Diseases*. Elk Grove Village, IL: American Academy of Pediatrics; 2006.

Amieva MR. Important bacterial gastrointestinal pathogens in children: A pathogenesis perspective. *Pediatr Clin North Am*. 2005;52:749–777.

Belshe RB, Edwards KM, Vesikari T, et al. Live attenuated versus inactivated influenza vaccine in infants and young children. *N Engl J Med*. 2007;356:685–696.

Burchett SK, Pizzo PA. HIV infection in infants, children, and adolescents. *Pediatr Rev*. 2003;24:186–194.

Caddle S. Enteroviruses. *Pediatr Rev*. 2003;24:186–194.

Casey JR, Pichichero ME. Metaanalysis of short course antibiotic treatment for group A streptococcal tonsillopharyngitis. *Pediatr Infect Dis J*. 2005;24:909–917.

Cavalcante SS, Mota E, Silva LR, et al. Risk factors for developing nosocomial infections among pediatric patients. *Pediatr Infect Dis J*. 2006;25:438–445.

Cheng TL. Staphylococcus epidermidis. *Pediatr Rev*. 2003;24:430–431.

Cherry JD. Epidemiology of pertussis. *Pediatr Infect Dis J*. 2006; 25:361–362.

Chesney PJ. Nontuberculous Mycobacteria. *Pediatr Rev*. 2002;23: 300–309.

Cornell T. International travel with infants and children. *Pediatr Rev*. 2005;26:306–307.

Durbin WJ. Pneumococcal infections. *Pediatr Rev*. 2004;25:358–359.

El-Kamary SS. Hepatitis A. *Pediatr Rev*. 2005;26:74–75.

Emerick K. Treatment of hepatitis C in children. *Pediatr Infect Dis J*. 2004;23:257–258.

English R. Cat-scratch disease. *Pediatr Rev*. 2006;27:123–128.

Fisher M, Hilinski J, Stephens DS. Adjuvant therapy for meningococcal sepsis. *Pediatr Infect Dis J*. 2005;24:177–178.

Goldman R. Escherichia coli. *Pediatr Rev*. 2006;27:114–115.

Gotoff SP. Group B streptococcal infections. *Pediatr Rev*. 2002;23: 381–386.

Hammerschlag MR. Chlamydia trachomatis and Chlamydia pneumoniae infections in children and adolescents. *Pediatr Rev*. 2004; 25:43–51.

Hillenbrand K. Antiviral therapy for influenza infections. *Pediatr Rev.* 2005;26:421–422.
Hyman EL. Syphilis. *Pediatr Rev.* 2006;27:37–38.
Jaggi P, Shulman ST. Group A streptococcal infections. *Pediatr Rev.* 2006;27:99–105.
Jantausch BA. Cephalosporins. *Pediatr Rev.* 2003;24:128–136.
Junker AK. Epstein-Barr virus. *Pediatr Rev.* 2005;26:79–85.
Kimberlin DW. Antiviral therapies in children: Has their time arrived? *Pediatr Clin North Am.* 2005;52:837–867.
Kimberlin DW. Diagnosis of herpes simplex virus in the era of polymerase chain reaction. *Pediatr Infect Dis J.* 2006;25:841–842.
Langley JM. Adenoviruses. *Pediatr Rev.* 2005;26:238–243.
Leach CT. Hepatitis A in the United States. *Pediatr Infect Dis J.* 2004;23:551–552.
Loeffler AM. Treatment options for nontuberculous mycobacterial adenitis in children. *Pediatr Infect Dis J.* 2004;23:957–958.
Long SS. Infant botulism and treatment with BIG-IV. *Pediatr Infect Dis J.* 2007;26:261–262.
Malik ZA. The penicillins. *Pediatr Rev.* 2006;27:471–473.
Mani CS, Murray DL. Rabies. *Pediatr Rev.* 2006;27:129–136.
Meissner HC. Reducing the impact of viral respiratory infections in children. *Pediatr Clin North Am.* 2005;52:695–710.
Moon TD, Oberhelman RA. Antiparasitic therapy in children. *Pediatr Clin North Am.* 2005;52:917–948.
Pong AL, Bradley JS. Guidelines for the selection of antibacterial therapy in children. *Pediatr Clin North Am.* 2005;52:869–894.
Posfay-Barbe KM, Wald ER. Listeriosis. *Pediatr Rev.* 2004;25:151–157.
Razzaq S, Schutze GE. Rocky Mountain spotted fever: A physician's challenge. *Pediatr Rev.* 2005;26:125–130.
Risko W. Infant botulism. *Pediatr Rev.* 2006;27:36–37.
Romero JR, Newland JG. Diagnosis of viral encephalitides: Nonzoonotic-associated viruses. *Pediatr Infect Dis J.* 2006;25:739–740.
Romero JR, Newland JG. Diagnosis of viral encephalitides: Zoonotic-associated viruses. *Pediatr Infect Dis J.* 2006;25:741–742.
Sabharwal V, Marchant CD. Fluoroquinolone use in children. *Pediatr Infect Dis J.* 2006;25:257–258.
Schutze GE. Ehrlichiosis. *Pediatr Infect Dis J.* 2006;25:71–72.
Steinbach WJ. Antifungal agents in children. *Pediatr Clin North Am.* 2005;52:895–915.
Steinbach WJ. Pediatric aspergillosis: Disease and treatment differences in children. *Pediatr Infect Dis J.* 2005;24:358–364.
Stevens DM. Giardiasis and cryptosporidiosis. *Pediatr Rev.* 2004; 25:260–261.
Tanz RR, Shulman ST. Chronic pharyngeal carriage of group A streptococci. *Pediatr Infect Dis J.* 2007;26:175–176.
Tay ET. Azole antifungal agents. *Pediatr Rev.* 2005;26:20–21.
Todd JK. Staphylococcal infections. *Pediatr Rev.* 2005;26:444–450.
Villavicencio EH. Acyclovir and ganciclovir. *Pediatr Rev.* 2005;26: 347–348.
Waggoner-Fountain LA, Grossman LB. Herpes simplex virus. *Pediatr Rev.* 2004;25:86–93.
Weinberg GA. Parainfluenza viruses: An underappreciated cause of pediatric respiratory morbidity. *Pediatr Infect Dis J.* 2006;25:447–448.
Weingarten-Arams J. Clindamycin. *Pediatr Rev.* 2002;23:149–150.
Wheeler JG, Simmons AL. Pertussis update. *Pediatr Infect Dis J.* 2005;24:829–830.
Wyatt J. Rabies—Update on a global disease. *Pediatr Infect Dis J.* 2007;26:351–352.

QUESTIONS

1. An 11-year-old patient with moderate persistent asthma presents to your office in late October for his regular health maintenance visit. He was seen about 1 year ago for an asthma check-up and was vaccinated against influenza at that visit. Which of the following lists vaccinations that should be administered to the patient at this visit?

A) Influenza, *Neisseria meningitidis,* booster tetanus-diphtheria-pertussis vaccine (adolescent preparation)
B) Influenza, and booster tetanus-diphtheria-pertussis vaccine (adolescent preparation)
C) Influenza and *Neisseria meningitidis*
D) *Neisseria meningitidis* and booster tetanus-diphtheria-pertussis vaccine (adolescent preparation)
E) No vaccinations are indicated at this time.

2. The tetravalent meningococcal conjugate vaccine is recommended for all of the following patients EXCEPT:

A) A 12-year-old male in the office for a health maintenance visit who has never been vaccinated against *N. meningitidis*
B) The 12-year-old classmates of a patient who has developed *N. meningitidis* serogroup B meningitis
C) A 15-year-old male who has never been vaccinated against *N. meningitidis*
D) A 14-year-old male entering high school who has never been vaccinated against *N. meningitidis*
E) A 17-year-old male who will be living in a college dormitory and has never been vaccinated against *N. meningitidis*

3. Which of the following statements regarding pneumococcal disease and vaccination is TRUE?

A) Immunogenicity of the heptavalent pneumococcal conjugate vaccine is limited in children under 24 months of age.
B) Universal vaccination against pneumococcal disease prior to the age of 24 months has resulted in a dramatic decrease in physician visits for otitis media.
C) Children who are appropriately vaccinated against pneumococcal disease are less likely to require tympanostomy tube placement.
D) Routine vaccination with the heptavalent pneumococcal conjugate vaccine has not resulted in a significant drop in invasive pneumococcal disease, because there has been a corresponding increase in invasive pneumococcal disease due to non-vaccine serotypes.
E) Routine vaccination with the heptavalent pneumococcal conjugate vaccine has not resulted in a significant drop in early pediatric bacteremia and meningitis, because there has been a corresponding increase in invasive *Haemophilus influenzae* disease.

4. Which of the following patients with an open wound should be vaccinated against tetanus at the initial visit for management?

A) An 8-month-old with two prior DTaP vaccinations
B) A 16-year-old with no documented diphtheria-tetanus vaccinations beyond his 5-year health maintenance visit
C) A 12-month-old who received DTaP vaccinations at ages 2, 4, and 6 months
D) A and B
E) A, B, and C

5. Which of the following statements regarding poliovirus is TRUE?

A) Wild poliovirus was successfully eradicated worldwide in the year 2000.
B) A poliovirus booster vaccine is recommended for patients who received only three doses of the oral poliovirus vaccine prior to adolescence.
C) Herd immunity is an important component of poliovirus disease prevention, as only about 80% of individuals who receive three doses of the inactivated poliovirus vaccine become immune.
D) Vaccine-associated paralytic poliomyelitis is a frequent complication of oral poliovirus vaccine administration.
E) No serious reactions or complications have been reported following administration of the modern inactivated poliovirus vaccine.

6. You are seeing a 14-year-old female in your office who is complaining of a sore throat and profound fatigue. Her illness started 1 week ago with a low-grade fever, headache, and throat pain. The fever and headache have now resolved and her sore throat is improving; however, her malaise has kept her from returning to school. On physical examination, she is afebrile with stable vital signs. You note scattered petechiae on her palate. Her spleen is mildly enlarged. Her skin appears normal, and she has no hepatomegaly or liver tenderness. Which of the following tests results is supportive of the diagnosis of infectious mononucleosis due to Epstein-Barr virus (EBV)?

A) Positive heterophile antibody test
B) Leukocytosis with an increased percentage of atypical lymphocytes
C) Elevated EBV viral capsid antigen IgG
D) A and B
E) A, B, and C

7. Which of the following statements regarding polysaccharide conjugate *Haemophilus influenzae* vaccines is FALSE?

A) The HbOC vaccine requires three doses for completion of the primary series.
B) Comvax may be used as the second dose of the primary vaccination series against hepatitis B, but the *Haemophilus influenzae* component of this combination vaccine does not count toward fulfillment of the primary Hib series.
C) The PRP-OMP requires two doses for completion of the primary series.
D) Any one of the following may be used as the 15 to 18 month booster shot for protection against *Haemophilus influenzae*: HbOC, PRP-T, PRP-OMP, and TriHIBit.
E) Comvax should not be administered to any infant younger than 6 months of age.

8. Administration of the varicella vaccine is indicated for which of the following patients?

A) A 10-year-old female with no history of disease or vaccination who was exposed to an individual with chicken pox 3 days ago
B) A 13-year-old female with no history of disease or vaccination
C) A 15-year-old female who has no history of disease or vaccination and was exposed to an individual with chicken pox 7 days ago
D) A, B, and C
E) A and B

9. A 9-year-old previously healthy male is rushed to the emergency department following a generalized tonic-clonic seizure. He was well until yesterday, when he developed a high fever and appeared ill. During the night, he became confused and agitated; emergency medical services was called when he developed right-sided spasms and weakness. The patient is lethargic but arousable in the emergency department. He has a fever of 40°C, respiratory rate of 24 breaths per minute, heart rate 144 beats per minute, and blood pressure 125/78. Which of the following test results is most likely to be present with a diagnosis of herpes simplex virus (HSV) encephalitis?

A) A markedly elevated cerebrospinal fluid white blood count with a predominance of neutrophils
B) Positive cerebrospinal fluid HSV viral cultures
C) Absolute red blood cell counts in the cerebrospinal fluid which decrease from tube 1 to tube 4
D) An electroencephalogram which demonstrates periodic lateralizing epileptiform discharges emanating from the temporal lobe
E) An unremarkable magnetic resonance imaging study of the brain

10. A 10-year-old boy who plays competitive soccer year-round presents to your office complaining of a low-grade fever, sore throat, loss of appetite, and "feeling tired." The patient is afebrile and has stable vital signs in the office. The physical examination reveals tender but discrete cervical lymphadenopathy, an erythematous pharynx, and grayish-white exudates on the tonsils. The spleen is palpable 4-cm below the left costal margin. A rapid heterophile antibody test is positive. In addition to supportive and symptomatic care, you are correct in communicating which of the following to the patient and his parent?

A) He may return to participation in organized contact sports when he has been without a fever for at least 72 hours.
B) He may return to participation in organized contact sports when he feels well enough to return to school.
C) He may return to participation in organized contact sports when his spleen is no longer palpably enlarged.
D) He may return to participation in organized contact sports when his lymphadenopathy has resolved.
E) He may return to participation in organized contact sports when he is no longer at significant risk for upper airway obstruction.

11. Which of the following patients is at greatest risk for the development of sensorineural hearing loss?

A) A 14-day-old infant with intrauterine growth retardation, hepatosplenomegaly, and CMV detected in the urine
B) A 14-day-old healthy asymptomatic infant with CMV detected in the saliva
C) A healthy asymptomatic infant with CMV detected in the saliva at 30 days of life following a negative test at 21 days of life
D) A healthy neonate born to a CMV-negative mother
E) A healthy neonate born to a CMV-positive mother

12. A 4-year-old boy has a history of unilateral swelling in his neck. He has no other symptoms. A single enlarged lymph node is palpated in the anterior cervical triangle. The child has no history of foreign travel, exposure to immigrants, or contact with recently released prison inmates. His chest radiograph is negative, but a purified protein derivative skin test is positive for induration at 12 mm. Which of the following is the most likely pathogen in this child?

A) *Mycobacteria tuberculosis*
B) Nontuberculous *Mycobacteria*
C) *Bartonella henselae*
D) *Aspergillosis*
E) *Pasturella multocida*

13. A 7-year-old male recently returned from an overnight camping trip in the North Carolina mountains. Three days following the trip, he develops a fever to 104°F. When you see him in the office the next day, he is complaining of a severe headache and photophobia. The physical examination is significant for blanching erythematous macules around the ankles and on the feet, with a few others scattered on the wrists. A complete blood count reveals a total white blood count of 7.0 X 10^3/mcL, with a differential of 60% neutrophils, 14% bands, and 36% lymphocytes. His hematocrit is 33%, with a platelet count of 45 X 10^3/mcL. Which of the following is the most appropriate choice for initial therapy in this patient?

A) Ceftriaxone and chloramphenicol
B) Ceftriaxone and tetracycline
C) Ceftriaxone and doxycycline
D) Ceftriaxone alone
E) Tetracycline alone

14. A 7-year-old patient diagnosed with Kawasaki disease is being treated with his first dose of intravenous immunoglobulin when he develops difficulty breathing, poor perfusion, and profound anxiety. The infusion is discontinued, and the patient responds to treatment for anaphylaxis. Which of the following is the most likely cause of his reaction?

A) Blood type incompatibility
B) Complement-mediated increase in vascular permeability
C) Disseminated intravascular coagulation
D) Undiagnosed selective IgA deficiency
E) Incorrect diagnosis of Kawasaki disease

15. A 35-year-old asymptomatic woman who has recently arrived in this country delivers a healthy newborn infant with a maturity rating of 37 weeks' gestation. On the second day of hospitalization, a purified protein derivative skin test placed on the mother at admission is read as "positive." Which of the following is the most appropriate immediate treatment of her asymptomatic infant, who has a negative chest radiograph?

A) No isolation from the mother is required at this time.
B) The infant should be isolated from the mother until the mother has started isoniazid.
C) The infant should be isolated from the mother until the mother has been on isoniazid for 7 days.
D) The infant should be started on isoniazid regardless of how the mother is treated.
E) The infant should be started on combination therapy regardless of how the mother is treated.

16. Which of the following cytokines is the primary chemotactic agent involved in attracting neutrophils to pathogenic organisms?

A) Interleukin-8
B) Interleukin-6
C) Interleukin-1
D) Interferon-alpha
E) Interferon-gamma

17. Which of the following illness-isolation precaution pairings is INCORRECT?

A) Measles—airborne precautions
B) Respiratory syncytial virus—airborne precautions

C) Adenovirus—droplet precautions
D) *E. coli* O157—contact precautions
E) Influenza—droplet precautions

18. A nurse has sustained a puncture wound with a needle contaminated with blood from a known HIV-positive adolescent. Which of the following is not part of the recommended protocol following needle-stick injuries?
A) The patient should be tested for hepatitis B.
B) The patient should be tested for hepatitis C.
C) The nurse's wound should immediately be covered in order to limit tissue agitation and discourage self-inoculation.
D) The nurse should be vaccinated against diphtheria and tetanus if not inoculated within the past 5 years.
E) The nurse should be tested for HIV immediately.

19. Which of the following medications is the most appropriate choice for prophylaxis against malaria in areas where drug resistance has not been detected?
A) Atovaquone-proguanil
B) Mefloquine
C) Sulfadoxone-pyrimethamine
D) Chloroquine phosphate
E) Quinine

20. Which of the following antiviral agents is recommended as prophylactic therapy to prevent CMV retinitis and blindness in the pediatric HIV-positive patient?
A) Zanamivir
B) Foscarnet
C) Cidofovir
D) Acyclovir
E) Ganciclovir

21. A healthy full-term infant is born to a woman who developed vesicular lesions consistent with primary varicella infection 3 days prior to delivery. Which of the following statements regarding varicella post-exposure prophylaxis in neonates is TRUE?
A) This infant should receive varicella-zoster immune globulin at birth and be vaccinated against varicella at the same age as his peers.
B) This infant should not receive varicella-zoster immune globulin because the maternal lesions did not develop during the period known to cause severe infection in the neonate (2 days before to 2 days after delivery).
C) This infant should be vaccinated against varicella at birth; however, this initial vaccination does not count toward fulfillment of the two-shot primary series.
D) This infant should receive varicella-zoster immune globulin and be vaccinated against varicella at birth.
E) This infant is likely to develop severe perinatal varicella-zoster infection with serious sequelae regardless of management.

22. A 9-month-old Asian infant is brought to the clinic by her foster mother because she has a cough, runny nose, and "a cold in her eyes." The patient appears uncomfortable but not toxic. Her temperature is 101.5°F. Weight is below the third percentile for age. Her length is at the 10th percentile, and her head circumference is at the 25th percentile. The physical examination is significant for marked conjunctival injection, copious mucoid nasal discharge, and small grayish-white spots with red centers scattered over her buccal mucosa bilaterally. Which of the following is the most appropriate management of this patient?
A) Immediate vaccination against measles PLUS measles immune globulin
B) Vitamin A supplementation and symptomatic care
C) Immediate vaccination against measles PLUS vitamin A supplementation
D) Measles immune globulin PLUS vitamin A supplementation
E) Vitamin A supplementation PLUS intravenous vancomycin and ceftriaxone

23. A 16-year-old young man comes to your clinic complaining of headache, right-sided earache, and facial pain. He has a temperature of 99.9°F. The physical examination is significant for bilateral clear, mobile tympanic membranes and normal canals. There is tenderness to palpation at the angle of the right jaw. You suspect mumps. Which of the following is the diagnostic study of choice for detecting infection with mumps virus?
A) Viral culture from a nasopharyngeal swab specimen
B) Viral culture from a urine specimen
C) Mumps IgM serology
D) Enzyme-linked immunosorbent assay of a nasopharyngeal swab specimen
E) Direct fluorescent antibody test of a sputum specimen

24. A 17-year-old male with T-cell leukemia has been exposed to rubella. Which of the following should be administered for post-exposure prophylaxis?
A) Standard intravenous immune globulin
B) Rubella-specific intravenous immune globulin
C) Immediate vaccination against rubella PLUS standard intravenous immune globulin
D) Immediate vaccination against rubella PLUS rubella-specific intravenous immune globulin
E) None of the above will prevent rubella in this patient.

25. Prophylaxis against respiratory syncytial virus is indicated for all but which of the following patients?
A) A 20-month-old male with bronchopulmonary dysplasia born at 32 weeks of gestation
B) A 9-month-old male with bronchopulmonary dysplasia born at 32 weeks of gestation

C) A 20-month-old currently healthy male born at 30 weeks of gestation
D) A 9-month-old male born at 30 weeks of gestation with tetralogy of Fallot
E) A 9-month-old currently healthy male born at 30 weeks of gestation

26. A 15-year-old previously healthy adolescent female presents to your office with complaints of right eye pain and blurry vision. She does not wear contacts or glasses. She had been well until 4 days ago, when she developed a fever to 102°F, malaise, mucoid rhinorrhea, and a cough. She awoke this morning with pain and tearing her right eye and unilateral blurry vision and photophobia. The physical examination is significant for folliculitis on inversion of the lower lid, lid swelling and erythema, conjunctival hyperemia, and right-sided preauricular lymphadenopathy. This clinical scenario is most consistent with infection with which of the following organisms?
A) Adenovirus
B) Echovirus
C) Parainfluenza virus
D) Influenza virus
E) Human immunodeficiency virus

27. Which of the following antigen/antibody profiles is consistent with chronic hepatitis B infection?

HBsAg: hepatitis B surface antigen
anti-HBs: hepatitis B surface antigen antibody
anti-HBc: hepatitis B core antigen antibody
HBeAg: hepatitis B envelope antigen
anti-HBe: hepatitis B envelope antigen antibody

A) HBsAg positive
anti-HBs negative
anti-HBc positive
HBeAg positive
anti-HBe negative
B) HBsAg positive
anti-HBs negative
anti-HBc positive
HBeAg positive
anti-HBe positive
C) HBsAg negative
anti-HBs negative
anti-HBc positive
HBeAg positive
anti-HBe negative
D) HBsAg positive
anti-HBs positive
anti-HBc negative
HBeAg positive
anti-HBe negative
E) HBsAg positive
anti-HBs positive
anti-HBc negative
HBeAg negative
anti-HBe negative

28. Which of the following statements regarding the use of foscarnet in pediatric patients is false?
A) Foscarnet is effective against herpes simplex virus.
B) Foscarnet is effective against cytomegalovirus.
C) Foscarnet is an acceptable alternative to acyclovir in immunocompetent adolescents with primary varicella-zoster virus infection.
D) Foscarnet is the drug of choice for HIV/AIDS patients with ganciclovir-resistant cytomegalovirus.
E) Serum creatinine and electrolyte levels should be monitored frequently in patients on foscarnet.

29. A 12-year-old previously healthy child was playing with his friends in the woods when they cornered a skunk in broad daylight. The skunk appeared injured and off-balance. The patient was bitten by the skunk on the forearm. The animal is not currently available for further evaluation. Which of the following is indicated for post-exposure prophylaxis?
A) Prophylaxis is unnecessary unless the animal remains at large for ≥7 days.
B) Post-exposure prophylaxis is unnecessary because rabies has never been recovered from a skunk.
C) Rabies vaccination today and on days 3, 7, 14, and 28
D) Rabies immune globulin and rabies vaccination today; rabies vaccination repeated on days 3, 7, 14, and 28
E) Rabies immune globulin today and on days 3, 7, 14, and 28

30. A 17-year-old female with newly-diagnosed HIV infection has a viral load of >100,000 copies. Which of the following statements concerning viral load is incorrect?
A) Viral load is a quantitative measure of free virus in the serum.
B) A viral load which exceeds 100,000 copies per mL is considered "high."
C) Patients with high viral loads are considered highly contagious.
D) The viral load is determined by HIV RNA PCR.
E) The viral load remains unchanged in optimally treated patients, but the HIV DNA PCR result approaches zero with optimal treatment.

31. A 20-month-old patient with failure to thrive and recurrent thrush has a positive HIV ELISA which is confirmed by Western blot. Which of the following statements regarding this patient is true?
A) There is no question that this patient is infected with HIV.
B) Maternal testing is unnecessary because the patient was probably infected after birth.

C) Viral-specific tests are required to determine if this patient is infected with HIV.
D) HIV testing is not indicated for this patient's asymptomatic older siblings.
E) This patient will be classified as having "severe immunosuppression" if the CD4+ count is <750 per mm^3.

32. Which of the following pairings regarding complications due to hepatitis is incorrect?
A) Hepatitis A—fulminant hepatitis
B) Hepatitis A—chronic persistent hepatitis
C) Hepatitis B—chronic persistent hepatitis
D) Hepatitis B—chronic active hepatitis
E) Hepatitis C—chronic active hepatitis

33. A 3-month-old infant presents with poor feeding and a weak cry several days after a weekend trip to his grandparents' rural home. There is no history of fever. His mother notes that he has not had a bowel movement since they returned from her parents' home. On physical examination, the patient is afebrile with stable vitals, but he is listless and hypotonic. His head rolls against his mother while he is being held upright. When specifically questioned, the mother denies feeding the infant honey, but does tell you that her father was plowing the side-fields next to the house the weekend that they were visiting in preparation for planting alfalfa hay. Which of the following laboratory results is most likely to be positive in this patient?
A) *Clostridium difficile* toxin assay of the stool
B) *Corynebacterium diphtheriae* toxin assay of the stool
C) *Clostridium botulinum* toxin assay of stool
D) *Clostridium tetani* exotoxin assay of the serum
E) *Staphylococcus aureus* toxin assay of the serum

34. A 2½-year-old previously healthy boy who presented to your office 4 days ago with cough and low-grade fever has been diagnosed with pertussis. When you phone the parents to give them the results, the mother tells you that his 5-month-old brother developed a similar cough yesterday which has now become persistent. The younger brother does not have the characteristic "whoop." He has not had any episodes of post-tussive emesis, cyanosis, or apnea. He is a former full-term infant with no significant past medical history. Which of the following is the most appropriate management of the infant at this stage of his illness?
A) Admission to the hospital for observation and supportive care; oral rifampin for 7 to 10 days
B) Admission to the hospital for observation and supportive care; oral azithromycin for 3 days
C) Admission to the hospital for observation and supportive care; oral erythromycin estolate for 7 to 10 days
D) Admission to the hospital for observation and supportive care; oral erythromycin estolate for 14 days
E) Oral erythromycin estolate for 14 days at home while on a home apnea monitor

35. A mother calls your office to report that her 16-month-old daughter brought a note home from preschool yesterday informing her parents that one of her classmates has been diagnosed with pertussis. The note instructed the parents to call her private physician regarding any necessary treatment. Her daughter is asymptomatic and up-to-date on her vaccinations. Which of the following is the most appropriate course of action regarding this patient?
A) Close observation at home while continuing to attend preschool
B) Close observation at home with isolation from preschool for 5 days
C) This child is not at risk for the development of pertussis because she has been adequately vaccinated.
D) This child is not at risk for the development of pertussis because she is not considered a close contact of the infected child.
E) Erythromycin estolate for 14 days or azithromycin for 5 days

36. Which of the following statements regarding the impact of routine use of the heptavalent pneumococcal conjugate vaccine is FALSE?
A) The addition of the heptavalent pneumococcal conjugate vaccine to the routine childhood immunization schedule has resulted in a significant decrease in total physician visits for otitis media.
B) The addition of the heptavalent pneumococcal conjugate vaccine to the routine childhood immunization schedule has resulted in a significant reduction in tympanostomy tube placement.
C) The addition of the heptavalent pneumococcal conjugate vaccine to the routine childhood immunization schedule has resulted in a significant decrease in total hospitalizations for *S. pneumoniae* pneumonia.
D) The addition of the heptavalent pneumococcal conjugate vaccine to the routine childhood immunization schedule has resulted in a significant decrease in total hospitalizations for *S. pneumoniae* meningitis.
E) The addition of the heptavalent pneumococcal conjugate vaccine to the routine childhood immunization schedule has not affected the incidence of *S. pneumoniae* pneumonia and meningitis caused by non-vaccine serotypes.

37. Which of the following studies is the test of choice for diagnosing *Haemophilus influenzae* type b meningitis?
A) Serum serology studies in conjunction with a CSF Gram stain demonstrating gram-positive coccobacilli
B) Latex agglutination antigen testing

C) Enzyme-linked immunosorbent assay
D) Direct fluorescent antibody testing
E) CSF culture

38. A 14-year-old previously healthy boy presents to the emergency department with a 1-day history of fever, chills, "feeling bad," and a rash. His temperature on presentation is 103.5°F, with a respiratory rate of 30 breaths per minute and a heart rate of 132 beats per minute. His blood pressure is 80/60. The physical examination is remarkable for an ill-appearing adolescent with wide-spread petechial lesions concentrated on the distal extremities and multiple areas of palpable purpura on the buttocks and legs. Initial laboratory results include an elevated white blood count, low-normal hemoglobin, and depressed platelet count. Gram stain of the peripheral blood demonstrates gram-negative diplococci. Which of the following organisms is most likely to be responsible for this patient's infectious illness?
A) *Haemophilus influenzae* type b
B) *Streptococcus pneumoniae*
C) *Neisseria meningitidis*
D) *Rickettsia rickettsii*
E) *Ehrlichia chaffeensis*

39. A 16-year-old female presents to the emergency department complaining of fever, vomiting, and diarrhea for 36 hours. Her vitals are as follows: temperature 103.9°F, respiratory rate 32 breaths per minute, heart rate 130 beats per minute, blood pressure 90/60 mm Hg. The physical examination is remarkable for a toxic-appearing adolescent female with hyperemia of the conjunctival and oral mucosa, a strawberry tongue, and generalized erythema of the skin. Which of the following antibiotic choices is most appropriate for initial therapy?
A) Vancomycin alone
B) Ceftriaxone alone
C) Vancomycin and cefuroxime
D) Vancomycin and clindamycin
E) Vancomycin and rifampin

40. A 23-month-old previously healthy girl is brought to your office by her mother because she has been exposed to "strep throat" at her school and is now complaining of "neck pain." She has no fever and is eating normally. On physical examination, the child's tonsils are mildly enlarged, but there is no pharyngeal erythema or inflammation. Several small, discrete, non-tender lymph nodes are palpable in the anterior cervical triangles bilaterally. Upon reviewing the child's history and physical findings, you decide that this child should not undergo rapid antigen testing for group A *Streptococcus* (GAS) pharyngitis because:
A) She is younger than 3 years of age, so she is not at risk for the development of acute rheumatic fever.
B) She is not a household contact of the infected individual.
C) She has no convincing evidence of GAS pharyngitis on exam.
D) A, B, and C
E) A and C

41. Methicillin-resistant *Staphylococcus* species are also most likely to be resistant to which of the following antibiotics?
A) Dicloxacillin
B) Vancomycin
C) Teicoplanin
D) Linezolid
E) Daptomycin

42. A 3-day-old former full-term infant with a history of a precipitous delivery presents to the emergency department with a chief complaint of fever. She was well until about 4 hours ago, when she became fussy and refused to feed. Her mother took a rectal temperature and reports that it was 100.8°F. The infant is still febrile in the emergency department. Other vital signs include a respiratory rate of 36 breaths per minute, heart rate 130 beats per minute, and blood pressure 84/50 mm Hg. The physical examination is significant for a bulging fontanelle. A lumbar puncture reveals cloudy fluid, with laboratory results as follows: CSF white blood count 2 X 10^3 per mcL (90% neutrophils); protein 65 mg per dL; glucose 40 mg per dL. Which of the following is the most appropriate empiric antibiotic regimen for this infant?
A) Cefotaxime
B) Ampicillin and cefotaxime
C) Ampicillin
D) Vancomycin and cefotaxime
E) Vancomycin and ampicillin

43. A 4-year-old patient is brought to your office on a weekend because he has an unusual rash. He has no other symptoms. His father initially noticed a red "bump" on his thigh a few days ago. This morning when he woke the child, he saw several large circular lesions in the same area. The physical exam is significant for a well-appearing young child with five "bull's-eye" lesions varying in diameter from 5 to 9 cm. Neither the father nor the child recalls a tick bite, but they do live next to a protected forested land area. Which of the following is the most appropriate initial management of this patient?
A) Ceftriaxone 50 mg per kg per day
B) Doxycycline 50 mg per kg per day

C) Amoxicillin 50 mg per kg per day
D) Doxycycline 50 mg per kg per day, with antibody titers to be drawn at this visit
E) Amoxicillin 50 mg per kg per day, with antibody titers to be drawn at this visit

44. Which of the following gastrointestinal pathogens is most likely to cause a pseudoappendicitis syndrome in an adolescent?
A) Non-typhoidal *Salmonella*
B) *Shigella* species
C) *Camphylobacter jejuni*
D) *Yersinia enterocolitica*
E) *Giardia lamblia*

45. A 17-year-old previously healthy young man with abdominal cramping and bloody diarrhea is diagnosed with non-typhoidal *Salmonella* gastroenteritis. He is afebrile and has no other symptoms. Which of the following antimicrobial agents is indicated for this patient?
A) Ampicillin
B) Trimethoprim-sulfamethoxazole
C) Chloramphenicol
D) Ceftriaxone
E) No antimicrobial therapy is indicated for this patient.

46. A 15-year-old previously healthy young lady presents with a 2-month history of epigastric discomfort and "feeling tired." She has taken over-the-counter antacids with no relief and has eliminated milk from her diet. A stool sample is positive for occult blood, and her hematocrit is 29%. Following additional studies, the patient is diagnosed with *Helicobacter pylori* infection and gastritis. Which of the following treatment regimens is indicated for first-line management of this patient?
A) Amoxicillin plus clarithromycin plus omeprazole
B) Tetracycline plus clarithromycin plus omeprazole
C) Ciprofloxacin plus clarithromycin plus omeprazole
D) Tetracycline plus clarithromycin plus lansoprazole
E) Ciprofloxacin plus clarithromycin plus lansoprazole

47. Two days after returning from a ski vacation, twin 8-year-old boys are brought to your office by their parents complaining of an itchy rash. The parents also have this rash, but the family members are otherwise asymptomatic. Yesterday, the children developed small itchy bumps scattered on the legs, trunk, arms, and abdomen and concentrated on the buttocks area. On examination, some of the papules are filled with pus, and a few on the buttocks have evolved into tender red nodules. Upon questioning, the mother tells you that the family used the resort's wooden hot tub on the last night of their stay, and that her rash seems to be worse in the areas that were covered by her bathing suit. This family's symptoms are most likely caused by which of the following organisms?
A) *Staphylococcus aureus*
B) *Pseudomonas aeruginosa*
C) Group A *Streptococcus*
D) Human papillomavirus
E) *Candida* species

48. Which of the following laboratory tests can be used to monitor response to treatment in a patient with secondary syphilis?
A) Venereal Disease Research Laboratory test (VDRL)
B) Rapid plasma reagin test (RPR)
C) Microhemagglutination assay (MHA-TP)
D) A and B
E) A, B, and C

49. A 16-year-old male HIV-negative patient in your clinic who has recently emigrated from Guatemala is diagnosed with active pulmonary tuberculosis. Which of the following is the most appropriate course of action regarding initial evaluation and treatment of his HIV-negative, asymptomatic 5-year-old sibling, who lives with him?
A) Placement of a Mantoux skin test; no treatment at this time
B) Placement of a Mantoux skin test; chest radiograph; no treatment at this time
C) Placement of a Mantoux skin test; chest radiograph; initiation of isoniazid therapy if both are negative
D) Placement of a Mantoux skin test; chest radiograph; initiation of isoniazid therapy if both are negative; isolation from school
E) Placement of a Mantoux skin test; chest radiograph; initiation of isoniazid therapy if both are negative; hospitalization

50. The addition of the beta-lactamase inhibitor clavulanic acid to amoxicillin results in increased activity against all of the following pathogens EXCEPT:
A) *Klebsiella pneumoniae*
B) *Proteus mirabilis*
C) Methicillin-sensitive *Staphylococcus aureus*
D) *Haemophilus influenzae*
E) *Pseudomonas aeruginosa*

51. Which of the following medications does not require dosing adjustment in patients with renal failure?
A) Nafcillin
B) Ampicillin
C) Ciprofloxacin
D) Acyclovir
E) Cephalexin

52. Which of the following cephalosporins has the greatest penetration into the cerebrospinal fluid?
A) Loracarbef
B) Cefotaxime
C) Cephalexin
D) Cefazolin
E) Cephalothin

53. Cefotaxime is preferred to gentamycin in the treatment of infections with *Haemophilus influenzae* type b (Hib) for which of the following reasons?
A) Gentamycin is not active against Hib.
B) Gentamycin requires blood level monitoring.
C) Cefotaxime is less toxic than gentamycin.
D) A and C
E) B and C

54. Which of the following statements regarding adverse effects related to macrolide antibiotic treatment is INCORRECT?
A) Erythromycin has been associated with the development of hypertrophic pyloric stenosis in infants.
B) Erythromycin should not be given to patients with pre-existing prolonged QT interval.
C) The most common side effects of macrolide use are gastrointestinal (nausea, vomiting, diarrhea).
D) Macrolide use has been associated with the development of kernicterus in infants.
E) All of the above are true.

55. Which of the following is the major serious adverse effect of imipenem?
A) Cardiotoxicity
B) Ototoxicity
C) Nephrotoxicity
D) Serum sickness
E) Lowering of the seizure threshold

56. The serum level of which of the following medications may be elevated into the toxic range when treatment is started with ciprofloxacin?
A) Phenytoin
B) Phenobarbital
C) Carbamazepine
D) Coumadin
E) None of the above are affected by concurrent administration of ciprofloxacin.

57. Which of the following antibiotic-serious adverse effect pairings is incorrect?
A) Chloramphenicol—gray baby syndrome
B) Ampicillin—kernicterus
C) Sulfonamides—toxic epidermal necrolysis
D) Tetracycline—dental staining
E) Erythromycin—hypertrophic pyloric stenosis

58. Which of the following medications is indicated as first-line therapy in patients with latent tuberculosis who are allergic to isoniazid?
A) Vancomycin
B) Chloramphenicol
C) Rifampin
D) Clindamycin
E) Ethambutol

59. Which of the following illnesses is virtually indistinguishable from Rocky Mountain spotted fever based on clinical course and physical examination?
A) Measles
B) Dermatomyositis
C) Systemic lupus erythematosus
D) Ehrlichiosis
E) Sporotrichosis

60. Which of the following is NOT a risk factor for the development of *Candida* infection?
A) Presence of an indwelling catheter
B) Broad-spectrum antibiotic use
C) Total parenteral nutrition
D) HIV/AIDS
E) Asymptomatic trichomoniasis

61. Flucytosine (5-FC) is inappropriate for use in all of the following patients EXCEPT:
A) A patient with renal failure
B) A patient who cannot tolerate oral medications
C) A patient with gastrointestinal malabsorption
D) A patient taking amphotericin B for treatment of invasive *Candida*
E) A patient with *Haemophilus influenzae* meningitis

62. Which of the following antifungal agents is the most appropriate medication for first-line treatment of meningitis due to *Histoplasma capsulatum*?
A) Fluconazole
B) Ketoconazole
C) Clotrimazole
D) Itraconazole
E) Miconazole

63. A mother brings her 15-month-old son to your office with complaints of watery diarrhea and cramping. About 3 weeks ago, two cases of giardiasis were reported in her son's day care center room. The patient is afebrile, and vital signs and a screening hematocrit are within normal limits. Following collection of the appropriate laboratory specimens, which of the following agents is most appropriate for treatment of this patient?
A) Ampicillin
B) Metronidazole
C) Cefotaxime
D) Fluconazole
E) Trimethoprim-sulfamethoxazole

64. A 3-year-old previously well girl is brought to the office for her second visit for fever in 1 month. She has no other symptoms but has been less active than usual for the past 2 weeks. She has gained no weight in the past three months. Her physical examination is significant for expiratory wheezing and hepatomegaly (liver edge palpable 3 cm below the right costal margin). Upon questioning, the father replies that about 3 months ago, the family took in a stray dog which has not yet been examined by a veterinarian. The dog has never been permitted inside the house. Infection with which of the following organisms is most consistent with this clinical scenario?
A) *Enterobius vermicularis*
B) *Giardia lamblia*
C) *Toxocara* roundworms
D) *Trichinella spiralis*
E) *Ascaris lumbricoides*

65. A 9-month-old former full-term infant presents to the emergency department in respiratory distress. He is currently undergoing evaluation for failure to thrive. Lung auscultation is negative for wheezing, rales, rhonchi, or focal findings. A chest radiograph demonstrates mild hyperinflation and diffuse interstitial perihilar infiltrates. The patient requires a 1 L flow of oxygen in the emergency department to maintain oxygen saturation within the normal range. He is admitted to the pediatrics unit. Following 48 hours of cefuroxime therapy, he still has an oxygen requirement, and a subsequent chest radiograph shows no improvement. Which of the following pathogens is the most likely cause of the respiratory illness in this patient?
A) *Chlamydophila pneumoniae*
B) *Streptococcus pneumoniae*
C) Methicillin-resistant *Staphylococcus aureus*
D) *Haemophilus influenzae*
E) *Pneumocystis jiroveci*

66. Management of infection with *Enterobius vermicularis* includes all of the following EXCEPT:
A) Confirmation of infection through demonstration of eggs in a stool sample
B) Oral mebendazole in a single dose, repeated 2 weeks later
C) Treatment of all household family members
D) Trimming fingernails to interfere with transmission
E) Bathing infected individuals upon rising in the morning

67. A 7-year-old patient is brought to the emergency department by the police following a report of possible sexual abuse. Which of the following methods of detection is appropriate for admission in a court of law as evidence of sexually-acquired *Chlamydia trachomatis*?
A) Nucleic acid amplification tests
B) *Chlamydia* culture
C) Fluorescent antibody staining
D) ELISA
E) IgM and IgG serologies

68. Which of the following diagnostic studies is most useful for documenting acute *Mycoplasma pneumoniae* infection in an adolescent?
A) Culture of sputum
B) Detection of acid-fast bacilli in a sputum sample
C) IgM antibody specific for *Mycoplasma pneumoniae*
D) Cold agglutinin titers
E) IgG antibody specific for *Mycoplasma pneumoniae*

69. A 3-year-old girl with fever and a rash is brought to the emergency department by her mother. Two days ago, the girl finished an antibiotic given to her by her primary care physician for a "sore throat." The physical examination is significant for swollen lymph nodes and pain with passive motion in her large joints. You suspect serum sickness. Which of the following medications is most closely associated with the development of serum sickness?
A) Nitrofurantoin
B) Penicillin G
C) Azithromycin
D) Cefaclor
E) Ciprofloxacin

70. Which of the following represents the percentage of patients allergic to penicillin who will also have a hypersensitivity reaction when given a cephalosporin?
A) 90%
B) 75%
C) 50%
D) 25%
E) ≤10%

71. You are providing a lecture about Epstein-Barr virus to a group of medical interns. In discussing diagnostic testing in a patient with suspected infectious mononucleosis, you would be correct in informing them of all the following expected laboratory results in patients of specific ages EXCEPT:
A) Absolute (>50%) lymphocytosis, all ages
B) >10% atypical lymphocytosis, all ages
C) Positive heterophile antibody, children younger than 3 years of age
D) Presence of viral capsid antigen-specific IgM, children older than 4 years of age
E) Positive heterophile antibody, children older than 8 years of age

72. You are providing a lecture about Epstein-Barr virus (EBV) to a group of medical interns. In discussing the epidemiology of the virus, you would be correct in informing them of all of the following EXCEPT:
A) Virtually all adults harbor latent EBV.
B) EBV is a herpesvirus.

C) Latent EBV resides in circulating B cells.
D) Congenital EBV is a common but benign occurrence.
E) EBV is transmitted through blood and saliva.

73. An 8-year-old previously healthy boy has clinical manifestations consistent with pharyngitis due to group A beta-hemolytic streptococci. A rapid streptococcal test is positive. In order to prevent both suppurative and nonsuppurative complications, appropriate antibiotic therapy should be initiated within how many days of the onset of symptoms?
A) 2 days
B) 3 days
C) 7 days
D) 9 days
E) 14 days

74. A 6-year-old girl has completed a 10-day course of oral penicillin V for group A beta-hemolytic streptococcal (GAS) pharyngitis. She initially presented with fever and sore throat and had a positive rapid streptococcal test. She is now asymptomatic. Her mother desires a throat culture to make sure her child is no longer infected with GAS. Which of the following is the most appropriate next course of action in this patient?
A) Obtain a throat culture for GAS if the child becomes symptomatic.
B) Obtain a throat culture for GAS at this time to document resolution of infection.
C) Obtain a throat culture for GAS at this time because the parent desires it.
D) Provide rifampin for the child to prevent carriage.
E) Counsel the mother to watch for blood in the child's urine.

75. A 5-year-old boy with an enlarged anterior cervical lymph node of three months duration is otherwise asymptomatic. Plain chest radiographs are normal, and a Mantoux skin test is reactive but not extensive enough to be classified as positive. Which of the following courses of action is indicated at this time?
A) A 3 to 6 month course of clarithromycin in combination with ethambutol
B) Open excision of the node and biopsy
C) Needle aspiration biopsy
D) Reevaluation in 1 month, or sooner if symptoms develop
E) A 4-week course of isoniazid in combination with rifampin

76. Antimicrobial therapy is indicated for the treatment of atypical *Mycobacteria* lymphadenitis in all of the following patients EXCEPT:
A) A 3-year-old boy who has undergone excisional biopsy of the node, with subsequent isolation of *Mycobacterium avium complex* organisms which are resistant to isoniazid
B) A 3-year-old boy who is HIV-positive and has undergone excisional biopsy of the node
C) A 4-year-old girl with a chronic drainage from an associated sinus tract
D) A 4-year-old boy with intraparotid adenitis
E) A 5-year-old girl with involvement of a node in close proximity to the facial nerve

ANSWERS

1. A	27. B	53. E
2. B	28. C	54. D
3. C	29. D	55. E
4. D	30. E	56. A
5. E	31. A	57. B
6. E	32. B	58. C
7. B	33. C	59. D
8. E	34. D	60. E
9. D	35. E	61. D
10. C	36. A	62. A
11. A	37. B	63. B
12. B	38. C	64. C
13. C	39. D	65. E
14. D	40. E	66. A
15. A	41. A	67. B
16. A	42. B	68. C
17. B	43. C	69. D
18. C	44. D	70. E
19. D	45. E	71. C
20. E	46. A	72. D
21. A	47. B	73. D
22. B	48. D	74. A
23. C	49. C	75. B
24. E	50. E	76. A
25. D	51. A	
26. A	52. B	

Endocrine Disorders

11

DISORDERS OF SEX DIFFERENTIATION

Persistent Müllerian Duct Syndrome

Male fetal masculinization occurs during a critical period between 8 and 12 weeks of gestation, the time of peak testosterone secretion by Leydig cells in the fetal testes. Müllerian-inhibiting substance (MIS) is a hormone secreted by the Sertoli cells in the fetal testis that prompts involution of the embryologic precursors of the internal duct system (the cervix, uterine, and fallopian tubes). *Persistent müllerian duct syndrome* is an autosomal recessive disorder in which MIS or MIS receptors are absent or otherwise nonfunctional. Affected patients have an XY chromosomal pattern and normal external genitalia, although the testes may not be fully descended. Patients with normal testes who retain patency of the vas deferens (e.g., patients whose gonads descend and thus do not have to be surgically removed) progress through typical puberty and have normal sexual function. Unfortunately, a significant minority of patients are infertile. Rudimentary fallopian tubes or a uterus may be discovered during incidental abdominal surgery.

Congenital Adrenal Hyperplasia

Congenital adrenal hyperplasia (CAH) consists of a group of autosomal recessive defects involving enzymes engaged in the conversion of cholesterol to aldosterone, cortisol, testosterone, and estradiol (Fig. 11-1). In the fetus, a block in the cortisol synthesis pathway leads to: (a) a compensatory increase in adrenocorticotropin (ACTH) secretion with resultant adrenal hyperplasia, and (b) overproduction of adrenal hormone precursors such as androgens. Over 90% of CAH results from *21-hydroxylase deficiency*. Patients with 21-hydroxylase deficiency do not produce sufficient end products of the glucocorticoid (cortisol) and occasionally mineralocorticoid (aldosterone) pathways. Even at birth, they have dramatically increased serum levels of *17-hydroxyprogesterone*. Many state newborn screening programs detect elevated 17-hydroxyprogesterone levels, but none screen for other varieties of CAH such as 11 β-hydroxylase deficiency (~6%).

The presentation of CAH depends in part on where the enzyme block occurs and which precursors accumulate. Patients may remain asymptomatic until physiologically stressed, develop signs of disease in adolescence or adulthood, or present with life-threatening adrenal crisis within days of birth. 21-Hydroxylase deficiency occurs in two forms:

- *Classic virilizing adrenal hyperplasia*—Females are born with varying degrees of virilization and ambiguous genitalia due to excess androgen production, resulting in diagnosis soon after birth. Male infants have normal genitalia at birth; early identification depends on newborn screening.
- *Salt-wasting form*—Patients with salt-wasting 21-hydroxylase deficiency who are not identified by ambiguous genitalia (females) or newborn screen present within the first month of life with failure to thrive, vomiting, dehydration, hyponatremia, hyperkalemia, and adrenal crisis (hypotension, shock).

CAH due to 21-hydroxylase deficiency and other enzyme defects may also present later in life if the genitalia are normal at birth:

- Females present in *childhood* with precocious pubic hair, clitoromegaly, and accelerated growth and skeletal maturation; in *adolescence* with oligomenorrhea and hirsutism; in *adulthood* with infertility; or at any time with unexplained hypertension.
- Males who do not have a salt-wasting form of CAH may present in childhood, with precocious pubic hair, phallic enlargement, and accelerated growth and skeletal maturation, or at any time with unexplained hypertension.
- Individuals of either gender may remain undiagnosed until physiologically stressed (e.g., infectious gastroenteritis), whereupon they rapidly develop hyponatremia, hyperkalemia, hypoglycemia, and shock.
- Excessive ACTH secretion is associated with subtle hyperpigmentation of the skin folds, scars, and genitalia.

Diagnosis rests on detection of elevated serum levels of precursors and inadequate cortisol production in the setting of clinical disease consistent with CAH. Patients with 21-hydroxylase deficiency have elevated serum 17-hydroxyprogesterone concentrations and elevated urinary pregnanetriol concentrations (a metabolite of 17-hydroxyprogesterone). Genetic testing is available for known mutations and is used for prenatal counseling and prenatal diagnosis (chorionic villus sampling, amniocentesis).

Adrenal insufficiency presents with hyponatremia, hyperkalemia, hypoglycemia, and circulatory collapse. *Adrenal*

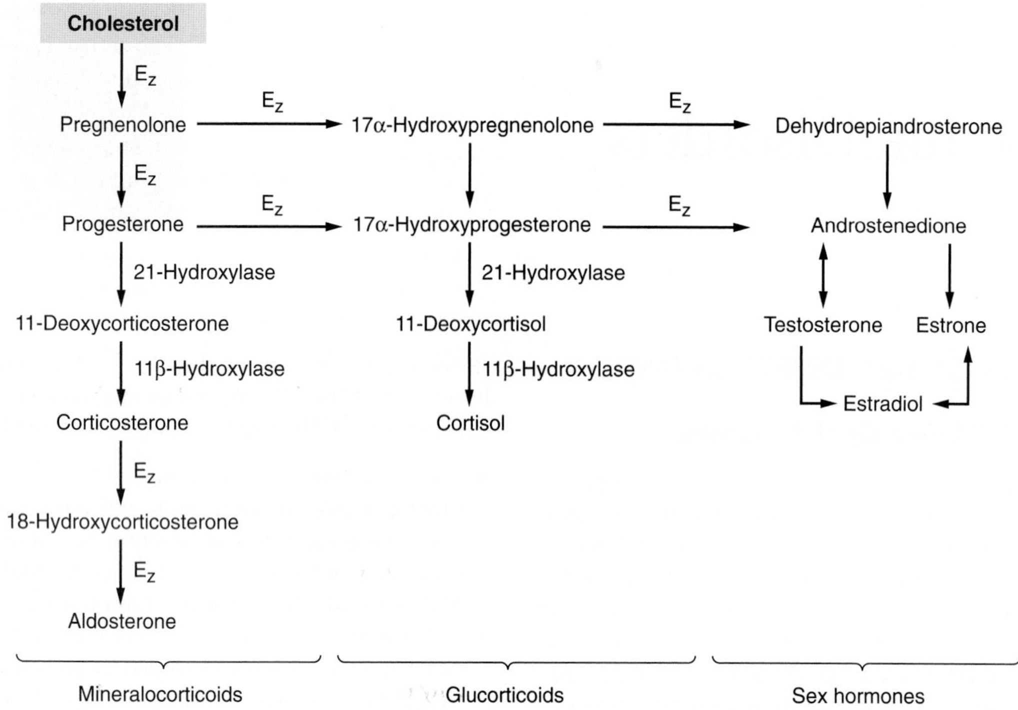

Figure 11-1 Enzymes (E_z) involved in the metabolism of cholesterol to aldosterone, cortisol, testosterone, and estradiol.

crisis is a medical emergency, regardless of age at presentation. Acute management consists of:

- *intravascular volume replenishment* (normal saline infusion, with glucose added as needed)
- *blood pressure normalization* (infusion as above; stress doses of intravenous hydrocortisone hemisuccinate)
- *correction* of electrolyte abnormalities (as discussed in Chapter 7)

Asymptomatic infants with positive newborn screens should have 17-hydroxyprogesterone and electrolyte levels drawn for confirmation as soon as possible. If results are consistent with CAH, hydrocortisone therapy is started immediately. Patients with a salt-wasting form of the disease also require maintenance mineralocorticoid medication and salt supplementation daily. Hydrocortisone doses are increased in times of stress and illness; increases in mineralocorticoid medications are not required because high-dose hydrocortisone has a mineralocorticoid effect.

Male Pseudohermaphroditism

Male pseudohermaphroditism is a rare disorder in which XY individuals are born with external genitalia consistent with females with mild virilization. Gonadal masses may be palpable distal to the inguinal ligaments. Most patients are found to have at least some degree of androgen insensitivity, which is inherited in an X-linked pattern. Many of these patients are unknowingly raised as women, with the abnormality eventually diagnosed as part of an evaluation for infertility or amenorrhea. *Five-α-reductase deficiency* and *17-ketosteroid reductase defects* may also present with male pseudohermaphroditism.

Female Virilization

In addition to CAH, virilization of the female fetus may result from prenatal exposure to androgens (danazol) or progestins (norethindrone). Exposure early in pregnancy is associated with labial fusion; clitoral enlargement is more likely if the exposure occurs during the last trimester. Virilization due to maternal androgen/progestin use typically resolves within a few months of birth.

DISORDERS OF STATURE

Short Stature

Proportionate short stature may represent a normal variant (genetic short stature, constitutional growth delay) or result from endocrine or other chronic disease (Table 11-1). Short patients with *dysmorphisms* are more likely to have genetic syndromes; skeletal dysplasias (see Chapter 19) cause *disproportionate short stature*. Evaluation for possible pathologic short stature should be undertaken in any patient:

TABLE 11-1

DIFFERENTIAL DIAGNOSIS OF SHORT STATURE

Normal Variants

Familial (genetic) short stature

- Generally normal or above average weight-for-height
- Height velocity normal
- No decline in height percentile
- Other family members are short.
- Child's growth curve is consistent with growth curves of other family members.
- Child's growth curve parallels the normal growth curve.
- Bone age equivalent to chronologic age

Constitutional growth delay

- Generally normal weight-for-height
- Height velocity normal
- Child is short for chronologic age during preadolescence.
- Puberty and growth spurt are delayed by 2 to 4 years when compared with peers.
- Height parallels the normal growth curve but begins to cross percentiles at typical age of puberty.
- Family history of growth and pubertal delay
- Individual experiences catch-up growth and attains expected adult height.
- Bone age is delayed 2 to 3 years but is consistent with height age (age at which patient's height would represent the 50th percentile).

Endocrine Disorders

- Deceleration in height velocity, with decline in height percentage
- *Excessive weight for height*, because weight growth velocity is preserved
- Bone age is generally somewhat delayed.
- Endocrinologic causes of short stature include hypothyroidism, growth hormone deficiency, Cushing syndrome

Chronic Systemic or Nutritional Disease

- Weight loss or inadequate weight gain followed by deceleration in height velocity
- Patients are typically underweight for height.

- with a height >2 standard deviations below the mean
- whose height percentile crosses two percentile lines (indicating deceleration in height velocity)
- whose height is obviously atypical in relation to his or her siblings
- whose height velocity is such that he or she is unlikely to attain expected adult height [average of parental heights, plus (for boys) or minus (for girls) 6.5 cm]

The evaluation of short stature includes:

- calculation of the weight-for-height measurement
- calculation of height velocity (minimum of 5 cm a year from age 4 years to the onset of puberty)
- comparing the child's height and weight curves to the growth curves of parents and siblings (when available)
- examination for any physical anomalies, dysmorphic features, or abnormalities suggesting systemic disease
- bone age (radiograph of the left hand and wrist), a measure of skeletal maturity. The bone age and chronologic age may be disparate by up to 2 years and still be normal, especially during adolescence.
- screening tests for chronic disease (renal, gastrointestinal, cardiac, pulmonary, metabolic, immunologic) if indicated based on results of history and physical examination

Growth hormone deficiency (GHD) may be congenital or acquired and may arise in isolation or as part of a larger pituitary hormone deficiency syndrome. Patients with *congenital GHD* begin to fall off their growth curves by about 9 months of age while maintaining their weight percentiles, making them appear chubby. There are three distinct forms of congenital GHD:

- GHD resulting from significant perinatal asphyxia
- GHD resulting from enzymatic or receptor mutations
- GHD associated with central nervous system (CNS) defects, midline facial malformations, and (in males) microphallus

Any condition that damages the hypothalamus or pituitary gland can result in *acquired GHD*, including space-occupying lesions and tumors (craniopharyngiomas, pituitary adenomas), trauma, infection, inflammation, radiation, or surgery. Idiopathic acquired GHD is also known to occur. Acquired GHD may cause decelerated height growth velocity anytime during childhood or adolescence. Bone age is typically delayed in affected patients.

Screening tests for GHD include insulin-like growth factor-1 (IGF-1) and insulin-like growth factor binding protein 3 levels. Random tests are not informative because growth hormone levels fluctuate throughout the day. The definitive diagnostic study is the growth hormone stimulation test. Growth hormone replacement is available for patients with documented deficiency.

Cushing syndrome is a specific constellation of clinical findings resulting from prolonged exposure to inappropriately elevated glucocorticoid levels. The most common signs of hypercortisolism are *weight gain* and *height growth deceleration*. Conditions associated with excessive production of endogenous cortisol include pituitary adenoma, adrenal tumors, adrenal hyperplasia, and ACTH-producing tumors. The exogenous steroids prednisone and prednisolone are often given in sufficient amounts over a long enough period of time to produce Cushing syndrome. Prominent signs and symptoms include obesity, fatigue and muscle weakness, headaches, alterations in mood, delayed sexual development, amenorrhea, moon facies (a rounded, flushed face with prominent cheeks), truncal obesity, buffalo hump, thin skin, striae, acne, acanthosis nigricans, and/or hirsutism. *Hypertension* is present in at least half of affected patients at diagnosis.

The 24-hour urine free cortisol measurement is a good screening test for hypercortisolism. Hyperglycemia is an associated finding. Bone age is typically delayed. Other laboratory studies that may be helpful include serum

TABLE 11-2
SYNDROMES ASSOCIATED WITH PATHOLOGIC TALL STATURE

Marfan Syndrome
- Autosomal dominant with variable penetrance
- Patient may have a personal/family history of lens subluxation, crowded dentition, scoliosis, mitral valve prolapse, or aortic root dilatation or dissection.
- Physical characteristics include a long, narrow face, pectus excavatum or carinatum, scoliosis, and disproportionately long arms and legs.
- Patients with Marfan syndrome are not always tall.

Klinefelter Syndrome
- Results from inheritance of at least one extra X chromosome in a male (e.g., XXY)
- Characterized by impaired androgen production
- Most affected individuals are not diagnosed until adolescence (tall stature, gynecomastia, small testes, pubertal delay) or adulthood (infertility).
- Physical characteristics include increased carrying angle at the elbow and relatively wide pelvis.
- Affected individuals tend to be less socially mature than their same-age peers, have particular difficulty with math, and suffer from low self-esteem.

Soto Syndrome
- Rare autosomal dominant condition characterized by overgrowth and advanced bone age in the early years of life
- Also called "cerebral gigantism"
- Physical examination may reveal dysmorphisms such as macrodolichocephaly, downward-slanting palpebral fissures, and pointed chin.
- Most patients have motor and speech delays but normal intelligence.

17-hydroxycorticosteroid and midnight serum cortisol concentrations, the dexamethasone suppression test, and the corticotrophin-releasing hormone stimulation test. Treatment consists of addressing the underlying cause of glucocorticoid excess (e.g., reducing steroid therapy if possible).

Tall Stature

Most tall stature is familial in origin, but Marfan, Klinefelter, and Soto syndromes are also associated with tall stature (Table 11-2). The evaluation of tall stature is similar to that for short stature. An additional value that often proves helpful is the predicated adult height; once this value and its relative percentile are calculated, the child's height percentile should be consistent with predicated adult height percentile.

PUBERTY

In males, the onset of puberty typically ranges from ages 9.5 to 13.5 years but may be occurring earlier, especially in the African-American population. *Testicular enlargement* (>2.5 mm prepubertal length) is the earliest sign of puberty, followed sequentially by *pubarche* (the start of pubic hair growth), *penile growth,* and *peak height velocity*. In females, the onset of puberty ranges from ages 8 to 13 years but may be occurring earlier, especially in the African-American population. *Breast budding* is the earliest sign of puberty, followed sequentially by *pubarche, peak height velocity,* and *menarche.* Normal puberty is discussed in Chapter 24.

Precocious Puberty

Precocious puberty is defined as the appearance of physical and hormonal signs of puberty before the age of 9 years in males and 8 years in females. Recent trends suggest that normal pubertal development may begin in girls as young as 6 to 8 years of age, especially in the African-American population. Obesity is associated with an earlier onset of puberty in girls. Precocious puberty initially results in tall stature, but final adult height is shorter than predicted due to premature closure of the growth plates. Children who undergo early pubertal development are more likely than their peers to experience teasing, psychological distress, and confusion related to their premature maturation.

Two conditions that may initially be misdiagnosed as precocious puberty are premature thelarche and premature pubarche. Both are benign and nonprogressive. *Premature thelarche* occurs in girls as young as 2 years of age. During normal pubertal development, breast budding is followed by pubarche within about 6 months. Sexual Maturation Rating (SMR) stage 3 breast development in a child without pubic hair or pubertal growth acceleration is consistent with isolated premature thelarche rather than precocious puberty. Most cases are idiopathic, but parents should be questioned about any possibility of an exogenous source of estrogen. *Premature pubarche* is the appearance of pubic hair in a girl younger than 8 years of age with no evidence of breast budding or acceleration of growth. It is thought to be due to increased secretion of androgens and may be associated with other signs of virilization including clitoromegaly, hirsutism, and acne. The suggested laboratory workup for suspected precocious puberty includes luteinizing hormone (LH), follicle-stimulating hormone (FSH), estradiol, testosterone, 17-OH progesterone, 11-deoxycortisol, human chorionic gonadotropin (HCG), thyroid function tests, and bone age.

Precocious puberty may be gonadotropin-dependent (central) or gonadotropin-independent (peripheral) (Table 11-3):

- *Central precocious puberty* (CPP) is caused by early maturation of the entire hypothalamic-pituitary-gonadal axis. The best screening test for CPP is a random LH level. CPP can be confirmed by measuring FSH and LH levels following stimulation with intravenous gonadotropin-releasing hormone (GnRH). CPP due to a space-occupying lesion of the CNS is often accompanied by headaches and visual field deficits. CNS imaging (computed tomography

TABLE 11-3
CAUSES OF CENTRAL AND PERIPHERAL PRECOCIOUS PUBERTY

Central Precocious Puberty
Idiopathic (most common cause in girls)
Central nervous system (CNS) tumors (most common cause in boys), particularly hypothalamic hamartomas and intracranial germ cell tumors
CNS trauma, radiation therapy, surgery, inflammation
CNS congenital anomalies (cysts, hydrocephalus)

Peripheral Precocious Puberty
Congenital adrenal hyperplasia
HCG-secreting tumors (liver, gonadal tumors)
Ovarian tumors
Adrenal tumors
Exposure to exogenous estrogen, testosterone
Severe hypothyroidism (rare)

or magnetic resonance imaging) is indicated for any patient with physical or laboratory evidence of CCP.

- *Peripheral precocious puberty* (PPP) results from elevation of sex steroid hormones independent of GnRH stimulation. Pelvic ultrasonography is indicated for girls with suspected PPP to look for ovarian cysts or tumors.

Precocious puberty generally responds to treatment or resolution of the underlying causative condition. GnRH analogs are available for patients with idiopathic CPP. Patients should be assessed every 3 to 6 months to evaluate the effectiveness of therapy.

Delayed Puberty

Delayed puberty is the absence of any signs of puberty by the age of 13 years in girls (breast budding by age 13 years or menarche delayed beyond the age of 16 or 3 years after the onset of breast development) or 14 years in boys (testicular enlargement). Discordant rates of genital and pubic hair development also warrant investigation. The differential diagnosis of delayed puberty includes *constitutional delay* (the most common cause in boys), dysfunction of the hypothalamus or pituitary gland (craniopharyngiomas, pituitary adenomas), prolactinomas, GHD, gonadal failure, hypothyroidism, chronic illness, undernutrition (including anorexia nervosa), and various genetic syndromes (Turner, Klinefelter, Prader-Willi, Kallmann). Once the testes begin to enlarge, most boys complete puberty within 3 to 5 years. Boys with delayed puberty who have documented delay in bone age and signs of early pubertal development do not require further workup unless there are signs or symptoms of underlying disease. Delayed puberty that is not a normal variant results in a final height in excess of predicted adult height.

Pubertal development may be stimulated upon resolution of the underlying condition. Hormone replacement is indicated for patients with inalterable deficiencies.

Gynecomastia

Pubertal gynecomastia is a relatively common development in males during adolescence, typically occurring during SMR stages 3 and 4. The mild enlargement of breast tissue results from temporary imbalance of the estrogen-testosterone ratio. Although obese males may appear to have breast enlargement, true gynecomastia involves glandular and stromal tissues. Palpable, often tender subareola breast tissue is present on examination but generally does not extend >2 cm beyond the areola in any direction. The condition may be uni- or bilateral. Pubertal gynecomastia is benign and generally resolves within 2 years; cases that persist beyond that time become fibrotic and are unlikely to regress but can be addressed with cosmetic surgery. The testes continue to enlarge at a normal rate when breast enlargement is due to pubertal gynecomastia.

Pathologic causes of gynecomastia are listed in Table 11-4. Further evaluation is indicated for male patients who:

- present with gynecomastia at any time other than puberty (except newborns)
- present with breast enlargement that begins during SMR stage 5
- present with macromastia (enlargement >4 cm in diameter)
- present with rapidly enlarging breast tissue

TABLE 11-4
PATHOLOGIC CAUSES OF GYNECOMASTIA IN MALES

Klinefelter syndrome
Liver disease (cirrhosis)
Androgen insensitivity
Testicular failure
Hyperthyroidism
Adrenal tumors
Estrogen-producing tumors
Kallmann syndrome (familial gynecomastia)
Medications
  Spironolactone
  Ketoconazole
  Digitalis
  Cimetidine
Drug use
  Anabolic steroids
  Marijuana

Further assessment is based on findings from the history and physical examination (e.g., drug history, testicular size). Exogenous testosterone is indicated for patients with low testosterone levels.

Breast Masses

Breast cancer is extremely rare in adolescent females. Most breast masses in this age group are due to normal nodular breast tissue (i.e., fibrocystic changes) or fibroadenomas. Benign breast tumors, such as lipomas, neurofibromas, and dermoid cysts, may occasionally present during adolescence. *Fibrocystic changes* often cause some degree of cyclic premenstrual breast tenderness or fullness. Examination of the breast reveals cordlike thickening or diffuse nodularity, which changes from cycle to cycle. *Fibroadenomas* are discrete, firm, mobile masses 2 to 4 cm in diameter that usually arise in isolation but may rarely be multiple or even bilateral. They are generally found in the lateral quadrants. Fibroadenomas are persistent in size and location and are not affected by the menstrual cycle. Other causes of breast masses in adolescents are listed in Table 11-5. Factors that increase the likelihood that a breast mass is malignant include a history of breast malignancy in multiple family members, particularly women younger than 50 years of age; a personal history of prior cancer (acute lymphoblastic leukemia, lymphoma, neuroblastoma, or rhabdomyosarcoma); and a history of radiation therapy to the chest. Examining the mass following subsequent menstrual cycles over 4 to 8 weeks may assist in diagnosis. Needle biopsy is the diagnostic procedure of choice; mammography is rarely helpful in adolescents.

THYROID DISORDERS

Hypothyroidism

Hypothyroidism is the most common endocrinologic cause of poor growth. Hypothyroidism in the pediatric population may be congenital or acquired. *Congenital hypothyroidism* is discussed in detail in Chapter 5. Most cases of *acquired hypothyroidism* occur in older children and adolescents and are autoimmune in origin (see "Hashimoto Thyroiditis" later in this chapter). Immune-mediated thyroiditis results from cellular infiltration, inflammation, and destruction of thyroid follicular cells. Patients with <25% residual gland function become hypothyroid. Signs and symptoms of acquired hypothyroidism are provided in Table 11-6. The presentation of acquired hypothyroidism in infancy is very similar to that of congenital hypothyroidism.

Hypothyroidism is diagnosed when the serum free thyroxine concentration (FT_4) is below the normal range for age. *Primary hypothyroidism,* caused by abnormalities in or absence of the gland itself, results in elevation of the serum thyroid-stimulating hormone (TSH) concentration. Hypothyroidism in the setting of a normal or depressed TSH generally indicates *central hypothyroidism* due to failure of the hypothalamus or pituitary gland. If the FT_4 test is not available, serum thyroxine (T_4) and triiodothyronine (T_3) resin uptake values may be substituted in order to estimate FT_4.

TABLE 11-5
BREAST MASSES IN THE ADOLESCENT FEMALE

Physiologic fibrocystic changes
Fibroadenomas
Breast abscesses (acute onset of tender mass with warmth and erythema of the overlying skin)
Hematoma (history of trauma, visible bruising)
Fat necrosis (history of trauma and a small, firm mass on physical examination that slowly resolves)
Breast cancer (presents as a hard, fixed lesion with or without overlying skin changes)

TABLE 11-6
CLINICAL MANIFESTATIONS OF HYPOTHYROIDISM

At All Ages:
Deceleration of linear growth
Short stature
Fatigue
Weakness
Constipation
Cold intolerance
Hair loss
Dry skin
Goiter
Easy bruising
Myxedema
Generalized swelling
Diminished deep tendon reflexes

Laboratory Results:
Hypochromic Anemia
Hyperlipidemia

In Children:
Delayed eruption and shedding of primary teeth
Pseudohypertrophy of arm and leg muscles
Precocious puberty
Breast development not followed by pubarche (girls)
Testicular enlargement not followed by pubarche (boys)

In Adolescents:
Delayed puberty
Galactorrhea (girls)
Menorrhagia

The T_3 resin uptake test (T_3RU) is also useful for diagnosing *thyroid-binding globulin* (TBG) *deficiency*. TBG deficiency presents as low T_4 and elevated T_3RU levels in a patient with a normal thyroid examination, normal TSH, and no signs or symptoms of hypothyroidism. No treatment is necessary.

Patients with hypothyroidism require thyroid hormone replacement with levothyroxine (L-thyroxine). Because of variability in absorption and metabolism, both FT_4 and TSH should be monitored frequently at the outset of therapy and yearly once normal values are achieved. Medications, diseases, and other factors that impact T_4 absorption are noted in Table 11-7. Most of the detrimental effects of hypothyroidism acquired after 3 years of age are reversible with adequate treatment. However, hypothyroidism that persists untreated for longer than 6 to 9 months results in linear growth attenuation and short stature, which may have a deleterious effect on final adult height. Children at high risk for the development of hypothyroidism should have heights, TSH, and FT_4 levels recorded yearly to ensure prompt diagnosis and treatment when necessary.

Hyperthyroidism

Hyperthyroidism is uncommon in pediatric practice; adolescents and adults are more often affected. The most common cause of hyperthyroidism is *Graves' disease*, the continual synthesis and release of thyroid hormone that results when circulating thyroid-stimulating immunoglobulin binds to TSH receptors on the gland. Graves' disease may occur in isolation or be associated with other autoimmune disorders. The signs, symptoms, and laboratory evaluation of hyperthyroidism are provided in Table 11-8. Hyperthyroidism may rarely present initially as *thyroid storm*, characterized by the acute onset of hyperthermia, hypertension, and altered mental status progressing to coma and, if untreated, death.

Children with Graves' disease are primarily treated with antithyroid medication (propylthiouracil, methimazole). Serious adverse drug effects are rare but include hepatitis, nephritis, vasculitis, arthritis, and agranulocytosis (severely decreased numbers of circulating neutrophils). Beta-blockers are prescribed to control blood pressure. Most patients can eventually be weaned off medications as the illness resolves. Radioiodine treatment and surgical removal of the gland are reserved for patients with resistant disease; both usually result in lifelong hypothyroidism. Radiotherapy is associated with an increased risk of thyroid carcinoma later in life; surgical resection may damage the recurrent laryngeal nerve or remove the majority of the parathyroid glands.

TABLE 11-7
FACTORS THAT IMPACT THYROXINE ABSORPTION AND NECESSITATE INCREASED DOSAGE

Iron supplements
Calcium supplements
Dietary fiber
Soy protein
Gastrointestinal malabsorption
- Celiac disease
- Inflammatory bowel disease

TABLE 11-8
DIAGNOSIS OF HYPERTHYROIDISM

Symptoms
Increased appetite
Heat intolerance
Excessive sweating
Palpitations
Diarrhea
Altered mood
Poor concentration
Oligomenorrhea or amenorrhea

Signs
Weight loss
Hypertension
Exophthalmos
Thyroid gland enlargement
Persistent sinus tachycardia
Hyperdynamic precordium
Flow murmurs
Bounding pulses
Tremor

Laboratory Evaluation
TSH (depressed)
FT_4 (elevated)
T_3 (elevated)

Hashimoto Thyroiditis

Hashimoto thyroiditis, also called *chronic lymphocytic thyroiditis*, is an autoimmune disorder characterized by lymphoid infiltration and destruction of the thyroid gland. The classic presentation is firm, painless enlargement of the thyroid gland (goiter); in fact, Hashimoto thyroiditis is the most common cause of goiter in adolescents. Most patients are clinically well and have normal function at diagnosis (normal T_4, normal T_3RU, increased TSH) but eventually become hypothyroid (decreased T_4, decreased T_3RU, increased TSH). Transient hyperthyroidism is not uncommon. The diagnosis is made through demonstration of circulating antithyroid autoantibodies (e.g., antibodies against thyroperoxidase or thyroglobulin). Chronic lymphocytic autoimmune thyroiditis occurs in isolation but also may be associated with other autoimmune disorders such as type 1 diabetes, Addison disease, rheumatoid arthritis, systemic lupus erythematosus, hypoparathyroidism, and autoimmune hepatitis. Patients with Down, Turner, and Klinefelter syndromes are disproportionately affected with Hashimoto thyroiditis.

Thyroid Masses

Thyroid masses may be cysts, tumors, or nodules. Benign masses include adenomas, colloid nodules, and most cysts. Masses at least 1 cm in diameter are readily palpable. A mass within the gland will move with the thyroid when the patient swallows. Most thyroid masses are benign, but malignant masses are clinically indistinguishable from benign growths. *Papillary and follicular carcinomas* comprise the vast majority of malignant thyroid growths in children. Factors that increase the risk of malignancy include a history of radiation therapy to the head and/or neck, fixture of the mass to underlying tissues, firmness, irregularity in shape, firm cervical lymphadenopathy on the same side as the mass, iodine deficiency, Hashimoto thyroiditis, and Graves' disease. Cysts may become painful due to rapid growth or hemorrhage, but other thyroid masses are generally nontender. Hoarseness and dysphagia are not uncommon. Occasionally hypo- or hyperthyroidism is present; however, both are rare in individuals with thyroid carcinoma. All patients with discrete thyroid masses should be referred to an endocrinologist for specialized evaluation and management.

The physical examination includes thorough characterization of the mass, evaluation for ipsilateral cervical lymphadenopathy, and visualization of the vocal cords if possible. Disordered vocal cord function increases the likelihood of malignancy. Laboratory assessment of thyroid function typically yields normal results. Thyroid masses are evaluated with technetium-99 or iodine-123 scintigraphy. Ultrasonography can differentiate a cyst from a nodule and guide fine-needle aspiration biopsy, which is the diagnostic study of choice for solitary nodules. Definitive diagnosis requires resection of the growth. Resection or total thyroidectomy with lymph node dissection may be indicated for confirmed malignancies. Survival rates for children exceed 90%.

PARATHYROID DISORDERS

The parathyroid glands regulate serum calcium levels within a narrow physiologic range. *Parathyroid hormone* (PTH) *deficiency*, which results in hypocalcemia and hyperphosphatemia, may be autoimmune or secondary to neck surgery or radioactive iodine treatment. Infants with classic *DiGeorge syndrome* who are born without parathyroid glands present with hypocalcemic seizures in the newborn period. *Pseudohypoparathyroidism* is an autosomal dominant disorder involving mutation of a stimulatory enzyme normally responsive to PTH. Children born to males with the disorder are short and stocky, with brachydactyly of the fourth digits of the hands and feet and mild mental retardation. Children born to affected females suffer from hypocalcemia and hyperphosphatemia as well.

DISORDERS OF THE ADRENAL GLAND

Addison disease is a state of *adrenal insufficiency* and inadequate adrenocortical hormone production resulting from hypoplasia or destruction of the adrenal glands. Most cases are autoimmune in origin, but infection [particularly human immunodeficiency virus (HIV) and tuberculosis], hemorrhage, malignant carcinoma, certain medications, and CAH can also lead to adrenal insufficiency. As is true for most autoimmune endocrine disorders, other immune-mediated conditions may also be present. Adrenal insufficiency is occasionally the presenting feature of *adrenoleukodystrophy*, a rare X-linked neurodegenerative disease.

Primary adrenal insufficiency is confirmed by a low cortisol level that does not respond to exogenous ACTH administration. The patient with a low initial level and a significant response to ACTH may have secondary hypocortisolism; neuroimaging is indicated under these circumstances. *Secondary hypocortisolism* is caused by abnormalities of hypothalamic or pituitary functioning due to CNS trauma, hemorrhage, infection, surgery, inflammation, or space-occupying lesions. Secondary adrenal insufficiency is not associated with salt-wasting or hyperpigmentation.

CAH presenting in infancy is discussed earlier in the chapter. Older children with adrenal insufficiency usually present with the gradual onset of any combination of the following: weight loss; weakness; headaches, poor concentration, or memory impairment; abdominal pain or constipation; myalgia and arthralgia; salt craving; and atypical seizures. Hyperpigmentation of skin folds and scars, loss of axillary and pubic hair, and vitiligo may be noted during the physical examination. Acute decompensation due to adrenal insufficiency presents with nausea, vomiting, diarrhea, abdominal pain, weakness, hypotension, shock, confusion, and coma. Hypoglycemia is invariably present and may be accompanied by ketosis. Patients with adrenal insufficiency and salt-wasting will have hyperkalemia with low serum sodium, chloride, and bicarbonate levels and elevation of blood urea nitrogen (prerenal azotemia). Spot plasma cortisol levels are generally quite low, even in the setting of acute stress and/or hypoglycemia.

Acute management of adrenal crisis and maintenance therapy for patients with adrenal insufficiency are provided in Table 11-9.

TYPE 1 DIABETES

Type 1 diabetes is a condition of *hyperglycemia* and *impaired blood glucose control* that results when an individual with an *inherited susceptibility* is exposed to an *environmental trigger*

TABLE 11-9
MANAGEMENT OF ADRENAL INSUFFICIENCY

Acute Adrenal Crisis
- Volume restoration with normal saline or other salt-containing fluids
- Intravenous hydrocortisone, preferably after obtaining blood for laboratory analysis of cortisol, ACTH levels
- Normalization of serum glucose level with glucose administration
- Correction of the precipitating condition

Maintenance Therapy
- Oral cortisone therapy, with double or triple dosing during periods of stress or illness
- Oral mineralocorticoid therapy (9α-fluorohydrocortisone)
- Immediate medical evaluation for any episode of emesis, and hospital admission for repeated vomiting

that precipitates immune-mediated destruction of pancreatic β-cells. Patients in the "prediabetic" stage have lost the first-phase insulin response and have abnormal intravenous glucose tolerance tests. Continued destruction results in the onset of clinical disease and abnormalities in oral glucose tolerance test results. Many patients enter a "honeymoon phase" soon after diagnosis during which they require very little or no supplemental insulin; however, insulin requirements generally begin to rise again within 1 to 2 years. Individuals with type 1 diabetes are at risk for the development of other autoimmune disorders such as Graves' disease, Hashimoto thyroiditis, Addison disease, and celiac disease.

In children, the onset of clinical disease may be acute [diabetic ketoacidosis (DKA)] or insidious. Classic symptoms include polyuria, polydipsia, polyphagia, and weight loss. In the presence of symptoms, the diagnosis can be made through demonstration of a random blood glucose >200 mg per dL. The management of type 1 diabetes is provided in Table 11-10. Baseline laboratory assessment in the newly diagnosed patient who is not in DKA includes a glucose tolerance test and islet/β-cell antibody assays (antibodies against insulin, glutamate decarboxylase, and tyrosine phosphatase IA2).

Diabetes has numerous serious vascular complications, including retinopathy, nephropathy, and neuropathy. The risk of complications increases with disease duration, poor glycemic control, family history of significant complications due to diabetes, hypertension, hyperlipidemia, and smoking.

TABLE 11-10
MANAGEMENT OF AND MAINTENANCE THERAPY FOR TYPE 1 DIABETES

Insulin Therapy

Continuous subcutaneous insulin infusion: administers a steady basal rate of insulin, with boluses programmed by the patient according to preprandial glucose levels; provides the best control of blood sugar when used correctly. This is currently the preferred method of insulin therapy. Hypoglycemic episodes are not uncommon during early use of infusion pumps. Conversely, patients who rely solely on pumps may present with the sudden onset of diabetic ketoacidosis due to pump blockage or failure.

Rapid-acting insulin: administered following meals in patients with unreliable food intake, such as small children

Short-acting insulin: administered immediately prior to meals

Intermediate-acting insulin: administered in the morning and at bedtime for longer control

Long-acting insulin

Basal insulin

Premixed ratios of the above are available in pen and autoinjector forms.

Conventional treatment of newly diagnosed diabetics involves the administration of three injections a day totaling 0.5 to 2 units per kilogram per day:

- ⅔ of total insulin dose in the morning; ⅓ short-acting, ⅔ intermediate-acting insulin
- ⅙ of total insulin dose before dinner, short-acting insulin
- ⅙ of total insulin dose at bedtime, intermediate-acting insulin

Blood Glucose Monitoring

Ideally, blood glucose levels should be determined several times a day, including before meals and snacks, at bedtime, and 2 hours after eating. Desirable preprandial values range from 70 to 150 mg per dL (higher in infants and toddlers).

Both the *dawn phenomenon* and the *Somogyi effect* can result in elevated morning blood glucose levels:

- Dawn phenomenon: occurs when hormones released in the early morning hours (cortisol, catecholamines, growth hormone) stimulate the liver to release large amount of glucose into the blood.

(*continued*)

TABLE 11-10
(continued)

- Somogyi effect: occurs in patients who take long-acting insulin preparations that drop their blood glucose too low, stimulating cortisol and catecholamine release with a resultant increase in blood sugar. The Somogyi effect is most commonly seen with early morning blood sugar levels but may occur at any time.
- If early morning hyperglycemia is due to the dawn phenomenon, 2 a.m. blood glucose levels gathered over several nights will trend *normal-to-high*; *low* levels at 2 a.m. are more consistent with the Somogyi effect.

Ketones should be monitored during periods of illness and persistent hyperglycemia.

Diet
Patients with type 1 diabetes require specialized individual nutrition plans and counseling regarding recommended daily caloric intake (total and distribution), percentages and sources of carbohydrates/fats/proteins, limitation of refined sugar intake, and symptoms and treatment of hypoglycemia.

Exercise
Regular exercise improves glucose control. Patients should know how to regulate caloric intake to prevent hypoglycemia during periods of increased activity.

Screening
Quarterly outpatient visits to include:

- *Glycosylated hemoglobin level* (HbA1c)—reflects glucose control over the past 2 to 3 months; normal range, 4% to 6%; desirable range for patients with type 1 diabetes, <7%. Diabetics with poor control have elevated HbA1c levels. Patients with relatively low HbA1c levels have a decreased risk of developing retinopathy, renal disease, and neuropathy.
- *Review* of recorded blood glucose levels and *adjustment* of insulin regimen as needed
- *Questions* regarding changes in medication, activity, diet, life circumstances
- *Physical examination*, with special attention to growth parameters, blood pressure, thyroid gland, abdomen, peripheral pulses, skin, and joints
- Yearly *laboratory assessment* for microalbuminuria and autoimmune thyroid disease; other screening tests to consider in select patients include urinalysis, creatinine, fasting lipid profile, and serum immunoglobulin A concentrations or tissue transglutaminase antibody to screen for celiac disease
- Yearly dilated *funduscopic examination* and detailed *neurologic examination*

Psychosocial/Educational Issues

- The patient should be assisted in accepting that he or she has a chronic disease that can result in serious health consequences, including death, if not properly controlled.
- Patients should be made aware that they are responsible for monitoring their own blood glucose levels and adjusting insulin doses.
- Patients should be counseled regarding how risk-taking behavior might impact their disease.
- Patients should be encouraged to maintain a healthy lifestyle, congratulated on treatment successes, and motivated to improve when possible.

About a quarter of patients with type 1 diabetes initially present in DKA. DKA should be suspected in any patient with vomiting, dehydration, abdominal pain, and altered mental status. The evaluation and management of DKA is outlined in Table 11-11. Patients with recurrent episodes of DKA may or may not have brittle disease; noncompliance is a more frequent determinant of repetitive hospitalization. *Cerebral edema* is the most serious complication of DKA and is associated with significant morbidity and mortality. Patients in DKA must be closely monitored for any signs or symptoms of neurologic compromise (headache, lethargy, pupillary changes, bradycardia, hypertension, seizures). Cerebral edema is occasionally a consequence of DKA treatment, presenting 6 to 12 hours after the initiation of therapy. The use of intravenous bicarbonate exacerbates hypokalemia and increases the risk of cerebral edema by causing the cerebrospinal fluid to become paradoxically acidotic. Its use should be reserved for the DKA patient with severe acidosis (pH <7.1) compromising cardiorespiratory function.

TABLE 11-11
EVALUATION AND MANAGEMENT OF DIABETIC KETOACIDOSIS

- Perform rapid assessment of patient's vital signs, hydration, mental status.
- Obtain bedside dextrose stick and send blood for measurements of electrolytes, glucose, urea nitrogen, venous pH, and complete blood count; monitor D-stick every 30 minutes, other labs every 2 to 4 hours until stable.
- Obtain urine for glucose, ketone measurements if possible.
- Begin infusion of 10 mL per kg normal saline over 30 to 60 minutes.
- Calculate deficit replacement over 36 to 48 hours plus composition and rate of maintenance fluids.
- Initiate insulin drip within 2 hours of presentation with goal of reducing blood glucose no more than 100 mg per dL per hour. Add glucose to fluids when blood glucose falls below 300 mg per dL.
- Add maintenance potassium to fluids when measured serum potassium falls within the normal range and patient has produced urine.

Hyperglycemic nonketotic hypertonicity may occasionally be mistaken for DKA, although patients are usually hypernatremic at presentation. The pathophysiology is similar to that for DKA, except that these patients do not seem to metabolize fat to produce the large amounts of ketones present in DKA. Altered sensorium progressing to coma is not uncommon and is related to the associated hypertonicity. Management is similar to that of DKA, except that hypotonic saline is used to correct the hypernatremia.

TYPE 2 DIABETES

The prevalence of type 2 diabetes, formerly called adult-onset diabetes or noninsulin-dependent diabetes, is increasing in the pediatric population as rates of childhood obesity rise. Whereas type 1 diabetes is essentially autoimmune in origin, type 2 diabetes is due to a combination of increased insulin resistance and inadequate insulin production/release. The best method of differentiating between type 1 and type 2 diabetes is measurement of islet cell and insulin autoantibodies. Otherwise, the laboratory criteria for the diagnosis of type 2 diabetes are identical to those for type 1 disease (Table 11-12).

Risk factors for the development of type 2 diabetes are listed in Table 11-13. Children with type 2 diabetes are usually asymptomatic at diagnosis, although there may be a history of mild polyuria and polydipsia. *Acanthosis nigricans* is a physical marker of insulin resistance. DKA is rare but does occur. The initial management of type 2 diabetes consists of diet and exercise. If this approach does not result in normalization of blood glucose within a few months, oral metformin is added to further decrease insulin resistance.

TABLE 11-12
LABORATORY DIAGNOSIS OF DIABETES (TYPES 1 AND 2)

Impaired glucose tolerance is indicated by:

- two fasting blood glucose concentrations between 100 and 126 mg per dL on separate occasions
- 2-hour post-oral glucose load blood glucose concentration between 140 and 200 mg per dL (normal: $<$140 mg/dL)

At least one of the following laboratory results must be present for a diagnosis of diabetes:

- random blood glucose concentration $\geq$200 mg per dL in the presence of symptoms
- two random blood glucose concentrations $\geq$200 mg per dL on separate occasions
- fasting blood glucose concentration $\geq$126 mg per dL in the presence of symptoms
- 2-hour post-oral glucose load blood glucose concentration $\geq$200 mg per dL

TABLE 11-13
RISK FACTORS FOR THE DEVELOPMENT OF TYPE 2 DIABETES IN CHILDHOOD

Obesity
Low level of physical activity
Family history of diabetes
African-American, Asian-American, Hispanic, or Native-American race
Female gender

METABOLIC SYNDROME

Metabolic syndrome, the combination of obesity, hypertension, insulin resistance, and dyslipidemia, is discussed in detail in Chapter 2.

DISORDERS OF CALCIUM AND PHOSPHATE METABOLISM

Hypocalcemia

Calcium is involved in muscle contractility and neuronal excitation. The body's homeostatic mechanisms restrict the serum calcium within a very narrow physiologic range. PTH, vitamin D, and calcitonin regulate calcium levels, which are also affected by imbalances in phosphorus and magnesium. Table 11-14 includes a partial list of conditions that may result in hypocalcemia. Clinical manifestations and suggested laboratory studies are provided in Table 11-15.

Early neonatal hypocalcemia is hypocalcemia that occurs within 72 hours of birth. Prematurity is the most common cause of early neonatal hypocalcemia, and up to a third of

TABLE 11-14
DIFFERENTIAL DIAGNOSIS OF HYPOCALCEMIA

Renal insufficiency
Liver disease
Hypoparathyroidism (hyperphosphatemia)
Pseudohypoparathyroidism
Vitamin D deficiency
Hypomagnesemia (amphotericin B, aminoglycosides, loop diuretics)
Sepsis
Toxic shock syndrome
Rhabdomyolysis
Tumor lysis syndrome
Medications
  Calcitonin
  Fluoride

TABLE 11-15
CLINICAL AND LABORATORY MANIFESTATIONS OF HYPOCALCEMIA

Symptoms
Vomiting
Paresthesias
Muscle weakness
Muscle spasms
Laryngospasm (stridor)
Irritability
Poor memory/concentration

Signs
Chvostek sign[a]
Trousseau sign[b]
Tetany
Seizures

Electrocardiogram
Prolonged QT interval

Suggested Laboratory Studies
Total serum calcium (normal range, 9.6 to 10.6 mg/dL)
Ionized serum calcium (normal range, 4.9 to 5.5 mg/dL)
Phosphorus
Magnesium
Parathyroid hormone
Alkaline phosphatase
Total protein, albumin
Amylase
Creatinine
Serum pH
25-hydroxycholecalciferol
1,25-dihydroxycholecalciferol

[a]Contraction of the ipsilateral mouth, nose, eye, and facial muscles elicited by tapping the facial nerve just anterior to the ear lobe below the zygomatic arch.

[b]Contraction of the carpal muscle following inflation of a blood pressure cuff around the upper arm for 2 minutes.

preterm infants are affected. Hypocalcemia is uncommon in term infants but may result from perinatal asphyxia or maternal diabetes. *Late neonatal hypocalcemia* presents at about 1 week of age due to high phosphate feedings (cow milk, evaporated milk).

Hypercalcemia

Hypercalcemia is less common than hypocalcemia in the pediatric population. Prolonged immobilization can lead to hypercalcemia in children due to the relatively high bone turnover caused by rapid growth. Other causes are listed in Table 11-16. Classic symptoms of hypercalcemia include polyuria, thirst, headache, nausea, anorexia, muscle weakness, and constipation. Treatment consists of saline diuresis and loop diuretics.

TABLE 11-16
DIFFERENTIAL DIAGNOSIS OF HYPERCALCEMIA IN CHILDREN

Primary hyperparathyroidism
Malignancy
Sarcoidosis
Hypervitaminosis D
Idiopathic hypercalcemia
Excessive intake of calcium

TABLE 11-17
COMPARISON OF LABORATORY RESULTS IN RICKETS DUE TO VITAMIN D DEFICIENCY OR FAMILIAL HYPOPHOSPHATEMIA

Vitamin D Deficiency	Familial Hypophosphatemia
Normal-to-low serum calcium	Normal serum calcium
Low serum phosphorus	Low serum phosphorus
Elevated serum alkaline phosphatase	Elevated serum alkaline phosphatase
Low serum 25-hydroxycholecalciferol	Normal serum 25-hydroxycholecalciferol
Elevated parathyroid hormone level	Normal parathyroid hormone level

Hypophosphatemia and Rickets

Rickets due to vitamin D deficiency is discussed in Chapter 2. Although the clinical manifestations of vitamin D rickets and familial hypophosphatemic rickets are virtually identical, laboratory studies can be used to differentiate the two condi-tions (Table 11-17). Familial hypophosphatemia may be X-linked or autosomal dominant. Treatment consists of oral phosphate supplementation combined with rapid-onset 1,25-dihydroxyvitamin D to prevent hypocalcemia.

SOURCES

Chianese J. Short stature. *Pediatr Rev*. 2005;26:36–37.
Foley TP. Hypothyroidism. *Pediatr Rev*. 2004;25:94–100.
Glaser N. Pediatric diabetic ketoacidosis and hyperglycemic hyperosmolar state. *Pediatr Clin North Am*. 2005;52:1611–1635.
Haller MJ, Atkinson MA, Schatz D. Type 1 diabetes mellitus: etiology, presentation, and management. *Pediatr Clin North Am*. 2005;52: 1553–1578.
Kaplowitz PB. Thyroid testing; when to worry (not often) and when to reassure. *Contemp Pediatr*. 2007;24:45–63.
Kaufman FR. Type 1 diabetes mellitus. *Pediatr Rev*. 2003;24:291–300.
Oberlin JM, Rogers WM, Fenton CL. Endocrine emergencies: recognizing signs and symptoms. *Pediatr Ann*. 2005;34:870–877.

QUESTIONS

1. A 14-month-old male undergoing removal of a right-sided intra-abdominal testis is found to have rudimentary internal duct structures (Fallopian tubes, uterus). The external genitalia appear normal, and both testes are normal in size. This clinical scenario is most consistent with which of the following disorders?
A) Persistent müllerian duct syndrome
B) Congenital adrenal hyperplasia
C) Klinefelter syndrome
D) Testicular feminization syndrome
E) Mosaic Turner syndrome

2. Which of the following physical findings is most likely to be noted in a newborn girl born to a woman who took danazol, a synthetic androgen, early in her pregnancy?
A) Ambiguous genitalia
B) Labial fusion
C) Gynecomastia
D) Galactorrhea
E) Leukorrhea

3. A full-term infant with ambiguous genitalia and clitoromegaly has a palpable 1-cm firm mobile mass in each inguinal canal just distal to the inguinal ligaments. Which of the following is the most likely karyotype of this infant?
A) 45 XO
B) 46 XX
C) 46 XY
D) 47 XYY
E) 47 XXY

4. A 2-week-old former full-term male infant is brought to the emergency department by his parents for progressive vomiting. He was well until 24 hours ago, when he fed poorly and spit up. Since then, he has continued to vomit, has had no stool, and has urinated only once in the past 12 hours. His birth weight was 3,080 g. Currently, he weighs 2,782 g. He is afebrile, but his heart rate is 140 beats per minute, and he is obviously clinically dehydrated. Serum electrolytes include: sodium 119 mEq per L; potassium 10.5 mEq per L; chloride 92 mEq per L; and bicarbonate 12 mEq per L. His glucose was 65 mg per dL by dextrose stick. Consultation with the state newborn screening laboratory is most likely to reveal which of the following abnormalities on this patient's screen?
A) Elevated concentration of methionine
B) Elevated concentration of phenylalanine
C) Elevated concentration of galactose-1-phosphate
D) Elevated concentration of 17-hydroxyprogesterone
E) Elevated concentration of vanillylmandelic acid (VMA)

5. The state newborn screening laboratory has just notified you that one of your patients has a screening result consistent with 21-hydroxylase deficiency. The infant is brought to your office for subsequent testing. He is asymptomatic but has a low serum sodium level and a slightly elevated potassium level. His serum 17-hydroxyprogesterone concentration is markedly elevated. In consultation with an endocrinologist, which of the following is most appropriate for initial management?
A) The patient should be admitted to the hospital, and intravenous hydrocortisone hemisuccinate should be administered as soon as he begins to vomit.
B) The patient should have outpatient electrolyte levels drawn daily, with hydrocortisone to be started when the serum potassium reaches 5.5 mEq per L.
C) The patient should have outpatient electrolyte levels drawn daily, with a synthetic mineralocorticoid to be started when the serum potassium reaches 5.5 mEq per L.
D) No further evaluation or treatment is indicated at this time.
E) The patient should be started on maintenance doses of hydrocortisone, a mineralocorticoid, and salt supplements.

6. A mother brings her 8-year-old daughter to your office because she has gained a significant amount of weight in the past 9 months. At that time, her weight was at the 50th percentile, with a height at the 75th percentile. Her weight is now greater than the 97th percentile, and she has only grown 1.75 cm. Her mother also tells you that she doesn't play outside with the neighborhood children as much because she feels "weak." She has not complained of headaches, changes in vision, fever, constipation, or cold intolerance. She is taking no medications. Her blood pressure in the office is above the 90th percentile for age. The physical examination reveals truncal obesity, moon facies, and mild acne. Bone age is 5 years 6 months. Which of the following screening tests is most likely to reveal the cause of her weight gain?
A) 24-hour urinary free cortisol level
B) Serum IgA level
C) Tissue transglutaminase antibody
D) Serum insulin-like growth factor-1
E) Serum insulin-like growth factor binding protein 3

7. A 16-year-old young man comes to your clinic for a regular health maintenance visit, his first appointment. His mother tells you that he is having difficulty with his schoolwork and has been suspended twice this year for fighting with peers. When questioned regarding concerns, he reluctantly tells you that he is worried that he has not started to "develop" yet. The physical examination reveals a tall, thin male without facial or axillary hair; bilateral gynecomastia; SMR stage 3 pubic hair; and testes and phallus consistent with prepubertal development. This patient's clinical findings are most likely due to which of the following?

A) Testicular feminization syndrome
B) Klinefelter syndrome
C) Persistent müllerian duct syndrome
D) 5-α-reductase deficiency
E) 17-ketosteroid reductase defect

8. You are examining a 15-year-old young lady with type 1 diabetes. You note that her thyroid gland is moderately enlarged and firm. There is no tenderness to palpation. The patient has no complaints of fatigue, cold intolerance, behavior changes, or weight gain or loss. Her thyroid-stimulating hormone levels have remained consistently within the normal range. This patient's goiter is most likely a result of which of the following?

A) Congenital thyroxine-binding globulin deficiency
B) Acquired thyroxine-binding globulin deficiency
C) Hashimoto thyroiditis
D) Graves' disease
E) Thyroid carcinoma

9. A 3-cm firm mass is detected in the right lobe of the thyroid gland in an asymptomatic 16-year-old patient during a regular health maintenance visit. Which of the following statements regarding this patient's condition is FALSE?

A) A history of radiation exposure increases the risk that the mass will be malignant.
B) Excisional biopsy is the diagnostic study of choice for determining if the nodule is malignant.
C) The mass will move with the thyroid when the patient swallows if it is within the gland.
D) Malignant and benign thyroid nodules can be reliably differentiated based on history and clinical presentation.
E) Firm cervical lymphadenopathy on the same side as the mass increases the likelihood that the nodule is malignant.

10. A 9-year-old girl presents to your office for a routine health maintenance visit. She has grown <2 cm in the past year. Her mother notes that the girl frequently seems fatigued and has developed persistent constipation. Which of the following laboratory values is (are) most helpful in evaluation for hypothyroidism in this patient?

A) Thyroid-stimulating hormone (TSH) alone
B) Thyroxine (T_4) alone
C) T_4 and triiodothyronine (T_3)
D) TSH and T_3 resin uptake
E) TSH and free T_4

11. A 16-year-old previously healthy adolescent develops persistent nausea, vomiting, diarrhea, and shakiness. Upon arrival at the emergency room, she has signs of significant dehydration on physical examination, and hyperpigmentation of skin lines, palms, and scars is noted. Her mother cannot tell you her daughter's baseline weight but does know that she has been losing weight and feeling tired for several months. Which of the following sets of laboratory values is most consistent with this patient's probable diagnosis?

A) Sodium 123 mEq per L
Potassium 7.1 mEq per L
Chloride 99 mEq per L
Dextrose stick 30 mg/dL
B) Sodium 123 mEq per L
Potassium 4.5 mEq per L
Chloride 99 mEq per L
Dextrose stick 30 mg per dL
C) Sodium 145 mEq per L
Potassium 7.1 mEq per L
Chloride 99 mEq per L
Dextrose stick 30 mg per dL
D) Sodium 123 mEq per L
Potassium 7.1 mEq per L
Chloride 120 mEq per L
Dextrose stick 30 mg per dL
E) Sodium 123 mEq per L
Potassium 7.1 mEq per L
Chloride 99 mEq per L
Dextrose stick 260 mg per dL

12. A 17-year-old patient with a non-salt-wasting form of congenital adrenal hyperplasia requires extraction of his wisdom teeth under general anesthesia. Which of the following plans of care is most appropriate for this patient?

A) Oral administration of stress-dose cortisone following surgery, with gradual weaning over 72 hours to his maintenance oral dose
B) Hospitalization for surgery and intravenous administration of stress-dose hydrocortisone until he can be weaned to his maintenance oral dose
C) Hospitalization for surgery and oral administration of stress-dose hydrocortisone until he can be weaned to his maintenance oral dose
D) Oral administration of stress-dose cortisone prior to and during surgery with gradual weaning over 72 hours to his maintenance oral dose
E) Outpatient surgery with no adjustment of oral cortisone dose

D) Celiac disease
E) Familial (genetic) short stature

26. An 11-year-old male is in your office for his routine health maintenance visit. He is concerned that he is becoming progressively shorter than his peers. His height is at the 10th percentile; 18 months ago, his height was at the 25th percentile. His weight has dropped from the 10th to the 5th percentile. His testes are slightly <2.5 cm in diameter, and no pubic or axillary hair is detected. The remainder of the physical examination is normal. He is adopted, and his family history is unknown. His bone age is delayed by 2 years and 6 months. Which of the following is the most likely cause of this patient's short stature?
A) Constitutional growth delay
B) Chronic disease
C) Undernutrition
D) Familial short stature
E) Endocrine disease

27. A mother brings her 7-year-old daughter to you because she is concerned about her child's progressive weight gain. The girl's weight is at the 75th percentile; 2 years ago, her weight was at the 75th percentile. Her height is at the 25th percentile; 2 years ago, it was at the 75th percentile. Her bone age is moderately delayed. Which of the following is most consistent with this patient's growth pattern?
A) Chronic systemic disease
B) Endocrine disease
C) Familial short stature
D) Constitutional growth delay
E) Excessive caloric intake

28. You are on-call when your outside laboratory notifies you that one of your partner's patients has a normal random serum insulin-like growth factor-1 (IGF-1) concentration. You review the 8-year-old patient's chart and note that your partner is concerned about possible acquired growth hormone deficiency. A normal random serum IGF-1 level:
A) rules out growth hormone deficiency
B) is not informative because growth hormone deficiency presents in the first year of life
C) is not informative because growth hormone level fluctuates throughout the day
D) is not informative because IGF-1 must be compared with insulin-like growth factor binding protein 3 to determine whether growth hormone deficiency is present
E) is not informative because alterations in IGF-1 levels are not associated with acquired growth hormone deficiency

29. You are seeing a 15-year-old male for his routine health maintenance visit. His family history is significant for lens subluxation in his father and mitral valve prolapse in a paternal uncle. His height is above the 95th percentile. On examination, he has upper and lower orthodontia, and his arms and legs are disproportionately long. This patient's tall stature is most likely caused by which of the following?
A) Soto syndrome
B) Klinefelter syndrome
C) Kallmann syndrome
D) Marfan syndrome
E) Familial tall stature

30. A 2-month-old boy with congenital hypothyroidism is on levothyroxine with stable serum thyroxine and thyroid-stimulating hormone levels. He is currently breast-fed, but his mother is going back to work. She is a vegetarian and prefers to start him on soy formula. Which of the following statements concerning the use of soy formula in this patient is true?
A) Soy protein should have no effect on serum thyroxine levels.
B) Soy protein may interfere with thyroid gland binding sites for thyroxine.
C) Soy protein may interfere with renal excretion of thyroxine.
D) Soy protein may increase gastrointestinal absorption of thyroxine.
E) Soy protein may decrease gastrointestinal absorption of thyroxine.

31. A 3-week-old, previously full-term male infant is brought to the emergency department for evaluation of his persistent vomiting. He has not regained his birth weight and is now not waking to feed. Vital signs include temperature 37.0°C, heart rate 180 beats per minute, and blood pressure 60/30 mm Hg. The patient is thin, lethargic, and obviously dehydrated. Serum electrolytes drawn with placement of intravenous access reveal hyponatremia, hyperkalemia, hypochloremia, and hypoglycemia. Which of the following studies is most likely to reveal the underlying abnormality in this patient?
A) Serum 17-hydroxyprogesterone concentration
B) Serum 17-hydroxycorticosteroid concentration
C) Serum 11-deoxycortisol concentration
D) Serum thyroxine concentration
E) Serum free thyroxine concentration

32. An 8-year-old boy who is in a medically induced coma following surgical evacuation of an epidural hematoma develops hyponatremia (serum sodium concentration 125 mEq/L). The serum potassium concentration falls within the normal range. Which of the following sets of urinary electrolyte findings suggests primary adrenal insufficiency rather than syndrome of inappropriate antidiuretic hormone as the etiology of the hyponatremia?

A) Sodium 70 mEq per L; potassium 50 mEq per L
B) Sodium 70 mEq per L; potassium 5 mEq per L
C) Sodium 10 mEq per L; potassium 5 mEq per L
D) Sodium 10 mEq per L; potassium 50 mEq per L
E) Sodium 50 mEq per L; potassium 60 mEq per L

ANSWERS

1. A
2. B
3. C
4. D
5. E
6. A
7. B
8. C
9. D
10. E
11. A
12. B
13. C
14. D
15. E
16. A
17. B
18. C
19. D
20. E
21. A
22. B
23. C
24. D
25. E
26. A
27. B
28. C
29. D
30. E
31. A
32. B

Gastrointestinal Disorders

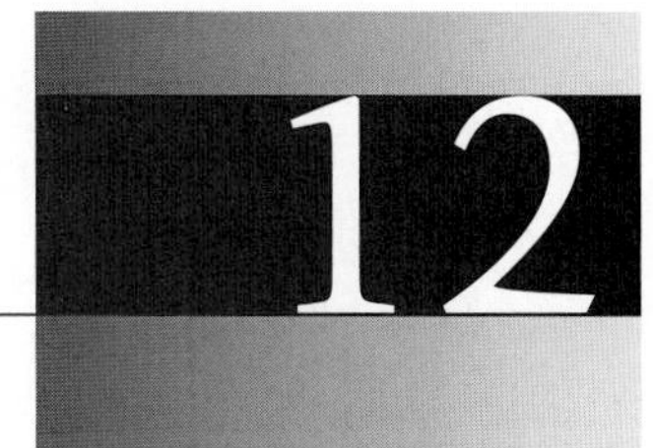

ACUTE ABDOMINAL PAIN

Acute abdominal pain may represent a *medical condition*, a *surgical emergency*, or *referred visceral pain* (Table 12-1). The majority of pediatric medical visits for acute abdominal pain are due to infection. Table 12-2 provides clinical and laboratory characteristics of several common and/or significant causes of abdominal pain in children, along with suggested imaging studies and treatment. Evaluation of the patient with acute abdominal pain begins with a careful history and physical examination, followed by judicious and targeted use of laboratory and radiographic studies:

- *History*—characterization of the pain, including onset, duration, location, radiation, severity, quality (e.g., colicky, cramping), temporal characteristics, and exacerbating and alleviating factors; associated symptoms (nausea, vomiting, anorexia, diarrhea, constipation, dysuria, joint pain, sore throat); ill contacts; recent diet history; history of previous laparoscopic or open abdominal surgery; past medical history; sexual history (in the adolescent); family history
- *Physical examination*—noting degree to which the pain limits the child's movement; auscultation for bowel sounds; palpation of the abdomen for guarding, rebound tenderness, mass; psoas/obturator signs; rectal, pelvic examination if appropriate
- *Laboratory assessment* and *radiographic studies* as indicated by results of history and physical examination

Findings on physical examination suggestive of peritoneal irritation due to a surgical abdomen include severe pain with walking or moving on the examination table, abdominal tenderness associated with distention or (more concerning) rigidity of the abdominal wall, and rebound tenderness. The acute management of patients with abdominal pain resulting from bowel obstruction or other surgical conditions consists of the following: decompression with a nasogastric tube; administration of appropriate replacement and maintenance fluids; diagnosis and treatment of electrolyte abnormalities; complete blood count, blood type, and cross-match; and surgical consultation/intervention.

TABLE 12-1
TYPICAL PATTERNS OF REFERRED PAIN

Right lower lobe pneumonia presenting with **right lower quadrant abdominal pain**
Gallbladder inflammation presenting with **right infrascapular pain**
Pancreatitis presenting with **posterior flank pain**
Ureteral stone presenting with **groin pain**
Rectal or gynecologic conditions presenting with **sacral pain**

CHRONIC RECURRENT ABDOMINAL PAIN

Recurrent abdominal pain was defined by Apley in 1958 as at least three episodes of pain over a 3-month period that are severe enough to limit activities and for which there is no organic explanation. The classic presentation involves a child with typical growth and normal physical examination who complains of recurrent periumbilical pain (unassociated with eating or stooling) that interferes with activities but resolves on its own and is not severe enough to cause nighttime wakening. Recently, recurrent functional abdominal pain has been subclassified into four separate disorders:

- *Functional abdominal pain*—nearly continuous abdominal pain for at least 3 months that interferes with daily functioning and is not associated with physiologic triggers (e.g., eating, defecation, menstrual cycle).
- *Irritable bowel syndrome* (IBS)—at least 12 weeks of pain over a 12-month period that has no medical explanation and at least two of the following: relief of pain with defecation; onset of pain associated with changes in stool frequency (>3 per day or <3 per week); and onset of pain associated with changes in stool character (much firmer or looser than usual; mucus in stool). Patients often complain of bloating and abdominal distension as well. IBS may be either constipation- or diarrhea-dominant.
- *Functional dyspepsia*—at least 12 weeks of upper abdominal pain (not relieved by defecation) over a 12-month period with no evidence of gastrointestinal pathology and no changes in stool frequency or character.
- *Abdominal migraine*—three or more paroxysmal episodes of midline abdominal pain lasting hours to days, with complete resolution to a pain-free state between episodes,

TABLE 12-2
EVALUATION OF ABDOMINAL PAIN IN THE PEDIATRIC PATIENT

Viral Gastroenteritis

Etiology

Rotavirus, enteric *adenovirus*, *enterovirus*, Norwalk virus

Symptoms

Mild-to-moderate fever and nonbloody emesis, followed by intermittent cramping, periumbilical or generalized abdominal discomfort; diarrhea (usually nonbloody, excepting rotavirus in infants). Typical duration, 2 to 10 days.

Signs

Physical findings consistent with dehydration may be present depending on the degree of fluid lost. Notable absence of toxic appearance, distention, guarding, rebound tenderness.

Laboratory Results

White blood count normal or slightly elevated without significant left shift; other laboratory results consistent with dehydration, when present. Immunoassay studies available for specific viral agents but usually unnecessary.

Radiographic Studies

None indicated

Treatment

Supportive care to prevent/manage dehydration. Caution against the use of antimotility agents in pediatric patients. Early refeeding (or continuation of regular feeds when possible) does not exacerbate the course of mild-to-moderate gastroenteritis and may actually decrease the duration of diarrhea.

Complications

Temporary secondary lactose intolerance following diarrheal illnesses characterized by abdominal cramping, distension, flatulence, and watery diarrhea

Bacterial Gastroenteritis

Etiology

Shigella, Salmonella, Campylobacter, Yersinia, Escherichia coli

Symptoms

Fever, abdominal pain, tenesmus; diarrheal stools frequently mixed with blood and mucus

Signs

Similar to those for viral gastroenteritis

Laboratory Results

Elevated white blood count with left shift; fecal leukocytes; identification of organism (which may or may not produce enterotoxin) via stool culture; sensitivity testing

Radiographic Studies

None indicated unless focal findings on abdominal examination

Treatment

Specific antimicrobial therapy may or may not be indicated based on the suspected or recovered pathogen (see Chapter 10)

Complications

Adjacent or hematogenous spread

Parasitic Gastroenteritis

See Chapter 10 (specifically, *Giardia lamblia*)

Appendicitis

Etiology

Bacterial invasion of an obstructed appendix

Symptoms

Vague periumbilical pain localizing to the right lower quadrant (McBurney point); fever; anorexia (note: retrocecal appendicitis presents with localized periumbilical pain and diarrhea)

Signs

Hypoactive bowel sounds; guarding, rebound tenderness; positive psoas and obturator signs

Laboratory Results

High-normal or elevated white blood count with left shift

Radiographic Studies

Computed tomography with contrast enema demonstrating thickened, inflamed appendix (most sensitive, specific diagnostic study); ultrasonography as initial screen in some cases; abdominal plain radiographs generally not helpful but may reveal an appendicolith

(*continued*)

TABLE 12-2
(continued)

Treatment
Surgical removal of the appendix
Complications
Perforation of the appendix with subsequent peritonitis (most common in young children)

Acute Pancreatitis
Etiology
Gallstones (adolescence); blunt trauma to the abdomen; idiopathic; infectious; drug associated (e.g., valproic acid); vasculitis
Symptoms
Acute, unremitting pain localized to the right upper quadrant or epigastric area with radiation to the back; pain worsens when the patient is supine; vomiting, anorexia; low-grade fever
Signs
Tenderness to palpation of the upper abdomen without peritoneal signs
Laboratory Results
Elevated serum lipase; elevated serum amylase (note: serum amylase may also be elevated in cases of biliary tract obstruction, appendicitis, and peritonitis); hypercalcemia and hyperlipidemia may precipitate acute pancreatitis in rare cases
Radiographic Studies
Abdominal ultrasonography (stones, enlarged pancreas); computed tomography
Treatment
Hospital admission; nasogastric suction; meperidine for pain control; supportive care; surgery occasionally required
Complications
Hypovolemic shock; hypocalcemia, hyperglycemia
Note: Recurrent/chronic pancreatitis may be due to genetic disease (*cystic fibrosis, hereditary pancreatitis*) and anatomic abnormalities (*pancreas divisum*, which interferes with ductal drainage, and *long common channel*, which results in activation of pancreatic enzymes within the pancreas).

Intussusception
Etiology
One portion of the bowel telescopes into another (most commonly invagination of the terminal ileum into the adjacent large bowel), resulting in obstruction; Meckel diverticulum or intestinal polyp may serve as a "lead point" in the older child, but the condition is usually idiopathic in younger children
Symptoms
Sudden onset of recurrent short episodes of severe pain alternating with virtually asymptomatic periods; vomiting; bloody "currant jelly" stools (50% to 70%); eventual weakness progressing to profound lethargy between episodes of pain
Signs
Palpation of the abdomen reveals moderately tender indistinct mass, usually in the right upper quadrant; absence of peritoneal signs
Laboratory Results
Stool positive for occult blood
Radiographic Studies
Air (preferred) or barium contrast enema diagnostic and often therapeutic; demonstrates filling defect, cupping, or coil-spring within the intussuscepted bowel
Treatment
Laparoscopic reduction is indicated for cases that do not resolve with contrast enema and those resulting in bowel perforation and/or shock
Complications
Pneumatosis intestinalis; intestinal perforation; shock
Note: Intussusception occurs most frequently in children younger than 2 years of age and is the most common cause of intestinal obstruction in young childhood beyond the neonatal period. The condition may follow a self-limited infectious illness such as gastroenteritis or viral upper respiratory symptoms.

(*continued*)

TABLE 12-2
(continued)

Midgut Volvulus/Malrotation

Etiology

Abnormal fixation of the mesentery allows a section of bowel and its arterial supply (superior mesenteric artery) to twist upon itself, resulting in strangulation of the vasculature and bowel necrosis within 2 to 4 hours

Symptoms

Acute onset of abdominal pain that does not abate; bilious emesis; bloody stools (late)

Signs

Mild-to-moderate distension; diffuse abdominal tenderness with guarding; occasionally, dilated loops of bowel are palpable

Laboratory Results

Metabolic acidosis; stool may be positive for occult or frank blood

Radiographic Studies

Flat and upright abdominal films with dilated loops of bowel overlying the liver shadow and little or no gas distal to the obstruction; "corkscrew" pattern on upper gastrointestinal series, which is the diagnostic study of choice

Treatment

Surgical correction (laparotomy with detorsion of the involved segment); intravenous antibiotic therapy is indicated due to the high risk of systemic infection with enteric organisms; total parenteral nutrition immediately following surgery (longer in patients status-post resection due to bowel necrosis)

Complications

Rapid progression to shock, bowel necrosis; death

Note: Midgut volvulus is most common in neonates and young infants but may rarely present in childhood and beyond. *Malrotation* refers to abnormal rotation of the fetal bowel outside the abdominal cavity; the upper gastrointestinal series demonstrates aberrant positioning of the ligament of Treitz and proximal jejunum. Malrotation predisposes to acute volvulus or chronic intermittent obstruction, characterized by periodic abdominal pain and vomiting. Malrotation may remain asymptomatic.

Postoperative Intestinal Obstruction

Etiology

Small bowel obstruction following abdominal surgery; usually due to the development of intestinal adhesions

Symptoms

Intermittent cramping abdominal pain; vomiting; decreased urine output (due to third-spacing)

Signs

Hyperactive bowel sounds; abdominal distension; diffuse abdominal tenderness; surgical scars

Laboratory Results

Variable and related to degree of dehydration

Radiographic Studies

Dilated loops of small bowel proximal to the obstruction on abdominal flat and upright radiographs; obtain computed tomography if questionable

Treatment

Observation on nasogastric suction; surgical intervention if no resolution

Complications

Shock, peritonitis, sepsis, wound dehiscence; death

Other conditions included in the differential diagnosis of acute abdominal pain:

group A streptococcal infection
gastritis
drug-induced dyspepsia
peptic ulcer disease
hepatitis
Fitz-Hugh-Curtis syndrome
cholecystitis
mesenteric lymphadenitis
incarcerated hernia
Crohn disease
ulcerative colitis
constipation
urinary tract infection
ureteropelvic junction obstruction
hydronephrosis
renal stones
pelvic inflammatory disease
ectopic pregnancy
ovarian or adnexal torsion
testicular torsion
traumatic injury
abdominal migraine
Henoch-Schönlein purpura
sickle cell crisis
malignancy

and at least two of the following: headache during painful episodes; photophobia during painful episodes; family history of migraines; unilateral headaches; and visual, sensory, or motor auras.

Contrary to earlier speculation, lactose intolerance and *Helicobacter pylori* infection are not associated with functional abdominal pain. *Lactose intolerance* presents with cramping abdominal pain, bloating, flatulence, and loose stools following the ingestion of dairy products. The diagnostic test of choice is the breath hydrogen test, which detects an elevation in breath hydrogen concentration after oral lactose administration in patients who are intolerant. Elimination of lactose from the diet, when associated with resolution of symptoms, can be both diagnostic and therapeutic. *H. pylori-associated peptic ulcer disease* (PUD) is discussed later in this chapter. In the absence of characteristic symptoms, routine testing for lactose intolerance and *H. pylori* infection is not indicated in patients with functional abdominal pain.

The differential diagnosis of chronic recurrent abdominal pain includes celiac disease, inflammatory bowel disease (IBD), PUD, lactose intolerance, chronic constipation, cholelithiasis, pancreatitis, malrotation, ovarian cysts, endometriosis, Mittelschmerz, and parasitic infections. However, no causative medical condition is identified in as many as 85% of children with recurrent abdominal pain. "Red flags" associated with an increased likelihood of organic disease include:

- age younger than 5 years
- family history of IBD or PUD
- constitutional symptoms (fever, weight loss, poor growth)
- repetitive vomiting, diarrhea, or bilious emesis
- pain that progressively increases in intensity or duration over time
- perianal disease (skin tags, fissures, ulcerations)
- pain that is referred to back or shoulders
- pain that awakens the patient from sleep
- organomegaly
- joint inflammation
- frankly bloody or guaiac-positive stools
- abnormal urinalysis, positive urine culture
- anemia, hypoalbuminemia, abnormal liver function tests, elevated erythrocyte sedimentation rate (ESR)

Patients with any of the above and those whose symptoms are not consistent with functional abdominal pain warrant further investigation for an identifiable organic cause of their pain.

The laboratory evaluation of recurrent abdominal pain should be guided by results of the history and physical examination. Baseline testing consists of a *complete blood count, urinalysis, and stool for occult blood*. Other studies that may be beneficial depending on clinical presentation include ESR; celiac screening studies; serum protein, albumin, and liver enzymes; and stool for fecal leukocytes, ova and parasites, and culture. Abdominal radiographs can confirm the diagnosis of constipation in any patient with a questionable history. Abdominal ultrasonography is appropriate in patients with lateralizing pain, for lower abdominal pain in adolescent females, and in patients with suspected renal disease. Signs and symptoms suggestive of IBD or PUD warrant referral to a gastroenterologist for endoscopy.

Management of recurrent abdominal pain of functional origin centers on symptom relief and return to normal functioning. Peppermint oil, an antispasmodic agent, has been used with some success in patients with functional abdominal pain. Approximately half of patients with IBS experience significant improvement with fiber supplementation. Second-line therapies include antispasmodic agents such as hyoscyamine, loperamide and other antidiarrheal drugs, cholestyramine, probiotics, and management of constipation when present. Colonoscopy is indicated for patients with IBS that does not respond to medical therapy. Functional dyspepsia often improves with H2-receptor antagonists or proton pump inhibitors. Abdominal migraines are treated in much the same way as classic migraine headaches; prophylaxis should be considered in patients with significant impairment.

UPPER GASTROINTESTINAL BLEEDING

Upper gastrointestinal (UGI) bleeding takes place proximal to the *ligament of Treitz* (which inserts into the distal portion of the duodenum). *Hematemesis* is usually a sign of UGI bleeding, although blood ingested during nasal or oropharyngeal bleeding may also result in bloody emesis. Newborn infants may vomit ingested maternal blood, which is differentiated through Apt testing. Certain foods and dyes in medication or candy resemble blood in emesis; bedside testing will identify true blood. *Melena* is a consistent finding in UGI bleeding, although massive UGI bleeding may result in bright red blood per rectum. The differential diagnosis of UGI bleeding includes esophageal varices, erosive esophagitis, Mallory-Weiss tear, gastritis, duodenitis, PUD, arteriovenous malformations, tumors, and bleeding disorders. Patients with UGI bleeding require hemovascular stabilization with fluid replacement and possibly transfusion. Ideally, laboratory specimens should be obtained at the time of IV placement for a complete blood count, coagulation studies, and blood typing and cross-matching. Patients with liver disease may require vitamin K or fresh frozen plasma to correct associated coagulopathies. Placement of a nasogastric tube confirms blood in the stomach and permits assessment of ongoing bleeding. Additional evaluation (ideally endoscopy) is delayed until the patient is stabilized.

Esophageal varices virtually always present with UGI bleeding and hematemesis, which is generally sudden in onset, severe, painless, and not preceded by vomiting. *Portal hypertension* (elevated pressure in the portal vein) is by far the most common cause of esophageal varices; the varices are a form of collateral circulation allowing blood flow from the portal vein into the systemic circulation.

Portal hypertension may be prehepatic, intrahepatic, or posthepatic in origin:

- *Portal vein thrombosis* (PVT) is an important cause of *prehepatic portal hypertension*. PVT is a known complication of umbilical vein catheterization in the neonate. Intra-abdominal infection, inflammation (Crohn disease), and generalized hypercoagulable states have been associated with PVT. A significant minority of cases are idiopathic.
- *Intrahepatic* causes of portal hypertension include cirrhosis, hepatitis (infectious, autoimmune), metabolic disorders, cystic fibrosis, hepatic fibrosis, and biliary disease. A history of liver disease suggests an intrahepatic abnormality.
- *Posthepatic* portal hypertension may result from thrombosis or elevated pressure in the hepatic vein, inferior vena cava, or right atrium (e.g., constrictive pericarditis, right-sided congestive heart failure).

Although hematemesis from bleeding esophageal varices is the most frequent presentation of portal hypertension, splenomegaly may be the sole presenting feature in some patients.

Abdominal ultrasonography with Doppler enhancement allows evaluation of the liver, portal vein flow, and associated structures and vessels. Somatostatin (or vasopressin) is administered to decrease portal blood flow and assist in initial stabilization if needed. Endoscopy is both diagnostic and therapeutic, allowing sclerosis or band ligation of any visible varices. Surgery is reserved for patients with unresponsive or recurrent bleeding. Propranolol, which reduces portal perfusion, is prescribed following initial management to decrease the risk of rebleeding.

LOWER GASTROINTESTINAL BLEEDING

Lower gastrointestinal (LGI) bleeding originates distal to the ligament of Treitz and presents as occult blood, melena, or bright red blood per rectum. An extensive differential diagnosis of LGI bleeding is included in Table 12-3. Since massive UGI bleeding can also produce hematochezia, passage of a nasogastric tube should be considered in patients with hematochezia to rule out UGI hemorrhage. In practice, however, the colon is the most likely source of bleeding seen with hematochezia. Examination of the anus is essential in any child who presents with rectal bleeding.

Young children with LGI bleeding who are hemodynamically compromised and/or anemic and those with significant comorbid conditions require urgent intervention, which is virtually identical to that for acute UGI bleeding. Further evaluation is deferred until the patient's condition is stabilized and depends on results of the history and physical examination.

Juvenile Polyps

Inflammatory polyps are a common cause of periodic painless bright red rectal bleeding in preschool-age children. The risk of malignant transformation is extremely low in isolated juvenile inflammatory polyps. However, the diagnosis should be verified by colonoscopy to remove the polyps, exclude more serious possibilities, and identify patients who require periodic colonoscopic screening (which includes *patients with four or more polyps, patients with recurrent rectal bleeding, and patients with a positive family history of juvenile polyposis*). Polyps rarely bleed enough to produce anemia.

Polyposis syndromes that do carry a risk of malignant transformation include *Peutz-Jeghers syndrome* (PJS) and familial adenomatous polyposis. PJS is an autosomal dominant condition consisting of numerous polyps scattered along the colon, small intestine, and stomach. Melanotic pigmentation of the lips, the buccal mucosa, and occasionally the palms and soles is a common finding. Intussusception is a known complication of PJS in children. At least half of adult patients with PJS develop malignancies of the gastrointestinal tract, breast, ovary, pancreas, or endometrium.

Familial adenomatous polyposis (formerly called Gardner syndrome) is an autosomal dominant condition in which patients develop multiple adenomas of the colon starting in the adolescent years, with an extremely high rate of malignant transformation to colorectal cancer that necessitates prophylactic colectomy in adulthood. Colonoscopy is recommended every 1 to 3 years.

TABLE 12-3
DIFFERENTIAL DIAGNOSIS OF LOWER GASTROINTESTINAL BLEEDING

Cow milk allergy
Volvulus with malrotation
Necrotizing enterocolitis
Crohn disease
Intussusception
Meckel diverticulum
Infectious colitis
Intestinal polyps
Ulcerative colitis
Henoch-Schönlein purpura
Hemolytic uremic syndrome
Hemorrhoids
Anal fissures
Abdominal or rectal trauma

Meckel Diverticulum

Meckel diverticulum typically presents with painless rectal bleeding manifesting as melena or brick/maroon-colored stools. Bleeding associated with Meckel diverticulum is most common in patients younger than 2 years but may occur at any age. The diverticulae are located in the distal ileum within 2 feet of the ileocecal valve, and the vast majority remains asymptomatic. Occasionally, a Meckel diverticulum presents with massive LGI bleeding, hypovolemia, and anemia. Abdominal tenderness is uncommon, but if present, it is usually noted in the right lower quadrant. Fever and fecal leukocytes are notably absent.

ABDOMINAL MASSES

The differential diagnosis of abdominal mass in the pediatric population varies according to age (Table 12-4).

VOMITING

Vomiting is a common pediatric complaint that prompts parents to seek medical attention. The leading diagnosis in all age groups is *infection* (Table 12-5). *Small bowel obstruction* often presents with vomiting; some conditions that predispose to obstruction of the small bowel include adhesions, malrotation with volvulus, incarcerated inguinal hernia, intussusception, and Crohn disease. Vomiting is a frequent complication of *cancer chemotherapy*; ondansetron, a selective serotonin receptor antagonist, is beneficial for treating postchemotherapy emesis.

Cyclical vomiting syndrome is an uncommon disorder thought to be an atypical variant of migraine. Patients present with a history of recurrent episodes of vomiting that are acute in onset and severe, usually lasting several hours. Diarrhea and photophobia may accompany the emesis. Between these episodes, the patient is completely asymptomatic for days or weeks at a time. Once organic disease has been ruled out, cyclic vomiting syndrome treatment is similar to that for migraine headaches.

TABLE 12-4
DIFFERENTIAL DIAGNOSIS OF ABDOMINAL MASS BY AGE

Neonate/Young Infant
Hydronephrosis (posterior urethral valves)
Cystic kidney disease
Wilms tumor
Ectopic kidney
Pyloric stenosis
Neuroblastoma

Older Infant/Child/Adolescent
Constipation
Intussusception
Abdominal or pelvic abscess
Pregnancy
Ovarian cyst, torsion, or mass
Hydrometrocolpos (distension of the uterus with retained fluids resulting from imperforate hymen)
Neuroblastoma
Renal tumor
Adrenal tumor
Lymphoma

TABLE 12-5
DIFFERENTIAL DIAGNOSIS OF VOMITING IN THE PEDIATRIC POPULATION

Neonate
Anatomic or surgical conditions of the intestinal tract

Infant
Gastroesophageal reflux
Metabolic disorders
Food intolerance
Allergies
Obstructive lesions
Renal disease
Sepsis

Toddler
Foreign body in the esophagus

Child
Reflux esophagitis
Peptic ulcer disease
Pancreatitis
Cholecystitis
Inflammatory bowel disease
Cyclic vomiting

Any Age
Brain tumors
Diabetes mellitus
Gastrointestinal obstructive lesions

Bilious Emesis

Bilious vomiting is consistent with small bowel obstruction distal to the ampulla of Vater, where bile passes into the bowel lumen midway through the duodenum. In the infant, vomiting bile is a medical emergency because of the possibility of malrotation with acute volvulus. Mild bilious emesis is occasionally associated with intestinal dysmotility following a viral infection.

Pyloric Stenosis

Pyloric stenosis is caused by hypertrophy of the musculature surrounding the pylorus, resulting in gastric outlet obstruction. Preterm neonates, infants with a positive family history, and males are at higher risk. The classic presentation is *projectile nonbilious emesis* beginning between the second and fourth weeks of life. The vomiting may be slowly progressive, resulting in poor weight gain, or sudden in onset, presenting with dehydration. Infants with pyloric stenosis remain hungry and feed eagerly but retain little of what they take in. Upper abdominal distension and visual gastric peristaltic waves are relatively common. Physical examination often reveals an olive-sized mass above and slightly to the right of the umbilicus. The loss of primarily gastric secretions in pyloric stenosis results in *hypochloremic metabolic alkalosis*, with hypokalemia developing as the kidney retains hydrogen ions in the place of potassium. The hypertrophied pylorus is easily identifiable on abdominal ultrasonography, the diagnostic study of choice. Following rehydration and correction of acid-base and electrolyte abnormalities, affected patients undergo surgical correction (pyloromyotomy) with complete resolution of vomiting.

Duodenal Atresia/Stenosis

Duodenal atresia is an anatomic obstruction resulting from nonpatency of the duodenal lumen. The condition is significantly more common in patients with Down syndrome and fetal alcohol syndrome. Duodenal atresia presents with bilious vomiting after feeds in the first day of life. The appearance of a "double-bubble" in the upper abdomen on an upright radiograph coupled with the absence of gas in the distal bowel strongly suggests duodenal atresia.

Duodenal stenosis, duodenal webs, and annular pancreas may all result in partial obstruction of the duodenal lumen. These conditions present in infancy or beyond, depending on the degree of obstruction. Typical signs and symptoms include nausea, vomiting, abdominal pain, and poor growth.

Antral Web

Antral webs are thin membranes found just proximal to the pylorus of the stomach. The presentation is similar to that of pyloric stenosis in infants, although the pylorus is normal in size and structure on ultrasound. Older children with antral webs develop intermittent nausea, vomiting, and abdominal pain. Surgical ablation results in complete resolution of symptoms.

DIARRHEA

Infectious Diarrhea

Gastrointestinal infection is the most common cause of diarrhea in all age groups. The most likely pathogens vary by age (Table 12-6). Specific infectious agents are discussed in detail in Chapter 10. Loperamide and other antidiarrheal medications are not indicated for the treatment of infectious gastroenteritis in children; retention of infectious fluid in the bowel may, in some cases, lead to toxic megacolon and/or local/systemic invasive disease.

TABLE 12-6
INFECTIOUS DIARRHEA: LIKELY PATHOGENS BY PATIENT AGE GROUP

Infants and Young Children

- Rotavirus, enteric adenovirus
- *Salmonella, Shigella, Campylobacter, Yersinia enterocolitica*
- *Giardia lamblia*

Older Children

- Norwalk virus
- *Escherichia coli, Salmonella, Campylobacter*
- *Giardia lamblia*

Adolescents and Adults

- Norwalk and Norwalk-like viruses
- *Campylobacter, E. coli, Salmonella, Shigella*

Noninfectious Diarrhea

Noninfectious diarrhea may be related to malabsorption syndromes, protein or carbohydrate intolerance, primary gastrointestinal abnormalities, food allergies, ingestions, or systemic disease. Most of these conditions are discussed in their respective chapters.

Complex carbohydrates are broken down into monosaccharides by amylase and intestinal enzymes. Deficiency of any of these enzymes produces carbohydrate malabsorption (Table 12-7).

TABLE 12-7
CARBOHYDRATE MALABSORPTION

Primary Carbohydrate Malabsorption

- Inherited deficiency of an intestinal enzyme involved in the breakdown of di- or trisaccharides
- *Congenital sucrase-isomaltase deficiency* (autosomal recessive)—presentation at approximately 6 months of age coincides with regular ingestion of starch- or sucrose-containing foods; higher prevalence in Canadian Indians and Greenland Eskimos; treated with dietary restriction and enzyme replacement
- *Congenital lactase deficiency* (autosomal recessive)—extremely rare disorder that presents with the institution of milk feedings in the first week of life; higher prevalence in the Finnish population
- *Adult-type lactase deficiency*—relatively common condition resulting from a steady decrease in lactase production beginning in childhood and progressing throughout adulthood; more common in Asian, American-Indian, and African-American populations, but also affects a significant minority of whites; may or may not cause symptoms of lactose intolerance; when present, symptom onset ranges from middle childhood to adulthood; treated with dietary restriction and enzyme replacement

Secondary Carbohydrate Malabsorption

- *Temporary lactose intolerance* resulting from an infectious (rotavirus, *Giardia*) or inflammatory condition (celiac disease) that damages the intestinal brush border. *Intractable diarrhea of infancy* (discussed on the next page).

Chronic Diarrhea

A partial list of disorders that cause chronic diarrhea in the pediatric population is provided in Table 12-8. Malnutrition,

TABLE 12-8
DIFFERENTIAL DIAGNOSIS OF CHRONIC DIARRHEA

Infancy
Intractable diarrhea of infancy
Gastrointestinal infection
Chronic nonspecific diarrhea (toddler's diarrhea)
Cystic fibrosis
Celiac disease[a]
Hirschsprung disease
Immunodeficiency syndromes or human immunodeficiency virus
Intestinal malrotation
Acrodermatitis enteropathica
Microvillus inclusion disease[a]
Congenital chloride diarrhea[a]
Congenital sodium diarrhea[a]
Factitious diarrhea
Children
Gastrointestinal infection
Cystic fibrosis
Celiac disease[a]
Irritable bowel syndrome
Crohn disease[a]
Ulcerative colitis[a]
Postinfectious diarrhea
Chronic cholestasis
Lactase deficiency[a]
Hirschsprung disease

[a]Bowel biopsy required for definitive diagnosis.

chronic disease, systemic illness, and immunodeficiencies increase the risk of chronic diarrhea and its complications.

Intractable diarrhea of infancy and chronic nonspecific diarrhea are two causes of chronic diarrhea in infants and very young children. *Intractable diarrhea of infancy* (IDI) is a more extreme form of secondary disaccharidase deficiency; destruction of the brush border and reduction of intake during an episode of infectious enteritis can severely limit the immature intestine's ability to digest and absorb nutrients, leading to variable degrees of feeding intolerance. IDI is more likely to occur in infants when oral intake during the initial illness is limited to hypotonic fluids (i.e., diluted juice). Affected patients have recurrent or persistent periods of watery diarrhea and grow poorly. Temporary parenteral nutrition is indicated for infants with failure to thrive and severe malabsorption in infancy, regardless of the cause of their chronic diarrhea. Intestinal biopsy should be considered for infants with diarrhea and malnutrition who do not respond to conservative interventions; however, this procedure carries a relatively high rate of perforation in young, malnourished infants.

Chronic nonspecific diarrhea (CNSD; also termed "toddler's diarrhea") presents between the ages of 9 and 24 months with explosive loose stools flecked with visible food particles that occur 4 to 12 times per day. Affected children have normal growth. Notably absent are frank or occult blood in the stool, fever, and anemia. Dietary factors that contribute to the persistence of CNSD include excessive intake of fluid, particularly fruit juices (apple and pear, which contain sorbitol), and low fat and fiber intake. The diagnosis of CNSD is usually clinically evident. In questionable instances, examination of the stool for pH, reducing substances, neutral fat, occult blood, and parasites may be informative and/or reassuring. Treatment consists of limiting overall fluid and specifically juice and sorbitol intake; increasing dietary fat and fiber; reassurance; and continued monitoring of growth. CNSD resolves spontaneously and is not thought to be associated with an increased risk of gastrointestinal disease later in life.

Bloody Diarrhea/Acute Colitis

Colitis, or inflammation of the colon, is evidenced by moderate generalized abdominal pain, bloody diarrhea, and fecal leukocytes on examination of the stool. Enteric bacterial infection is a common cause of acute colitis; in these cases, symptoms are typically of brief duration, and the patient is febrile. Culture of the stool and examination for ova and parasites should assist in diagnosis. Other causes of colitis in the child and adolescent include:

- pseudomembranous colitis caused by *Clostridium difficile* (history is positive for current or recent antibiotic therapy)
- amebiasis due to *Entamoeba histolytica* (higher likelihood in patients with history of travel to or recent emigration from a developing country, institutionalized patients, and males who have sex with males)
- IBD, particularly ulcerative colitis
- immune-mediated inflammatory process (Behcet syndrome)
- celiac disease
- eosinophilic gastroenteritis (abdominal pain and postprandial vomiting in the setting of anemia and peripheral eosinophilia)
- vasculitis (Henoch-Schönlein purpura, hemolytic-uremic syndrome)

CONSTIPATION

Constipation is the infrequent and/or difficult passage of hard stools. Chronic constipation causes overextension of the smooth muscle of the colon, resulting in functional ileus. Other complications of persistent constipation include overflow diarrhea, impaction, anal fissures and rectal bleeding, urinary retention and urinary tract infections, and abdominal pain. The most common cause of pediatric constipation beyond the neonatal period is *encopresis* (intentional withholding), which often begins during toilet training or a period of constipation. Organic causes of constipation are provided in Table 12-9. Even when the history is questionable, constipation is clearly evident on an abdominal radiograph. Dietary and behavior changes are usually sufficient to improve stooling habits. Children with impacted feces may respond to enemas or oral GoLYTELY; manual disimpaction is a last resort. The long-term use of enemas and stimulants should be avoided.

Encopresis is defined as voluntary withholding of stool with eventual stooling in inappropriate places (i.e., anywhere other than the toilet). The majority of encopresis is associated with functional constipation and resulting overflow diarrhea. The affected child presents with a history of difficult or painful stooling. Concomitant enuresis may indicate neurologic dysfunction or an associated urinary tract infection due to poor hygiene or bladder outlet obstruction. A digital rectal examination must be performed at least once during the evaluation of a child with encopresis in order to assess rectal and anal tone. Rectal fissures can be both a cause and consequence of stool withholding.

Delayed toilet training and toilet refusal may occasionally be mistaken for encopresis. Management of the three conditions is virtually identical when constipation is present. Treatment is adjusted based on the developmental age of the child and the severity and duration of constipation. Initial counseling is often beneficial for alleviating stress the child may be feeling related to shame, embarrassment, or anxiety about inappropriate stooling and proposed treatments. The most effective programs employ both pharmacologic and behavioral interventions. Laxative therapy with oral bisacodyl, suppositories, and enemas is appropriate for children ages 7 years and older. Oral therapy (polyethylene glycol, senna, or bisacodyl) alone is indicated for younger children and those with histories of anal or rectal trauma. Once the large bowel is free of stool, the child is placed on the toilet at scheduled times throughout the day (usually following breakfast and dinner) for a variable length of time, depending on age and attention span. Mineral oil or polyethylene glycol is administered to keep the stool soft and regular. Relapse is common and should be anticipated.

Encopresis that is not associated with constipation is more likely to result from underlying pathology or psychosocial stressors (e.g., abuse). Patients with difficult or painful stooling that is present from birth and accompanied by abdominal distention, emesis, recurrent enterocolitis, and/or failure to thrive should be evaluated for Hirschsprung disease. Detection of a tight segment of terminal bowel on digital examination is consistent with this diagnosis. Primary encopresis without constipation may respond to behavior therapy alone; laxatives are not indicated.

TABLE 12-9
ORGANIC CAUSES OF CONSTIPATION

Dietary
Low-fiber diet
Inadequate fluid intake

Gastrointestinal
Hirschsprung disease
Anal stenosis
Rectal abscess
Stricture following necrotizing enterocolitis (NEC)
Cystic fibrosis/meconium ileus
Anorectal dysfunction following pull-through surgery

Drugs or Toxins
Lead
Narcotics
Phenothiazines
Vincristine
Anticholinergic drugs

Neuromuscular
Meningomyelocele
Tethered spinal cord
Infant botulism
Prune belly syndrome

Metabolic
Hypokalemia
Hypercalcemia

Endocrine
Hypothyroidism

Other
Collagen vascular disease
Anxiety
Child abuse[a]

[a] Suppositories and enemas are avoided in the treatment of encopresis patients with suspected physical or sexual abuse.

JAUNDICE

Bilirubin is a product of the breakdown of heme-containing proteins from senescent red blood cells and other sources. Free (*unconjugated*) bilirubin is released into the plasma and binds to albumin for transport to the liver, where the majority is *conjugated* to form bilirubin glucuronide, a water-soluble molecule that can be excreted with bile salts and eventually eliminated in the feces. Excessive bilirubin in the blood accumulates in the skin and sclerae; the visible yellowish discoloration is termed *jaundice*. Physiologic and pathologic jaundice in the neonate is discussed in Chapter 5. Infectious hepatitis, the most common cause of acute hyperbilirubinemia in a previously well child, is included in Chapter 10. Some of the more common causes of unconjugated and conjugated hyperbilirubinemia in the infant and child are listed in Table 12-10. Primarily

TABLE 12-10
JAUNDICE IN THE INFANT AND CHILD

Infants ≥2 Months of Age
Unconjugated hyperbilirubinemia
Hemolytic disorders
Cystic fibrosis
Pyloric stenosis
Hypothyroidism
Sepsis
Drugs
Conjugated hyperbilirubinemia
Infection
  Viral hepatitis
  Toxoplasmosis
  Syphilis
Total parenteral nutrition
Drugs[a]
Disorders of carbohydrate metabolism
  Galactosemia
  Glycogen storage disease (I and IV)
  Hereditary fructose intolerance
Disorders of protein metabolism
  Tyrosinemia
Disorders of lipid metabolism
  Niemann-Pick disease
  Gaucher disease
Inherited genetic disorders
  Down syndrome
  Turner syndrome
  Alpha-1-antitrypsin deficiency
  Cystic fibrosis
Intrahepatic biliary obstruction
  Alagille syndrome (hereditary form of biliary atresia associated with peripheral pulmonary artery stenosis)
Extrahepatic biliary obstruction
  Biliary atresia
Older Children and Adolescents
Unconjugated hyperbilirubinemia
Hemolytic disorders
Gilbert disease
Crigler-Najjar syndrome
Conjugated hyperbilirubinemia
Viral, parasitic liver infections
Liver abscess
Cirrhosis
Primary or metastatic hepatic carcinoma
Medications/drugs[a]
Wilson disease
Hemochromatosis
Reye syndrome
Cholelithiasis
Cholecystitis
Choledochal cyst
Cholangitis
Dubin-Johnson syndrome
Total parenteral nutrition

[a]Minocycline, chlorpromazine, sulfa drugs, acetaminophen, phenytoin, isoniazid.

unconjugated hyperbilirubinemia is typically caused by an *excessive biliary load*. Conjugated hyperbilirubinemia is more likely to be due to *hepatic disease, impaired bile secretion, or cholestasis* (obstruction of bile flow from the liver, evidenced by acholic stool and hepatomegaly). A suggested evaluation of conjugated hyperbilirubinemia is provided in Figure 12-1.

Gilbert Disease

Gilbert disease results from any of a number of inherited defects in the enzyme uridine diphosphate-glucuronyltransferase, which facilitates the conjugation of bilirubin to a water-soluble molecule within the liver. The mild elevation in unconjugated bilirubin due to a modest reduction in conjugation capacity is manifested by scleral icterus, which is more noticeable in the morning. There are no other signs and symptoms, and liver function remains normal. The condition is chronic but not progressive; no therapy is indicated beyond education and reassurance.

While Gilbert disease is due to a decreased amount of a functionally normal enzyme, patients with *Crigler-Najjar syndrome* produce an abnormal form of uridine diphosphate-glucuronyltransferase. The infantile form of Crigler-Najjar syndrome is fatal in the first year of life; a milder form of the disease that presents in middle childhood is amenable to treatment with phenobarbital.

Alpha-1-Antitrypsin Deficiency

Although only 10% to 15% of children with alpha-1-antitrypsin deficiency develop liver disease, this autosomal recessive condition is the most common inherited cause of conjugated hyperbilirubinemia and the most common cause of *early-onset emphysema* in young adults. Onset and severity of disease are variable. Affected neonates present with intrauterine growth retardation, early jaundice from direct hyperbilirubinemia, hepatomegaly, and laboratory evidence of cholestasis and elevated serum transaminase concentrations. Older children may have severe liver involvement or only mildly increased transaminase levels. Most patients who present beyond the neonatal period experience a slow resolution of their hepatic disease, but a significant minority of patients progress to end-stage liver disease. Cholestasis in the setting of a liver biopsy specimen that stains positive for periodic acid-Schiff granules suggests a storage disorder such as alpha-1-antitrypsin deficiency or glycogen storage disease.

HEPATOMEGALY

Hepatomegaly, defined as a liver that is overly large for age, may be caused by any of the following processes:

- Passive congestion of the liver from heart failure or hepatic venous obstruction (enlarged, tender liver)
- Inflammation/infection (enlarged, tender liver)

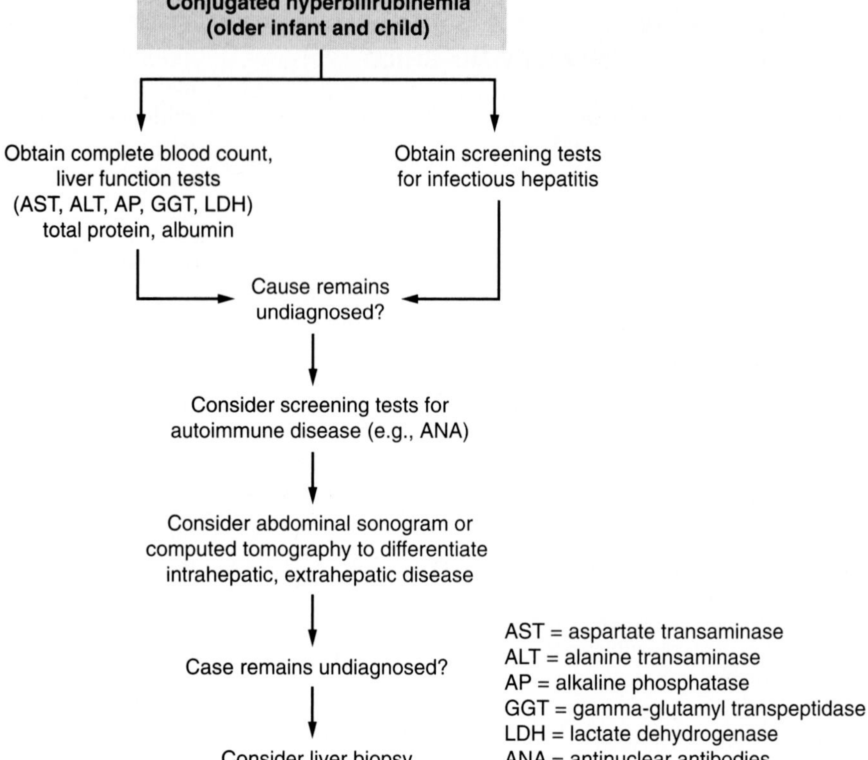

Figure 12-1 Evaluation of conjugated hyperbilirubinemia.

- Infiltration by tumor (enlarged, tender liver)
- Storage disorder (enlarged, nontender liver)
- Cirrhosis (enlarged or shrunken, firm, fibrotic liver with associated splenomegaly)

The liver edge is normally palpable below the costal margin in the young infant; however, a palpable liver edge is unusual beyond the age of 12 months. Other signs of hepatomegaly include palpation of the left liver lobe beyond the midline and an excessively firm organ. Percussion of the liver span provides a more reliable measure of size than extension below the costal margin. This is especially true in the setting of lung hyperinflation. Conditions associated with isolated hepatomegaly and hepatosplenomegaly are listed in Table 12-11.

Autoimmune Hepatitis

Autoimmune hepatitis is an immune-mediated disorder characterized by chronic hepatocellular inflammation, necrosis, and eventual progression to cirrhosis. This disorder has occasionally been associated with chronic minocycline administration. Affected patients have laboratory evidence of compromised liver function, including markedly elevated transaminases, hyperbilirubinemia, coagulopathy, and hypoalbuminemia. The hallmark of autoimmune hepatitis is an elevated total protein concentration despite low albumin levels, signifying elevation of the immunoglobulin fraction. The diagnosis is established by liver biopsy, which must be delayed in patients with ineffective coagulation. Early diagnosis and treatment with corticosteroids and azathioprine positively affect outcome.

Hemochromatosis

Hemochromatosis is an inherited disorder that results in accumulation of iron in parenchymal organs. Hepatomegaly, bronzing of the skin, and joint pain are the most common initial clinical features. Presentation is rare in pediatric age groups but does occur. Genetic testing for the mutant gene is available; occasionally, liver biopsy may be necessary.

Wilson Disease

Wilson disease is an autosomal recessive disorder of copper metabolism that results in accumulation of copper within the liver and brain. The disease presents in late childhood or adolescence with hepatomegaly, jaundice, or fulminant hepatitis. Kayser-Fleischer rings (caused by copper deposition in the limbic area of the cornea) are virtually pathognomonic for Wilson disease. An elevated hepatic copper concentration in a biopsy specimen confirms the diagnosis.

Reye Syndrome

Reye syndrome is a constellation of clinical manifestations resulting from acute liver failure and encephalopathy.

TABLE 12-11
DIFFERENTIAL DIAGNOSIS OF HEPATOMEGALY AND HEPATOSPLENOMEGALY

	Isolated Hepatomegaly	Hepatosplenomegaly
Infection	■ Viral hepatitis ■ Chronic active hepatitis ■ Chronic persistent hepatitis ■ Liver abscess ■ Amebiasis ■ Ascariasis	■ Epstein-Barr virus ■ Cytomegalovirus ■ Congenital rubella ■ Congenital syphilis ■ Congenital toxoplasmosis ■ Tuberculosis ■ Visceral larva migrans ■ Malaria ■ Cat-scratch disease
Liver disease	■ Cirrhosis ■ Hepatic fibrosis ■ Autoimmune hepatitis	■ Cirrhosis ■ Portal hypertension
Biliary tract obstruction	■ Biliary atresia ■ Gallstones ■ Alagille syndrome	
Metabolic disorders	■ Galactosemia ■ Hereditary fructose intolerance ■ Glycogen storage disease ■ Alpha-1-antitrypsin deficiency	■ Tyrosinemia ■ Niemann-Pick disease ■ Gaucher disease
Neoplasms	■ Hepatic tumors	■ Leukemia ■ Lymphoma ■ Neuroblastoma
Cardiac conditions	■ Congestive heart failure ■ Pericardial tamponade	
Collagen vascular disorders		■ Systemic lupus erythematosus
Medications/drugs	■ Acetaminophen ■ Ethanol ■ Isoniazid	■ Valproate ■ Phenytoin ■ Anabolic steroids
Trauma	■ Liver injury	■ Isolated splenomegaly with splenic injury
Other	■ Total peripheral nutrition ■ Cystic fibrosis ■ Hemochromatosis ■ Wilson disease ■ Reye syndrome	

The classic presentation involves a school-age child with vomiting, altered mental status, and hepatomegaly who has a history of recent viral infection treated with aspirin. Suggestive laboratory findings include elevated serum ammonia and transaminase concentrations, prolonged prothrombin and partial thromboplastin times, hypoglycemia, and elevated anion gap metabolic acidosis. Reye syndrome is essentially a clinical diagnosis. The goals of treatment are normalization of coagulopathy and electrolyte imbalances and prevention of increased intracranial pressure.

HEPATIC FAILURE AND TRANSPLANTATION

Liver failure ensues when damage to the organ becomes severe enough to interfere with normal function. The early stage of liver dysfunction is characterized by jaundice, hepatomegaly, and elevation of serum transaminase concentrations (e.g., alanine aminotransferase, lactate dehydrogenase). Hypoglycemia, hyponatremia, and hypoalbuminemia are consistent with a diagnosis of hepatic failure. Prolongation of prothrombin and partial thromboplastin times (coagulopathy) suggests imminent hepatic failure, preceding symptoms of encephalopathy by a few days to weeks. Coagulopathy that occurs in the setting of normal platelet levels and is unresponsive to vitamin K administration is usually of hepatic origin. Hepatic encephalopathy develops as liver function further deteriorates; irritability and confusion give way to progressive disorientation, delirium, hyperreflexia, and eventually coma, decerebrate or decorticate posturing, and death.

Liver transplantation is considered a viable option for pediatric patients with severe irreversible hepatic disease, including biliary atresia, alpha-1-antitrypsin deficiency, autoimmune hepatitis, and metabolic disease involving the liver. Complications include organ rejection, graft failure, and infection. Patients who do not have a willing living related donor are placed on the waiting list for a cadaveric liver; age, serum bilirubin concentration, albumin level, and growth rate affect ranking priority.

DISORDERS OF THE ESOPHAGUS

Esophageal Foreign Body

Foreign body ingestion is most common between the ages of 9 months and 5 years. Clinical presentation ranges from asymptomatic to life-threatening respiratory distress. When present, symptoms are generally gastrointestinal or respiratory in character:

- *Gastrointestinal manifestations*: dysphagia, pain with swallowing/eating, drooling, gagging, vomiting, pain
- *Respiratory manifestations*: choking, cough, stridor, wheezing

Treatment depends on object location and type, symptoms/respiratory compromise, and estimated duration of entrapment. Rigid esophagoscopy is the removal technique of choice.

- Objects causing respiratory symptoms must be removed.
- Objects located in the upper third of the esophagus must be removed due to risk of aspiration.
- Objects that do not pass into the stomach within 12 to 24 hours must be removed.
- Button batteries and sharp objects must be removed, regardless of placement within the esophagus.

Gastroesophageal Reflux

Gastroesophageal reflux (GER) is the retrograde flow of gastric material into the esophagus due to low esophageal sphincter tone. *Gastroesophageal reflux disease* (GERD) may result from severe or persistent GER at any age, as manifested by irritability, vomiting, hematemesis, esophagitis, failure to thrive, recurrent respiratory problems, or dysphagia due to stricture formation (esophageal irritation, inflammation, erosion, and UGI bleeding). The typical presentation of GER is age related:

- Infants present with effortless vomiting, which resolves in most patients during the first year of life. More severe or persistent GER is associated with irritability, poor growth, pain and arching of the back with feeding, *Sandifer syndrome* (spasmodic torsion of the neck and opisthotonic posturing resembling seizure activity), anemia, and occasionally respiratory signs such as stridor, wheezing, or recurrent pneumonia. When GERD is suspected in an infant, a UGI radiographic series is the initial study of choice. Endoscopy and/or pH probe monitoring may be appropriate in selective patients. Thickening feeds and upright prone positioning following feeding are beneficial for the majority of infants with GERD. Medical therapy consists of H2-receptor blockers and/or proton pump inhibitors and, less commonly, metoclopramide (a prokinetic agent). Nissen fundoplication is reserved for patients with persistent inflammation.
- Older children and adolescents with GER are less likely to vomit. Complaints of epigastric pain, burning, and/or "heartburn" are the most common symptoms. The esophageal pH probe study is the preferred method of diagnosis, although a trial of medication is reasonable in the patient with a history and physical examination consistent with GER. Changes in diet (limiting chocolate, caffeine, spicy foods, and peppermints) and lifestyle (weight reduction, limiting alcohol intake and cigarette smoke exposure) reduce symptoms in the majority of patients who are compliant. Antacids provide short-term relief but should never be used in infants and small children. *Proton pump inhibitors* (omeprazole, lansoprazole) are more effective than *H2-receptor antagonists* (cimetidine, ranitidine, famotidine) in most patients, but the two classes of drugs may be used in combination. Long-term therapy is usually necessary in older children and adolescents due to low rates of spontaneous resolution. *Erosive esophagitis*, when present, is initially treated with a proton pump inhibitor; a prokinetic agent is added if inflammation persists beyond 2 months of treatment.

PEPTIC ULCER DISEASE

PUD is erosive disruption of the lining of the stomach or duodenum resulting from contact with acidic gastric secretions. PUD should be suspected when abdominal pain is primarily epigastric, when it awakens the child from sleep, and when it is associated with anorexia, nausea, recurrent vomiting, iron deficiency anemia, or gastrointestinal bleeding. A majority of patients with PUD also have *H. pylori* infection (discussed in detail in Chapter 10), but approximately one third have idiopathic disease or risk factors such as chronic nonsteroidal anti-inflammatory treatment. Medical therapy to eradicate the organism is indicated for patients with duodenal ulcers and *H. pylori* infection; however,

TABLE 12-12
MEDICAL THERAPY FOR PEPTIC ULCER DISEASE

Drug Class	Examples	Mechanism of Action	Indications	Key Points
Proton pump inhibitors (PPIs)	Omeprazole Lansoprazole	Blocks H^+ (proton) production within the gastric parietal cell	GERD PUD *H. pylori* infection Nonulcer dyspepsia	qd, bid dosing Optimally should be taken 30 minutes prior to breakfast on an empty stomach
H2-receptor antagonists	Cimetidine Ranitidine Famotidine	Partially block gastric parietal cell acid production by competing with histamine receptors on the parietal cell membrane	Second-line therapy for GERD, PUD, nonulcer dyspepsia	
Antacids	Sodium bicarbonate Calcium, magnesium salts	Neutralize gastric acid	Acute symptomatic relief of reflux, dyspepsia symptoms not associated with inflammatory changes	
Sulfate-aluminum complex	Sucralfate	Coats the inflamed area and creates a protective barrier	Treatment and prevention of peptic ulcers, GERD Not effective in treating PUD or GERD as monotherapy	May cause constipation May reduce bioavailability of fluoroquinolones, ketoconazole, warfarin Contraindicated in patients with renal failure (results in increased plasma aluminum levels)
Synthetic prostaglandin	Misoprostol	Stimulates mucus production to maintain the integrity of the protective mucin glycoprotein-bicarbonate layer	Used to prevent PUD in high-risk patients, such as those on chronic NSAID therapy Not useful in the acute treatment of bleeding peptic ulcers	Common adverse side effects: nausea, diarrhea Less common adverse side effects: abdominal pain, constipation Contraindicated in pregnancy Use has been largely supplanted by PPIs

qd, once a day; bid, twice a day; NSAID, nonsteroidal anti-inflammatory drug.

elimination of *H. pylori* from the gastrointestinal tract appears to have no significant beneficial effect for patients with isolated gastritis or dyspeptic symptoms. Antibiotic therapy for *H. pylori* infection is presented in Chapter 10. Medications appropriate for PUD treatment are discussed in Table 12-12.

GALLBLADDER DISEASE

Biliary Atresia

Hepatomegaly, direct hyperbilirubinemia, and laboratory evidence of *cholestasis* in an infant younger than 2 months of age suggest *biliary atresia*. In fact, one third of infants in this age group with conjugated hyperbilirubinemia have biliary atresia. Other causes of neonatal cholestasis include anatomic, infectious, and metabolic diseases. The workup of direct hyperbilirubinemia in the neonate is provided in Chapter 5 but reviewed here:

- Cultures and serologies to rule out *infectious* etiologies (congenital infections, bacterial sepsis)
- Studies to rule out *metabolic disease* (urine for reducing substances, organic acids; serum amino acids, iron studies; alpha-1-antitrypsin level)
- Testing for *cystic fibrosis*
- *Abdominal ultrasonography* (when biliary atresia is present, the gallbladder is typically shrunken or not visible; a normal-appearing gallbladder makes biliary atresia unlikely)

- *Radionuclide scintigraphy* (a tracer is normally taken up in the liver; if biliary atresia is present, none of the tracer is excreted into the bowel; however, cholestasis from other causes in the setting of a normal, patent biliary system results in delayed uptake in the liver but normal excretion into the bowel)

Cholecystitis

Cholecystitis, or inflammation of the gallbladder, is associated with jaundice in approximately 15% of patients. Most cases of cholecystitis are due to *gallstones* in the *cystic duct*; a small minority of cases are *acalculous* in origin. Risk factors include positive family history, female gender, obesity or rapid weight loss, hyperlipidemia, diabetes, contraceptive use, biliary stasis due to prolonged fasting, and total parenteral nutrition. *Hemolytic disease* is a relatively common cause of cholelithiasis in children. Acute cholecystitis presents with fever, vomiting, and abdominal pain that becomes constant and severe, often radiating to the right scapula. Right upper quadrant fullness and/or a palpable gallbladder may be present on examination. Abdominal ultrasonography is the diagnostic study of choice when cholecystitis is suspected. Initial therapy consists of intravenous hydration, pain control, and administration of a broad-spectrum antibiotic in patients with fever. If the condition is secondary to cholelithiasis, the stones are removed via endoscopy or surgery prior to discharge.

Stones that lodge in the common bile duct result in hepatobiliary obstruction characterized by upper abdominal pain, jaundice, and elevation of serum conjugated bilirubin, alkaline phosphatase, and gamma-glutamyl transpeptidase concentrations. Following removal of the stone(s), hyperbilirubinemia may persist for up to 1 month. Normalization of serum bilirubin levels should be verified by serial testing.

INFLAMMATORY BOWEL DISEASE

Crohn disease (CD) and *ulcerative colitis* (UC) are chronic inflammatory conditions of the gastrointestinal tract. Both disorders are polygenic in origin; the disease manifests in an individual with an inherited predisposition who is then exposed to an environmental trigger. The incidence of CD peaks in late adolescence; the disorder may present significantly earlier in highly susceptible individuals but is rare in young children. CD is thought to be more common in certain ethnic groups (Northern Europeans, Ashkenazi Jews). Exposure to cigarette smoke and family history of a first-degree relative with IBD also increase the risk of the disease. The rate of UC diagnosis peaks in the 15- to 35-year age group, but the disorder afflicts individuals of all ages. First-degree relatives of patients with IBD are at greater risk for the development of UC, but the connection is not as pronounced as that for CD.

The presenting features, laboratory evaluations, treatment plans, and prognoses of CD and UC are provided in Table 12-13.

MALABSORPTION

Optimal absorption of nutrients depends on the interplay of the pancreas and hepatobiliary and gastrointestinal systems. Most digestion and absorption takes place in the proximal small intestine; bile acids and vitamin B_{12} are absorbed in the terminal ileum.

Malabsorption may result from any of the following (Table 12-14):

- Deficiency of digestive enzymes
- Damage to the intestinal villi
- Short bowel syndrome (inadequate absorptive surface)

Signs of malabsorption include:

- chronic diarrhea—not all patients with malabsorption have chronic diarrhea, but most do. Stools are often malodorous and contain excessive amounts of fat, carbohydrate, and/or protein.
- weight loss, failure to thrive
- malnutrition—edema, decreased muscle mass, large belly, easy bruising, rickets

Laboratory investigation in the patient with suspected malabsorption is guided by results of the history and physical examination. Suggested tests are listed in Table 12-15.

PERITONITIS

Peritonitis is infection of the *serosal membrane* lining the abdominal cavity and *fluid* contained within the abdomen.

- In *primary (spontaneous) peritonitis*, the infecting organism reaches the abdominal cavity through hematogenous or lymphatic spread. Patients with nephrotic syndrome are particularly susceptible to spontaneous bacterial peritonitis, usually involving *Streptococcus pneumoniae*. Third-generation cephalosporins are appropriate for the empiric treatment of primary peritonitis.
- Gastrointestinal flora is usually responsible for *secondary peritonitis*, which may result from perforation of the gastrointestinal tract or abscess formation. Appropriate initial antibiotic therapy includes any of the following: a second- or third-generation cephalosporin, a fluoroquinolone in combination with metronidazole, or a broad-spectrum penicillin with anaerobic activity.
- Patients who undergo regular peritoneal dialysis are subject to the development of *chronic (tertiary) peritonitis*. Empiric therapy is guided by Gram stain results of peritoneal fluid and local resistance patterns.

TABLE 12-13
INFLAMMATORY BOWEL DISEASES: CROHN DISEASE AND ULCERATIVE COLITIS

	Crohn Disease (CD)	Ulcerative Colitis (UC)
Clinical manifestations (more often chronic in onset but may be acute)	**Abdominal pain** (varies in location depending on area of involvement; generally milder than that with UC) **Diarrhea** (occult blood, melena, or occasionally bright red blood per rectum) **Fever**[a] **Anorexia**[a] **Weight loss/growth delay/deceleration of height velocity**[a] (may precede gastrointestinal manifestations by up to a year) **Pubertal delay**[a] **Perianal disease**[a] (skin tags, fistulae, bleeding, abscesses) **Recurrent oral aphthous ulcers**	*Mild-to-moderate disease* **Diarrhea** (melena, hematochezia) **Tenesmus** **Abdominal pain** (may awaken child from sleep) *Severe disease* **Weight loss** **Cramping abdominal pain** **Diffuse abdominal tenderness** **Fever** **Tachycardia**
Additional extraintestinal manifestations (may accompany or precede gastrointestinal symptoms)	Arthralgia/arthritis Erythema nodosum Uveitis Iron deficiency anemia	
Suggested laboratory workup	Complete blood count with differential Serum total protein, albumin Liver function tests (evaluation for sclerosing cholangitis, autoimmune hepatitis) Stool for culture, ova and parasites pANCA (perinuclear antineutrophil) ASCA (anti-*Saccharomyces* antibody) ompC (antibody to the outer membrane of *Escherichia coli*)	
Laboratory parameters	Leukocytosis Anemia Thrombocytosis Hypoalbuminemia Elevated acute phase reactants (erythrocyte Sedimentation rate, C-reactive protein) Positive pANCA (10%) Positive ASCA or ompC (60–70%)	*Mild disease* Normal or mild anemia with slightly elevated acute phase reactants (APR) *Moderate disease* Moderate leukocytosis, mild anemia, elevated APR *Severe disease* Leukocytosis with significant left shift, anemia, elevated APR, hypoalbuminemia
Suggested radiographic workup	*Upper gastrointestinal series with small bowel follow-through* to ascertain location and extent of lesions in the small bowel (nodular changes, thickened wall of the terminal ileum in CD) *Double-contrast barium/air enema* to ascertain location and extent of lesions in the colon (risk of perforation in severe disease) *Upper endoscopy with biopsy* allows further evaluation of esophageal, gastric, and upper intestinal involvement and yields biopsy specimens *Colonoscopy with biopsy* to determine extent of disease, presence of skip lesions, involvement of terminal ileum; biopsy specimens	
Endoscopy, colonoscopy results	Involvement anywhere along the gastrointestinal tract from the mouth to the anus (most commons areas: terminal ileum and cecum) Rectal sparing Regional inflammation (skip lesions) Involvement of the terminal ileum (typically)	Continuous inflammatory involvement extending variable distance proximally from the rectum No involvement of the terminal ileum or small bowel No perianal involvement

(*continued*)

TABLE 12-13
(continued)

	Crohn Disease (CD)	Ulcerative Colitis (UC)
Biopsy results	Patchy areas of transmural inflammation Noncaseating granulomas (1/3 of CD patients)	Continuous area of mucosal inflammation Mucosal granularity
Treatment	Nutritional support (patients with disease of the terminal ileum cannot absorb vitamin B_{12}) **Induction of remission** (mild-to-moderate disease): 5-Aminosalicylates (mesalamine, sulfasalazine) Antibiotics (metronidazole, cyclosporine) **Induction of remission** (moderate-to-severe disease): Corticosteroids (intravenous if no response to oral therapy) 6-Mercaptopurine (MP), azathioprine methotrexate Infliximab (monoclonal antibody to tumor necrosis factor) **Maintenance**: 6-MP, azathioprine Methotrexate Infliximab **Surgery** not curative (most patients eventually relapse), but indicated for failure of medical therapy, obstruction, intra-abdominal abscess, fistulae	Nutritional support **Induction of remission** (mild-to-moderate disease): 5-Aminosalicylates **Maintenance** (mild-to-moderate disease): 5-Aminosalicylates **Induction of remission** (moderate-to-severe disease): Corticosteroids (intravenous if no response to oral therapy) 6-MP, azathioprine Cyclosporine Infliximab **Maintenance** (moderate-to-severe disease): 6-MP, azathioprine Infliximab UC is surgically curable (total proctocolectomy with ileal-anal anastomosis); **Surgery** indicated for failure of medical therapy, need for recurrent transfusions, dysplasia, malignant transformation
Complications	Sclerosing cholangitis Autoimmune hepatitis Toxic megacolon	
Prognosis	Slightly increased lifetime risk of colorectal cancer	Significantly increased lifetime risk of colorectal cancer (necessitates periodic surveillance colonoscopy)

[a]Any of these features may be the sole presenting symptom of inflammatory bowel disease.

ABDOMINAL TRAUMA

Emergency evaluation of the patient with abdominal trauma depends in part on the mental status of the patient and whether there is associated significant head trauma. In the alert, hemodynamically stable trauma patient without a history of head injury who is complaining of abdominal pain, computed tomography with oral and intravenous contrast is the diagnostic study of choice. Children who require emergent surgical intervention (i.e., those who are hemodynamically unstable or require a neurosurgical procedure for associated head trauma) instead undergo diagnostic peritoneal lavage in the operating room due to time considerations. Immediate laparotomy is indicated for patients with open abdominal wounds (e.g., gunshot wounds) and those with blood or bile obtained on diagnostic peritoneal lavage. Abdominal ultrasonography has a growing role in the evaluation of pediatric trauma patients; however, computed tomography is generally preferred in patients who are hemodynamically stable because the enhanced detail provides more accurate information for decisions regarding further management and prognosis.

The sudden onset of severe pain localized to the left upper quadrant following blunt trauma suggests splenic rupture,

TABLE 12-14
MALABSORPTIVE CONDITIONS OF CHILDHOOD

Pancreatic Insufficiency

Causes

Cystic fibrosis (see Chapter 13)—pancreatic insufficiency, hepatobiliary disease. Gastrointestinal manifestations in infancy include meconium ileus, cholestasis. Older children may present with chronic liver disease, recurrent pancreatitis, or rectal prolapse in absence of respiratory symptoms. Oral pancreatic enzyme replacement is available.

Shwachman syndrome—autosomal recessive disorder; associated pancytopenia due to bone marrow dysfunction

Chronic Cholestasis

Causes

Biliary atresia—steatorrhea (fat malabsorption) leads to poor growth, chronic malnutrition, fat-soluble vitamin deficiencies (most notably vitamins E and K)

Alagille syndrome—chronic cholestasis associated with peripheral pulmonic stenosis

Intestinal Villous Injury

Causes

Celiac disease—mucosal injury resulting from autoimmune response to dietary gluten, found in wheat, rye, and barley products. Symptom severity ranges; presentation may include any of the following: diarrhea, constipation, or bulky stools; poor growth/significant malnutrition; irritability; signs of malabsorption. Screening tests for celiac disease are included in Table 12-15; diagnosis rests on characteristic biopsy results from small bowel lesions and positive response to a gluten-free diet.

Crohn disease

Giardiasis (see Chapter 10)

Postinfectious diarrhea

Short Bowel Syndrome

Causes

Congenital intestinal anomalies

Surgical resection—patients susceptible to poor growth, steatorrhea, carbohydrate malabsorption, electrolyte imbalances, trace mineral deficiencies. Managed with parenteral nutrition and slow progression of enteral feeds. Bacterial overgrowth may undermine success of enteral feedings; condition is suggested by hydrogen breath test and confirmed (if necessary) by culture of duodenal fluid.

---

particularly when accompanied by tachypnea, tachycardia, and hypotension of variable severity. Patients with splenomegaly resulting from infectious mononucleosis (Epstein-Barr virus) are at increased risk for splenic rupture. Once again, computed tomography with contrast is the most appropriate study for the hemodynamically stable trauma patient with suspected splenic rupture. Minor splenic lacerations often resolve without surgical intervention, but children with splenic rupture or major lacerations resulting in hemodynamic compromise require surgical repair.

TABLE 12-15
LABORATORY ASSESSMENT FOR POSSIBLE MALABSORPTION

Stool Studies

Fecal fat (fat malabsorption)

Reducing substances in the stool (carbohydrate malabsorption)

Stool alpha-1-antitrypsin (excessive enteric protein loss)

Stool cultures, ova and parasites

Stool for occult blood

Studies to Evaluate Nutritional Status

Complete blood count

Serum total protein, albumin

Serum electrolytes, calcium, phosphorus

Serum vitamin B_{12}, folate, iron

Serum 25-hydroxyvitamin D, vitamins E and A concentrations; prothrombin time

Studies to Evaluate for Systemic/Liver Disease

Erythrocyte sedimentation rate (ESR)

Liver enzymes

Serum bilirubin

Studies to Screen for Celiac Disease[a]

Serum antigliadin immunoglobulin (Ig) G, IgA

Serum antiendomysial IgA

Serum antitissue transglutaminase IgA

Total serum IgA concentration

Studies to Screen for Cystic Fibrosis

Sweat chloride test

Studies to Screen for Carbohydrate Malabsorption, Bacterial Overgrowth

Hydrogen breath test

Studies to Evaluate Condition of Intestinal Villi

Endoscopy

---

[a]Positive screen consists of either of the following: ≥1 positive antibody test without evidence of IgA deficiency or positive IgG antigliadin antibody test plus IgA deficiency in the setting of positive family history or consistent clinical presentation.

SOURCES

Arnold LD. Ingested and aspirated foreign bodies: making sure that what went in comes out. *Contemp Pediatr.* 2006;23:32–44.

Braganza SF. Gastroesophageal reflux. *Pediatr Rev.* 2005;26:304–305.

Chandler JC, Gauderer MW. The neonate with an abdominal mass. *Pediatr Clin North Am.* 2004;51:979–997.

DeGennaro BA, Jacobson S. Abdominal pain. In: Harwood-Nuss AL, Wolfson AB, Linden CH, et al., eds. *The clinical practice of emergency medicine.* 3rd ed. Philadelphia: Lippincott Williams & Wilkins; 2001:9–12.

Harb R, Thomas DW. Conjugated hyperbilirubinemia: screening and treatment in older infants and children. *Pediatr Rev.* 2007;28:83–91.

Judd RH. Chronic nonspecific diarrhea. *Pediatr Rev.* 1996;17:379–384.

Keating JP. Chronic diarrhea. *Pediatr Rev.* 2005;26:5–14.

McCollough M, Sharieff GQ. Abdominal pain in children. *Pediatr Clin North Am.* 2006;53:107–137.

Michail S. Gastroesophageal reflux. *Pediatr Rev.* 2007;28:101–110.

Rasquin-Weber A, Hyman PE, Cucchiara S, et al. Childhood functional gastrointestinal disorders. *Gut.* 1999;45:60–68.
Saps M, Li BU. Chronic abdominal pain of functional origin in children. *Pediatr Ann.* 2006;35:246–258.
Silbermintz A, Markowitz J. Inflammatory bowel diseases. *Pediatr Ann.* 2006;35:268–274.
Skae CC. Esophageal foreign bodies. *Pediatr Rev.* 2005;26:34–35.
Suwandi E, Ton MN, Schwarz SM. Gastroesophageal reflux in infancy and childhood. *Pediatr Ann.* 2006;35:259–267.
Thiessen PN. Recurrent abdominal pain. *Pediatr Rev.* 2002;23:39–47.
Wegener S, Colleti JE, Van Wie D. Pediatric blunt abdominal trauma. *Pediatr Clin North Am.* 2006;53:243–256.
Zeiter DK, Hyams JS. Recurrent abdominal pain in children. *Pediatr Clin North Am.* 2002;49:53–71.

QUESTIONS

1. Which of the following is a typical pattern for referred visceral pain in the abdomen?
A) Right lower quadrant pain with right lower lobe pneumonia
B) Posterior flank pain with gallbladder inflammation
C) Right infrascapular pain with pancreatitis
D) Sacral pain with rectal inflammation
E) Right upper quadrant pain with ureteral stones

2. A mother brings her 8-year-old son to your office with a chief complaint of abdominal pain. The pain started 24 hours ago and has grown progressively worse. It was initially generalized but has localized to the right lower quadrant. The patient had one episode of nonbloody, nonbilious emesis yesterday. He has had no stool today. He has not eaten today, and his urine output is moderately decreased. He denies dysuria. His mother carried him into the office, and he refuses to walk due to the pain. The physical examination reveals a well-nourished, well-developed child curled up on his side on the table, in obvious pain. His temperature is 100.7°F, and he is slightly tachycardic, but otherwise, his vitals are within normal limits. No abdominal distension is noted; bowel sounds are hypoactive. Tenderness is localized to the right lower quadrant, and guarding is present. Which of the following conditions is the most likely cause of this child's pain?
A) Acute colitis
B) Appendicitis
C) Ulcerative colitis
D) Pyelonephritis
E) Pancreatitis

3. One of your patients, a 9-year-old boy, presents to the local emergency department with a 24-hour history of abdominal pain that was initially periumbilical but now has localized to the right lower quadrant. His temperature is 99.7°F, heart rate is 106 beats per minute, respiratory rate is 20 breaths per minute, and blood pressure is normal. He is in obvious pain and lies still on his side curled up on the examining table. The patient's hematocrit is 34%; the white blood count is $11.7 \times 10^3/\mu L$, with a mild left shift. Which of the following studies is most appropriate for definitive evaluation of the appendix in this patient?
A) Abdominal laparotomy
B) Abdominal ultrasonography
C) Computed tomography
D) Plain film radiography
E) Magnetic resonance imaging

4. A 12-year-old, markedly obese female presents to your office following the acute onset of constant, severe upper abdominal pain radiating to her back. She denies any history of antecedent trauma, dysuria, diarrhea, or sexual activity. She is afebrile; vital signs are unremarkable beyond mild tachycardia. While in your office, she has two episodes of bilious, nonbloody emesis. There is no obvious abdominal distension on physical exam. Her pain is localized to the upper abdominal area. She has no flank pain. A rectal examination is negative for tenderness and occult blood. Which of the following conditions is the most likely cause of this patient's pain?
A) Cholecystitis
B) Acute small bowel obstruction
C) Malrotation with gastric volvulus
D) Acute pancreatitis
E) Acute hepatitis

5. Which of the following sets of laboratory results is most consistent with acute pancreatitis?
A) Hypocalcemia, hypoglycemia
B) Hypercalcemia, hypoglycemia
C) Elevated serum direct bilirubin, hypercalcemia
D) Elevated serum indirect bilirubin and serum transaminases
E) Elevated serum lipase and amylase concentrations

6. Which of the following inherited conditions is the most common cause of chronic/recurrent pancreatitis in adolescents?
A) Cystic fibrosis
B) Biliary atresia
C) Wilson disease
D) Annular pancreas
E) Diabetes mellitus

7. An 18-month-old female presents to the urgent care center with an 8-hour history of intermittent crying episodes due to "stomach pain." The episodes occur four to five times an hour and last for 2 to 3 minutes. Initially, the patient was asymptomatic between

episodes; however, she is becoming progressively more listless even when the pain is not present. She has thrown up three times since the pain began, but the emesis is not described as bloody or bilious. She has had one loose, brown stool. Examination of the abdomen reveals diffuse tenderness with localization to the right side and an indistinct mass in the right upper quadrant. There is some guarding but no evidence of rebound tenderness. A rectal examination yields scant stool positive for occult blood. Which of the following is the most likely cause of this patient's pain?
A) Small bowel obstruction
B) Intussusception
C) Appendicitis
D) Viral gastritis
E) Inflammatory polyps

8. A 24-month-old boy with no significant past medical history presents with recurrent short episodes of abdominal pain, vomiting, and "currant jelly" stools. Which of the following radiographic studies is preferred for initial evaluation of this patient?
A) Plain film abdominal radiography
B) Abdominal ultrasonography
C) Air contrast enema
D) Barium contrast enema
E) Meckel scan

9. A 6-day-old former full-term infant with an unremarkable perinatal course presents following two episodes of bilious emesis in the past hour. On physical examination, the infant is irritable and obviously uncomfortable. He is afebrile but moderately tachycardic. Both blood pressure and respiratory rate are in the upper range of normal for age. The abdominal examination is remarkable for moderate distension and diffuse abdominal tenderness with guarding. Stool obtained via rectal examination is positive for occult blood. Which of the following conditions is the most likely cause of this infant's vomiting?
A) Biliary atresia
B) Hyperammonemia
C) Intussusception
D) Midgut volvulus
E) Cow milk allergy

10. Which of the following radiographic results is most consistent with malrotation and midgut volvulus?
A) Pneumatosis intestinalis
B) Nonspecific ileus pattern on flat and upright abdominal radiographs
C) Dilated loops of small bowel on flat and upright radiographs
D) Coil-spring pattern on barium contrast enema
E) Upper abdominal "corkscrew" pattern on upper gastrointestinal series

11. *Helicobacter pylori* infection of the gastrointestinal tract is conclusively linked to the development of which of the following?
A) Nonulcerative dyspepsia
B) Peptic ulcer disease
C) Irritable bowel syndrome
D) A and B
E) A, B, and C

12. A 7-year-old boy presents with nearly continuous mild-to-moderate diffuse abdominal pain for 3½ months that interferes with his after-school activities and has occasionally caused him to miss school. The pain is not affected by eating or defecation. There is no history of vomiting, diarrhea, or disturbed sleep. The patient continues to grow along his established weight and height curves. Examination of the abdomen reveals normal bowel sounds; no tenderness, masses, or distension are noted. The rectal examination is nontender, and the sample obtained is negative for occult blood. This patient's clinical manifestations are most consistent with which of the following conditions?
A) Irritable bowel syndrome
B) Functional abdominal pain
C) Ulcerative colitis
D) Crohn disease
E) Functional dyspepsia

13. An adolescent female presents with recurrent abdominal pain over a 12-month period (>1 episode/month). The onset of the pain coincides with changes in stool frequency (>3/day) and character (diarrheal stools occasionally mixed with mucus). She often feels bloated during these episodes, which may last for 3 to 5 days. The pain, which is diffuse and mild-to-moderate in severity, does not restrict her activities, is not affected by diet, and is temporarily relieved by defecation. She has been evaluated at the local urgent care center on multiple occasions; none of the visits has resulted in a definitive medical diagnosis. Which of the following conditions is most likely responsible for this patient's pain?
A) Lactose intolerance
B) Functional abdominal pain
C) Irritable bowel syndrome
D) Functional dyspepsia
E) Abdominal migraine

14. A 7-year-old patient is brought to your office by his father for evaluation of recurrent abdominal pain. The child has suffered four episodes of intense midline abdominal pain lasting 4 to 6 hours at a time over the past 4 months. The only thing that seems to help with the pain is going to sleep in a dark room. The father is frustrated because the child seems to be able to tell when he is going to have the pain and becomes very agitated if he is away from home at the time. There is no history of vomiting or diarrhea, and growth parameters are consistent with established curves. The physical examination is within normal limits. The patient is on no medications, but his mother takes ergotamine as needed. Which of the following conditions is the most likely cause of this child's recurrent abdominal pain?

A) Functional abdominal pain
B) Irritable bowel syndrome
C) Malrotation
D) Abdominal migraine
E) Lactose intolerance

15. Which of the following signs or symptoms suggests the possibility of an organic cause of recurrent abdominal pain?

A) Age younger than 5 years
B) Family history of peptic ulcer disease
C) Perianal skin tags
D) Pain that progresses in frequency over time
E) All of the above

16. You are seeing an 8-year-old, recently emigrated Korean girl at the free clinic for a well-child examination and immunizations. Through an interpreter, her mother tells you that the girl develops abdominal pain, bloating, and loose stools following the ingestion of the free breakfasts and lunches offered at her school. You suspect adult-type lactase deficiency. Which of the following is most appropriate for the diagnosis of lactose intolerance in this patient, who has no insurance?

A) Elimination of dairy products from the child's diet, a symptom diary, and re-evaluation in 2 weeks
B) Breath hydrogen test
C) Stool for reducing substances
D) Stool lactase levels
E) Stool for occult blood

17. A 6-month-old infant presents with irritability, vomiting, and jaundice coinciding with the onset of ingestion of baby foods. Hepatosplenomegaly is noted on the physical examination. Laboratory assessment reveals an elevated direct bilirubin concentration. This patient is most likely afflicted with which of the following hereditary conditions?

A) Galactosemia
B) Fructose intolerance
C) Glycogen storage disease type 1
D) Glycogen storage disease type 4
E) Congenital sucrase-isomaltase deficiency

18. Which of the following therapeutic interventions should be administered prior to any endoscopic procedure in a patient with liver disease and severe hematemesis?

A) Rehydration with intravenous fluids
B) Correction of any electrolyte abnormalities
C) Correction of coagulopathy with fresh frozen plasma
D) All of the above
E) None of the above; emergent endoscopy with banding or sclerosis of bleeding sites is the most effective therapy for stabilizing the patient.

19. Which of the following procedures should be carried out in any patient presenting with hematochezia and signs of hemodynamic instability?

A) Placement of a nasogastric tube to rule out massive upper gastrointestinal hemorrhaging
B) Examination of the anus
C) Intravenous fluid administration
D) A, B, and C
E) B and C

20. The parents of a 15-month-old boy witnessed him swallow a plastic button enclosing a small battery. A flat plate radiograph reveals that the object has passed into the patient's stomach. Which of the following is a true statement regarding the recommended treatment of this patient?

A) The object poses no risk to the patient because it is not located in the proximal third of the esophagus.
B) The object poses no risk to the patient because it has passed into the stomach.
C) The object should be removed as soon as possible.
D) The object should be removed from the stomach if it does not pass through the pyloric sphincter within 48 hours.
E) The parents should monitor the patient's stool for the next 10 days and notify their pediatrician if the object does not pass within that time.

21. A 4-year-old institutionalized child with severe mental retardation and cerebral palsy due to extended perinatal asphyxia develops irritability and hematemesis. Enteral feeds through a gastrostomy tube account for all of her caloric needs. Following a thorough evaluation, you conclude that the patient has significant gastroesophageal reflux disease, including esophageal erosions. Which of the following medications is the best choice for initial therapy of gastroesophageal reflux disease in this patient?

A) Omeprazole
B) Magnesium hydroxide
C) Famotidine
D) Metoclopramide
E) Bethanechol

22. A 2-year-old patient develops severe cramping abdominal pain and diarrheal stools mixed with blood a week after spending the day in the "kiddie" pool at a local water park. She is admitted to the hospital for observation and intravenous hydration. Over the next 3 days, the patient becomes progressively oliguric.

Pertinent laboratory results include the following: blood urea nitrogen, 60 mg per dL; serum creatinine, 2.5 mg per dL; and hematocrit, 22%. Which of the following enteric pathogens is most likely responsible for this patient's diarrheal illness?
A) *Shigella dysenteriae*
B) Enterohemorrhagic *Escherichia coli*
C) Enterotoxigenic *E. coli*
D) Enteropathogenic *E. coli*
E) *Salmonella typhi*

23. A 2-month-old infant who has received no medical care since discharge from the newborn nursery is admitted to the hospital for evaluation and management of failure to thrive. The physical examination reveals an irritable, cachectic male infant with a 3/6 systolic ejection heart murmur. The intern on call sends a stool sample that is positive for *Clostridium difficile* toxin. Which of the following statements regarding this patient's laboratory result is true?
A) Three separate stool samples must be positive for *C. difficile* toxin in a patient in this age group in order to conclusively diagnose toxin-mediated disease.
B) The detection of *C. difficile* toxin by immunoassay of a gross stool sample is not informative unless the toxin is isolated from organisms gathered from the patient's stool.
C) Infection with *C. difficile* is unlikely to be the cause of this patient's failure to thrive.
D) Invasive *C. difficile* disease can result in systemic toxin production and a hyperdynamic state.
E) This patient is at risk for the development of toxic megacolon.

24. A 15-month-old patient presents with a parental complaint of several diarrheal stools per day that often overflow her diaper. The stool is watery and flecked with recognizable food particles. The patient does not seem to be bothered by the stools, which are nonbloody. She is a well-nourished, well-developed, active little girl. Her vital signs are all within normal limits. Examination of the abdomen is unremarkable, and stool collected from the diaper is negative for occult blood. Which of the following is the most likely cause of this patient's diarrhea?
A) Noninfectious intractable diarrhea of infancy
B) Sucrase-isomaltase deficiency
C) Milk protein allergy
D) Chronic nonspecific diarrhea of early childhood
E) Parasitic gastroenteritis

25. You have diagnosed chronic nonspecific diarrhea of early childhood ("toddler's diarrhea") in a 16-month-old patient. Which of the following interventions has proven most successful in producing symptomatic improvement in patients with this condition?
A) Loperamide
B) Diphenoxylate with atropine
C) Decreased dietary fiber intake
D) Decreased dietary fat intake
E) Decreased dietary sorbitol intake

26. A 15-year-old previously healthy adolescent presents to your office with a chief complaint of "yellow eyes," which are more noticeable upon wakening. He denies sexual activity and drug use and feels otherwise healthy. There is no history of foreign travel and no known exposure to blood products. The physical examination is significant for mild scleral icterus; findings are otherwise normal. The patient's total serum bilirubin level is elevated at 2.5 mg per dL, with a direct fraction of 0.2 mg per dL. Serum transaminase concentrations are within normal limits. This patient's jaundice is most likely due to which of the following conditions?
A) Gilbert syndrome
B) Crigler-Najjar syndrome
C) Gaucher syndrome
D) Viral hepatitis
E) Autoimmune hepatitis

27. A 4-month-old infant presenting with jaundice and hepatomegaly is found to have an elevated direct fraction of serum bilirubin and elevated serum transaminase concentrations. The family history is significant for early-onset emphysema in his father (age 30 years) and paternal uncle (age 34 years). Which of the following conditions is the most likely cause of this patient's jaundice?
A) Crigler-Najjar syndrome
B) Alpha-1-antitrypsin deficiency
C) Congenital cytomegalovirus infection
D) Congenital rubella infection
E) Galactosemia

28. A 3-week-old infant born at 35 weeks of gestation develops jaundice. The examination is significant for shortened phalanges and a continuous, high-pitched, 3/6 murmur that radiates to the axillae. This patient's jaundice and cardiac murmur are presenting characteristics of which of the following disorders?
A) Alpha-1-antitrypsin deficiency
B) Cystic fibrosis
C) Alagille syndrome
D) Prune belly syndrome
E) Congenital hypothyroidism

29. Kayser-Fleischer rings in an adolescent with jaundice and hepatomegaly are virtually pathognomonic for which of the following conditions?
A) Reye syndrome
B) Gilbert disease
C) Hemochromatosis

D) Wilson disease
E) Autoimmune hepatitis

30. Which of the following laboratory tests should be included on initial screening for celiac disease?
A) Serum antigliadin IgG, IgA concentrations
B) Serum antiendomysial IgA
C) Serum antitissue transglutaminase IgA
D) A and B
E) A, B, and C

31. A previously well 10-year-old boy presents to the emergency department for evaluation of abdominal pain. He was well until last night, when he vomited once before bed and complained that his stomach hurt. When he awoke this morning, he had a temperature of 38.7°C. He does not want to eat or drink. Examination of the abdomen reveals mild distension and hypoactive bowel sounds. Which of the following additional physical findings is most suggestive of a surgical abdomen?
A) Rigidity of the bowel wall
B) Guaiac-positive stool
C) Right lower quadrant tenderness
D) Pain with urination
E) Refusal to ambulate

32. A 5-year-old boy who was an unrestricted back seat passenger in a car involved in a motor vehicle accident is brought to the emergency room complaining of abdominal pain. Vital signs are stable, the patient is awake and alert, and there is no history or evidence of head trauma. The abdomen is not distended, but bowel sounds are hypoactive, and palpation produces diffuse tenderness and rebound tenderness. Which of the following is the most appropriate next step in the evaluation of this patient's abdominal pain?
A) Computed tomography of the abdomen without contrast
B) Computed tomography of the abdomen with contrast
C) Ultrasonography of the abdomen
D) Flat plate and upright plain radiographs of the abdomen
E) Diagnostic peritoneal lavage

33. A 16-year-old male who is a victim of physical assault is brought to the emergency department complaining of severe left upper quadrant pain. He is tachycardic and has mild hypotension. Urinalysis is negative for blood. Following stabilization of airway, breathing, and circulation, which of the following tests is most appropriate for the evaluation of this patient's abdominal pain?
A) Ultrasonography of the abdomen
B) Flat plate and upright plain radiographs of the abdomen
C) Computed tomography of the abdomen with contrast
D) Computed tomography of the abdomen without contrast
E) Diagnostic peritoneal lavage

34. Which of the following laboratory abnormalities is most suggestive of imminent liver failure and hepatic encephalopathy?
A) Elevated serum alanine aminotransferase concentration
B) Elevated serum lactate dehydrogenase concentration
C) Elevated serum indirect bilirubin concentration
D) Prolonged prothrombin time
E) Diminished serum albumin concentration

35. A 5-year-old girl is brought to your office by her mother because she is complaining of dysuria. Palpation of the abdomen is significant for firm masses in the left lateral quadrants thought to be due to hard stool. Examination of the external genitalia reveals foul-smelling debris in the folds between the labia majora and minora without erythema or disruption of the hymen or surrounding tissues. A clean-catch mid-void urine sample is positive for leukocyte esterase and nitrites. This patient's dysuria is most likely due to which of the following?
A) Voluntary withholding of urine
B) External irritation
C) Constipation
D) Poor hygiene
E) A urinary tract infection

36. Which of the following regimens is most effective in the treatment of encopresis?
A) Counseling, pharmacologic therapy for evacuation of the bowel, and behavioral intervention
B) Biofeedback, pharmacologic therapy for evacuation of the bowel, and behavioral intervention
C) Pharmacologic therapy for evacuation of the bowel and biofeedback
D) Counseling and pharmacologic therapy for evacuation of the bowel
E) Pharmacologic therapy for evacuation of the bowel and behavioral intervention

37. A 4-year-old patient is referred to you for evaluation of his encopresis. According to his mother, evacuation of stool has been "problematic" since birth, and although he has been continent of urine for over a year, he continues to regularly soil his underwear. The patient's weight is at the 10th percentile, and his height is at the 25th percentile. No external abnormalities are noted, but a tight ring of terminal bowel is detected on

digital examination. This patient's incontinence of stool is most likely due to which of the following?
A) Encopresis
B) Hirschsprung disease
C) Delayed toilet training
D) Toilet refusal
E) Spina bifida occulta

38. A 6-year-old boy with no significant past medical history presents with his fourth episode of severe vomiting within the past 3 months. Which of the following questions on history is most likely to differentiate organic disease from cyclical vomiting syndrome?
A) Is there a family history of migraine headaches?
B) Does the vomiting keep the child from attending school?
C) Is the patient asymptomatic between the periods of vomiting?
D) Is the vomiting painful?
E) Is the vomiting interfering with activities of daily living?

ANSWERS

1. A	14. D	27. B
2. B	15. E	28. C
3. C	16. A	29. D
4. D	17. B	30. E
5. E	18. E	31. A
6. A	19. D	32. B
7. B	20. C	33. C
8. C	21. A	34. D
9. D	22. B	35. E
10. E	23. C	36. A
11. B	24. D	37. B
12. B	25. E	38. C
13. C	26. A	

Respiratory Disorders

13

RESPIRATORY SIGNS AND SYMPTOMS

Tachypnea

Respiratory rate varies with changes in activity and arousal. Normal respiratory rates in children decrease with advancing age (Table 13-1). Ideally, breaths should be counted for a full minute when determining the rate of breathing. Minute ventilation is directly proportional to both tidal volume and respiratory rate; breathing faster increases minute ventilation. The World Health Organization defines *tachypnea* as respiratory rate:

- >60 breaths per minute in patients younger than 30 days
- >50 breaths per minute in patients 2 to 12 months of age
- >40 breaths per minute in patients 1 to 5 years of age

Tachypnea in children may result from many different processes, including fever and anxiety. A compensatory increase in respiratory rate is often noted in patients with pulmonary disease (e.g., asthma exacerbation, pneumonia), metabolic acidosis, or congestive heart failure. *Hyperventilation syndrome* is a rare disorder of unknown etiology occurring mostly in adolescents. Affected individuals experience recurrent episodes of rapid breathing in the absence of any underlying metabolic need. Resultant hypocapnia produces the clinical symptoms of distal extremity and facial paresthesias, dizziness, chest tightness, and palpitations. While the presentation is similar to that of anxiety attacks, episodes of dysfunctional breathing due to hyperventilation syndrome resolve spontaneously rather than in response to reassurance that the symptoms are benign in nature.

TABLE 13-1
NORMAL RESPIRATORY RATES IN CHILDREN

Age	Normal Range (breaths/min)
Neonate	30 to 60
1 to 36 months	28 to 40
6 to 12 months	23 to 30
1 to 4 years	18 to 28
4 to 8 years	14 to 22
8 to 12 years	13 to 20
>12 years	12 to 18

Cough

Upper respiratory infection is by far the most common cause of acute cough in the pediatric population. Preschool-age children normally suffer from four to ten viral upper respiratory infections a year. Although caretakers often administer *cough suppressants* to young children with colds, most have no proven effect on symptoms and are potentially harmful. Based on available evidence, a U.S. Food and Drug Administration advisory panel recommended that cough and cold preparations not be marketed for use in children younger than 6 years of age (Table 13-2). Parents should be counseled that cough suppressants are of limited or no benefit in children; if they choose to give them, they should use single-ingredient preparations to decrease the likelihood of double-dosing and toxicity. Cough suppressants should not be given to a child whose cough is believed to result from asthma or bacterial/viral pneumonia. Nonpharmacologic interventions for cough include use of a humidifier, bulb suctioning, nasal saline drops, and elevation of the child's upper body and head.

TABLE 13-2
COUGH SUPPRESSANTS IN CHILDREN

Antitussives
- Dextromethorphan (nonnarcotic)—does not appear to suppress cough in young children
- Hydrocodone, codeine (narcotics)—act centrally and may suppress cough in some children; sedation also contributes to decreased coughing

Expectorants
- Help thin secretions so that they are more readily expelled from the respiratory tract
- Guaifenesin is used in pediatric preparations
- No proven benefit in children

Decongestants
- Provide symptomatic relief in older children
- Adjunctive therapy in younger patients with sinusitis
- Use of topical decongestants (e.g., oxymetazoline) for >72 hours results in considerable rebound congestion

Antihistamines
- Diphenhydramine, chlorpheniramine, promethazine
- Do not suppress cough directly, but sedative effect may result in less coughing
- Antihistamines are not appropriate for acute symptom control in asthmatic patients

The differential diagnosis of chronic/recurrent cough in children is rather broad. Chronic cough is defined as cough that persists for longer than 8 weeks. Table 13-3 lists several conditions to consider in the differential diagnosis of chronic cough and provides distinguishing clinical characteristics. Children with chronic cough should receive posteroanterior and lateral chest radiographs, pulmonary function testing, and diagnostic studies for cystic fibrosis (CF). Further evaluation is guided by pertinent information gathered from the history, physical examination, and initial screening tests.

Intact sensation, normal efferent vagal propagation, and adequate muscle strength must be present in order to generate an effective cough. Conditions that may result in cough suppression or weak, ineffective cough include thoracic and/or

TABLE 13-3
DIFFERENTIAL DIAGNOSIS OF CHRONIC/RECURRENT COUGH IN CHILDREN

Asthma
- Cough may be the predominant or even sole presenting feature of asthma.
- Cough-variant asthma is defined as recurrent cough due to bronchial hyperresponsiveness that is not associated with wheezing or chest tightness.
- Cough-variant asthma is exacerbated at night, during periods of physical activity, and with episodic upper respiratory infections.

Gastroesophageal Reflux (GER)
- Cough may be the predominant or even sole presenting feature of GER.
- Cough usually follows feeding rather than occurring during feeding.
- Cough due to GER may worsen when the patient is in the supine position.
- GER usually becomes symptomatic by 2 months of age and resolves by age 12 months.

Chronic Sinusitis
- Cough results from persistent postnasal drip.
- Cough is generally worse when the patient lies down and first thing in the morning.

Viral Infections
- Patients with viral pneumonia may cough for several weeks following resolution of the infection.
- Chronic cough is more likely to occur with viral respiratory infections that destroy the ciliated respiratory epithelium.

Pertussis
- Duration of cough is typically 3 to 4 weeks but may persist for ≥2 months.

Atypical Pneumonia
- *Mycoplasma* pneumonia is typically accompanied by fever, headache, and/or malaise.
- Condition is unusual in children under 3 years of age.

Tuberculosis (discussed in Chapter 10)

Allergic Rhinitis
- Cough due to allergic rhinitis is usually accompanied or superseded by allergic ocular and nasal manifestations.
- Cough results from persistent postnasal drip.

Aspiration
- Cough occurs during feedings.

Foreign Body Aspiration
- Classic symptoms include cough, wheezing, and focal decreased breath sounds.
- Cough is abrupt in onset and persistent.
- Foreign body aspiration is an uncommon cause of cough beyond the age of 3 years.

Cystic Fibrosis
- Cystic fibrosis is part of the differential diagnosis of chronic cough in the pediatric population regardless of age.
- Cough is usually accompanied by poor growth.

Tracheoesophageal Fistulas
- Cough is present from birth.
- Cough occurs during feedings.
- There may be a history of polyhydramnios during the pregnancy.

Psychogenic/Habitual Cough
- Cough has a voluntary component.
- Cough is not present at night (as opposed to cough due to medical conditions).
- Cough improves or disappears when the patient is distracted.
- More common in school-age children and adolescents.

Asthma, GER, and sinusitis account for >90% of chronic cough in infants and children.

respiratory muscle weakness (e.g., Becker-type muscular dystrophy), pain, cerebral palsy, vocal cord paralysis, central nervous system disease, neurodegenerative disease, and thoracic and/or spinal deformities. Of note, neither laryngomalacia nor pectus excavatum interferes with the cough reflex.

Stridor

Stridor is a harsh, high-pitched breathing sound superimposed over typical-sounding respirations. It signals narrowing and partial obstruction of the upper airway (larynx, extreme proximal trachea). Stridor is usually limited to inspiration but may also be expiratory or biphasic. The pattern of stridor suggests (but is not definitive of) the location of the obstruction:

- Isolated *inspiratory stridor* results from partial obstruction of the pharynx, glottis, or subglottis.
- Partial obstruction of the proximal intrathoracic trachea causes *expiratory stridor*.
- *Biphasic stridor* is due to extrathoracic proximal tracheal obstruction or fixed obstruction at the level of the vocal cords.

The differential diagnosis of stridor is extensive. Conditions that produce stridor and their typical presentations are provided in Table 13-4. Stridor is best evaluated through direct laryngoscopy with or without bronchoscopy. Plain radiographs of the neck and chest, including lateral views, should be considered for initial screening. Management decisions are dictated by the causative condition.

Stridor accompanied by open-mouth breathing, drooling, dysphagia, and/or the need to maintain an upright position in order to breath signals severe airway obstruction with impending loss of airway patency.

Wheezing

Wheezing is a high-pitched expiratory noise that results from airway narrowing inferior to the vocal cords. Wheezing may be *generalized* (diffuse) or primarily *localized*:

- Asthma, CF, gastroesophageal reflux, and recurrent bronchiolitis present with recurrent generalized wheezing.
- Localized wheezing is more likely in cases of foreign body aspiration and extrinsic compression of the lower trachea or bronchi by a vascular ring or tumor.

Extrinsic compression of the lower trachea is characterized by recurrent wheezing exacerbated by feeding, crying, and flexion of the neck. Recurrent wheezing associated with congenital anomalies typically begins in the neonatal period. Patients with CF or asthma often begin wheezing later in the first year of life. Recurrent wheezing secondary to tracheoesophageal fistula and gastroesophageal reflux is temporally related to feeding periods. Other conditions that may cause repetitive wheezing include cardiac disease and immune disorders.

If the diagnosis is not suggested by a careful history and thorough physical examination, initial screening tests for recurrent wheezing include chest radiographs, sweat test, and possibly barium swallow to assess for a vascular ring, aspiration, or gastroesophageal reflux. Further assessment (e.g., serum immunoglobulins, echocardiography, bronchoscopy) is guided by the results of the additional screening tests.

Respiratory Failure

Respiratory failure is diagnosed on the basis of measured arterial blood gas tensions [arterial partial pressure of carbon dioxide ($PaCO_2$) >50 mm Hg (normally ~40 mm Hg); arterial partial pressure of oxygen (PaO_2) <60 mm Hg (normally ~100 mm Hg); or both]. Signs of impending respiratory failure include tachypnea, accessory muscle use, hypoxia, fatigue, altered level of consciousness, cyanosis, and diminished skeletal tone. Adequate respiration is dependent on intact central nervous system respiratory drive, normal peripheral nerves and communication at the neuromuscular junction, airway patency, and adequate lung ventilation and perfusion. If respiratory drive is intact, the patient will appear anxious and actively distressed. By contrast, a patient in failure due to hypoventilation may be somnolent but is not generally in discomfort. *Hypercapnia* (increased $PaCO_2$) is the hallmark of hypoventilation but is usually neither clinically evident nor physiologically harmful until the tension exceeds 80 to 90 mm Hg. Acute hypercapnia produces agitation and confusion, headache, flushing, and tachycardia, with progression to central nervous system depression and/or cardiopulmonary arrest. *Hypoxemia* (decreased PaO_2) can be caused by hypoventilation, ventilation-perfusion mismatch, or shunting. Much smaller changes in PaO_2 produce significant respiratory distress, irreversible organ and tissue damage, and cardiopulmonary arrest. Complications of chronic hypoxia include *polycythemia, pulmonary hypertension*, and *cor pulmonale.*

Oxygen saturation measurement is not an acceptable method of determining the presence of respiratory failure or monitoring response to treatment. Patients in respiratory failure can maintain normal or near-normal oximetry measurements with minimal supplemental oxygen despite significant hypoxemia, hypoventilation, and hypercapnia. Oximetry results must be interpreted with caution in patients with carboxyhemoglobin (carbon monoxide poisoning), methemoglobin (oxidizing drugs, toxin exposures), and sickle cell disease. Arterial blood gas and acid-base measurements are the only accepted indicators of the adequacy of gas exchange.

Management decisions are guided by whether the respiratory failure is acute, chronic, or chronic with superimposed acute failure. *Acute respiratory failure* is by far the most common cause of cardiac arrest in the pediatric population and requires emergency evaluation and management of airway, breathing, and circulation (see Chapter 29). Oxygen is

TABLE 13-4
DIFFERENTIAL DIAGNOSIS OF STRIDOR

Acute Laryngotracheobronchitis
- Primarily inspiratory stridor
- Most common in children 6 months to 2 years of age
- Usually caused by parainfluenza, but also respiratory syncytial virus, influenzae, and adenovirus
- Stridor results from subglottic edema
- Associated with barky cough

Bacterial Tracheitis
- Most common in children younger than age 3 years

Laryngomalacia
- Most common cause of congenital stridor
- Stridor begins in the neonatal period (4 to 6 weeks of age)
- Stridor is worse when supine and disappears when prone
- Stridor exacerbated by crying, feeding

Laryngeal Web
- Partial failure of embryonic airway recanalization
- Most are positioned at the vocal cords
- Stridor from birth
- Weak cry, biphasic stridor

Laryngeal Foreign Body (aspiration)
- Rapid onset of persistent inspiratory or biphasic stridor
- Absent cough
- Voice may also be lost
- More common in children younger than 3 years of age

Subglottic Stenosis
- Associated with (prolonged) intubation in the neonatal period (or thereafter)
- Inspiratory or biphasic stridor
- Symptoms present anytime in the first few years of life
- Congenital subglottic stenosis involves incomplete recanalization of the subglottis and cricoid rings

Subglottic Inflammation
- Often results from chronic gastroesophageal reflux

Vocal Cord Paralysis
- Stridor may be inspiratory or biphasic
- Respiratory distress uncommon unless paralysis affects both vocal cords
- Presents with noisy breathing, respiratory difficulties from birth
- Stridor does not change with adjustment of positioning (supine vs. prone)
- Associated with central nervous system abnormalities (Arnold-Chiari malformation, increased intracranial pressure)
- Associated with trauma during cardiac or intrathoracic surgery (e.g., ligation of patent ductus arteriosus)

Acquired Vocal Cord Dysfunction
- Most common in older children and adolescents
- May mimic asthma
- Worse with exercise

Vascular Rings
- Noisy breathing from birth or early infancy

Anaphylaxis
- Inspiratory stridor and hoarseness
- Usually associated with hypotension, hives, facial edema

administered to maintain PaO_2 at or above 95%. Patients with insufficient ventilation require bag-mask ventilatory support. Tracheal intubation is indicated for the individual who can no longer protect the airway, who has apnea or severe hypoventilation, who is at risk for imminent respiratory failure due to respiratory muscle fatigue, or who presents in cardiopulmonary arrest. Any patient with acute respiratory failure should be transported to an emergency department or intensive care unit as soon as possible for specialized care.

Acute decompensation is uncommon in patients with *chronic respiratory failure* unless they develop unrelated illnesses. Clinical manifestations of chronic respiratory failure include disordered sleep, morning headaches, daytime somnolence, altered mentation, and cardiomegaly. Treatment is aimed at reversing the underlying pathophysiology and/or improving respiratory function through:

- assistance with airway clearance (chest physiotherapy, clearance assistance devices) for patients with thick secretions (CF) or neuromuscular disease (muscular dystrophy)
- pharmacologic anti-inflammatory therapy if needed (for patients with asthma or airway inflammation)
- prompt and aggressive management of fever (which increases oxygen requirement)
- the judicious use of supplemental oxygen—maintenance of near-normal oxygen saturation (92%) can prevent or potentially reverse the sequelae of chronic hypoxia (pulmonary hypertension, cor pulmonale). However, in patients with chronic hypercapnia, the respiratory drive is maintained primarily through hypoxia; when this stimulus is removed with supplemental oxygen, hypoventilation and severe hypercapnia develop and may progress to apnea.
- ventilatory support with positive pressure nasal or face mask ventilation or tracheostomy, which is reserved for patients with refractory or untreatable disease

APNEA

Apnea is defined as cessation of breathing for ≥20 seconds or a pause of shorter duration accompanied by cyanosis, pallor, hypotonia, or bradycardia. Apnea is categorized as primarily *central*, primarily *obstructive*, or *mixed*.

- Central apnea is due to depression of the central nervous system respiratory drive. It is most common in neonates and young infants. Intracranial hemorrhage, increased intracranial pressure, sepsis, pneumonia, meningoencephalitis, necrotizing enterocolitis, hypoglycemia, severe anemia, closed head trauma, and hypoxia are all possible causes of central apnea. In patients with central apnea, no chest wall movement is noted during the apneic episode.
- Obstructive apnea is caused by partial or complete obstruction of the airway. Since the respiratory drive remains intact, the apneic episode is characterized by choking sounds and obvious movement of the chest wall in an attempt to draw air into the lungs. Obstructive apnea is typically diagnosed in older children but may occur at any age. Large tonsils and/or adenoids, nasal polyps, macroglossia, neck flexion, subglottic stenosis, and laryngomalacia have all been associated with obstructive apnea.
- Mixed apnea has both central and obstructive elements. This type of apnea generally requires polysomnography for diagnosis.

Periodic breathing is the presence of episodic brief respiratory pauses associated with minimal changes in heart rate and oxygen saturation. Periodic breathing is a normal variant in young infants; diagnostic procedures are unnecessary, and the condition gradually disappears within the first 3 months of life.

Apnea of prematurity may occur in infants born prior to 37 weeks of gestation and is thought to be a mixed type of apnea due to immaturity of respiratory centers in the brain and low airway tone. This type of apnea presents between 2 and 7 days of life. Caffeine stimulates the central nervous system and has been proven to significantly reduce the number of apneic episodes due to prematurity. Isolated apnea of prematurity should resolve by the age of 37 weeks postconception. Apnea that is noted on the first day of life, occurs in infants >36 weeks postconception, requires aggressive resuscitation measures, is associated with cyanosis, and/or recurs is more likely to be secondary to an underlying pathologic condition.

Premature infants also may develop apnea in response to *anemia*. Anemia reduces oxygen carrying capacity, resulting in tissue hypoxia despite normal oxygen saturation. Although most premature infants with anemia do not present with apnea, anemia should be suspected in patients with resting tachycardia and/or tachypnea, pallor, and poor weight gain. Transfusion to a hematocrit ≥30% typically correlates with resolution of the apneic episodes. *Joubert syndrome* is a rare autosomal recessive condition of disordered brain growth that presents in the neonatal period with central apnea and nystagmus.

The presentation of obstructive apnea is often nonspecific. Snoring, choking, and gagging while sleeping, poor growth, developmental delay, and behavioral problems have all been observed in patients with obstructive apnea. Although expensive and time consuming, *polysomnography* is the study of choice for evaluating apnea in the older child. Polysomnography provides information concerning chest wall movement, air flow, oxygen saturation, heart rate, and number and duration of apneic episodes. Obstructive sleep apnea is discussed in detail later in the chapter.

Exercise Intolerance

Many conditions are associated with exercise intolerance in the pediatric patient (Table 13-5). The two most common are poor physical conditioning and asthma. Exercise intolerance may also be the presenting manifestation of interstitial lung disease or vocal cord dysfunction. If the patient's history and physical examination do not point to a specific etiology, the first diagnostic intervention is a trial of β-agonist therapy prior to exercise. Pulmonary function testing during exercise challenge is indicated if symptoms do not significantly improve or resolve with bronchodilators.

TABLE 13-5
PARTIAL DIFFERENTIAL DIAGNOSIS OF EXERCISE INTOLERANCE

Condition	Clinical Characteristics	Results of Pulmonary Function Testing during Exercise
Poor conditioning	Onset of shortness of breath within minutes of exercise without associated wheezing or stridor; reluctance to exercise	Normal lung function
Exercise-induced asthma	Coughing, shortness of breath, and/or wheezing after 5 to 6 minutes of exercise, with gradual improvement after 20 to 30 minutes of rest; asymptomatic at other times	Restrictive lung function following exercise challenge
Vocal cord dysfunction	Wheezing and/or inspiratory stridor with exercise	Distinctive changes in lung function
Anemia	Associated fatigue in the absence of exercise	Normal lung function, but may be unable to complete study
Neuromuscular disease	Typically presents in infancy or early childhood; associated fatigue in the absence of exercise; physical examination findings	Normal lung function (unless respiratory muscles are involved), but usually unable to complete study
Cardiac disease	Typically presents in infancy; associated fatigue in the absence of exercise; physical examination findings	Variable; patients often too young for this type of evaluation

Hemoptysis

Hemoptysis (coughing up blood) is uncommon in children. It may be relatively benign or signal life-threatening disease. The differential diagnosis of hemoptysis in children is broad and varies by age (Table 13-6), with CF being the most common cause in older children.

The first step in the evaluation and management of the patient with hemoptysis is assessment of the stability of airway, breathing (including oxygenation), and circulation. Areas of compromise must be addressed prior to further diagnostic procedures. Thereafter, the source of bleeding should be identified. The observed blood may originate in the nasal passages, mouth, throat, bronchi, lung parenchyma, or gastrointestinal tract. Gastrointestinal bleeding is typically bright red or resembles coffee grounds, with an acidic pH. In contrast, pulmonary bleeding is red, frothy, and alkaline in pH. Informative history and physical examination results and suggested laboratory studies are provided in Table 13-7. Fortunately, hemoptysis in children usually resolves spontaneously before a significant amount of blood is lost. Diagnostic bronchoscopy is indicated for pulmonary bleeding that is massive (>240 mL in 24 hours) and/or ongoing. Patients with blood loss sufficient to produce hypotension benefit from blood transfusion.

Cyanosis

Cyanosis is discussed in detail in Chapter 14.

Clubbing

Digital clubbing is loss of the nail angle due to blunting and soft tissue enlargement of the distal digit. Subtle evidence of clubbing may be noted by 3 months of age in children with congenital disease. Clubbing is associated with cardiac and pulmonary disease as well as disorders involving other organ systems:

- *Congenital heart defects* that produce right-to-left intracardiac shunting present with chronic hypoxia and clubbing. Polycythemia is often noted as well.
- *Chronic pulmonary conditions*, most commonly CF, are associated with the development of clubbing. Recurrent wheezing, chronic cough, and failure to thrive are additional manifestations of pulmonary involvement.
- Although the mechanism of action is unknown, *gastrointestinal disorders* may also cause clubbing (ulcerative colitis, Crohn disease, biliary atresia, cirrhosis).
- Clubbing is associated with *malnutrition* and poor growth in underdeveloped countries; undernutrition due to *chronic disease* may rarely also result in clubbing.

TABLE 13-6
DIFFERENTIAL DIAGNOSIS OF HEMOPTYSIS IN CHILDREN

Cystic fibrosis[a]
Congenital heart disease[b,c]
Bacterial pneumonia[b,c]
Trauma (common cause at any age)
Foreign body[d]
Coagulopathy/hemorrhagic disorder[b]
Vasculitis[a]
Bronchiectasis
Bronchogenic cyst[c]
Hemosiderosis[a]
Pulmonary embolus
Tumor
Arteriovenous malformations
Factitious hemoptysis

[a]More common in older children.
[b]More common in neonates.
[c]More common in infants.
[d]More common in toddlers.

TABLE 13-7
HISTORY, PHYSICAL EXAMINATION, AND SUGGESTED LABORATORY STUDIES IN THE PEDIATRIC PATIENT WITH HEMOPTYSIS

History
Onset of bleeding (acute, subacute, chronic)
Fever
Cough
Dyspnea
Recurrent pneumonias
Adequacy of growth

Physical Examination
Wheezing
Rales
Crackles
Cyanosis
Clubbing
Pallor

Suggested Laboratory and Diagnostic Studies
Complete blood count
Coagulation studies
Serum chemistry
Blood type and cross-match
Sputum sample for Gram stain, culture
Urinalysis
Serum blood urea nitrogen/creatinine
Chest radiographs
Computed tomography of the chest
Bronchoscopy

- *Familial clubbing* is an isolated disorder of no known significance.

DIAGNOSTIC TECHNIQUES

Spirometry

Spirometry, or measurement of air volume and flow rate, is an invaluable tool in the evaluation of lung function. The most important objective measures of pulmonary function provided by spirometry include forced vital capacity (FVC) and volume of forcibly expired air within 1 second (FEV^1). Spirometry assists in differentiating between obstructive and restrictive disease (Table 13-8). Patients with asthma are periodically evaluated with spirometry to assess compliance with and effectiveness of therapy. Of note, spirometry testing does not measure total lung volume, functional residual capacity, adequacy of gas exchange, diffusion capacity, oxygenation, or exhaled hydrogen or nitric oxide concentrations.

Blood Gas Testing

Although capillary and venous blood gas testing are useful under certain circumstances, arterial blood gas measurement is the preferred method for determining adequacy of pulmonary function. Regardless of the source of the sample, the blood pH and partial pressures of oxygen and carbon dioxide are measured directly, with subsequent calculation of serum bicarbonate and base deficit or excess values. Arterial samples are more difficult to obtain and painful for the patient, but they are the only reliable method of determining whether hypoxemia is present. Venous and capillary samples can be used to approximate arterial pH, $PaCO_2$, and bicarbonate values in most patients, although capillary measurements are unreliable in patients with poor perfusion, peripheral vasoconstriction, hypothermia, or hypovolemia.

Oxyhemoglobin Saturation

Pulse oximetry is a measure of the arterial hemoglobin saturation. Although generally a reliable noninvasive indicator

TABLE 13-8
SPIROMETRY: OBSTRUCTIVE vs. RESTRICTIVE DISEASE

Lung Measurement	Obstructive Disease	Restrictive Disease
FVC	Decreased	Normal to decreased
FEV_1/FVC	<75 to 80%	Normal
FEV_1	Decreased	Decreased

Obstructive lung disease—asthma, cystic fibrosis, emphysema, or bronchiectasis.
Restrictive lung disease—interstitial fibrosis, sarcoidosis, scoliosis, or progressive neuromuscular disease (Becker-type muscular dystrophy).

of oxygenation, pulse oximetry does have several limitations that must be noted in the care of children with pulmonary disease:

- Correlation of hemoglobin saturation with arterial PaO_2 is less reliable under circumstances that shift the oxygen dissociation curve (temperature changes, acid-base balance disturbances, 2,3-diphosphoglycerol content in erythrocytes, increased fetal hemoglobin).
- Pulse oximetry provides no assessment of ventilation.
- Arterial hemoglobin saturation values may remain deceptively elevated in the setting of ventilation-perfusion mismatching, and clinical improvement in aeration often results in a transient reduction in pulse oximetry readings.

Chest Radiograph

Plain radiographs of the chest are part of the initial evaluation of any patient with suspected pulmonary disease and/or respiratory distress. The radiographic characteristics of different pulmonary abnormalities are presented under their respective headings.

UPPER AIRWAY DISORDERS

Laryngomalacia

Laryngomalacia is a dynamic reversible airway disorder that causes raspy breathing but is otherwise usually benign. Flaccidity of the epiglottis and surrounding structures permits prolapse into the glottis during inspiration, resulting in inspiratory stridor. Stridor due to laryngomalacia usually presents in the second month of life, although, in severe cases, it may begin shortly after birth. The stridor becomes more pronounced with agitation, crying, and upper respiratory infections; it is worse when the patient is supine and noticeably improves or resolves when the infant is prone. Feeding is generally unaffected unless the obstruction is severe. When the history and physical examination are consistent with mild uncomplicated laryngomalacia, no further evaluation is necessary. If the diagnosis is in doubt, laryngomalacia is confirmed through direct laryngoscopic visualization of the prolapsing (often omega-shaped) epiglottis during inspiration. Laryngomalacia resolves spontaneously by 1 to 2 years of age in the vast majority of cases. Surgical correction is reserved for patients with severe obstruction. Most laryngomalacia is congenital in origin, although the disorder has also been associated with gastroesophageal reflux and generalized neuromuscular weakness.

Vocal Cord Dysfunction

The vocal cords are contained within the larynx. Congenital *vocal cord paralysis* (VCP) may be uni- or bilateral and is usually diagnosed in infancy:

- Unilateral VCP produces a weak cough, hoarse cry, and noisy breathing from birth; occasionally, inspiratory stridor will be present as well. Infants with unilateral VCP rarely develop respiratory distress.
- Bilateral VCP results in inspiratory or biphasic stridor that is often accompanied by tachypnea, retractions, difficulty feeding, and cyanotic spells.

A key feature differentiating VCP from laryngomalacia is response to positioning; noisy breathing associated with VCP is the same whether the child is in the supine or prone position. Congenital VCP may be due to central nervous system anomalies, atrial enlargement, or birth trauma (e.g., traumatic forceps delivery). Paralysis is confirmed by laryngoscopy.

VCP may be *acquired* later in life secondary to neurologic or cardiac abnormalities, throat surgery, trauma, or infection.

Vocal cord dysfunction involves paradoxic closure of the vocal cords during expiration. It is more common in females and most noticeable when the patient is exercising or anxious. Although characteristic expiratory flow loop changes on spirometry are suggestive, direct laryngoscopic visualization of inappropriate cord closure is necessary to confirm the diagnosis.

Croup

Croup is a constellation of respiratory signs associated with temporary upper airway obstruction. The classic symptoms of croup (*inspiratory stridor* and a barky, seal-like, nonproductive *cough*) result from narrowing of the laryngeal structures and/or proximal trachea. Croup may be infectious or spasmodic in origin:

- *Acute laryngotracheobronchitis* (infectious croup) is the most common cause of upper airway obstruction in young children beyond the neonatal period. The majority of cases result from infection with *parainfluenza* virus, although influenza, adenovirus, and respiratory syncytial virus can also cause croup. Typically, a 1- to 3-day period of low-grade fever, rhinorrhea, and mild cough is followed by the sudden onset of inspiratory stridor and the characteristic barking cough, often during the night. Hypoxia is unusual, even among patients brought to the emergency department in respiratory distress. Infectious croup is generally a clinical diagnosis. Subglottic narrowing (the "*steeple sign*") may or may not be appreciated on an anteroposterior chest radiograph. Administration of systemic steroids results in significant improvement within hours. Nebulized epinephrine is reserved for the patient with moderate-to-severe respiratory distress.
- *Spasmodic croup* is much less common than infectious croup and is thought to be allergic in origin. There are no preceding or associated symptoms such as fever or rhinorrhea. Spasmodic croup resolves within a few hours without specific treatment.

Epiglottitis

Epiglottitis is decreasing in incidence but remains a potentially life-threatening condition. Incidence peaks in the

3- to 5-year age group. Inflammation and edema of the epiglottis and surrounding tissues result in acute and rapidly progressive upper airway narrowing with a very real risk of complete obstruction and cardiopulmonary arrest. The classic presentation involves an upright, toxic-appearing child with high fever, stridor, significant respiratory distress, and drooling with the chin thrust forward. Dysphagia is universally present. Painful and/or frightening procedures should be avoided because they may precipitate total airway obstruction. Patients with suspected epiglottitis and respiratory distress should be intubated in a controlled environment (i.e., the operating room or intensive care unit) by experienced medical personnel prior to additional evaluation. A lateral neck radiograph demonstrating edema of the epiglottis ("thumb sign") can be helpful in patients with less severe disease. The incidence of epiglottitis has decreased substantially due to routine childhood vaccination against *Haemophilus influenzae* type b. Empiric antibiotic therapy effective against *H. influenzae* and *Streptococcus pneumoniae* is administered until culture and sensitivity results become available. Examples of effective regimens include intravenous cefotaxime alone, ceftriaxone alone, or ampicillin and sulbactam.

LOWER AIRWAY DISORDERS

Vascular Anomalies

Vascular rings are an important, often overlooked cause of airway obstruction. Aberrant vasculature arising from the aorta completely encircles both the trachea and esophagus. Although vascular rings occur relatively infrequently, three of the more common types are described in Table 13-9.

Patients with vascular rings are often misdiagnosed with recurrent croup, bronchiolitis, or asthma. Airway symptoms are exacerbated by intercurrent viral upper respiratory infections and may initially respond to bronchodilator therapy, further clouding the clinical picture. The predominant manifestations of vascular rings are directly related to tracheal and esophageal compression:

- Recurrent inspiratory or biphasic stridor and/or wheezing, which may be more pronounced when feeding
- Coughing with feeds
- Recurrent pneumonias
- Slow feeding, frequent regurgitation
- Dysphagia with solids
- Aspiration pneumonia

The radiologic hallmark of vascular ring is *esophageal indentation* noted on posteroanterior or lateral views of the barium swallow. Radiographs may be of value for noting tracheal deviation and determining "sidedness" of the aortic arch, but more often, they are normal or provide only nonspecific evidence of air trapping and hyperinflation. A pulsatile indentation is usually evident in the trachea on bronchoscopy. High-resolution computed tomography of the chest with contrast allows definitive assessment of the vessels composing the ring and surrounding vasculature. Echocardiography is indicated for all patients with confirmed vascular rings due to the risk of associated intracardiac lesions.

TABLE 13-9
VASCULAR RINGS

Double Aortic Arch
- Most common form of vascular ring
- Compresses both trachea and esophagus
- Typically diagnosed in the neonatal period or early infancy due to more severe compression
- May present with respiratory distress and/or difficult intubation on the first day of life; occasionally found during evaluation of an infant intubated for pneumonia who repeatedly fails trials of extubation
- Low incidence of intracardiac pathology

Right Aortic Arch with Left Ligamentum Arteriosum
- Second most common form of vascular ring
- Compresses both trachea and esophagus
- Diagnosis often delayed until late infancy or beyond due to less severe compression
- May present as recurrent stridor or wheezing
- Ten percent of patients have associated intracardiac defects

Pulmonary Sling
- Left pulmonary artery arises from the right pulmonary artery
- Onset of respiratory symptoms during the first postnatal month
- High incidence of associated tracheal abnormalities (tracheomalacia, tracheal stenosis or web)
- Fifteen percent to 30% of patients have associated intracardiac defects
- Barium swallow is the diagnostic study of choice for determining the presence of pulmonary slings (anterior indentation of the esophagus on the lateral projection is diagnostic)

Supportive treatment is appropriate for patients with mild symptoms, in the hopes that respiratory symptoms will improve or resolve with growth. Obstruction associated with double aortic arch, right-sided aortic arch with left ligamentum arteriosum, and pulmonary sling usually worsens over time despite adequate growth. Although surgery may be completely curative, a small minority of patients suffer variable degrees of ongoing (albeit diminished) airway obstruction.

Tracheomalacia

Tracheomalacia is similar to laryngomalacia in that it is a dynamic airway disorder caused by flaccidity of respiratory structures (in this case, the cartilage comprising the rings of the tracheal wall). The condition may be congenital (idiopathic) or associated with tracheoesophageal fistula, gastroesophageal reflux, bronchopulmonary dysplasia, Down syndrome, or chronic mechanical ventilation. Congenital tracheomalacia typically presents in the second month of life with expiratory wheezing that is exacerbated by agitation, crying, upper respiratory infections, and supine positioning.

Feeding may be problematic. The wheezing improves or resolves when the patient is placed in the prone position; bronchodilator therapy is not helpful and may even worsen the symptoms. In contrast to laryngomalacia, tracheomalacia may be complicated by cyanotic spells and/or complete airway obstruction. Tracheomalacia is suggested by history and physical examination and confirmed with fluoroscopy of the airway. Patients with tracheomalacia often require placement of a tracheostomy tube.

Tracheitis

Bacterial tracheitis is a serious infection of the airway that results in tracheal edema and sloughing of purulent airway lining. *Staphylococcus aureus* is often the causative organism. The illness begins with a cough that becomes increasingly productive over several days, accompanied by consistently rising fevers. Expiratory stridor may develop, but there is a notable absence of dysphagia and drooling. The sudden onset of toxicity and severe respiratory distress often necessitate short-term endotracheal intubation and mechanical ventilation. The anteroposterior chest radiograph may demonstrate ragged tracheal borders. Treatment consists of removal of tracheal debris through the endotracheal tube or via bronchoscopy. Epinephrine and steroids offer no benefit. Broad-spectrum antibiotic therapy effective against *S. aureus*, *Moraxella catarrhalis*, and nontypeable *H. influenzae* should be administered until culture and sensitivity results are available. Bacterial tracheitis usually arises in isolation but may rarely complicate acute viral laryngotracheobronchitis.

Congenital Malformations

Congenital malformations of the lung may remain asymptomatic or present with respiratory distress, recurrent wheezing (due to bronchial compression), and/or lung infection. *Hypoplastic lung* and *cystic adenomatoid malformation* are two of the more common congenital malformations of the lung.

- Hypoplastic lung—may be isolated or associated with renal agenesis, congenital obstruction of the urinary tract, or diaphragmatic hernia. Presentation depends on the severity of hypoplasia, ranging from severe respiratory distress in the newborn period to recurrent or chronic tachypnea, cough, cyanosis, and/or dyspnea in older children.
- Cystic adenomatoid malformation—a cystic mass of abnormal lung tissue found within the lung parenchyma. It is identifiable on prenatal ultrasound, but more than half of cases resolve prior to birth. Cystic adenomatoid malformation presents with respiratory distress in the newborn period or persistent/recurrent pneumonia in older infants and children, depending on the size and location.

Bronchiolitis

Bronchiolitis is discussed in detail in Chapter 10.

Aspiration Syndromes

Aspiration is the accidental inspiration of foreign material into the respiratory tract. Commonly aspirated substances include foreign bodies (food, coins, small toys), saliva, and refluxed gastric contents. The presentation may be obvious or subtle, acute, or chronic, but virtually always consists of some combination of the following:

- Episodic choking and gagging
- Episodic cyanosis
- Episodic apnea and/or bradycardia
- Recurrent wheezing unresponsive to β-agonist therapy
- Recurrent pneumonia and/or bronchitis
- Chronic cough
- Feeding difficulties
- Excessive drooling
- Failure to thrive

Foreign body aspiration (FBA) is most common in children 1 to 3 years of age. Aspiration of the object may or may not be witnessed. FBA should be suspected in any young patient with the abrupt onset of coughing and wheezing, especially if the symptoms persist despite intervention and focal findings are present on lung auscultation. Children commonly respond to the initial aspiration event with choking, gagging, and/or paroxysmal coughing but may then become asymptomatic for a variable period of time. Eventually, patients develop chronic symptoms such as recurrent wheezing, chronic cough, pneumonia, or hemoptysis. Radiograph findings on plain chest films (inspiratory and expiratory) depend on the location and type of obstruction:

- Focal atelectasis—no air flow into or out of the space
- Focal air trapping and hyperinflation—ball-valve obstructive effect (air can enter during inspiration, but the space becomes fully obstructed on expiration)
- Normal chest radiographs—most aspirated objects are radiolucent. If the aspirated object does not obstruct airflow, both inspiratory and expiratory films may be normal.

Normal chest radiographs do not rule out FBA. Bronchoscopy is required for definitive diagnosis and removal of the object.

Although their presentations may be similar, aspiration due to *disordered swallowing* is treated differently than aspiration resulting from *gastroesophageal reflux*:

- *Swallowing dysfunction* is often associated with static neurodevelopmental disorders (e.g., cerebral palsy), progressive neuromuscular or central nervous system disease, and oropharyngeal anomalies (cleft palate). The presence of a tracheostomy tube does not prevent aspiration. The modified barium swallow is the study of choice to assess the presence and severity of swallowing abnormalities. Specialized occupational therapy techniques have been beneficial for many patients. Total gastrostomy feeding is required in severe cases.

- Severe *gastroesophageal reflux* predisposes to aspiration of regurgitated stomach contents. An upper gastrointestinal series (with or without a swallow study) and pH probe test are indicated for patients with suspected gastroesophageal reflux disease. Radionuclide tracers (the milk scan, among others) can be used to document aspiration of stomach contents. The management of gastroesophageal reflux disease is provided in Chapter 12.

Aspiration pneumonia is most common in patients who are acutely or chronically incapable of protecting their airways (e.g., patients with neuromuscular impairment or anatomic abnormalities of the airway or proximal gastrointestinal tracts; patients who are heavily sedated for medical procedures or following drug use or alcohol intoxication). Healthy, immunocompetent, neurologically intact patients who develop aspiration pneumonia are hospitalized for observation but generally do not require antibiotic therapy or systemic corticosteroids. Penicillin is indicated for patients with significant or progressive respiratory disease. Unresponsive disease may require culture of tracheal aspirates to identify resistant or unusual organisms.

Bronchiectasis

Bronchiectasis is the irreversible enlargement and distortion of bronchi and bronchioles. Bronchiectasis may be diffuse or localized:

- CF is the most common cause of *diffuse bronchiectasis* in children. The differential diagnosis also includes primary ciliary dyskinesia, allergic bronchopulmonary aspergillosis, immunodeficiency syndromes, and tuberculosis infection.
- Lobar pneumonia and FBA may both be complicated by *localized bronchiectasis.*

A cough productive of copious sputum (with or without hemoptysis) is the most prominent symptom of bronchiectasis. Focal wheezing and/or rales are appreciated on auscultation of the lungs. The chest radiograph is significant for atelectasis and focal or generalized cystic areas within the parenchyma. The diagnosis of bronchiectasis is confirmed through computed tomography of the chest. Long-term management includes any combination of the following as needed: chest physiotherapy, bronchodilators, supplemental oxygen, and prophylactic or episodic antimicrobial medications.

PARENCHYMAL DISEASE

Pneumonia

Pneumonia is defined as infection of the lung parenchyma. Probable pathogens differ by age (Table 13-10). Pneumonia in the newborn is covered in Chapter 5. In infants and young children, the clinical sign most closely associated with pneumonia is *tachypnea*. Febrile children younger than 2 years of age who are not tachypneic are unlikely to have pneumonia. Fever increases the respiratory rate slightly less than 10% per Celsius degree above normal. Pneumonia should be suspected in the young febrile patient with a respiratory rate exceeding that expected, especially when the tachypnea is accompanied by flaring, retractions, and/or other signs of increased work of breathing.

Bacterial pneumonia in infants 1 to 6 months of age usually presents with the acute onset of fever, a wet-sounding cough, and tachypnea. Grunting, retractions, nasal flaring, and cyanosis are appreciated in patients with severe disease. Auscultation of the chest rarely reveals focal changes in this age group, even when significant consolidation is confirmed through radiography. Blood cultures may detect the causative organism; urine and cerebrospinal fluid should be cultured as well in infants younger than 90 days of age. Hospitalization is indicated for all infants ≤ 6 months of age with suspected bacterial pneumonia. Empiric therapy with cefuroxime is appropriate until culture and sensitivity results are available. Patients should complete a 10-day course of antibiotics but may be switched to an oral agent prior to hospital discharge. Respiratory viruses are known to cause severe pneumonia in this age group, which may require intense respiratory support and be slow to resolve.

Preschool-age children with pneumonia are typically febrile and tachypneic. Cough may or may not be present, but rhinorrhea and sore throat are not prominent symptoms. Focal findings on auscultation of the lungs are more consistent with bacterial pneumonia; diffuse wheezing or crackles suggests viral or *Mycoplasma* pneumonia. Evaluation of the young child with suspected bacterial pneumonia includes a complete blood count, blood cultures, and plain radiographs of the chest. Bacterial infections are more likely to result in consolidated lobar infiltrates, whereas diffuse interstitial infiltrates suggest viral or atypical pneumonia. Sputum cultures are difficult to obtain and of little value in this age group due to high rates of colonization of the upper airway. Hospitalization for supportive care and intravenous antibiotic therapy is indicated for the patient who appears toxic, is markedly tachypneic, and/or requires oxygen. Ambulatory patients should be followed daily until afebrile and significantly improved.

Pneumonias caused by *Mycoplasma* and *Chlamydophila pneumoniae* are more common than bacterial pneumonia in school-age children and adolescents; the diagnosis and treatment of these pathogens is discussed in detail in Chapter 10. Patients in this age group with bacterial pneumonia usually present with the acute onset of high fever and productive cough. Focal findings on lung auscultation are more reliable indicators of bacterial pneumonia in this age group. Signs consistent with consolidation include crackles/rales, increased transmission of whispered syllables, dullness to percussion, and tactile fremitus. The best method of identifying a causative organism in this age group is the sputum culture; samples with >25 leukocytes and <25 squamous epithelial

TABLE 13-10
COMMON CAUSES OF INFECTIOUS PNEUMONIA BY AGE

1 to 6 Months	6 Months to 5 Years	School Age/Adolescent
Streptococcus pneumoniae[a]	*Streptococcus pneumoniae*[a]	*Mycoplasma pneumoniae*
Staphylococcus aureus	*Moraxella catarrhalis*	*Chlamydophila pneumoniae*
Moraxella catarrhalis	*Haemophilus influenzae*	*Streptococcus pneumoniae*
Haemophilus influenzae	*Staphylococcus aureus*	*Haemophilus influenzae*
Bordetella pertussis	*Neisseria meningitidis*	*Staphylococcus aureus*
Chlamydia trachomatis[b]	*Mycoplasma pneumoniae*	*Mycobacterium tuberculosis*
Ureaplasma urealyticum[b]	Group A streptococci	Respiratory viruses[d]
Cytomegalovirus[b]	*Mycobacterium tuberculosis*	
Respiratory viruses[c]	Respiratory viruses[d]	

[a]Most common cause of bacterial pneumonia in this age group.
[b]Perinatal infections that often do not present with pneumonia until after 1 month of age.
[c]Respiratory syncytial virus, influenza, parainfluenza, and adenovirus.
[d]Adenovirus and influenza.

cells per low-power field are appropriate for culture. Indications for hospitalization are similar to those for the younger child.

Patients with pneumonia who have underlying neuromuscular disease are at significant risk for respiratory failure due to decreased strength reserves. Acute decompensation can lead to apnea. Such patients require close monitoring of oxygenation through pulse oximetry or arterial blood gas analysis. Bedside spirometry measurements of FVC can detect early fatigue and predict subsequent respiratory compromise. Intubation and mechanical ventilation should be considered for the patient with a significant decrease in FVC.

Documenting resolution of radiographic abnormalities with follow-up chest films is unnecessary for immunocompetent children with community-acquired pneumonias. Infiltrates may persist for a month or more but resolve completely within 2 to 3 months. Repeat studies are indicated for patients with persistent dyspnea, constitutional or systemic symptoms, or abnormal findings on physical examination. Dyspnea on exertion related to bacterial pneumonia may persist for up to 2 to 3 months but should gradually and consistently improve. It is not unusual for the cough associated with viral or atypical pneumonia to last 3 months or longer, but this too should progressively clear over time.

Recurrent pneumonia may be the presenting feature of an underlying anomaly or chronic disease (e.g., CF, ciliary dyskinesia, immunodeficiency, allergic bronchopulmonary *Aspergillus*, tracheoesophageal fistula, gastroesophageal reflux aspiration, malignancy).

Pleural effusion is a not uncommon complication of bacterial pneumonia. *S. pneumoniae* infection is most commonly associated with parapneumonic pleural effusions; *Mycoplasma*, *S. aureus*, and respiratory viruses account for a significant minority. *S. aureus* pneumonia, in particular, may cause large pleural effusions filled with infected fluid (*complicated parapneumonic effusion* or *empyema*). Small effusions are usually clinically irrelevant. Large effusions result in dyspnea, increased work of breathing, orthopnea, and, if massive, cyanosis and respiratory failure. Auscultation of the chest reveals decreased breath sounds and decreased vocal fremitus over the fluid-filled area, which is dull to percussion. *Empyema* is suggested by persistence of fever despite appropriate antimicrobial therapy. Pleural fluid obtained via thoracentesis demonstrates >10,000 white blood cells per L, with a predominance of polymorphonuclear cells. Complicated parapneumonic effusions are managed with intravenous broad-spectrum antibiotics and prompt drainage and chest tube placement to prevent the development of loculation and fibrosis. Asymptomatic uncomplicated parapneumonic effusions resolve spontaneously with no long-term sequelae.

Lung abscess and pneumatocele are two complications of pneumonia most closely associated with *S. aureus* infection. In immunocompetent individuals, *lung abscesses* are treated with intravenous antibiotics until radiographic resolution of the abscess; drainage is unnecessary. Anaerobic bacterial abscesses are more common in immunodeficient or neurologically impaired children. *Pneumatoceles* are small air-filled sacs that develop in the setting of acute pneumonia. They are usually asymptomatic and resolve spontaneously; rare cases are complicated by pneumothorax.

Acute Respiratory Distress Syndrome Secondary to Drowning

Regardless of the initial response to submersion (laryngospasm, aspiration), *acute respiratory distress syndrome* (ARDS) is the most common pulmonary sequelae of near drowning.

ARDS may be defined as pulmonary edema in absence of volume overload or ventricular dysfunction that manifests as bilateral pulmonary infiltrates and impaired oxygenation. The natural progression of ARDS is as follows:

- *Exudation*—Increased capillary permeability floods the lungs with fluid. This state is characterized by the acute development of respiratory failure, which may be the initial presentation, evolve over several hours, or herald acute decompensation following a period of apparent recovery. In the spontaneously breathing patient, ARDS should be suspected in the setting of increasing hypoxia unresponsive to high supplemental oxygen concentrations and diffuse pulmonary infiltrates on chest radiograph. Hypoxemia and decreased lung compliance are observed in the ventilated patient.
- *Inflammation*—Alveolar-capillary membrane damage results in alveolar fibrosis and secondary surfactant deficiency, further compromising adequacy of gas exchange.
- *Resolution*—Some patients achieve full recovery; others are left with variable degrees of residual pulmonary fibrosis. Long-term sequelae include exertional dyspnea, chronic hypoxemia, and clinically significant reductions in lung volume and compliance.

Supplemental oxygen and ventilatory support form the foundation of ARDS management. Persistent ARDS may respond to high-dose systemic steroids. Antibiotics are not routinely indicated unless the patient has fever, leukocytosis, and chest radiograph findings consistent with bacterial pneumonia.

Reliable predictors of outcome include water temperature, duration of submersion, degree of aspiration, and effectiveness of early resuscitation efforts. Submersion for >5 minutes in warm water associated with significant aspiration and minimal response to initial cardiopulmonary resuscitation (CPR) virtually always results in major disability or death. Children who are rescued prior to the development of cardiopulmonary arrest or who respond to resuscitation attempts within 10 minutes (i.e., have palpable pulses at the scene) have the best prognosis. Those who remain in a coma for > 24 hours after rescue rarely recover. Patients who are severely hypothermic after resuscitation (<28°C) should undergo active internal warming using extracorporeal life support. Passive warming (with blankets) is inadequate, and warming with external heat sources may precipitate vasodilatation and cardiovascular collapse. Mild hypothermia may be managed with rewarming of the head and trunk only, which minimizes the risk of peripheral vasodilatation. Mild hypothermia (>32°C) in the first 24 hours may be beneficial for resuscitated patients who remain comatose.

Plain radiographs of the chest should be obtained in any victim of near drowning, although the results are often nonspecific, and the extent of pulmonary damage does not necessarily correlate with radiographic findings. The patient who does not require resuscitation, has a normal physical examination and normal blood oxygenation after a 6- to 8-hour period of observation, and has a reliable caregiver may be discharged; all others should be admitted for continued observation and supportive care.

The development of ARDS is not limited to drowning. Any injury that directly or indirectly injures the lung, including pneumonia, aspiration, trauma, burns, smoke inhalation, sepsis, fat embolism, disseminated intravascular coagulation, and massive blood product transfusion may result in ARDS. As opposed to cases associated with drowning, ARDS associated with other causes may develop hours to days after the initial insult. Although the mortality rate in patients with ARDS is relatively high, most patients succumb to complications of their underlying illnesses (e.g., multiorgan failure, sepsis).

BRONCHOPULMONARY DYSPLASIA

Bronchopulmonary dysplasia (BPD) is a chronic respiratory disorder that can develop in infants who are dependent on supplemental oxygen and mechanical ventilation for a prolonged (>28 days) or specific (at or around 36 weeks postconception) time period. BPD is more prevalent among former preterm infants but can occur in term infants as well. Specific clinical and radiologic features are required for diagnosis. Patients with BPD have decreased lung compliance, ventilation-perfusion mismatch, and increased airway resistance. The most significant long-term sequelae of BPD are *chronic hypoxemia* and *poor growth:*

- Patients with moderate-to-extensive pulmonary changes often need supplemental oxygen while asleep, active, or feeding. Some infants require oxygen at all times. Infection with childhood respiratory pathogens is associated with recurrent wheezing in infants with BPD, who may experience severe exacerbation of their underlying pulmonary illness. *Cor pulmonale* is a known complication of chronic or recurrent BPD-associated hypoxemia.
- Poor growth in infants with BPD may be due to insufficient oxygenation, increased work of breathing, oromotor dysfunction/aversion, and/or gastroesophageal reflux, all of which are more prevalent in this population. Nutritional counseling and growth monitoring are necessary for optimal developmental outcome. Patients with BPD typically require additional caloric intake to meet energy requirements for maintenance and growth.

Infants with BPD experience very gradual improvement. Noticeable clinical impairment beyond the age of 36 months is rare. However, abnormalities persist at the alveolar level, and functional deficits can be detected on spirometry for years. Infants with BPD also have an increased risk of developing asthma later in life.

ASTHMA

Asthma is discussed in detail in Chapter 9.

CYSTIC FIBROSIS

CF is an autosomal recessive, multisystem disease characterized by disordered exocrine gland function. The prevalence is highest in whites. Seventy percent of patients have the ΔF508 mutation on chromosome 7. The gene product is a cell membrane protein that functions as a cyclic adenosine monophosphate (cAMP)-activated chloride channel on the epithelial cells of the respiratory tract, pancreas, sweat and salivary glands, intestines, and reproductive system. This channel is nonfunctional in patients with CF, so chloride remains sequestered inside the cell. Sodium and water are drawn into the cell to maintain ionic and osmotic balance, resulting in relative dehydration at the cell surface and abnormally viscid secretions.

Presenting signs and symptoms of CF are listed in Table 13-11. All levels of the respiratory tract may be affected, including the nasal passages, sinuses, and lower airways. Nasal polyps in any pediatric patient should prompt further testing for CF. Opacification of the sinuses and sinusitis are extremely common. Mucus stasis and ineffective clearance lead to bacterial colonization and frequent pneumonias. Typical early childhood pathogens include *S. aureus* and *H. influenzae*. Colonization with *Pseudomonas aeruginosa* occurs in late childhood or early adolescence; over 90% of patients eventually acquire *P. aeruginosa*, which is not eradicated. Colonization with *Burkholderia cepacia* is a particularly ominous development associated with accelerated pulmonary deterioration and death.

Gastrointestinal manifestations include pancreatic insufficiency, bowel obstruction and rectal prolapse, diabetes, and hepatic cirrhosis. Interference with normal pancreatic enzyme secretion results in decreased fat absorption and steatorrhea; parents may notice that the child's stools are large, bulky, foul smelling, and greasy, with visible fat droplets. Consequences of steatorrhea include failure to thrive and deficiencies in fat-soluble vitamins. Later, stool becomes extremely dense, predisposing to distal intestinal obstruction. Failure to thrive is the most common manifestation of CF in infants and children. Near-normal growth can often be achieved with pancreatic enzyme replacement, fat-soluble vitamin supplements, and high-calorie, high-protein diets. Nasogastric or gastrostomy tube feedings may be instituted if oral intake is inadequate. In the neonate, *meconium ileus* is virtually pathognomonic for CF.

Classic diagnostic findings in CF include an elevated sweat chloride concentration, pancreatic insufficiency, and chronic pulmonary disease. The *sweat chloride level* remains the initial diagnostic test of choice. A level >60 mEq per L is considered abnormal. Genetic and prenatal testing is now available for the most common gene mutations. Recurrent lower airway infection results in bronchiectasis, fibrosis, parenchymal loss, and the characteristic "bleb" formation noted on chest radiographs. Pulmonary function tests demonstrate mostly *obstructive* and some *restrictive* changes. Fat droplets can be visualized in a fresh stool sample stained with acidified Sudan red; steatorrhea is confirmed through calculation of the coefficient of fat absorption.

TABLE 13-11 CLINICAL MANIFESTATIONS OF CYSTIC FIBROSIS

Chronic Sinopulmonary Disease

Persistent colonization/infection with pathogens typical of CF lung disease, including:

- *Staphylococcus aureus*
- *Pseudomonas aeruginosa*
- Nontypable *Haemophilus influenzae*
- *Burkholderia cepacia*
- *Stenotrophomonas maltophilia*

Cough and sputum production

Wheezing and air trapping

Radiographic abnormalities

Evidence of obstruction on spirometry

Digital clubbing

Chronic sinus disease

  Nasal polyps

  Radiographic changes

Intestinal Disease

Meconium ileus

Prolonged jaundice in the neonatal period

Exocrine pancreatic insufficiency

Endocrine pancreatic insufficiency (diabetes)

Distal intestinal obstruction

Rectal prolapse

Recurrent pancreatitis

Chronic hepatobiliary disease manifested by clinical and/or laboratory evidence of:

- Focal biliary cirrhosis
- Multilobular cirrhosis

Failure to thrive (protein-calorie malnutrition)

Hypoproteinemia–edema

Fat-soluble vitamin deficiencies (A, D, E, K)

Genitourinary Abnormalities

Obstructive azoospermia (infertility) in males

Metabolic Abnormalities

Salty skin

Salt-loss syndromes

Acute salt depletion (hyponatremic, hypochloremic dehydration)

Recurrent heat stroke

Chronic metabolic alkalosis

The management of pulmonary CF is multifocal. Chest physical therapy, exercise, and frequent coughing are helpful in mobilizing secretions. Bronchodilators and anti-inflammatory medications relax smooth muscle walls, decrease airway reactivity, and curb tissue destruction. Nebulized recombinant human deoxyribonuclease breaks down thick

DNA complexes present in mucus. Alternate months of regular inhaled tobramycin may be indicated for patients infected with *Pseudomonas*. More recently, azithromycin has been proven to be effective as a possible immune modifier. Frequent disease exacerbations are triggered by viral or bacterial infections and are managed with aggressive chest physical therapy, postural drainage, and antibiotics, which may be taken orally or inhaled if the exacerbation is mild and the organisms are susceptible. Usually, however, bacterial infections require treatment with an intravenous aminoglycoside (e.g., tobramycin) and semisynthetic penicillin or cephalosporin, depending on organism sensitivities.

The following are three important pulmonary complications of CF:

- *Hemoptysis* is an alarming development that may occur during pulmonary exacerbations in long-standing disease. Frequent coughing and inflammation lead to erosion of the walls of bronchial arteries in areas of bronchiectasis, and expectorated sputum becomes streaked with blood. Arterial embolization is indicated for frank blood loss of >500 mL in 24 hours (or >300 mL/day for 3 days).
- *Spontaneous pneumothorax* is characterized by the sudden onset of severe chest pain and difficulty breathing. Placement of a chest tube results in rapid re-expansion, but approximately half of pneumothoraces recur unless sclerosed. Sclerosis is avoided if at all possible because lung transplantation becomes more difficult after this procedure.
- Progressive obstruction and hypoxia in advanced disease lead to chronic *pulmonary hypertension* and *cor pulmonale*. For CF patients with a life expectancy limited to 1 to 2 years, lung transplantation is a potentially viable option.

PRIMARY CILIARY DYSKINESIA

Primary ciliary dyskinesia (PCD) is a disorder of mucociliary clearance resulting from abnormalities in proteins composing the dynein arms of the respiratory cilia. Various presentations of PCD are provided in Table 13-12. The diagnosis is made via electron microscopy (ultrastructural defects of the cilia, missing dynein arms) and functional studies (mucociliary clearance tests).

TABLE 13-12
CLINICAL MANIFESTATIONS OF PRIMARY CILIARY DYSKINESIA

Any Age
Dextrocardia
Situs inversus (50%)

Infancy
Unexplained tachypnea
Persistent or recurrent atelectasis
Recurrent pneumonia
Family history of primary ciliary dyskinesia

Childhood
Chronic/recurrent sinusitis
Chronic secretory otitis media
Persistent otorrhea through ventilation tubes
Recurrent pneumonia
Bronchiectasis
Nasal polyps
Clubbing

Adults
Infertility (males)

EXTRATHORACIC DISORDERS

Pleural Fluid

In the chest, the parietal and visceral lung pleura form a potential space lubricated with a small amount of fluid. Movement of fluid between the plural and intravascular spaces is governed by Starling forces. Fluid is primarily absorbed from the pleural space across the parietal membrane. Pleural effusion can result from any process that increases filtration into the space (increased capillary permeability or hydrostatic pressure) or interferes with absorption. By far, the most common cause of pleural effusion in the pediatric population is *parapneumonic effusion* due to subpleural pneumonia.

Clinical presentation ranges from asymptomatic to severe, life-threatening respiratory distress and cardiovascular instability, depending on the amount of fluid in the pleural space. The earliest symptom of pleural effusion is often focal chest pain on deep inspiration or cough (pleurisy). As more fluid accumulates, the pain resolves and is replaced by dyspnea, orthopnea, and worsening cough and fever. Physical signs include decreased breath sounds over the affected area, dullness to percussion, and decreased vocal fremitus. Hypoxemia and hypercarbia are noted on blood gas analysis.

Plain radiographs of the chest with the patient in the upright and lateral decubitus positions are the best screening study for detecting excess fluid in the pleural space. Blunting of the costophrenic angle is the earliest radiographic sign. The lateral decubitus view provides information about the quality (fluid vs. loculated) and quantity of the effusion and permits evaluation of the lung parenchyma. Small, asymptomatic pleural effusions require no specific treatment. Thoracentesis is indicated for patients with shifting pleural effusions who have persistent fever, toxicity, hypoxia, mediastinal shift, infection with specific organisms (*S. aureus, S. pneumoniae*), or involvement of >25% of a lung field. Surgical management is necessary for effusions that are loculated, persistent, or recurring. Specific criteria for placement of a chest tube with ongoing drainage include the following:

- pH of pleural fluid ≤7.2
- Glucose concentration of pleural fluid <40 mg per dL
- Lactate dehydrogenase concentration of pleural fluid > 1,000 IU per mL
- Bacterial organisms present on Gram stain of pleural fluid
- Foul-smelling or purulent pleural fluid

The appearance and composition of pleural fluid usually suggest the pathologic process underlying fluid accumulation (Table 13-13). Categorization of the fluid as "transudate" or "exudate" is less closely tied to specific disorders in children than it is in adults.

A *chylothorax* is an accumulation of pleural fluid with a high concentration of lipids. Disruption of the thoracic duct allows triglyceride-rich chyle fluid to enter the pleural space. Thoracic surgery and trauma to the chest are the most common causes of chylothorax, but nontraumatic processes may also interfere with thoracic duct drainage. T lymphocytes are found in abundance in chyle fluid, which has an electrolyte composition similar to that of plasma. The protein concentration is typically >3 g per dL. Management consists of chest tube drainage and limiting dietary fat intake to medium-chain triglycerides.

TABLE 13-13
PLEURAL FLUID: TRANSUDATE OR EXUDATE?

Gross Appearance of the Fluid
Pale yellow—transudate
Purulent—empyema
Milky white opalescent—chyle
Bloody—vascular erosion

	Transudate	Exudate
Underlying process	Relationship between hydrostatic and oncotic pressures favors filtration in excess of absorption	Inflammation of the pleural surface or impaired lymphatic drainage interferes with absorption
Example	Congestive heart failure	Infection of the pleura
	Laboratory Parameters	
Protein concentration	<3 g/dL	≥3 g/dL
Lactate dehydrogenase (LDH) concentration	<2/3 LDH	>2/3 LDH
pH	>7.45 (or greater than blood pH)	<7.3

Pneumothorax

Pneumothorax occurs when air enters the pleural space, usually as a result of a tear in the lung space adjacent to the visceral pleura. Trauma, resuscitation, and intubation with mechanical ventilation are some leading causes of pneumothorax in children. *Tension pneumothorax* presents with tachypnea, chest pain, splinting, hypoxia, respiratory distress, and diminished breath sounds on the affected side of the chest, which is hyperresonant to percussion. Immediate needle decompression is indicated, followed by placement of a chest tube. Further evaluative studies (chest radiograph, blood gas analysis) are delayed until the patient is stabilized. Decompression usually results in immediate improvement. Positive pressure ventilation is contraindicated until correct placement of the chest tube is confirmed. If necessary, tension pneumothorax is confirmed by an upright expiratory film of the chest demonstrating mediastinal shift to the unaffected side. Adequately ventilated patients who suddenly decompensate should be extubated and ventilated via bag-valve mask. If this maneuver does not result in respiratory stabilization, the most likely cause is pneumothorax.

Spontaneous pneumothorax occurs in patients with CF, asthma, and Marfan syndrome. Adolescents who inhale cocaine are also at risk.

Flail Chest

Flail chest is the paradoxic movement of a localized area of the chest wall resulting from the traumatic fracture of multiple ribs, with each affected rib broken in at least two places. The now-isolated segment of ribs and attached musculature sinks inward with inspiration and bows outward with expiration. Splinting in response to pain may produce airway edema and limit air movement on the affected side. Trauma victims with obvious flail chest should be placed with the injured area downward in order to optimize chest wall movement and ventilation of the uninjured side. Flail chest accompanied by traumatic pneumothorax or hemothorax may require additional intervention. Isolated flail chest typically resolves without complication with respiratory physiotherapy and adequate control of pain.

Pectus Excavatum

Pectus excavatum is the anteroposterior narrowing of the thoracic cavity due to inward depression of the sternum. It is usually an isolated defect but occurs more commonly among children with Marfan syndrome. Pectus excavatum is not typically associated with measurable changes in thoracic volume, impaired cough, or exercise intolerance, although severe deformity may result in minor restrictive functional changes. The presence of a loud systolic murmur over the pulmonic area is related to positioning against the sternum rather than valvular abnormalities. Surgical correction is unnecessary but may be employed for cosmetic purposes.

PULMONARY HYPERTENSION AND COR PULMONALE

Pulmonary hypertension is abnormally high blood pressure in the pulmonary arteries (mean pulmonary artery pressure >25 mm Hg at rest). Idiopathic pulmonary hypertension is uncommon; most cases involve an underlying pathologic process (Table 13-14). Increased pressure damages both the small pulmonary arteries responsible for gas exchange (leading to chronic hypoxia) and the large pulmonary arteries, which stiffen and narrow, further exacerbating the hypertension. As the right ventricle pumps against increased pressure, it becomes thickened and enlarged, eventually progressing to heart failure. *Cor pulmonale* (congestive heart failure secondary to pulmonary hypertension and right ventricular overload) is suggested by signs of right-sided heart failure, including:

- easy fatigability
- systemic edema
- hepatomegaly
- jugular venous distension
- prominence of the precordial impulse
- a loud single or narrowly split second heart sound
- a systolic murmur at the cardiac apex that radiates to the left axilla

Electrocardiography demonstrates right axis deviation, T-wave inversion in the limb leads (right ventricular strain), and a pure R wave in lead V_1. Right ventricular hypertrophy and systolic/diastolic pressure can be assessed by Doppler echocardiography. Cardiac catheterization is required to measure pulmonary artery pressure and the resistance and reactivity of the pulmonary vasculature. Progressive pulmonary hypertension, chronic hypoxia, and right-sided heart failure eventually culminate in death but are potentially reversible if recognized and addressed.

TABLE 13-14
CONDITIONS THAT PLACE PATIENTS AT RISK FOR THE DEVELOPMENT OF PULMONARY HYPERTENSION

Congenital heart disease resulting in right-to-left shunting
- Ventricular septal defect
- Atrial septal defect
- Patent ductus arteriosus

Congenital heart disease resulting in increased pulmonary venous pressure
- Mitral stenosis
- Pulmonary vein stenosis
- Total anomalous pulmonary venous return

Cyanotic congenital heart disorders
- Transposition of the great vessels
- Truncus arteriosus

Lung disease
- Upper airway obstruction
- Bronchopulmonary dysplasia
- Cystic fibrosis

Pulmonary thromboembolism

Sickle cell disease

Autoimmune disorders

Portal hypertension

SLEEP DISORDERS

Obstructive sleep apnea (OSA), also called obstructive sleep-disordered breathing, consists of recurrent partial or complete upper airway obstruction during sleep. Obstruction with hypoventilation may be due to hypertrophied adenoids and/or tonsils, craniofacial anomalies, macroglossia, neuromuscular or genetic diseases associated with decreased airway tone, and obesity. The detrimental effects of OSA are not limited to disordered sleep. Recurrent hypoxia and hypercapnia during sleep eventually result in pulmonary hypertension and, if undiagnosed, cor pulmonale. Obese patients with OSA have increased rates of systemic hypertension and stroke.

One of the earliest symptoms of OSA is excessive daytime sleepiness. Other symptoms directly related to obstruction and poor sleep include snoring, gasping/choking/apneic episodes during sleep, frequent nighttime awakenings, enuresis, morning headaches, and hyperextension of the neck during sleep. Behavior changes such as concentration problems, learning difficulties, hyperactivity, and mood alteration are obvious but may seem unrelated to disordered sleep. Although the physical examination is often normal, many children have evidence of one or more of the following: obesity or inadequate growth, Down syndrome, mouth breathing, hyponasal speech, dysmorphic facial features, nasal polyps or septal deviation, cleft palate, and enlarged tonsils. Laboratory abnormalities are unusual, but screening studies in patients with long-standing disease may reveal polycythemia, compensated respiratory acidosis, hypertrophied adenoids on lateral neck films, and right ventricular hypertrophy. The gold standard for diagnosis is polysomnography, which detects chest wall motion, nasal air flow, heart rate, and oxygen saturation. The addition of pH probe or electroencephalogram monitoring may be indicated for some patients. Unfortunately, polysomnography is expensive and time consuming. If the diagnosis of OSA is obvious from the history and physical examination, polysomnography is generally unnecessary, even in patients scheduled for removal of tonsils and adenoids. However, polysomnography is indicated when the diagnosis is uncertain, the patient is neurologically impaired, the patient is very young, or there is an underlying disease that might complicate surgical intervention.

Hypoventilation associated with OSA has become the most common indication for surgical removal of the tonsils and adenoids. The vast majority of affected children experience resolution of their symptoms following surgery. Most patients with OSA tolerate surgery well; however, as a group, OSA patients are at increased risk for several surgical complications, including pulmonary edema, laryngospasm, apnea, and pneumonia. *Postobstructive pulmonary edema* is an uncommon complication associated with surgical removal of the tonsils and adenoids in patients with severe, long-standing OSA.

Continuous positive airway pressure (CPAP) during sleep is reserved for patients with OSA who do not have tonsillar/adenoidal hypertrophy and patients who are considered at risk for surgical complications. Tracheostomy should be considered for children who do not tolerate CPAP.

APPARENT LIFE-THREATENING EVENTS/SUDDEN INFANT DEATH SYNDROME

Sudden infant death syndrome (SIDS) has been defined by a subcommittee of the National Institutes of Health as "the sudden death of an infant . . . which is unexplained by history and in which a thorough postmortem evaluation fails to demonstrate an adequate cause of death." The same committee defined an apparent life-threatening event (ALTE) as "an episode that is frightening to the observer and is characterized by some combination of apnea, color change, change in muscle tone, choking, or gagging." In many cases of ALTE, the caregiver reports believing that the infant was dying or would have died without intervention. The differential diagnosis of ALTE is extensive and includes:

- idiopathic (apnea of infancy)
- infection: respiratory (particularly respiratory syncytial virus, pertussis), systemic (sepsis), meningitis
- metabolic disease
- gastroesophageal reflux
- aspiration
- seizures
- cardiac arrhythmias
- abuse

The medical evaluation of ALTE is considered in Table 13-15.

Home monitoring is rarely indicated for infants with a history of ALTE because, although monitoring can document episodes of apnea, bradycardia, or hypoxia, neither ALTE nor any of the aforementioned diagnoses increases the risk of death due to SIDS.

The incidence of SIDS peaks between 3 and 5 months of age. Known risk factors for SIDS are included in Table 13-16. Home monitoring is often employed in an attempt to prevent SIDS in patients with known risk factors; however, the incidence of SIDS in monitored patients is not statistically different than the incidence in unmonitored patients.

TABLE 13-15
EVALUATION OF THE INFANT WITH AN APPARENT LIFE-THREATENING EVENT

Event History—Attempt to Obtain a Full Characterization of the Event

- Description of the episode
- Duration of the episode
- Intervention during the episode
- History of any changes in skin color (cyanosis, mottling, pallor)
- History of choking, gagging, or vomiting just prior to event
- Time elapsed between last feeding and event
- History of fever, congestion, other symptoms/signs of possible infection
- Any noted respiratory effort or chest movement during event
- Muscle tone during event (posturing, hypotonia)
- Any noted rhythmic body or eye movements
- Appearance of infant following resolution of event

Past Medical History

- Pre- and perinatal histories
- Comorbidities

Family History

- History of unexplained sudden death in infants or children
- History of genetic, cardiac, metabolic, endocrine, and neurologic diseases of childhood

Physical Examination

Subsequent assessment is guided by pertinent results of the above and generally takes place during a hospital stay for continuous monitoring unless the event was mild (required no intervention) and the history and physical examination are reassuring.

TABLE 13-16
RISK FACTORS FOR SUDDEN INFANT DEATH SYNDROME

Prone sleeping
Prematurity
Low birth weight
Intrauterine growth retardation
Male gender
Lower socioeconomic status
Age 3 to 5 months during winter
Maternal smoking during pregnancy and infancy
Young maternal age
Limited maternal education
Single motherhood
Multiple gestation
Inappropriate bedding materials
Potentially obstructive objects in crib

Note: Apnea of prematurity, apnea of infancy, and history of apparent life-threatening event are not risk factors for sudden infant death syndrome.

SOURCES

Adam HM. Apnea. *Pediatr Rev.* 2003;24:32–34.

American Academy of Pediatrics Task Force on Sudden Infant Death Syndrome. The changing concept of sudden infant death syndrome: diagnostic coding shifts, controversies regarding the sleeping environment, and new variables to consider in reducing the risk. *Pediatrics.* 2005;116:1245–1255.

Belamarich PF. Recognizing and diagnosing pancreatic insufficiency in infants. *Pediatr Rev.* 2002;23:69–70.

Bloomfield D. Tachypnea. *Pediatr Rev.* 2002;23:294–295.

Cover RA, Spahn JD. Treating the wheezing infant. *Pediatr Clin North Am.* 2003;50:631–654.

Efrati O, Barak A. Pleural effusions in the pediatric population. *Pediatr Rev.* 2002;23:417–426.

Fallot A. Respiratory distress. *Pediatr Ann.* 2005;34:885–892.

Farrell PA, Weiner GM, Lemons JA. SIDS, ALTE, apnea, and the use of home monitors. *Pediatr Rev.* 2002;23:3–9.

Guilbert T, Krawiec M. Natural history of asthma. *Pediatr Clin North Am.* 2003;50:523–538.

Kelly HW. The assessment of childhood asthma. *Pediatr Clin North Am.* 2003;50:593–608.

Mack E. Co-oximetry. *Pediatr Rev.* 2007;28:73–73.

Kelly LF. Pediatric cough and cold preparations. *Pediatr Rev.* 2004;25:115–123.

National Institutes of Health Consensus Development Conference of Infantile Apnea and Home Monitoring, Sept 29–Oct 1, 1986. Consensus Statement. *Pediatrics.* 1987;79:292–299.

Pope J, McBride J. Respiratory failure in children. *Pediatr Rev.* 2004;25:158–164.

Rafei K, Lichenstein R. Airway infectious disease emergencies. *Pediatr Clin North Am.* 2006;53:215–242.

Sherman J. Evaluating a chronic cough: history often solves the mystery. *Contemp Pediatr.* 2006;23:36–46.

Szefler SJ. Identifying the child in need of asthma therapy. *Pediatr Clin North Am.* 2003;50:577–591.

Vicencio AG, Parik S. Laryngomalacia and tracheomalacia: common dynamic airway lesions. *Pediatr Rev.* 2006;27:e33–e35.

QUESTIONS

1. Which of the following awake, alert patients is tachypneic?

A) A 1-day-old infant with a respiratory rate of 70 breaths per minute
B) A 2-month-old infant with a respiratory rate of 45 breaths per minute
C) An 18-month-old infant with a respiratory rate of 25 breaths per minute
D) A 6-year-old child with a respiratory rate of 20 breaths per minute
E) A 10-year-old child with a respiratory rate of 17 breaths per minute

2. Which of the following statements regarding pharmacologic therapy for cough in young children is FALSE?

A) Parents who give cough suppressants to their children should be counseled to purchase single-ingredient preparations.
B) Cough suppressants are safe and efficacious in preschool-age children with viral pneumonia.
C) Cough suppressants should not be administered to a young child whose cough is thought to be due to asthma.
D) Cough suppressants should not be administered to a young child whose cough is thought to be due to bacterial pneumonia.
E) Antihistamines do not suppress cough directly, but their sedative effects may result in less coughing.

3. An 8-year-old boy is brought to your office by his mother with a complaint of chronic cough. He was diagnosed with bacterial pneumonia 6 months ago that resolved with a course of oral antibiotics. He is currently on no medications. His cough is loud, nonproductive, and persistent throughout the day. His mother has been called several times in the past month to pick him up from school due to his coughing. Upon questioning, she tells you that he sleeps through the night with no cough. Which of the following conditions is most likely to be the cause of this patient's chronic cough?

A) Allergic rhinitis
B) Chronic sinusitis
C) Habitual cough
D) Viral pharyngitis
E) *Mycoplasma* pneumonia

4. A mother brings her 3-year-old daughter to your office with a chief complaint of chronic cough. She tells you that the child's cough "is driving us all crazy" because it occurs intermittently throughout the night, interfering with the patient's (and everyone else's) sleep. The mother also notices the cough when the child plays at the park or runs around the yard. She has not noted any wheezing, rhinorrhea, or conjunctivitis. The physical examination is significant for a well-nourished, well-develop child with normal lung and chest findings. The chest radiograph demonstrates no abnormalities. Which of the following conditions is most likely to be the cause of this patient's chronic cough?

A) Foreign body aspiration
B) Allergic rhinitis
C) Habitual cough
D) Asthma
E) Cystic fibrosis

5. A 24-month-old Caucasian patient is brought to your office by his foster mother with a chief complaint of chronic cough. The child has no documented past medical history except an immunization record that documents that he has received his 2-, 4-, and 6-month vaccinations. The foster mother noticed the cough on the day the boy was placed in her home, and it has continued for the past month. The child coughs frequently while in the office but does not seem bothered by his symptoms. His height is at the 25th percentile, and his weight is at the 10th percentile. The chest examination is remarkable for generalized faint crackles that partially clear with coughing. Which of the following are appropriate initial screening tests for this child's chronic cough?

A) Venous blood gas, posteroanterior and lateral chest radiographs
B) Sweat testing, HIV testing
C) Posteroanterior and lateral chest radiographs, spirometry
D) Posteroanterior and lateral chest radiographs, sweat testing, spirometry
E) Posteroanterior and lateral chest radiographs, sweat testing

6. A 12-month-old male born at 28 weeks of gestation is in an intensive occupational therapy feeding program to address his oromotor dysfunction and aversion to oral feeding. He has a tracheostomy due to postintubation subglottic stenosis and requires oxygen only at night. He will tolerate oral stimulation and food placed in his mouth but immediately begins to choke when swallowing is induced. Which of the following statements regarding this patient's feeding difficulties is FALSE?

A) The presence of the tracheostomy makes aspiration with swallowing highly unlikely.
B) The choking and discomfort associated with gastroesophageal reflux usually occurs after, rather than during, a feeding.
C) Foreign body aspiration is an unlikely cause of this patient's feeding symptoms.
D) Increasing the amount of oral feeds may increase this patient's risk of recurrent pneumonia.
E) Tracheoesophageal fistula is part of the differential diagnosis for this patient.

7. An 18-month-old previously healthy boy suddenly begins to gag, choke, and forcefully cough at his sitter's house. By the time the parents arrive, the child has recovered but is irritable. There is no recent history of fever, rash, rhinorrhea, or cough, and no one else in the family is sick. In the emergency department, vital signs are unremarkable beyond a respiratory rate of 36 breaths per minute; lung auscultation is significant for faint right-sided expiratory wheezing, and inspiratory and expiratory films (though difficult to obtain) are read as negative. Which of the following is the most appropriate next step in the management of this patient?

A) Controlled intubation in the operating room, with subsequent transfer to the intensive care unit
B) Bronchoscopy in the operating room
C) Observation for 4 to 6 hours in the emergency room
D) Admission to the hospital overnight, with repeat chest radiographs 12 and 24 hours after the initial incident
E) Aerosolized bronchodilator therapy and systemic corticosteroids

8. A 3-year-old boy previously well until hospitalized 6 weeks ago for right middle lobe pneumonia is brought to the emergency department by his parents for a high fever and difficulty breathing. Based on the history and physical examination, you suspect the child has pneumonia again and order a chest radiograph, which is consistent with right middle lobe pneumonia. In questioning the parents further, you discover that the patient has been afebrile since the first episode of pneumonia but continues to cough off and on during the day and night. Which of the following conditions is most likely to be the cause of this child's recurrent pneumonia?

A) Congenital cardiac disease
B) Immunodeficiency syndrome
C) Foreign body aspiration
D) Hypoplastic lung
E) Cystic adenomatoid malformation

9. A 2-month-old former full-term infant presents to your office with a fourth episode of wheezing. His mother states that she believes he has been wheezing "off and on" since the first week of life. The wheezing is exacerbated by crying. The infant is afebrile and has a respiratory rate of 56 breaths per minute. He has full expiratory wheezes that are more pronounced on the right. Beta-agonist therapy does not result in complete resolution of the wheezing. Which of the following is the most likely cause of this child's recurrent wheezing?

A) Gastroesophageal reflux
B) Bronchogenic cyst
C) Cystic fibrosis
D) Congenital structural anomaly
E) Reactive airway disease

10. A 10-year-old obese child with asthma is brought to the emergency room in respiratory distress. His initial pulse oximetry reading is 90%. The physical examination is significant for diffuse inspiratory and expiratory wheezing and moderate accessory muscle use. He also has dental malocclusion, an elongated lower face, and a narrowed arch in the roof of the mouth. He is treated with supplemental oxygen, aerosolized bronchodilators, and systemic corticosteroids. His oxygen saturation improves to 98%, but he becomes progressively more

lethargic. Which of the following is the most likely cause of this patient's changing level of consciousness?
A) Undiagnosed underlying cardiac defect
B) Ventilation-perfusion mismatch
C) Increased intracranial pressure
D) Fatigue
E) Hypoventilation due to decreased respiratory drive

11. Which of the following arterial blood gas measurements is most consistent with acute respiratory compromise superimposed on chronic respiratory failure?
A) pH 7.28; $PaCO_2$ 70 mm Hg; PaO_2 50 mm Hg; HCO_3^- 34 mEq per L
B) pH 7.24; $PaCO_2$ 60 mm Hg; PaO_2 50 mm Hg; HCO_3^- 24 mEq per L
C) pH 7.35; $PaCO_2$ 60 mm Hg; PaO_2 50 mm Hg; HCO_3^- 34 mEq per L
D) pH 7.24; $PaCO_2$ 70 mm Hg; PaO_2 90 mm Hg; HCO_3^- 34 mEq per L
E) pH 7.40; $PaCO_2$ 40 mm Hg; PaO_2 98 mm Hg; HCO_3^- 24 mEq per L

12. An 18-month-old boy is brought to the emergency department following closed head trauma due to a fall from a second story window. A Glasgow Coma Scale score of 7 results in intubation in the emergency room. The patient has symmetric chest rise and good breath sounds bilaterally. He continues to undergo bag-valve mask ventilation in preparation for transport to the intensive care unit, with oxygen saturation of 96%. However, within several minutes, he becomes agitated and flushed, and his heart rate increases to 155 beats per minute. Which of the following conditions is the most likely cause of this child's clinical signs following intubation?
A) Migration of the endotracheal tube into the right mainstem bronchus
B) Carbon dioxide retention (hypercapnia)
C) Pneumothorax
D) Hypoxia
E) Pericardial tamponade

13. A mother brings her 11-year-old daughter to your office because the girl has developed exercise intolerance over the past few months. The girl tells you that she begins wheezing within a minute or two of beginning exercise in physical education class; this has been confirmed by the instructor. The wheezing gradually resolves upon rest. She has had no palpitations, light-headedness, or syncope. There is no change in appetite, no fatigue, and no constitutional symptoms. She is doing well academically and socially. There is no past medical or family history of asthma. The physical examination is remarkable for a well-nourished, well-developed female with Tanner SMR stage 2 breast development. Chest, lung, and cardiac examinations are within normal limits. You prescribe two puffs of an albuterol inhaler prior to exercise, which does not result in improvement of the child's symptoms. Which of the following is the most appropriate next step with regard to this girl's exercise intolerance?
A) Prohibit any further exercise and refer to a pediatric cardiologist.
B) Obtain an electrocardiogram.
C) Schedule pulmonary function testing during exercise challenge.
D) Obtain an echocardiogram.
E) Encourage physical workouts with a trainer, with gradually increasing intensity.

14. An infant born as a result of an uncomplicated vaginal delivery at 36$\frac{4}{7}$ weeks of gestation develops recurrent apnea associated with cyanosis on the first day of life. He responds to vigorous stimulation. Which of the following factors does not increase the likelihood that his apnea is due to an underlying pathologic condition?
A) Associated cyanosis
B) Presentation on the first day of life
C) Multiple apneic episodes
D) Initiation of breathing with vigorous stimulation
E) Patient age

15. A 3-day-old infant born at 33 weeks of gestation is one of triplets. She has an apneic episode lasting 18 seconds associated with bradycardia. Initial radiologic and laboratory results are negative for infection and cardiac and pulmonary abnormalities. The physical examination is normal. You decide this patient's apnea is most likely due to apnea of prematurity. In discussing this condition with the girl's parents, you are correct in telling them each of the following EXCEPT:
A) Apnea of prematurity is thought to be due to immaturity of respiratory centers in the brain.
B) Treatment with caffeine usually reduces the number of apneic episodes due to apnea of prematurity.
C) Apnea of prematurity typically resolves when the patient reaches a postconceptual age of 37 weeks.
D) Apnea of prematurity does not increase the risk of death due to sudden infant death syndrome (SIDS).
E) Apnea of prematurity presents any time during the first week of life.

16. A 5-week-old infant born at 27 weeks of gestation has two episodes of apnea in 12 hours. Both respond to stimulation. In reviewing the patient's chart, you note that her weight gain has slowed over the past week, and her heart and respiratory rates are trending up for the past 4 days despite pulse oximetry measurements in excess of 94%. On physical examination, the infant appears pale, but no other abnormalities are noted. Which of the following potential causes of apnea is most consistent with this patient's clinical picture?

A) Anemia of prematurity
B) Apnea of prematurity
C) Periodic breathing
D) Sepsis
E) Joubert syndrome

17. After witnessing two unsuccessful attempts to obtain an arterial sample for blood gas measurement, a medical student working with you asks why arterial sampling is preferable to capillary blood gas measurement. You are correct in telling him all of the following EXCEPT:
A) Arterial blood gas measurement is the most direct, reliable, and objective method of assessing the adequacy of oxygenation.
B) Capillary samples are not useful for approximating arterial pH and partial pressure of carbon dioxide.
C) Capillary blood gas measurement is unreliable in patients with vasoconstriction.
D) Capillary blood gas measurement is unreliable in patients with hypothermia.
E) Capillary blood gas measurement is unreliable in patients with poor perfusion.

18. You are lecturing a group of residents about different forms of pulmonary function testing. In regard to spirometry, you are correct in telling them all of the following EXCEPT:
A) Spirometry measures air volumes and rates of flow.
B) Spirometry can be used to differentiate obstructive pulmonary disease from restrictive pulmonary disease.
C) Values obtained through spirometry testing can be used to calculate total lung volume and functional residual capacity.
D) Periodic spirometry testing in asthmatic patients provides an objective measure of the effectiveness of treatment.
E) Spirometry does not provide information about diffusion capacity.

19. A 15-year-old female with known asthma presents to the emergency department in obvious respiratory distress. Her vital signs are as follows: temperature, 37.0°C; heart rate, 130 beats per minute; and respiratory rate, 42 breaths per minute. Her pulse oximetry reading is 94%. The physical examination is significant for diffuse bilateral inspiratory and expiratory wheezing and retractions. She receives multiple aerosolized bronchodilator treatments and intravenous solumedrol. Within 40 minutes of her arrival, she feels much improved. Her respiratory rate has decreased to 25 breaths per minute, and she has decreased work of breathing. Pulse oximetry measures 91% without supplemental oxygen. Which of the following is the most likely cause of this patient's drop in arterial hemoglobin saturation?

A) Respiratory fatigue
B) Respiratory failure
C) Pneumonia
D) Ventilation-perfusion mismatch
E) Pneumothorax

20. Which of the following pairings of conditions and radiographic signs is incorrect?
A) Vascular ring—esophageal indentation on barium swallow
B) Bacterial tracheitis—ragged tracheal air column on plain neck/chest radiograph
C) Epiglottitis—thumb sign on lateral neck radiograph
D) Acute laryngotracheobronchitis—steeple sign on plain neck/chest radiograph
E) Bronchiectasis—hyperinflation and air-fluid levels

21. A father brings his 7-year-old son to the emergency department for high fevers and difficulty breathing. The child was well until he woke up this morning with fever and a sore throat. He has refused to eat anything due to the pain. Throughout the day, he has had increasing difficulty breathing. Vital signs are as follows: temperature, 40°C; heart rate, 140 beats per minute; and respiratory rate, 38 breaths per minute. Physical examination reveals a toxic-appearing well-nourished male in obvious respiratory distress, sitting upright and drooling with his lower jaw thrust forward. Which of the following is the most appropriate next course of action in this patient?
A) Immediate transfer to the operating room for controlled intubation
B) Immediate rapid-induction intubation in the emergency room
C) Portable lateral neck radiograph to assess for a "thumb" sign
D) Admission to the intensive care unit for intravenous ampicillin-sulbactam and possible intubation
E) Supplemental oxygen, intramuscular solumedrol, and aerosolized epinephrine

22. A mother brings her 6-month-old infant to your office because he consistently chokes and gags with solid feeds. He has always been a slow bottle feeder, which is frustrating to the mother, but he cannot seem to tolerate solid feedings. He has had three episodes of wheezing with upper respiratory infections; the wheezing was minimally responsive to bronchodilator therapy. A chest radiograph demonstrates subtle tracheal deviation. You suspect compression of the trachea and esophagus, possibly due to a vascular ring. Which of the following studies will provide the most definitive diagnostic information?
A) Barium swallow
B) High-resolution computed tomography of the chest with contrast
C) Echocardiography

D) Bronchoscopy
E) Arteriography

23. A 7-day-old infant is brought to your office for her 1-week check-up by her parents. You note that the patient has a weak, hoarse-sounding cry and noisy inspiratory breathing. Her parents tell you that she always sounds this way, although her breathing is worse during feedings. They have not noted any color changes such as pallor or duskiness. The infant's respiratory rate is within normal limits, and she appears comfortable, with no retractions or flaring. Her noisy breathing does not change with changes in positioning (supine vs. prone). Which of the following is the most likely cause of this patient's noisy breathing?
A) Laryngomalacia
B) Bilateral vocal cord paralysis
C) Unilateral vocal cord paralysis
D) Tracheomalacia
E) Acquired vocal cord dysfunction

24. A 14-year-old female tennis player with no significant past medical history is brought to your office by her mother for a chief complaint of exercise intolerance. She was diagnosed with exercise-induced asthma 3 weeks ago at an urgent care center. However, correct use of a metered-dose inhaler has not resulted in improvement in her symptoms. She complains of wheezing within minutes of beginning sprints for tennis practice, although now she is so afraid of having difficulty breathing that she begins to wheeze and feel short of breath while changing for practice. She is asymptomatic at other times and has no complaints of weight loss, palpitations, lightheadedness, syncope, or fatigue. The physical examination is significant for a well-nourished, well-developed female with normal lung and cardiac findings. Which of the following conditions is the most likely cause of this patient's exercise intolerance?
A) Exercise-induced asthma
B) Moderate persistent asthma
C) Anxiety attacks
D) Vocal cord dysfunction
E) Vocal cord paralysis

25. A woman brings her 4-month-old grandson to your clinic for evaluation of his "noisy breathing." The child's parents are on vacation in another part of the country. The grandmother is concerned because, although the child always has noisy breathing, it seems worse to her now that he also has a cold. In reviewing the patient's chart, you note that your partner diagnosed the infant with laryngomalacia at his 2-month health maintenance visit based on history and physical examination alone. Today, the physical examination is significant for a well-nourished, well-developed infant with clear rhinorrhea and inspiratory stridor. Vital signs, including the respiratory rate, are stable and within normal limits, and the patient's oxygen saturation is 96% to 97%. The lungs are clear, and there is no evidence of accessory muscle use. The stridor disappears when the patient is placed in the prone position. The remainder of the examination is unremarkable. Which of the following conditions is the most likely cause of this patient's stridor?
A) Vascular ring
B) Asthma
C) Allergic rhinitis
D) Tracheomalacia
E) Laryngomalacia

26. A 6-month-old infant with a clinical diagnosis of laryngomalacia presents to your office for her routine health maintenance visit. Her mother reports that she has been taking longer and longer to bottle feed. In the past 2 months, her weight percentile has fallen from the 25th to the 10th percentile, and her length percentile has minimally declined. The physical examination is unchanged from previous visits. Which of the following is the most appropriate next step in the management of this patient?
A) Refer the patient to a pediatric otolaryngologist for direct laryngoscopic visualization of the airway.
B) Increase the caloric density of the formula, begin supplementing with pureed foods, and recheck weight in 1 week.
C) Order a barium swallow study.
D) Obtain anteroposterior and lateral neck and chest radiographs.
E) Thicken feeds with cereal twice daily and recheck weight in 1 week.

27. A 7-year-old boy with no significant past medical history is brought to the emergency department with wheezing and respiratory distress. He was well until 3 days ago, when he began coughing and developed a fever. The cough and fever have consistently worsened since that time. When the child woke about an hour ago, his cough was paroxysmal and productive, and he had trouble breathing. Vital signs in the emergency department include: temperature, 40°C; heart rate, 120 beats per minute; respiratory rate, 36 breaths per minute; and a pulse oximetry reading of 93%. The physical examination is significant for a well-nourished, well-developed male lying on his side on the gurney in obvious respiratory distress, with marked accessory muscle use. Diffuse wheezes are appreciated on expiration. Which of the following conditions is the most likely cause of this patient's respiratory distress?
A) Epiglottitis
B) Bacterial tracheitis
C) Asthma exacerbation
D) Bronchial pneumonia
E) Foreign body aspiration

28. Which of the following clinical findings is the most sensitive and specific for pneumonia in children under 2 years of age?
A) Generalized rales
B) Cough
C) Tachypnea
D) Fever
E) Tachycardia

29. A mother brings her 3-year-old daughter to the office for evaluation of her high fever. The girl was well until 3 days ago, when she developed a cough. Yesterday, her temperature climbed to 38.5°C, and she had trouble eating and finding a comfortable position. Her vital signs in the office are as follows: temperature, 39.5°C; heart rate, 115 beats per minute; respiratory rate, 42 breaths per minute; and pulse oximetry reading of 95%. Crackles and decreased breath sounds are appreciated at the right lung base. A chest radiograph is consistent with a consolidated lobar infiltrate. Which of the following pathogens is most likely to be responsible for this child's pneumonia?
A) Adenovirus
B) *Staphylococcus aureus*
C) *Haemophilus influenzae*
D) *Streptococcus pneumoniae*
E) *Moraxella catarrhalis*

30. A 12-year-old boy with Duchenne muscular dystrophy develops bacterial pneumonia and is hospitalized for intravenous antibiotic therapy and supportive care. Which of the following antimicrobial choices is most appropriate for empiric treatment in this patient?
A) Ampicillin-sulbactam
B) Cefotaxime
C) Cefuroxime
D) Vancomycin
E) Piperacillin-tazobactam

31. You are lecturing to a group of medical residents about the importance of determining the causative organism in cases of bacterial pneumonia. You would be correct in telling them all of the following EXCEPT:
A) Sputum cultures should be obtained from all patients 2 years of age or older if possible.
B) Infants younger than 90 days of age with suspected bacterial pneumonia should receive blood, urine, and cerebrospinal fluid cultures.
C) A sputum sample is appropriate for analysis if there are <25 squamous epithelial cells and >25 leukocytes per low-power field.
D) The workup of suspected bacterial pneumonia in an 18-month-old child includes a complete blood count, blood culture, and chest radiographs.
E) Pleural fluid gathered via thoracentesis for a symptomatic effusion should routinely be sent for culture.

32. You are lecturing a group of medical student about acute respiratory distress syndrome (ARDS) in children. You are correct in telling them which of the following?
A) Children with a prior episode of ARDS are at increased risk for the development of asthma.
B) Children with a prior episode of ARDS are at increased risk for the development of pulmonary fibrosis.
C) Children with a prior episode of ARDS are at increased risk for the development of bronchiectasis.
D) Children with a prior episode of ARDS are at increased risk for the development of emphysema.
E) There are no long-term sequelae associated with the diagnosis of ARDS.

33. A 13-year-old male who is determined to hold his breath longer than his brother is unconscious when he is pulled from the pool by his father. He responds to rescue breathing and within 45 seconds is conscious and breathing on his own. His father estimates that he was under water for a maximum of 2 minutes. The boy's physical examination, pulse oximetry reading, and chest radiographs are all unremarkable. Which of the following statements regarding further management of this child is true?
A) The boy may be discharged home with follow-up in his pediatrician's office tomorrow.
B) The boy may be discharged home and observed by his parents for the next 6 to 8 hours.
C) The boy should be admitted to the hospital for close observation and supportive care as needed.
D) The boy should be observed in the emergency room for 6 to 8 hours and allowed to go home if his physical examination and pulse oximetry readings remain normal.
E) The boy should be admitted to the hospital for further evaluation to rule out any underlying cardiac arrhythmia and ascertain the degree of neurologic compromise resulting from his near drowning.

34. An 8-year-old boy was walking on the frozen pond beside his house with a friend when he fell into the water. He was immersed for an estimated 5 minutes before his father was able to locate him and pull him up. Cardiopulmonary resuscitation was initiated at the scene. When paramedics arrived, the child had spontaneous pulse and respirations. In the emergency room, he is awake, lethargic, and shivering. Vital signs are as follows: rectal temperature, 34°C; heart rate, 70 beats per minute; respiratory rate, 17 breaths per minute; blood pressure, 90/60 mm Hg; and pulse oxygenation of 95% on 2 L of flow via face mask. His pupils are slightly dilated and sluggish, and deep tendon reflexes are diminished in the extremities. The cardiac monitor displays a regular rhythm with narrow QRS complexes. Which of the following is the most appropriate management of this patient's hypothermia?

A) Passive rewarming using heavy blankets
B) External rewarming using electric blankets
C) External rewarming via immersion in warm water
D) External rewarming limited to the head and trunk
E) Core rewarming via peritoneal lavage

35. Patients with cystic fibrosis are at risk for deficiencies in all of the following vitamins EXCEPT:
A) Vitamin A
B) Vitamin D
C) Vitamin E
D) Vitamin K
E) Vitamin B_6

36. A mother brings her 9-month-old daughter to your clinic for her routine health maintenance visit. The girl is a former full-term infant with an unremarkable perinatal course. Since her 6-month visit, the child's weight percentile has declined from the 50th to the 10th percentile, and her length percentile has declined from the 50th to the 25th percentile. Her mother is concerned about her child's frequent stools, which she describes as "greasy, pale like oatmeal, with a horrible smell." The mother is convinced that the change in the character of her daughter's stools is related to starting baby food at age 6 months. On physical examination, the patient is thin and irritable; no other abnormalities are noted. Which of the following is the most likely cause of this child's poor growth?
A) Pancreatic insufficiency
B) Congenital infection
C) Metabolic disease
D) Intractable diarrhea of infancy
E) Hereditary fructose intolerance

37. A father brings his 3-year-old son to your office with "another sinus infection." In reviewing the patient's chart, you note that he has had four sinus infections requiring treatment with antibiotics in the past 6 months. Today, the boy's temperature is 38.5°C. The physical examination is significant for copious purulent rhinorrhea, clear lung fields bilaterally, and displacement of the cardiac point of maximal impulse to the right. Which of the following conditions is the most likely cause of this child's recurrent sinusitis?
A) Cystic fibrosis
B) Primary ciliary dyskinesia
C) X-linked agammaglobulinemia
D) Chronic granulomatous disease
E) Common variable immunodeficiency

38. A 9-year-old boy with chest pain and fever is brought to your office by his mother. He was well until 3 days ago, when he developed a fever to 39°C and a cough. Two days ago, your partner diagnosed him with right-sided bacterial pneumonia based on history and physical examination and prescribed amoxicillin-clavulanic acid. The fever has not diminished, and last night, the child began complaining that the right side of his chest hurt. In the office, he is febrile and tachypneic to 36 breaths per minute, with a pulse oximetry reading of 95%. His chest examination is significant for dullness to percussion on the right, with diminished breath sounds and decreased vocal fremitus. Plain chest radiographs in the upright and lateral decubitus positions reveal free-flowing fluid in the pleural space. Which of the following is the most appropriate management of this patient?
A) Hospitalization for intravenous cefuroxime and clindamycin and drainage of the fluid via thoracentesis
B) Hospitalization for intravenous cefuroxime and clindamycin and thoracentesis every 12 hours until the fluid does not reaccumulate
C) Hospitalization for intravenous cefuroxime and clindamycin and placement of a chest tube for ongoing drainage
D) Hospitalization for intravenous cefuroxime and clindamycin and placement of a chest tube for ongoing drainage if the patient experiences respiratory decompensation
E) Hospitalization for intravenous cefuroxime and clindamycin and placement of a chest tube for ongoing drainage if fluid from an initial thoracentesis has a pH <7.4

39. A 5-year-old girl arrives at the emergency department via ambulance following a motor vehicle crash. She is awake and alert and complaining of pain on the right side of her chest. Vitals are as follows: temperature, 37°C; heart rate, 100 beats per minute; respiratory rate, 40 breaths per minute; and pulse oximetry of 95%. The chest examination is significant for dullness to percussion on the right, with diminished breath sounds and decreased vocal fremitus. Chest radiographs are consistent with pleural effusion. Fluid obtained during thoracentesis is pearly white. Which of the following is the most likely cause of this child's effusion?
A) Pericardial tamponade
B) Complicated parapneumonic effusion
C) Renal contusion
D) Disruption of the thoracic duct
E) Pneumomediastinum

40. A 15-year-old girl is intubated in the emergency department following narcotic overdose. Oxygenation initially improves with bag-valve mask ventilation, and breath sounds are appreciated bilaterally. Approximately 10 minutes later, her oxygen saturation precipitously falls. Removal of the endotracheal tube and ventilation via mask does not improve her respiratory status. Which of the following conditions is most likely responsible for her acute respiratory decompensation?

A) Obstruction of the endotracheal tube
B) Equipment failure
C) Displacement of the endotracheal tube into the right mainstem bronchus
D) Pneumomediastinum
E) Pneumothorax

41. The mother of a 12-year-old boy who is in your office for his routine health maintenance visit tells you that she is worried about how his chest deformity is affecting his health. When questioned, it is clear that the boy is embarrassed by his moderate pectus excavatum. You are correct in telling the boy and his mother all of the following EXCEPT:
A) Pectus excavatum is associated with exercise intolerance.
B) Pectus excavatum does not impair one's ability to generate an adequate cough.
C) Pectus excavatum is more common in patients with Marfan syndrome.
D) Pectus excavatum can be surgically altered for cosmetic purposes.
E) The murmur commonly associated with pectus excavatum is not due to valvular insufficiency.

42. A mother brings her 12-year-old daughter with Down syndrome to your office because the girl seems to be more fatigued and less active over the past several weeks. Vital signs are within normal range today. The physical examination is significant for an overweight female with obvious stigmata of Down syndrome, jugular venous distension, a prominent precordial impulse, single loud second heart sound, and hepatomegaly. She has pitting edema of her lower extremities. You note in her chart that an initial echocardiogram in the neonatal period demonstrated normal cardiac anatomy and function. Which of the following is most consistent with this child's clinical picture?
A) Left-sided heart failure
B) Cor pulmonale
C) Progressive neuromuscular disease
D) Undiagnosed congenital heart disease
E) Hypertrophic cardiomyopathy

43. A 5-year-old patient with Crouzon syndrome is diagnosed with obstructive sleep apnea (>5 apneic events per hour on polysomnography). Which of the following is most appropriate for initial intervention in this patient?
A) Removal of the tonsils and adenoids
B) Tracheostomy placement
C) Continuous positive airway pressure
D) Supplemental oxygen at night
E) Echocardiography

44. A 7-year-old boy with no significant past medical history has enlarged tonsils on physical examination and hypertrophied adenoids on a plain film of the lateral neck. His parents bring you a videotape of the child taken while he is sleeping. The 15-minute segment shows loud snoring interspaced with four episodes of extended silence followed by choking and gasping. Which of the following is the most appropriate next step in the management of this patient?
A) Schedule the patient for polysomnography.
B) Arrange for the patient to have overnight pulse oximetry monitoring.
C) Advise against supine or side positioning for sleeping.
D) Obtain a referral for surgical removal of tonsils/adenoids.
E) Nasal continuous positive airway pressure at night

45. All of the following are considered risk factors for sudden infant death syndrome EXCEPT:
A) male gender
B) low birth weight
C) prematurity
D) maternal smoking during pregnancy
E) apnea of prematurity

46. You are lecturing a group of medical students about sudden infant death syndrome (SIDS) and apparent life-threatening event (ALTE). You are correct in telling them which of the following?
A) A history of ALTE does not increase an infant's risk of SIDS.
B) All infants with a reliable history of ALTE should be sent home with apnea/bradycardia monitors.
C) Periodic breathing is a risk factor for ALTE.
D) Infants with ALTE who have normal past medical histories and physical examinations may be discharged home from the emergency department once follow-up has been arranged.
E) The incidence of SIDS peaks at 6 months of age.

47. Which of the following factors is associated with the best prognosis for return to normal neurologic functioning in a young child who is the victim of a near drowning?
A) Presence of coma for <12 hours following resuscitation
B) Palpable pulses at the scene
C) Close proximity of a tertiary care center
D) Near drowning in cold rather than warm water
E) Aspiration of minimal fluid

48. A 16-year-old who was an unrestrained front-seat passenger in a car involved in a side-impact collision is noted to have paradoxic movement of the right side of the chest at the scene. There was no loss of consciousness

or trauma to the head, and the patient is awake and alert but in pain. Which of the following is indicated in this patient during transport to the emergency department?

A) Needle decompression of the right pleural space
B) Needle evacuation of the right pleural space
C) Placement of the patient with the right side down and administration of oxygen
D) Bag-mask ventilation with the patient in the "sniffing" position
E) Binding of the chest with an elastic bandage to limit chest wall movement

ANSWERS

1. A
2. B
3. C
4. D
5. E
6. A
7. B
8. C
9. D
10. E
11. A
12. B
13. C
14. D
15. E
16. A
17. B
18. C
19. D
20. E
21. A
22. B
23. C
24. D
25. E
26. A
27. B
28. C
29. D
30. E
31. A
32. B
33. C
34. D
35. E
36. A
37. B
38. C
39. D
40. E
41. A
42. B
43. C
44. D
45. E
46. A
47. B
48. C

Cardiovascular Disease

14

CARDIOVASCULAR SIGNS AND SYMPTOMS

Chest Pain

Chest pain in healthy children is rarely due to cardiovascular disease; musculoskeletal, respiratory, and gastrointestinal conditions are much more common (Table 14-1). Cardiovascular pain complexes include:

- pericardial pain—results from inflammation of the pericardium; typically sharp, substernal, positional (improved upon sitting up and/or leaning forward, worse when lying down); may be severe; often accompanied by fever or laboratory evidence of inflammation
- angina/ischemia—rare in children; most common in patients with congenital or acquired anomalies of the coronary arteries; described as pressure or burning sensation; may radiate to the neck, shoulder, or arm; typically occurs during activity and improves with rest; may be a symptom of coronary vasospasm in patients who use cocaine or methylenedioxymethamphetamine [MDMA (Ecstasy)]
- acute aortic dissection—severe sharp anterior chest or back pain; suggested by patient or family history of Marfan or Ehlers-Danlos syndrome.

Findings on history and physical examination that warrant further evaluation for a cardiovascular etiology are included in Table 14-2. Pain that is brief, sharp, and transient, or pain that increases with inspiration, is more likely to be musculoskeletal or pulmonary in origin. If the physical examination is normal and the history suggests a noncardiac cause, reassurance and follow-up constitute the most appropriate management. Screening studies for chest pain with worrisome characteristics include chest radiograph (CXR), electrocardiogram (ECG), echocardiogram (ECHO), and serum troponin and acute-phase reactant levels.

Syncope

Syncope is the sudden, temporary loss of consciousness and postural tone resulting from transient and reversible generalized cerebral ischemia. The primary objective of the physician is determination of whether the fainting is due to benign or potentially life-threatening conditions. Neurocardiogenic (vasovagal, neurally-mediated) syncope is by far the most common cause of syncope in older children and adolescents. Fainting is brought on by sudden standing or standing for long periods of time, emotional stress, or the sight of blood or other viscerally-noxious stimuli. The syncopal event is often preceded by light-headedness, dizziness, sweating, weakness, nausea, pallor, clamminess, confusion, and/or altered visual or acoustic perception. Symptoms resolve completely when the patient lies down. When it occurs, the loss of consciousness is short-lived (seconds-to-minutes in duration), with the patient returning to normal mental status almost immediately. Neurocardiogenic syncope is not associated with sudden cardiac death; if the syncope is recurrent, salt tablets and fluid therapy may be beneficial. Other noncardiogenic disorders that may present with syncope include hyperventilation, anxiety attacks, hypoglycemia, anemia, breath-holding spells, seizures, and malingering.

Although syncope is rarely associated with significant disease, life-threatening conditions known to cause sudden cardiac death may initially present with syncope (prolonged QT syndrome, hypertrophic cardiomyopathy, congenital or acquired coronary artery abnormalities, aortic or pulmonic stenosis, cardiac structural defects, second- or third-degree heart block, supraventricular tachycardia, ventricular tachycardia or fibrillation). Factors that suggest a possible cardiovascular mechanism for syncope include:

- family history—sudden cardiac death, arrhythmias, myocardial disease, Marfan syndrome, deafness (Jervell/Lange-Nielsen syndrome of prolonged QT syndrome associated with deafness)
- past medical history—Kawasaki disease, Marfan or Turner syndromes
- history of present illness—exercise-induced syncope, palpitations

An ECG is indicated for *any* patient who presents with a syncopal episode. Cardiology consultation is recommended when the syncope is atypical for vasovagal syncope and/or when an arrhythmia is identified on ECG. Additional assessment may include any of the following: ECHO, exercise stress testing, 24-hour Holter monitoring, electroencephalogram (EEG) or computed tomography (CT) of the brain. Tilt table testing is reserved for definitive diagnosis of neurocardiogenic syncope in the patient

TABLE 14-1
DIFFERENTIAL DIAGNOSIS OF PEDIATRIC CHEST PAIN

Musculoskeletal—Pain is typically sharp, superficial, sternal or parasternal; pain is present at rest and exacerbated by deep inspiration.

Examples:
Chest wall strain
Trauma
Costochondritis
Precordial catch syndrome (acute onset of sharp, left-sided pleuritic chest pain lasting several seconds)

Respiratory—Sharp peripheral or posterior chest pain localized to the area of underlying lung or pleural pathology; often accompanied by tachypnea or other respiratory manifestations.

Examples:
Asthma
Exercise-induced bronchospasm
Chronic cough
Pleurodynia
Pneumonia
Pleural effusion
Empyema
Bronchitis
Pneumothorax
Pneumomediastinum
Pleural effusion
Pulmonary embolism

Gastrointestinal—Deep, often burning pain in substernal or medial lower chest area; timing may be associated with eating.

Examples:
Gastritis
Esophagitis
Gastroesophageal reflux

Psychogenic—Often inconsistent with typical pain/symptom complexes.

Examples:
Anxiety attacks
Fictitious

Hematologic

Example:
Sickle cell crisis

Idiopathic

Cardiac

Examples:
Hypertrophic cardiomyopathy
Pericarditis
Pericardial effusion
Pneumopericardium
Coronary artery insufficiency or arteritis
Myocardial ischemia or infarction
Myocarditis
Dissecting aortic aneurysm

TABLE 14-2
FINDINGS SUGGESTIVE OF CARDIAC PATHOLOGY IN PATIENTS WITH CHEST PAIN

Family History
Hypertrophic cardiomyopathy
Arrhythmias
Marfan or Turner syndrome
Sudden premature cardiac death (prior to the age of 40 years)

Past Medical History
Kawasaki disease
Congenital heart disease
Acute rheumatic fever

History of Present Illness
Pain radiating to the back, neck, shoulders, or left arm*
Pain that is frequent or constant, dull, or pressure-like*
Squeezing or visceral chest discomfort*
Exertional chest pain*
Exertional syncope*
Exercise intolerance
Pain-associated syncope*
Dyspnea*
Sense of impending doom*

Physical Examination
Tachypnea
Pathologic murmur*
Increased precordial activity*
Abnormal second heart sound*
Gallop rhythm*
Pericardial friction rub*

Laboratory Assessment
Diminished oxygen saturation with or without pain

*Presence of this sign or symptom warrants urgent cardiology referral and complete restriction of all exertional activity until a thorough cardiovascular investigation is completed.

with recurrent syncope, a questionable history, and normal ECG results.

Athletes who faint during exercise are prohibited from engaging in practice or competition until a full cardiovascular investigation has been completed.

Palpitations

Heart palpitations may be benign (sinus tachycardia) or related to underlying arrhythmias (atrial fibrillation, ventricular tachycardia). CXR and ECG are indicated for patients who report palpitations; further assessment is guided by the results of history, physical examination, and screening tests. Additional studies to consider include ECHO, 24-hour Holter monitoring, and exercise stress testing. A history of palpitations necessitates a thorough evaluation to rule out arrhythmias prior to athletic participation.

Murmur

Heart murmur is a frequent finding in the pediatric population; as such, perhaps no other cardiac sign results in more parental anxiety and diagnostic uncertainty for the clinician.

Murmurs result from turbulent blood flow. They are characterized based on the following:

- Intensity (loudness) of the murmur (graded on a scale of 1 through 6)
- Timing of the murmur (systolic, diastolic, continuous, ejection)
- Location of the murmur or its greatest intensity
- Radiation of the murmur
- Pitch of the murmur

Recognition of an innocent heart murmur (noisy flow through a structurally normal heart) can save the patient's family needless worry. Innocent murmurs typically:

- are relatively quiet (1-2/6)
- decrease in intensity when the patient moves from the supine to the upright position
- occur during systole
- are located over the left sternal border
- radiate to the upper left or right sternal areas
- are low-pitched, vibratory

Innocent murmurs are often initially heard when the patient is febrile or anemic. The characteristics of several innocent murmurs are provided in Table 14-3. No further evaluation is indicated for a heart murmur consistent with a known innocent murmur in a patient with a negative history and normal findings on physical examination. Several murmurs associated with underlying cardiovascular pathology are described in Table 14-4. Isolated diastolic murmurs are always pathologic.

Congestive Heart Failure

Congestive heart failure (CHF) is the final common pathway resulting when the heart becomes unable to meet perfusion requirements necessary for normal metabolic

TABLE 14-3
INNOCENT HEART MURMURS

Still's murmur—mid-systolic $2^{3}/_{6}$ low-pitch vibratory murmur heard best at the left lower sternal border; loudest in the supine position; age range 3 years to adolescent

Pulmonary flow murmur—medium-to-high-pitch $^{2}/_{6}$ systolic ejection murmur located at the left upper sternal border; age range 8 to 14 years

Peripheral pulmonic stenosis—high-frequency murmur heard throughout the precordium and loudest in the periphery (axillae); radiates to the back; age range birth to 6 months (pathologic in older infants and children)

Venous hum—continuous, low-pitch murmur best heard just above the right clavicle with radiation into the neck; disappears when pressure is placed on the ipsilateral internal jugular vein

TABLE 14-4
MURMURS ASSOCIATED WITH CARDIOVASCULAR PATHOLOGY

Aortic stenosis—harsh systolic murmur located at the right upper sternal border which may be accompanied by a systolic click

Aortic regurgitation—early diastolic decrescendo murmur, which is loudest when the patient is leaning forward in the sitting position

Mitral stenosis—a diastolic murmur located in the left axilla

Mitral regurgitation—apical, holosystolic murmur of mid-grade intensity radiating to the left axilla

Mitral valve prolapse—mid-to-late systolic click, which may be associated with a late-systolic, high-pitch crescendo diastolic murmur located at the cardiac apex. The click is earlier and the murmur longer with the patient standing; in the supine knee-to-chest position, the click is later and the murmur abbreviated in duration.

Tricuspid regurgitation—pansystolic murmur located at the left sternal border, which increases in intensity with inspiration; accompanied by an S_3

TABLE 14-5
CAUSES OF CONGESTIVE HEART FAILURE BY AGE

Birth
Severe tricuspid insufficiency
Severe pulmonary insufficiency
Large systemic arteriovenous fistulas

First Month of Life
Transposition of the great arteries
Patent ductus arteriosus (small, preterm infants)
Hypoplastic left heart syndrome
Total anomalous pulmonary venous return
Critical aortic stenosis
Critical pulmonic stenosis
Coarctation of the aorta (weeks 2 to 4)

One to 6 Months of Age
Endocardial cushion defects
Large ventricular septal defects
Patent ductus arteriosus

function. Congenital heart defects are the most common cause of CHF in the pediatric population. Myocardial insults that interfere with ventricular function, such as infection, inflammation, or infarction, can also lead to CHF. The diagnosis of CHF is based on clinical presentation. Signs and symptoms of progressive CHF include lethargy/sleepiness, poor feeding, poor growth or weight loss, sweating, tachypnea, tachycardia, gallop rhythm (i.e., S_3), hepatomegaly, and occasionally wheezing. Conditions which result in ventricular pressure and/or volume overload eventually lead to ventricular dilation and dysfunction and, if not reversed, inadequate tissue perfusion and cardiogenic shock (discussed below).

CHF which develops in the first few weeks of life is usually related to closure of the ductus, which typically occurs shortly after birth but may be delayed in the setting of hypoxia. Table 14-5 lists the most common congenital cardiac defects associated with the development of CHF. Due to the young infant's minimal reserves, accurate and timely diagnosis of congestive heart failure in this age group is paramount. Immediate management of patients who have CHF associated with closure of the ductus consists of continuous infusion of *prostaglandin* E_1 (PGE1). Definitive surgical repair is delayed at least until the infant's cardiovascular status stabilizes.

CHF resulting from left-to-right volume overload responds to treatment with diuretics such as furosemide. If the shunting is due to a structural defect, surgical repair is indicated when maximal pharmacologic therapy cannot support adequate growth. Digoxin may be administered in an attempt to improve myocardial contractility and ventricular function. Cardiogenic pulmonary edema which does not respond to pharmacologic intervention necessitates mechanical ventilatory support. Providing positive airway pressure, in the form of positive end airway pressure or continuous positive airway pressure, is the most effective method of improving oxygenation in patients with cardiogenic pulmonary edema.

Congenital Heart Disease

Congenital Heart Defects Associated with Known Syndromes

Congenital heart defects may arise in isolation or be part of multisystem inherited or congenital disorders (Table 14-6).

The Ductus Arteriosus and the Role of Prostaglandin E_1

The ductus arteriosus closes by the end of the first day of life in the majority of term infants, although prolonged patency is not uncommon in the setting of hypoxia. Persistence of flow through the ductus beyond a week of age is considered abnormal. Patent ductus arteriosus (PDA) is a frequent occurrence in preterm infants, with the prevalence rising as the gestational age at birth decreases. PDA increases pulmonary blood flow, leading to pulmonary edema, increased pulmonary artery pressure, left heart dilation, and episodic hypoperfusion of the cerebral and gastrointestinal systems. Clinical signs of PDA include bounding pulses, tachypnea, and a continuous "machinery" murmur best heard beneath the left clavicle. In the setting of normal platelet counts and renal function, intravenous indomethacin is the initial therapy of choice for PDA. Surgical ligation is indicated for lesions which do not resolve with medical treatment.

TABLE 14-6
SYNDROMES ASSOCIATED WITH CONGENITAL CARDIAC DEFECTS

Syndrome	Congenital Cardiac Defect
DiGeorge (22q11 deletion) syndrome	VSD, interrupted aortic arch, tetrology of Fallot, truncus arteriosus, pulmonary atresia (conotruncal defects)
Fetal alcohol syndrome	VSD, ASD
Trisomy 18	VSD with associated pulmonary and/or aortic valve defects
Trisomy 21	Endocardial cushion defects (ASD, VSD, complete AV septal defect)
Turner syndrome	Coarctation of the aorta, bicuspid aortic valve

VSD, ventricular septal defect; ASD, atrial septal defect; AV, atrioventricular.

PGE1 is a naturally-occurring vasodilator found in the body. Continuous infusion of PGE1 causes the ductus arteriosus to re-open or remain open. The widespread use of PGE1 has eliminated the need for emergency palliative therapy in many infants with congenital heart defects. In the fetus, blood flows right-to-left across the ductus due to high pulmonary vascular resistance and relatively lower systemic vascular resistance. After birth, systemic pressure exceeds pulmonary pressure, and flow across the ductus reverses to left-to-right. PGE1 is administered in the setting of lesions which require continued left-to-right shunting (pulmonary atresia) or right-to-left shunting (hypoplastic left heart syndrome, critical coarctation of the aorta, critical aortic stenosis) to support peripheral or pulmonary perfusion. PGE1 permits medical management of hypoxemia and deferment of corrective surgery until the patient is stabilized.

Cardiogenic Shock

The primary cause of cardiogenic shock in the neonate is a congenital heart lesion wherein systemic blood flow is dependent on patency of the ductus arteriosus. Three of the more common cardiac defects which predispose an infant to cardiogenic shock include critical aortic stenosis, coarctation of the aorta, and hypoplastic left heart syndrome (discussed later in this chapter). As the ductus closes, systemic perfusion drops, leading to metabolic acidosis, poor perfusion, and shock. Neonates with cardiogenic shock present with diminished peripheral pulses, prolonged capillary refill, oliguria, and lethargy. Intravenous PGE1 is instrumental in maintaining patency of the ductus and should be initiated in any neonate with suspected congenital heart disease who presents in shock.

Cyanotic Disease

Acrocyanosis is transient bluish discoloration of the distal extremities and occasionally the perioral region caused by peripheral vasoconstriction in response to cold or vasomotor instability. Acrocyanosis is a normal finding in infants up to 2 months of age; if growth remains adequate and the physical examination is reassuring, no additional evaluation is necessary. In contrast, central cyanosis involves the mucous membranes, skin, and nail beds. Cyanosis becomes clinically evident when the absolute concentration of deoxygenated hemoglobin reaches at least 3 g per dL or, in the infant with a normal hematocrit, when oxygen saturation drops below 75%. Polycythemic infants develop cyanosis at higher oxygen saturation levels, anemic infants at lower ones (if at all). Cyanosis may also be noted at higher oxygen saturations in the setting of acidosis, hypoventilation, or fever.

Cyanosis can result from cardiac defects, pulmonary disease, hematologic conditions, and metabolic abnormalities. The cardiac causes of cyanosis in the neonate are detailed in Table 14-7. Tetralogy of Fallot and transposition of the great arteries account for 3/4 of all congenital cyanotic heart disease in children. The goal of the initial evaluation of a cyanotic infant is determination of whether the cyanosis is cardiac or noncardiac in origin (Table 14-8). Cyanotic infants require immediate assessment and stabilization of airway, breathing, and circulation (see Chapter 29). Continuous intravenous PGE1 should be initiated in any unstable infant with suspected congenital heart disease. In newborns with mixing lesions or defects that have ductal-dependent pulmonary or systemic blood flow, PGE1 acts to maintain patency of the ductus arteriosus until definitive surgical repair is possible. The rare patient that becomes progressively more unstable after the initiation of PGE1 likely has a defect associated with obstruction of flow from the pulmonary veins or left atrium.

Patients with congenital heart defects that cannot be repaired and those patients who are undergoing staged repairs may continue to be cyanotic. Eisenmenger physiology is a form of cyanotic congenital heart disease in which patients with irreversible pulmonary hypertension due to unrepaired intracardiac shunts develop persistent cyanosis as left-to-right intracardiac shunting is replaced by right-to-left shunting due to elevated pulmonary vascular resistance. Regardless of the cause, chronic cyanosis leads to polycythemia, which increases a patient's risk of stroke. Cerebrovascular accidents in patients with cyanotic disease may be venous or arterial, thrombotic or embolic. Cardiac defects which predispose the patient to right-to-left shunting provide the necessary flow pattern for paradoxic embolism, in which the thrombus originates in the venous system but crosses into the systemic circulation due to the shunt. In addition, patients with congenital cyanotic heart disease have a greater risk of cerebrovascular accident due to "relative anemia." Hemoglobin concentrations in the normal range cannot carry sufficient oxygen to meet metabolic demand in these patients, predisposing to ischemic events.

TABLE 14-7
CYANOTIC CONGENITAL HEART DISEASE

Cardiac Defect	Anatomy	Flow Pattern	Typical Presentation	Physical Examination Findings	Findings on Chest Radiograph	Findings on Electrocardiogram	Treatment	Additional Points of Interest
Ductal-Dependent Mixing Lesions								
Truncus arteriosus	Coronary, systemic, and pulmonary arteries originate from a single vessel arising from the base of the heart; almost always accompanied by a VSD	Complete mixing of systemic, pulmonary venous blood in the truncal vessel	Nonspecific cardiac murmur, minimal cyanosis at birth Congestive heart failure within weeks	Systolic ejection murmur at the left sternal border; single second heart sound; widened pulse pressure; bounding arterial pulses	Marked cardiomegaly, increased pulmonary vascular markings Absence of thymic shadow if associated with DiGeorge syndrome	Biventricular hypertrophy	Surgical repair in the neonatal period	Associated with 22q11 microdeletion (DiGeorge, velocardiofacial syndromes)
D-transposition of the great arteries	Aorta arises from the right ventricle, pulmonary artery arises from the left ventricle	Parallel pulmonary, systemic circuits Mixing lesion is necessary for survival (PFO, PDA, ASD, or VSD)	Tachypnea, severe cyanosis developing in the first several days of life	Loud, single second heart sound Systolic murmur consistent with VSD or pulmonic stenosis	Cardiomegaly, increased pulmonary vascular markings "Egg-shaped" silhouette	Right-axis deviation, right ventricular hypertrophy	PGE1 infusion Surgical repair (arterial switch) in the first week of life	Second most common form of cyanotic congenital heart disease Most common cyanotic condition presenting in the neonatal period
Total anomalous pulmonary venous return	Pulmonary veins drain into the right atrium rather than the left atrium Mixing lesion is necessary for survival	Two variants: *with* obstruction of pulmonary flow (pulmonary hypertension); *without* obstruction of pulmonary flow (increased pulmonary blood flow)	With obstruction: severe cyanosis and respiratory distress in the neonatal period Without obstruction: mild cyanosis at birth; progressive congestive heart failure	With obstruction: loud, single or narrowly split second heart sound Without obstruction: active precordium with right ventricular heave, wide and fixed split second heart sound with accentuated pulmonic component, systolic ejection murmur at the left upper sternal border	With obstruction: normal heart size, increased pulmonary vascular markings Without obstruction: right-sided cardiomegaly, increased pulmonary vascular markings	With obstruction: right ventricular hypertrophy Without obstruction: right-axis deviation, right ventricular hypertrophy	With obstruction: emergent corrective surgery in the newborn period Without obstruction: Elective repair in early infancy prior to the onset of congestive heart failure	PGE1 is contraindicated, as additional blood flow from the ductus will add to an already flooded pulmonary circuit

(continued)

TABLE 14-7
(continued)

Cardiac Defect	Anatomy	Flow Pattern	Typical Presentation	Physical Examination Findings	Findings on Chest Radiograph	Findings on Electrocardiogram	Treatment	Additional Points of Interest
Ductal-Dependent Pulmonary Blood Flow								
Tricuspid atresia	Complete absence of connection between the right atrium and right ventricle	Blood is shunted through a PFO/ASD to the left atrium, and left side of the heart provides both pulmonary (oxygenated) and systemic (deoxygenated) venous return	Severe cyanosis in the newborn period upon closure of the ductus, OR progressive cyanosis, tachypnea, poor feeding, and congestive heart failure in the first two weeks of life	Holosystolic murmur and/or continuous murmur of PDA	Normal heart size and decreased pulmonary vascular markings OR, if congestive heart failure, cardiomegaly and increased pulmonary vascular markings	Superior-axis deviation and left ventricular hypertrophy	PGE1 infusion Staged surgical correction	Isolated tricuspid atresia is rare.
Tetralogy of Fallot	VSD Pulmonary stenosis (with right ventricular outflow obstruction) Right ventricular hypertrophy Large overriding ascending aorta	Right-to-left shunting across the VSD and decreased pulmonary blood flow	Characteristic murmur is usually noted prior to the onset of cyanosis Cyanosis, the timing and severity of which depend on the degree of right ventricular outflow obstruction Severe obstruction results in ductal-dependent flow and cyanosis within hours of birth Patients with less severe obstruction do not develop cyanosis until later in infancy	Right ventricular heave, loud systolic ejection murmur at left upper sternal border (pulmonary stenosis murmur), single second heart sound Tet spells: decreased or absent murmur (due to decreased or absent pulmonary blood flow); dyspnea/ hyperpnea, cyanosis	Normal heart size, decreased pulmonary vascular markings "Boot-shaped" heart	Right-axis deviation, right ventricular hypertrophy	Tet spells: Vagal maneuvers (knee-chest positioning, or squatting in older children), supplemental high-flow oxygen, morphine sulfate; intravascular volume expansion and vasoconstrictors (intravenous phenylephrine) if necessary Surgical repair in the first 3-6 months of life or following first tet spell	The most common form of cyanotic congenital heart disease May be associated with 22q11 microdeletion Periodic "tet spells," caused by temporarily increased right ventricular outflow obstruction, present with the sudden onset of progressive cyanosis and tachypnea/hyperpnea, severe hypoxia, low

(*continued*)

TABLE 14-7
(continued)

Cardiac Defect	Anatomy	Flow Pattern	Typical Presentation	Physical Examination Findings	Findings on Chest Radiograph	Findings on Electrocardiogram	Treatment	Additional Points of Interest
			Hypercyanotic episodes ("tet spells"): distress, crying, inconsolability, hyperpnea, and increasing cyanosis					cardiac output, and agitation lasting minutes to hours. Often occur in the morning or during eating, hot weather, exercise, or during times of dehydration (gastroenteritis) or fever. Spells usually resolve spontaneously but may progress to hypoxia, metabolic acidosis, loss of consciousness, convulsions, and death
Ebstein anomaly	Tricuspid valvular defect, right atrial enlargement, right ventricular hypoplasia	Tricuspid regurgitation; majority of pulmonary blood flow through the ductus	Severe disease: cyanosis and congestive heart failure in the first few days of life Mild disease: presentation in childhood with fatigue, exercise intolerance, palpitations, and/or mild cyanosis with clubbing	Fixed, widely-split second heart sound, gallop rhythm, blowing holosystolic murmur at the left lower sternal border	Extreme cardiomegaly, right atrial enlargement, decreased pulmonary vascular markings	Right bundle branch block with right atrial enlargement; possibly SVT or delta wave (Wolff-Parkinson-White syndrome)	Severe disease: PGE1 infusion, digoxin Defect cannot be corrected surgically; palliation or heart transplantation indicated	Extremely rare Associated with Wolff-Parkinson-White syndrome

(continued)

TABLE 14-7
(continued)

Cardiac Defect	Anatomy	Flow Pattern	Typical Presentation	Physical Examination Findings	Findings on Chest Radiograph	Findings on Electrocardiogram	Treatment	Additional Points of Interest
Ductal-Dependent Pulmonary Blood Flow								
Hypoplastic left heart syndrome	Hypoplasia of the left ventricle, aortic valve stenosis, mitral valve stenosis, coarctation of the aorta	Left-to-right shunting through ASD; right ventricle supplies pulmonary artery and systemic blood flow, which is completely ductal-dependent	Congestive heart failure, cardiogenic shock upon closure of the ductus If there is a PFO, tachypnea from the first day of life with progressive congestive heart failure Moderate cyanosis, tachycardia, tachypnea, pulmonary rales, hepatomegaly, diminished peripheral pulses	Right ventricular heave, single loud second heart sound, systolic ejection murmur at the left lower sternal border	Cardiomegaly, pulmonary edema	Right ventricular hypertrophy, poor R wave progression across the precordial leads	PGE1 infusion Staged surgical palliation beginning in the first week of life Heart transplantation	
Interrupted aortic arch	Discontinuous aortic arch	Systemic blood flow dependent on ductal patency	Pulmonary edema, congestive heart failure, cardiogenic shock upon closure of the ductus	Mottled or grey appearance of the lower body; diminished lower extremity pulses	Cardiomegaly, increased pulmonary vascular markings	Right ventricular hypertrophy, nonspecific ST-T wave changes	PGE1 infusion Surgical repair via end-to-end anastomosis	Associated with 22q11 microdeletion syndrome

VSD, ventricular septal defect; PFO, patent foramen ovale; PDA, patent ductus arteriosus; ASD, atrial septal defect; SVT, supraventricular tachycardia.

TABLE 14-8
INITIAL EVALUATION OF THE CYANOTIC INFANT

Preductal (right upper extremity) and Postductal (lower extremity) Oxygen Saturation Measurement

- *Differential cyanosis* is present when the preductal saturation is higher than the postductal saturation. Congenital cardiac defects resulting in differential cyanosis include persistent pulmonary hypertension of the newborn, interrupted aortic arch, critical coarctation of the aorta, and critical aortic stenosis.
- *Reverse differential cyanosis* is present when the preductal saturation is higher than the postductal saturation. Transposition of the great arteries can result in reverse differential cyanosis.

Four Extremity Blood Pressure Measurements

- A systolic blood pressure in the upper extremities >10 mm Hg higher than the systolic pressure in the lower extremities suggests arch hypoplasia, coarctation of the aorta, or other lesions with ductal-dependent flow.

Chest Radiograph

- Evaluation of the size and shape of the heart and whether pulmonary vasculature is increased or decreased (see individual defects).

Electrocardiogram

- Objective measure of heart rate and well as rhythm, axis, intervals, and wave forms (see individual defects).

Hyperoxia Test

- Hyperoxia testing is indicated for all neonates with resting pulse oximetry readings <95%, visible cyanosis, or circulatory collapse.
- Preductal (right radial) arterial blood gas measurement is obtained when the infant is breathing 100% oxygen under a head hood.
- A PaO_2 measurement >200 mm Hg on 100% oxygen essentially rules out cyanotic cardiac disease as a cause of the cyanosis; however, acyanotic heart disease may still be present
- A PaO_2 measurement between 50 to 150 mm Hg on 100% oxygen suggests a cardiac defect with complete mixing and unrestricted pulmonary blood flow (truncus arteriosus, unobstructed total anomalous pulmonary venous return, hypoplastic left heart syndrome, double-inlet single ventricle with mild pulmonic valve stenosis).
- A PaO_2 measurement <50 mm Hg on 100% oxygen indicates either a cardiac defect with parallel circulation or a mixing lesion with restricted pulmonary blood flow (D-transposition of the great arteries, Ebstein anomaly, tricuspid atresia, Tetralogy of Fallot, pulmonary atresia, pulmonary stenosis).
- Pulse oximetry measurements are not adequate for interpretation of the hyperoxia test.

If the results of these initial tests are consistent with cardiogenic cyanosis, an echocardiogram and cardiology referral are warranted.

Permanent sequelae from cyanotic congenital heart disease can include developmental delay, poor school performance, and difficulty with attention and learning. In fact, the majority of children with cyanotic congenital heart disease have some degree of cognitive disability. Factors which appear to affect the severity of the impairment include degree of preoperative hypoxia, cardiac bypass time, and postoperative complications. Children with histories of cyanotic congenital heart disease and abnormal neurologic findings have poorer cognitive outcomes than those with normal neurologic examinations; the latter group still fairs worse than patients with acyanotic heart disease or defects which do not require surgical intervention.

Acyanotic Disease

Acyanotic congenital defects can be categorized by their effects on pulmonary blood flow and pressure (Table 14-9):

- Increased pulmonary blood flow (left-to-right shunts)—ASD, VSD, PDA, and common atrioventricular canal
- Pulmonary venous hypertension—coarctation of the aorta, aortic valve stenosis
- Normal or decreased pulmonary blood flow—pulmonary valve stenosis

An important subset of acyanotic heart diseases is composed of conditions involving the critical left heart obstructive lesions (critical aortic stenosis, critical coarctation of the aorta, cyanotic defect hypoplastic left heart syndrome). In these lesions, systemic blood flow is dependent on the patent ductus arteriosus. As the ductus closes, patients who have critical left obstructive lesions present with poor feeding and tachypnea, which progresses to profound CHF when ductal patency is lost. Initiation of PGE1 is indicated to provide blood flow from the unobstructed right ventricle and pulmonary arteries through the ductus. The fraction of inspired

TABLE 14-9
ACYANOTIC CONGENITAL HEART DISEASE

Cardiac Defect	Anatomy	Flow Pattern	Typical Presentation	Physical Examination Findings	Findings on Chest Radiograph	Findings on Electrocardiogram	Treatment	Additional Points of Interest
Right-to-Left Shunting with Increased Pulmonary Blood Flow								
Atrial septal defect	*Ostium secundum* (mid-atrial defect) *Ostium primum* (lower atrial defect) *Sinus venosus* (atrial defect at the junction of the superior or inferior vena cava)	Left-to-right shunting through the ASD Right atrial, ventricular enlargement	Usually asymptomatic Congestive heart failure in infants May present with exercise intolerance in older children	Right ventricular heave; loud first heart sound; fixed, widely-split second heart sound; systolic ejection murmur at the left upper sternal border, mid-diastolic murmur at right lower sternal border	Cardiomegaly, increased pulmonary vascular markings	Right ventricular hypertrophy Right-axis deviation (secundum defects) Extreme left-axis deviation (primum defects) Possibly SVT due to atrial enlargement	Spontaneous closure may occur in the first year of life Digoxin and diuretics for congestive heart failure Trans-catheter closure Surgical closure	Risk of paradoxic embolism Subacute bacterial endocarditis prophylaxis is indicated for all but ostium secundum defect
Ventricular septal defect	Defect in the septum between the ventricles (five types are muscular, inlet, conoseptal hypoplasia, conoventricular, malalignment)	Restrictive VSD (small defect): left-to-right flow through the defect, with normal pulmonary blood flow and pulmonary vascular resistance Nonrestrictive VSD (large defect): direction of shunt is determined by ratio of pulmonary vascular resistance to systemic resistance	Small defect: no symptoms Large defect: congestive heart failure, poor growth	Small defect: loud, harsh, holosystolic murmur heard best at the mid-to-lower left sternal border Large defect: murmur shortens and softens, increased intensity of the second heart sound	Small defect: normal chest radiograph Large defect: cardiomegaly, increased pulmonary vascular markings	Small defect: normal electrocardiogram Large defect: left atrial and bi-ventricular hypertrophy	Small defect: most close spontaneously during childhood. No treatment is necessary. Large defect: management of congestive heart failure; surgical closure	The most common congenital heart defect

(continued)

TABLE 14-9
(continued)

Cardiac Defect	Anatomy	Flow Pattern	Typical Presentation	Physical Examination Findings	Findings on Chest Radiograph	Findings on Electrocardiogram	Treatment	Additional Points of Interest
Common atrioventricular canal	Endocardial cushion defect with ASD, VSD, and disordered septation of the tricuspid and mitral valves	Left-to-right shunting through the ASD and VSD, resulting in pulmonary hypertension over time	Presents in early infancy with congestive heart failure, tachypnea, dyspnea, and failure to thrive	Blowing holosystolic murmur at the left lower sternal border; fixed, widely-split second heart sound	Cardiomegaly, increased pulmonary vascular markings	Superior-axis deviation	Management of congestive heart failure Surgical repair prior to irreversible changes in the pulmonary vasculature	Complete heart block is a rare complication of surgical repair
Patent ductus arteriosus	Abnormal persistence of the ductus arteriosus, which connects the aorta and left pulmonary artery	Left-to-right shunting as pulmonary resistance falls after birth; if pulmonary vascular pressure exceeds systemic pressure, flow is reversed	Small PDA: asymptomatic, but may present later in childhood or adulthood Large PDA: congestive heart failure, poor growth	Small PDA: Continuous "machinery" murmur beginning after first heart sound, peaking at second heart sound, and trailing off in diastole; heard best in the left infraclavicular area Large PDA: murmur as above, plus widened pulse pressures, bounding pulses, palmar pulses	Small PDA: no abnormalities Large PDA: cardiomegaly, increased pulmonary vascular markings	Small PDA: no abnormalities Large PDA: if long-standing, left ventricular and atrial hypertrophy	Small PDAs often close in the first month of life. If persistent, indomethacin Surgical ligation	Higher incidence in premature infants
Pulmonary Venous Hypertension								
Coarctation of the aorta	Narrowing of the aorta at the level of the ductus,	Flow continues through the aorta unless there is critical narrowing, in	Presentation depends on severity of narrowing;	Nonspecific systolic ejection murmur at the heart apex, referred to the back	Mild narrowing: no abnormalities Moderate-to-severe narrowing: enlarged aortic knob	Mild narrowing: no abnormalities Moderate-to-severe narrowing: right ventricular	PGE1 infusion for patients with critical narrowing	Consider Turner syndrome when coarctation of the aorta occurs in a female.

(*continued*)

TABLE 14-9
(continued)

Cardiac Defect	Anatomy	Flow Pattern	Typical Presentation	Physical Examination Findings	Findings on Chest Radiograph	Findings on Electrocardiogram	Treatment	Additional Points of Interest
	often associated with patent ductus arteriosus or aortic and/or mitral valve abnormalities	which case systemic flow is ductal-dependent	ranges from asymptomatic to irritability, difficulty feeding, and poor growth to circulatory collapse if narrowing is critical	Femoral/dorsalis pedis pulses may be weak, delayed, or absent; upper extremity hypertension		hypertrophy in the infant; left ventricular hypertrophy if diagnosis delayed until childhood	Balloon dilation angioplasty or surgical reanastomosis	Hypertension is a long-term complication following surgical correction, requiring regular monitoring of pressures and pulses in upper and lower extremities
Aortic stenosis	Thickened, rigid aortic valvular tissue domes in systole; valve is usually bicuspid	Normal direction of flow, but increased pressures generated by the left ventricle result in hypertrophy and decreased left ventricular function over time	Presentation depends on severity of stenosis and preserved left ventricular function; ranges from asymptomatic to circulatory collapse upon closure of the ductus	Harsh, high-pitch systolic ejection murmur best heard at the right upper sternal border; murmur is preceded by an ejection click	Cardiomegaly with varying degrees of pulmonary edema depending on residual left ventricular function	Left ventricular hypertrophy	PGE1 infusion for critical aortic stenosis with ductal-dependent systemic blood flow Balloon valvuloplasty	Balloon valvuloplasty is usually complicated by chronic aortic regurgitation, necessitating eventual valve replacement
Normal or Decreased Pulmonary Blood Flow								
Pulmonic stenosis	Dome-shaped pulmonic valve with small central opening; associated with post-stenotic dilatation of the main pulmonary artery	Normal direction, decreased flow volume; or, if stenosis is critical, right-to-left shunting through a PFO	Asymptomatic unless stenosis is critical, which presents with dyspnea on exertion and angina	Ejection click which varies with inspiration accompanied by harsh systolic ejection murmur heard best at the left upper sternal border	Normal heart size, normal pulmonary vascular markings Enlargement of the pulmonary artery segment	Right-axis deviation, right ventricular hypertrophy	PGE1 infusion for critical pulmonic stenosis which is ductal-dependent Balloon valvuloplasty	Balloon valvuloplasty reserved for patients with increasing right ventricular pressures and/or right-sided congestive heart failure

oxygen should be minimized in these patients to avoid vasodilation of the pulmonary vasculature, which further reduces the amount of blood available to the systemic system.

Infectious and Postinfectious Diseases

Infective Endocarditis

Infective endocarditis consists of infection and inflammation of the endocardium, the endothelial lining of the inner surfaces of the heart. It is thought that turbulent blood flow causes endocardial injury and thrombus formation; organisms subsequently infect the thrombus during an episode of bacteremia. The most frequently recovered pathogens are noted in Table 14-10.

Risk factors for the development of infective endocarditis include:

- underlying rheumatic heart disease
- prosthetic valve or conduit
- indwelling central venous catheter
- intravenous drug use
- prior heart surgery, such as repair of a congenital heart defect
- congenital heart defect (lesions which allow mixing of oxygenated and deoxygenated blood; left-sided obstructive lesions; stenotic or regurgitant valves)
- ongoing immunosuppressant therapy
- poor dental hygiene

The onset of infective endocarditis may be acute or insidious. Symptoms include fever, night sweats, weight loss, malaise, chest pain, dyspnea, nausea/vomiting, abdominal pain, arthralgia, myalgia, and occasionally hematuria. An evolving heart murmur is the most consistent finding in patients with infective endocarditis, followed by splenomegaly and petechiae. Other cutaneous manifestations, such as Osler nodes, splinter hemorrhages, and Janeway lesions typically appear late in the course of illness (as do Roth spots). Diagnosis rests on blood cultures which are positive for pathogens known to cause infective endocarditis in a patient with positive echocardiogram findings (vegetations, newly diagnosed valvular regurgitation). Obtaining multiple sets of blood cultures at different points in time increases the likelihood of identifying the causative organism; specimen draws need not coincide with febrile episodes. The transthoracic echocardiogram is thought to be superior to a transesophageal study in children due to the high incidence of right-sided lesions in this patient population, but negative studies do not rule out infective endocarditis.

Antimicrobial treatment is delayed, if possible, until the causative organism is identified. Empiric management consists of combination intravenous therapy with two bactericidal antibiotics. Once the pathogen and its sensitivities are known, the patient should receive at least 4 to 8 weeks of high-dose antibiotic treatment (longer for *S. aureus*). Surgical intervention may be indicated for severe disease. The potential complications of infective endocarditis are significant and widespread. The most frequent include heart failure (right- or left-sided), arrhythmias, and embolic events involving the brain or lungs, resulting in infarction or infection. Patients with chronic bacterial endocarditis may develop elevated immunoglobulin levels or immune complex-mediated disease (thrombocytopenia, glomerulonephritis).

The American Heart Association recommends subacute bacterial endocarditis prophylaxis for any patient with a heart defect (excluding ostium secundum atrial septal defect and mitral valve prolapse without regurgitation) who is undergoing one of the following procedures:

- Surgery or procedures involving dental or gingival tissues, including extractions, placement of orthodontic bands, root canals, and (in many cases) routine cleaning
- Surgery or procedures involving the upper respiratory tract (tonsillectomy, adenoidectomy, bronchoscopy)
- Surgery or procedures involving the gastrointestinal tract (including endoscopy)
- Surgery or procedures involving the genitourinary tract (including cystoscopy)

Acceptable prophylaxis consists of oral amoxicillin 50 mg per kg (to a maximum of 2 g) taken one hour prior to the procedure. Patients who are allergic to penicillin may substitute clindamycin, cephalexin, cefadroxil, azithromycin, or clarithromycin.

TABLE 14-10
THE MICROBIOLOGY OF INFECTIVE ENDOCARDITIS

Streptococcus Viridans
- Generally nonpathogenic oral flora
- Most common in patients who have recently undergone dental procedures

Staphylococcus Aureus
- Often cultured from patients with indwelling catheters or prosthetic valves

***Enterococcus* Species**
- More commonly cultured from patients who have recently undergone gastrointestinal or genitourinary procedures

Pseudomonas Aeruginosa, Serratia Marcescens
- Associated with intravenous drug use

Additional Organisms
- *Streptococcus bovis*
- *Haemophilus influenzae*
- *Actinobaccillus actinomycetemcomitans*
- *Cardiobacterium hominis*
- *Eikenella* species
- *Kingella kingae*
- Fungal pathogens

Rheumatic Fever

Acute rheumatic fever (ARF) follows inadequately treated group A streptococcal pharyngitis by 2 to 4 weeks. ARF is an important cause of acquired heart disease in the pediatric population. Incidence peaks in middle childhood and adolescence. Recurrence is common in patients who are noncompliant with prophylactic antibiotics. The criteria required for diagnosis are presented in Chapter 10 in Table 10-16. Carditis (involving a single or multiple layers of the heart) and prolonged PR interval are major and minor diagnostic criteria, respectively. The carditis of ARF affects primarily the mitral valve, or less commonly the aortic valve, resulting in permanent regurgitation and eventual (mitral) stenosis. The characteristic murmurs of mitral and aortic regurgitation are provided in Table 14-4.

The management of ARF consists of:

- antibiotic therapy to eradicate the infective organism (group A beta-hemolytic *Streptococcus*)
- anti-inflammatory agents—high-dose aspirin therapy for several weeks; steroids for patients with moderate-to-severe carditis and congestive heart failure
- limitation of activity during the acute phase of illness

An echocardiogram is indicated for any patient diagnosed with ARF. ECHO with Doppler and color flow mapping provides information regarding cardiac anatomy and inflammation, myocardial function, valvular structure, and, if present, pericardial effusion.

Myocarditis

Myocarditis is the most significant cause of congestive heart failure in pediatric patients with previously normal hearts. Inflammation of the myocardium may follow a nonspecific febrile (presumably viral) respiratory or gastrointestinal illness but usually is asymptomatic and resolves spontaneously. The clinical presentation of symptomatic myocarditis may include any of the following: chest pain, abdominal pain, malaise, fatigue, exertional or resting dyspnea, nausea/vomiting, and tachycardia. Severe or focal myocarditis may result in arrhythmias (most commonly supraventricular tachycardia, heart block, ventricular tachycardia) or global myocardial dysfunction. The presence of ventricular arrhythmia, congestive heart failure, and/or cardiogenic shock is associated with significant morbidity and mortality; surviving patients often require heart transplantation.

The electrocardiogram is the preferred study for evaluating the presence of myocarditis and associated arrhythmias. Tachycardia and low-voltage QRS complexes are consistent with the diagnosis; more severe disease produces ST-T wave changes. Ventricular function should be assessed by echocardiogram. Serum cardiac troponin and fractionated creatinine kinase levels are elevated in the presence of myocardial injury and, while not specific for myocarditis, are used to monitor progression or resolution of the disease.

Disease of the Pericardium

Pericarditis is inflammation of the pericardium, a thin layer of specialized connective tissue surrounding the outer surface of the heart. It may be idiopathic or due to viral, bacterial, or tuberculosis infection; recent cardiac surgery; Kawasaki disease; autoimmune disorders (particularly systemic lupus erythematosus); acute rheumatic fever; kidney failure; or certain medications. Pericarditis presents with sharp, often severe substernal chest pain which is worse when the patient is lying down. The condition is usually accompanied by fever or laboratory evidence of inflammation.

Pericardial effusions are associated with many of the same conditions which cause pericarditis. Accumulation of enough fluid compresses the heart and prohibits effective filling and contraction (cardiac tamponade). Smaller effusions present with vague symptoms of abdominal discomfort or fullness, anorexia, and intermittent vomiting. Signs and symptoms of cardiac tamponade include tachypnea, sinus tachycardia, decreased intensity of peripheral pulses upon inspiration (pulsus paradoxus), diminished heart tones, jugular venous pulsations, and ultimately cardiogenic shock. An enlarged cardiac shadow on CXR is the timeliest method of identifying a large pericardial effusion. Urgent pericardiocentesis is indicated to relieve the compression. Smaller effusions often respond to anti-inflammatory agents.

Postpericardiotomy syndrome is an uncommon complication of open heart surgery. Postoperative inflammation results in the accumulation of sterile fluid in the pericardial space, usually within 6 weeks of the operation. The presentation and complications of postpericardiotomy syndrome are identical to those of pericardial effusion resulting from other processes.

Kawasaki Syndrome

The presentation, management, and prevention of cardiac complications of Kawasaki syndrome are discussed in Chapter 21.

Rate, Rhythm, and Ischemic Disorders

Premature Atrial Contraction

The cardiac impulse stimulating premature atrial contractions (PACs) is initiated from outside the sinus node and occurs earlier than the normal sinus impulse. Premature atrial beats can be conducted with normal QRS complexes, aberrant QRS complexes, or not conducted at all ("blocked" P waves). Isolated atrial ectopy, characterized by asymptomatic nonconducted PACs, is common in the healthy fetus and newborn, presenting as intermittent pauses in an otherwise normal cardiac rhythm (Figure 14-1). It is not associated with structural or functional cardiac abnormalities. Close inspection of the ECG should reveal premature P waves within the ST segment of the QRS complex that precedes the pause. Infants with very frequent atrial ectopic beats may develop atrial bigeminy (conduction of every other atrial contraction), a form of bradycardia without changes in respiratory pattern, color, perfusion, or pulses. Stimulation of the infant produces sinus tachycardia, overdriving the atrial ectopy and resulting in a normal ventricular rate.

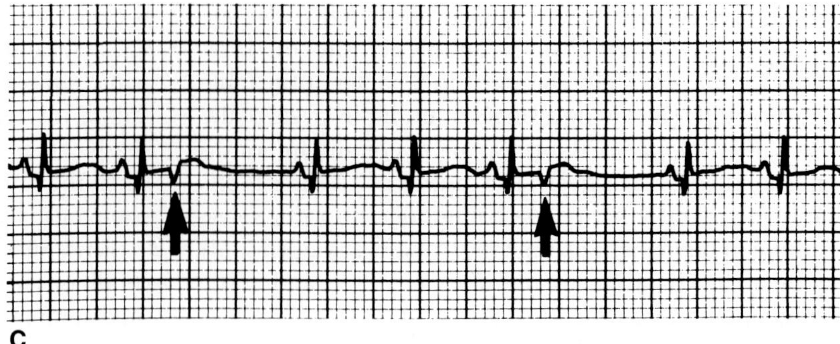

Figure 14-1 ECG demonstrating isolated atrial ectopy or premature atrial contractions. (From Flyer DC. *Nadas' Pediatric Cardiology* with permission.)

Premature Ventricular Contraction

Early spontaneous depolarization of the ventricles produces a wide QRS complex which is not associated with any preceding P wave (Figure 14-2). Premature ventricular contractions are uncommon in neonates but are usually benign.

Supraventricular Tachycardia

Paroxysmal supraventricular tachycardia (SVT) is a dysrhythmia which originates in the atria and perpetuates through a closed loop composed of atrial muscle tissue, the ventricular His-Purkinje system, and an aberrant atrioventricular (AV) connection. The electrical impulse may be propagated through the AV node with retrograde conduction through the accessory pathway, or the impulse may proceed in the reverse fashion. SVT produces a narrow QRS complex rhythm with rates between 240 and 300 beats per minute (Figure 14-3). Untreated SVT results in cardiopulmonary failure with a real risk of significant morbidity and mortality. Carotid massage is used to break the rhythm in adults but is contraindicated in children. Temporary interruption of impulse conduction through the AV node can be achieved with intravenous (push) adenosine; virtually all patients convert to normal sinus rhythm with this intervention. Common adverse effects (bronchospasm, flushing) are generally very brief. Atrial fibrillation is a rare complication of adenosine infusion; a DC cardioverter should be on hand whenever this treatment is employed.

Most patients can tolerate SVT for variable durations (minutes to hours) before becoming overtly symptomatic. Signs and symptoms in the infant include irritability, tachypnea, pallor, and diminished peripheral pulses. Older children complain of palpitations, shortness of breath, and diaphoresis.

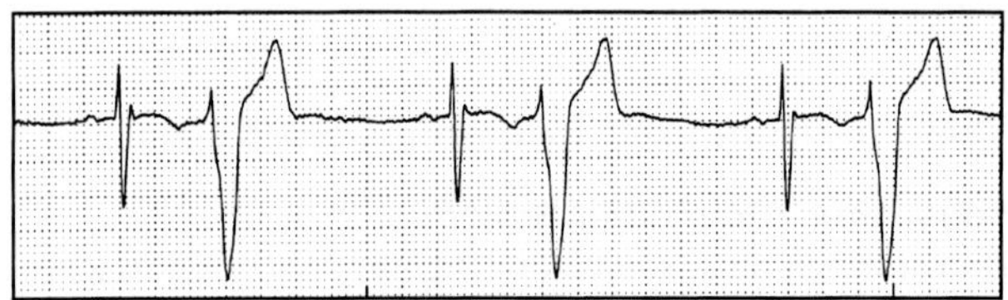

Figure 14-2 ECG demonstrating premature ventricular contractions. (From Cloherty JP. *Manual of Neonatal Care.* 6th ed. Philadephia: Lippincott Williams & Wilkins; 2008 with permission.)

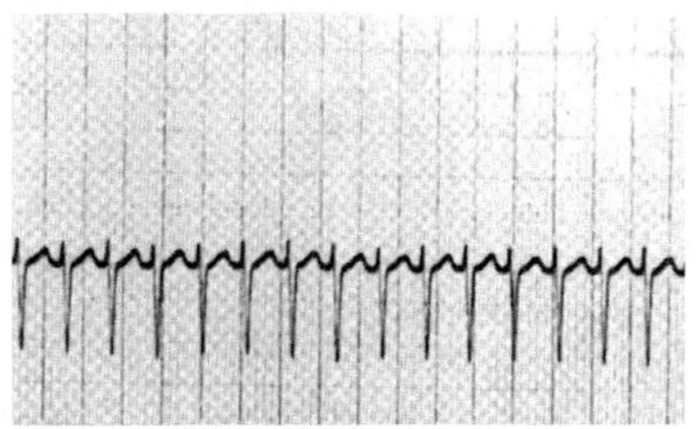

Figure 14-3 ECG demonstrating supraventricular tachycardia. (From Rogers M. *Handbook of Pediatric Intensive Care.* 3rd ed. Philadephia: Lippincott Williams & Wilkins; 1998 with permission.)

Ventricular Tachycardia

Ventricular tachycardia is defined by the presence of more than two premature ventricular beats occurring in a row at a rate faster than the sinus rate (Figure 14-4). Sustained ventricular tachycardia leads to cardiovascular collapse.

Second-Degree Heart Block

Second-degree heart block results from conduction delay within the AV node which may be:

- progressive—in Mobitz type I block, nonconducted P waves are preceded by a gradual increase in the PR interval (the Wenckebach phenomenon). QRS morphology is normal (Figure 14-5). This type of heart block may occur in athletically conditioned adolescents due to enhanced vagal tone.

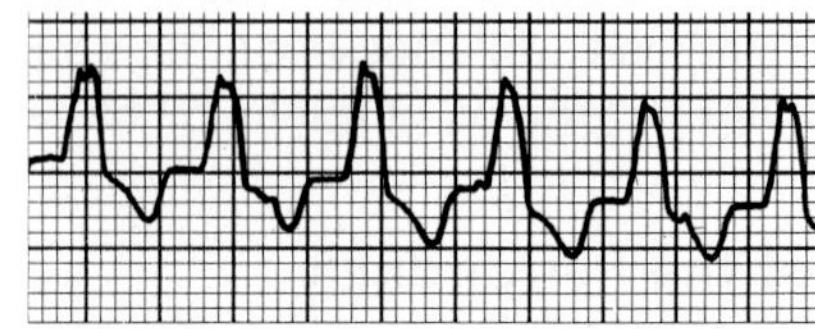

Figure 14-4 ECG demonstrating ventricular tachycardia. (From Fleisher GR. *Atlas of Pediatric Emergency Medicine.* Philadephia: Lippincott Williams & Wilkins; 2003 with permission.)

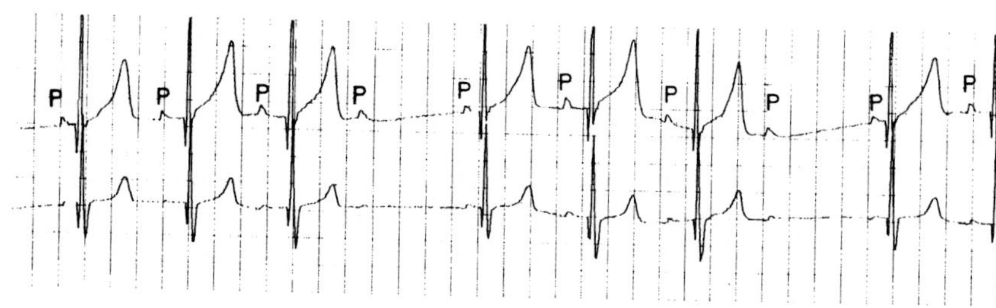

Figure 14-5 ECG demonstrating Mobitz type I second-degree heart block. (From Allen HG. *Moss and Adams' Heart Disease in Infants, Children, and Adolescents.* 7th ed. Philadelphia: Lippincott Williams & Wilkins; 2008 with permission.)

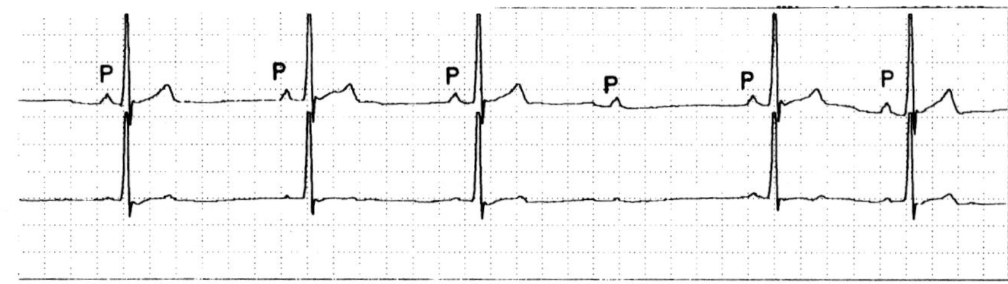

Figure 14-6 ECG demonstrating Mobitz type II second-degree heart block. (From Allen HG. *Moss and Adams' Heart Disease in Infants, Children, and Adolescents.* 7th ed. Philadelphia: Lippincott Williams & Wilkins; 2008 with permission.)

- consistent—Mobitz type II block is rare in childhood and is usually associated with abnormal QRS wave forms (Figure 14-6). Mobitz type II may progress to complete heart block.

Complete Heart Block

Complete heart block is rare beyond the neonatal period. Fetal complete heart block occurs in infants of mothers with systemic lupus erythematosus who produce anti-Ro and/or anti-La antibodies. The measured (ventricular) heart rate in the affected fetus varies between 40 to 80 beats per minute in the second half of pregnancy and after birth. An ECG clearly demonstrates a ventricular rate which is generated independently and disassociated from the atrial rate (120 to 180 beats per minute) (Figure 14-7).

Wolff-Parkinson-White Syndrome

Wolff-Parkinson-White (WPW) is a syndrome of ventricular pre-excitation associated with supraventricular tachycardia and sudden cardiac death due to ventricular fibrillation. ECG findings include a shortened PR interval and early depolarization of the QRS complex (the delta wave, Figure 14-8). Patients with WPW often present with syncope and/or palpitations. Digoxin is generally contraindicated in patients with WPW.

Long QT Syndrome

Long QT syndrome is an isolated arrhythmia which is not associated with underlying structural abnormalities. Affected patients present with recurrent syncope, palpitations, or occasionally seizures, and often have a family history of sudden cardiac death. ECG abnormalities include prolonged QT interval, ST-T wave changes, and at times significant bradycardia (Figure 14-9). Patients with long QT syndrome are at risk for ventricular tachycardia, torsades de pointes, ventricular fibrillation, cardiac arrest, and sudden death. Although a significant reduction in arrhythmic events is noted when beta-blocker therapy is instituted with propranolol or atenolol, neither drug eliminates arrhythmias entirely. Placement of a pacemaker is indicated for patients at high risk for sudden cardiac death.

Superior Vena Cava Syndrome

When superior venous vessels become obstructed, venous stasis and increased lymphatic pressure lead to generalized facial and/or neck edema and localized dusky cyanosis. The swelling may be sudden but is usually insidious in onset. Superior vena cava (SVC) syndrome can occur with caval obstruction secondary to intravenous lines, pacemaker leads, or masses. SVC syndrome which

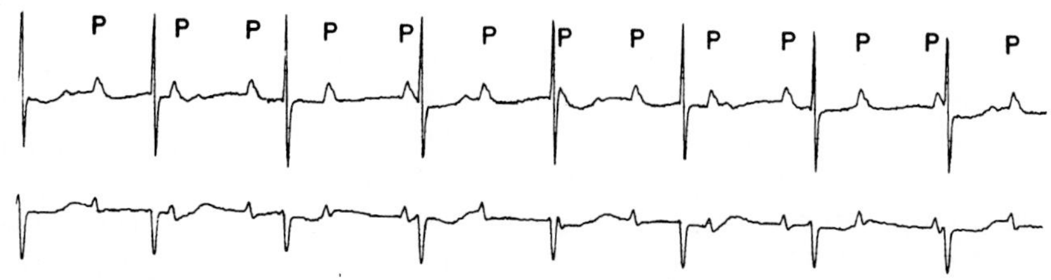

Figure 14-7 ECG demonstrating complete heart block in an infant born to a mother with systemic lupus erythematosus. (From Allen HG. *Moss and Adams' Heart Disease in Infants, Children, and Adolescents.* 7th ed. Philadelphia: Lippincott Williams & Wilkins; 2008 with permission.)

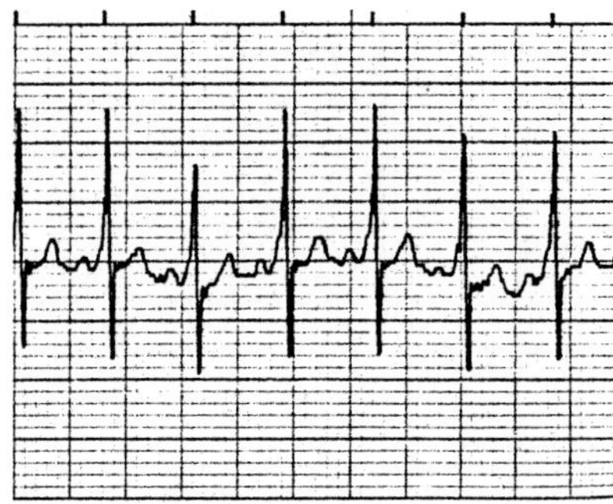

Figure 14-8 ECG demonstrating the delta wave in Wolff-Parkinson-White syndrome. (From Fleisher GR. *Atlas of Pediatric Emergency Medicine*. Philadephia: Lippincott Williams & Wilkins; 2003 with permission.)

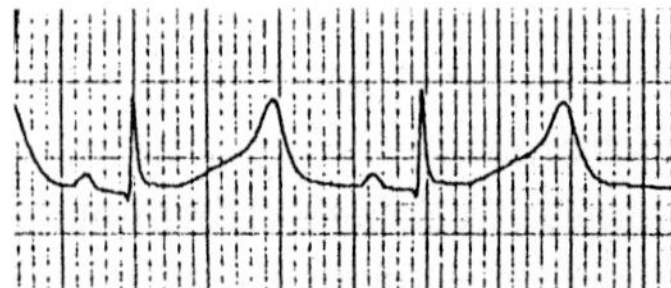

Figure 14-9 ECG demonstrating long QT syndrome. (From Fleisher GR. *Atlas of Pediatric Emergency Medicine*. Philadephia: Lippincott Williams & Wilkins; 2003 with permission.)

is accompanied by anorexia, weight loss, fatigue, and/or fevers or other constitutional symptoms suggests a cancerous tumor as the cause of the obstruction. Adolescents with mediastinal lymphoma may initially present with superior vena cava syndrome; the mass is evident on CXR. Computed tomography of the chest permits visualization of the superior venous structures and surrounding tissues and evaluation of tumor size and pattern of extension.

SOURCES

Berger S, Kugler J, Thomas JA, et al. Sudden cardiac death in children and adolescents: Introduction and overview. *Pediatr Clin North Am*. 2004;51:1201–1209.

Bush DM. Evaluating cardiovascular presentations: What does an electrocardiogram have to offer? *Pediatr Ann*. 2005;34:858–869.

Doniger SJ, Sharieff GQ. Pediatric dysrhythmias. *Pediatr Clin North Am*. 2006;53:85–105.

Hoyer A, Silberbach M. Infective endocarditis. *Pediatr Rev*. 2005;26: 394–400.

Marino BS, Fine KS. Cardiology. In: Marino BS, Fine KS, eds. *Pediatric Blueprints*. Philadelphia, PA: Lippincott Williams & Wilkins; 2007: 22–52.

Marone BJ. Hypertrophic cardiomyopathy in childhood. *Pediatr Clin North Am*. 2004;51:1305–1346.

Menashe V. Heart murmurs. *Pediatr Rev*. 2007;28:e19.

Rudolph AM. Heart failure—A historical perspective. In: Shaddy R, Wernovsky G, eds. *Pediatric Heart Failure*. Taylor and Francis Group; 2005:1–24.

Silberbach M, Hannon D. Presentation of congenital heart disease in the neonate and young infant. *Pediatr Rev*. 2007;28: 123–131.

QUESTIONS

1. You are called to the newborn nursery to evaluate an infant with dysmorphic facial features. The child has upward slanting palpebral fissures, bilateral epicanthal folds, a flat nasal bridge, and a protruding tongue. While you are examining the neonate, you note transient cyanosis of the lips and mucous membranes. The pulse oximetry reading on room air is 65%. Which of the following cardiac defects is most likely to be present on echocardiography?

A) Complete atrioventricular septal defect
B) Tetralogy of Fallot
C) Pulmonic stenosis
D) Interrupted aortic arch
E) Aortic stenosis

2. You are called to the newborn nursery to evaluate a 3-day-old former full-term infant born via elective Caesarian section. The infant has become progressively tachycardic and tachypneic over the past hour. On physical examination, he is lethargic, pale, and clearly ill. Extremities are cool to the touch, with prolonged capillary refill and diminished pulses. Vital signs include a heart rate of 176 beats per minute, respiratory rate 75 breaths per minute, and blood pressure 50/palpable. Which of the following is the most important immediate intervention for reversing shock in this child?

A) Rapid administration of 20 mL per kg normal saline
B) Intravenous prostaglandin E1
C) Intubation and endotracheal epinephrine
D) Thoracentesis of the chest
E) Hemodialysis

3. You are called to the nursery to evaluate a newborn infant with cyanosis. Arterial blood gas measurement obtained with the patient breathing 100% oxygen under a head hood yields the following results: pH 7.36; PaO_2 65 mm Hg; $PaCO_2$ 36 mm Hg. The results of this patient's hyperoxia test are most consistent with which of the following?

A) Tetralogy of Fallot
B) Critical pulmonic stenosis
C) Truncus arteriosus
D) D-transposition of the great arteries
E) Ebstein anomaly

4. You are called to the newborn nursery to evaluate a 12-hour-old infant with tachypnea. The full-term neonate is the product of an uncomplicated pregnancy and delivery; his birthweight is appropriate for gestational age. The patient has a respiratory rate of 68 breaths per minute and a heart rate of 160 beats per minute. Cyanosis is present in the hands and feet and around the mouth, with subtle cyanosis of the mucous membranes. A loud, single second heart sound and a holosystolic murmur located at the left lower sternal border are appreciated on cardiac auscultation. Which of the following congenital heart defects is most likely to be the cause of this patient's clinical manifestations?
A) Ventricular septal defect
B) Ebstein anomaly
C) Hypoplastic left heart syndrome
D) Transposition of the great arteries
E) Tetralogy of Fallot

5. A 6-week-old former full-term infant is brought to the emergency department by his parents, who are concerned about his breathing and coloring. They note that over the past 24 hours he has been irritable and feeding poorly. The infant is afebrile, with a heart rate of 180 beats per minute and a respiratory rate of 80 breaths per minute. The physical examination is significant for obvious cyanosis, a right ventricular heave, and a single second heart sound. Following intubation, a chest radiograph to document placement of the endotracheal tube reveals a "boot-shaped" heart. Which of the following diagnoses is most consistent with this infant's clinical picture?
A) Pulmonic stenosis
B) Hypoplastic left heart syndrome
C) Truncus arteriosus
D) Total anomalous pulmonary venous return
E) Tetralogy of Fallot

6. A 5-month-old infant with known tetralogy of Fallot presents to the emergency department with rapid breathing. Her physical examination is significant for a respiratory rate of 90 breaths per minute; a heart rate of 180 beats per minute; cyanosis of the hands, feet, and perioral area; and a loud, single second heart sound. No murmur is appreciated. Given your diagnosis (hypercyanotic episode), which of the following initial interventions are most appropriate?
A) Administering oxygen and placement of the patient in the knee-to-chest position
B) Administering oxygen and beginning infusion of prostaglandin E_1
C) Administering oxygen and preparation for emergent balloon angioplasty
D) Administrating oxygen and intravenous epinephrine
E) Administering oxygen and delivering aerosolized epinephrine

7. A 6-month-old infant with isolated tetralogy of Fallot underwent successful surgical repair of her condition 72 hours ago. Her physical examination is significant for mild but persistent clonus of the lower extremities. Her parents have questions for you regarding her expected neurodevelopmental outcome. In preparing to meet with them, you are correct in noting all of the following EXCEPT:
A) The infant may manifest difficulty with attention and learning when she attends school.
B) The incidence of cognitive impairment in children with repaired cyanotic congenital heart disease is not significantly different than the incidence in children with repaired acyanotic congenital heart disease.
C) Children with a history of repaired cyanotic congenital heart disease have an increased risk of cognitive impairment if they have persistent neurologic sings following surgical correction.
D) The infant should be closely monitored for signs of neurodevelopmental delay.
E) The majority of children with cyanotic congenital heart disease have some degree of cognitive impairment.

8. Which of the following is the most common long-term sequela in patients with repaired coarctation of the aorta?
A) Aortic regurgitation
B) Re-stenosis
C) Hypertension
D) Aortic dissection
E) Pulmonary hypertension

9. A 15-year-old adolescent with no significant past medical history comes to your office with a chief complaint of chest pain. The pain started about four days ago. She describes the pain as sharp left parasternal chest pain which occurs off and on throughout the day for 5 to 7 minutes at a time. During the episodes, her breathing becomes very shallow due to the pain. The episodes are not associated with exercise. A maternal uncle died of a heart attack 18 months ago at the age of 42 years. The physical examination is remarkable for a well-nourished well-developed female in no acute distress. Vital signs are stable, and pulse oximetry measures 98%. No cardiac or pulmonary abnormalities are noted on examination. The pain is reproducible on deep palpation of the area. Which of the following conditions is most consistent with this patient's presentation?
A) Gastroesophageal reflux
B) Pleurodynia
C) Pericardial effusion
D) Costochondritis
E) Myocarditis

10. One of your patients, an 8-year-old boy with an isolated ostium secundum atrial septal defect who is allergic to penicillin, has cracked a tooth in a bicycle accident. He is scheduled for dental repair this afternoon. Which of the following prophylactic choices is most appropriate for this patient?

A) Oral clindamycin 20 mg per kg (maximum 600 mg) taken 1 hour prior to the procedure
B) Oral clarithromycin 15 mg per kg (maximum 500 mg) taken 1 hour prior to the procedure
C) Oral azithromycin 15 mg per kg (maximum 500 mg) taken 1 hour prior to the procedure
D) Oral cephalexin 50 mg per kg (maximum 2 g) taken 1 hour prior to the procedure
E) Subacute bacterial endocarditis prophylaxis is not indicated for this patient.

11. A 15-year-old patient with no significant past medical history presents to your office about 30 minutes after fainting during a school choral recital. She had been standing on the platform for about 40 minutes when she suddenly began to feel lightheaded, dizzy, nauseous, and sweaty. She fell forward onto another singer, who caught her and lowered her to the floor. She regained consciousness within seconds with no residual confusion. Vital signs and pulse oximetry are within normal limits. The physical examination is normal. Which of the following is the best next step in the management of this patient?

A) Obtain an electrocardiogram.
B) Reassure the patient that her symptoms are consistent with vasovagal syncope, a benign condition.
C) Begin salt tablets and recommend increased oral fluid intake prior to recitals.
D) Refer the patient for an urgent cardiology consultation.
E) Schedule the patient for an outpatient electroencephalogram.

12. A 16-year-old adolescent with Ehler-Danlos syndrome is in your office for her routine health maintenance visit. Her cardiac examination is significant for a mid-systolic click, followed by a high-pitch crescendo murmur, which ends with the second heart sound. The click is heard earlier in systole when the patient is standing; lying in the knee-chest position produces a delay in the timing of the click. This patient's murmur is most likely due to which of the following valvular abnormalities?

A) Mitral valve stenosis
B) Mitral valve prolapse
C) Tricuspid valve stenosis
D) Aortic stenosis
E) Bicuspid aortic valve

13. A 10-year-old girl with no significant past medical history presents to your office with a chief complaint of fever and is diagnosed with influenza. During her physical examination, you note a mid-systolic 3/6 low pitch vibratory murmur heard best at the left lower sternal border. The murmur was louder when the girl was lying down than when she was sitting up. Which of the following is the most appropriate next step in the evaluation of this patient's heart murmur?

A) Electrocardiogram
B) Echocardiogram
C) No further evaluation is needed.
D) Cardiology consultation
E) Calculate the arm span-height ratio.

14. Which of the following syndrome-congenital heart defect pairings is incorrect?

A) Trisomy 21—endocardial cushion defect
B) Fetal alcohol syndrome—ventricular septal defect
C) Turner syndrome—coarctation of the aorta
D) Marfan syndrome—transposition of the great vessels
E) DiGeorge syndrome—conotruncal defects

15. Compromised patients with which of the following cyanotic congenital heart lesions will not improve and may even worsen with administration of prostaglandin E_1?

A) Hypoplastic left heart syndrome
B) Interrupted aortic arch
C) Tricuspid atresia
D) Transposition of the great arteries
E) Total anomalous pulmonary venous return

16. You are examining a 1-month-old infant during her routine health maintenance visit. Her mother states that she is doing well at home, and a review of her chart confirms that she continues to gain weight and length along her growth curves. Her cardiac examination is significant for a continuous "machinery" murmur best heard in the left infraclavicular area. There is no widening of the pulse pressures. Palmar pulses are absent. Which of the following is most likely to be the cause of this patient's murmur?

A) Patent ductus arteriosus
B) Venous hum
C) Peripheral pulmonic stenosis
D) Still's murmur
E) Coarctation of the aorta

17. A 17-year-old adolescent presents to the emergency department with fever, malaise, night sweats, abdominal pain, and vomiting. Track marks are noted on both his arms, and the patient admits to shooting heroin on a regular basis. The patient is diagnosed with infective endocarditis. Empiric antibiotic therapy should provide coverage against which of the following organisms?

A) *Pseudomonas aeruginosa*
B) *Serratia marcescens*
C) *Staphylococcus aureus*
D) A and B
E) A, B, and C

18. An 8-year-old boy in your practice was diagnosed with group A streptococcal pharyngitis 3 weeks ago following a positive rapid antigen test. He presents today with fever and significant pain in his left knee and right wrist. His temperature in the office is 39.0°C, with a heart rate of 120 beats per minute, respiratory rate 28 breaths per minute, and stable blood pressure. A serpentine, slightly raised erythematous rash is noted on his trunk and extremities. The remainder of the examination is significant for a well-nourished, well-developed male with normal cardiac and lung findings and tenderness of the left knee and right wrist without erythema, warmth, or swelling. Which of the following tests is indicated in the further assessment of this patient?

A) Antistreptolysin titers
B) AntiDNAse B titers
C) Echocardiography
D) Pharyngeal culture for group A *Streptococcus*
E) Electrocardiography

19. A 15-year-old previously healthy adolescent presents to the urgent care center where you are working with a 1 week history of malaise and intermittent vomiting. His vital signs in the office are as follows: temperature 38.0°C; heart rate 90 beats per minute; respiratory rate 40 breaths per minute; blood pressure 80/50 mm Hg. The examination is significant for diaphoresis, rales in the lower lungs fields bilaterally, a palpable liver edge three finger-breadths below the right costal margin, weak peripheral pulses, and a heart rate too rapid to count on cardiac auscultation. This patient's tachycardia is most likely secondary to which of the following?

A) Acute hypovolemia
B) Atrial septal defect
C) Coronary arteritis
D) Supraventricular tachycardia
E) Pericardial effusion

20. A 4-year-old patient with a history of recent gastroenteritis presents to the emergency department with complaints of intermittent vomiting, abdominal discomfort, and "just not looking right," according to his parents. The triage nurse palpates irregular peripheral pulses, but the cardiac monitor demonstrates narrow complex sinus tachycardia. His physical examination is significant for tachypnea, rales in the lung bases bilaterally, diminished heart sounds, jugular venous pulsations, and pulsus paradoxus. Which of the following interventions is indicated to address this patient's signs and symptoms?

A) Thoracentesis with placement of a chest tube
B) Pericardiocentesis
C) External cardiac pacing
D) Intravenous adenosine
E) Intravenous epinephrine

21. A 9-year-old girl with dilated cardiomyopathy is on maximal pharmacologic intervention for her congestive heart failure. The development of cardiogenic pulmonary edema necessitates intubation and mechanical ventilation. Despite this additional respiratory support, arterial oxygenation saturation slowly but steadily declines over the next several hours. Breaths sounds are equal bilaterally, and no pneumothorax is noted on portable chest radiograph. Which of the following changes in ventilatory settings will be most effective in improving this patient's oxygenation?

A) Increasing positive end expiratory pressure
B) Increasing respiratory rate
C) Decreasing tidal volume
D) Decreasing inspiratory time
E) Decreasing mean airway pressure

22. A previously well 16-year-old adolescent presents to the emergency department with a 3-day history of cough and rhinorrhea, followed by progressive "breathlessness" over the past few hours. His temperature is elevated to 38.3°C, and he is tachypneic and tachycardic. The physical examination is significant for weak peripheral pulses and prolonged capillary refill. Extremities are cool. Jugular venous distensions are noted. Inspiration produces a 15 mm Hg drop in systolic blood pressure compared with pressure during expiration. This patient's clinical manifestations are most consistent with which of the following conditions?

A) Hypertrophic cardiomyopathy
B) Pericardial tamponade
C) Infectious pericarditis
D) Inflammatory pericarditis
E) Myocardial infarction

23. A 13-year-old girl who is trying out for the middle school track team faints during practice and is transported to the emergency department by ambulance. A coach who witnessed the event states that she remained unconscious for "less than a minute" and was responsive and appropriate upon "waking." Vital signs are stable in the emergency department. An electrocardiogram is obtained and pictured below. This patient's syncope most likely resulted from which of the following? (See next page.)

A) First-degree heart block
B) Wolff-Parkinson-White syndrome
C) Prolonged QT syndrome
D) Second-degree heart block, Mobitz type I
E) Second-degree heart block, Mobitz type II

24. A newborn infant has a persistent ventricular heart rate of 50 to 70 beats per minute. An EKG is obtained (see next page). This patient's arrhythmia is most likely related to the presence of which of the following in the mother?

A) LE cells
B) Antiphospholipid antibodies

C) Anti-Sm antibody
D) Anti-Ro and anti-La antibodies
E) Anti-nuclear antibody

25. A 5-month-old infant presents to the emergency department for evaluation of his irritability. He was well until about 3 hours ago, when he suddenly became fussy. Attempts to feed the infant are disrupted by tachypnea. At presentation, the patient is afebrile, with vital signs as follows: heart rate 240 beats per minute (by monitor); respiratory rate 60 beats per minute; blood pressure 76/45 mm/Hg. Oxygen saturation is 96% to 98% on room air. The physical examination is significant for an irritable, pale infant with palpable pulses in all four extremities and prolonged capillary refill time. The cardiac monitor demonstrates tachycardia with a narrow QRS complex. Which of the following interventions is indicated in this patient?
A) Endotracheal intubation and instillation of 1:10,000 epinephrine
B) External DC cardioversion
C) Carotid massage
D) Adenosine via intravenous drip
E) Adenosine via intravenous push

ANSWERS

1. A	10. E	19. D
2. B	11. A	20. B
3. C	12. B	21. A
4. D	13. C	22. B
5. E	14. D	23. C
6. A	15. E	24. D
7. B	16. A	25. E
8. C	17. E	
9. D	18. C	

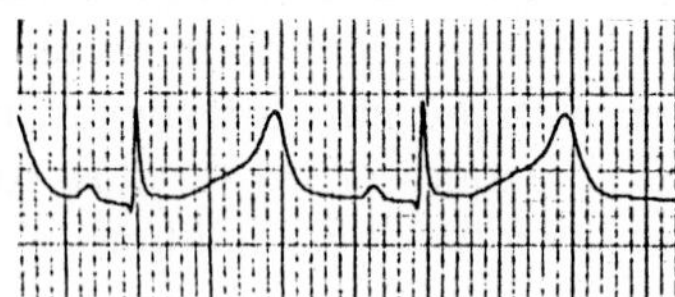

Strip for Question 23

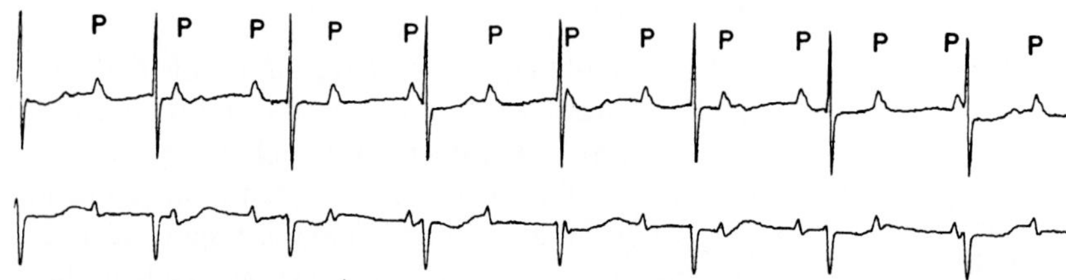

Strip for Question 24

Disorders of the Blood and Neoplastic Disorders

15

ANEMIA

Anemia is defined as a hemoglobin concentration (or hematocrit), which is two or more standard deviations below the mean for age and gender. Mean hemoglobin and hematocrit levels and normal ranges are provided in Table 15-1. Anemia may be categorized as primarily normocytic, microcytic, macrocytic, or hemolytic. As a group, microcytic conditions comprise the majority of childhood anemia. Screening studies, which along with history and physical examination findings help differentiate among the different disorders, are listed in Table 15-2. All are widely available and relatively inexpensive. Figure 15-1 provides an algorithm summarizing a practical approach to the evaluation of anemia in the pediatric patient.

Normocytic Anemia

Transient Erythroblastopenia of Childhood

Transient erythroblastopenia of childhood (TEC) is an acquired, transient red cell aplasia resulting from bone marrow suppression. Although the etiology is unknown, the condition is often preceded by a viral illness. TEC occurs most commonly in young children beyond the age of 12 months. Fatigue and progressive pallor may be the only presenting features, but many patients are also found to have tachypnea and tachycardia related to the anemia. Screening studies are consistent with a severe normocytic anemia and reticulocytopenia in the absence of other hematologic and biochemical abnormalities. Transfusion is indicated for patients with hemoglobin concentrations <5 g per dL. The vast majority of affected children recover without complication.

Anemia of Chronic Disease

Anemia is often associated with chronic disease (inflammatory bowel disease, renal failure, juvenile idiopathic arthritis, malignancy). Patients with anemia of chronic disease typically have normal body stores of iron but are unable to mobilize it and generate sufficient red blood cells. The cells are typically normocytic, but a minority of patients have microcytic anemia. The hemoglobin concentration normalizes upon resolution of the underlying illness.

Microcytic Anemia

Microcytic anemia is often asymptomatic, discovered incidentally on a routine screen or complete blood count obtained for other purposes. The two most common causes of microcytic anemia are iron deficiency anemia and thalassemia minor.

TABLE 15-1
HEMATOLOGIC MEANS AND NORMAL RANGES BASED ON AGE

	Hemoglobin (g/dL)		Hematocrit (%)		MCV		WBC		Percentage Neutrophils
Age	Mean	Range	Mean	Range	Mean	Lowest Acceptable	Mean	Range	Mean
Term infant	16.7	13.6 to 20.0	55	43 to 65	110	>102	18.1	9 to 30	60 (range 40 to 80)
1 month	14	10 to 18	43	31 to 53	104	85	10.8	5 to 19.5	35
6 to 24 months	12	10.5 to 13.5	36	33 to 39	78	70	11.3	6 to 17.5	33
2 to 6 years	12.5	11.5 to 13.5	37	34 to 40	81	75	9.5	5.5 to 15.7	50
6 to 12 years	13.2	11.0 to 16.0	39	35 to 40	86	76	8.3	4.5 to 14	54
>12 years (M)ale (F)emale	M 15 F 14	M 14 to 18 F 12 to 16	M 45 F 41	M 35 to 47 F 36 to 45	80	78	7.6	4.7 to 11	60

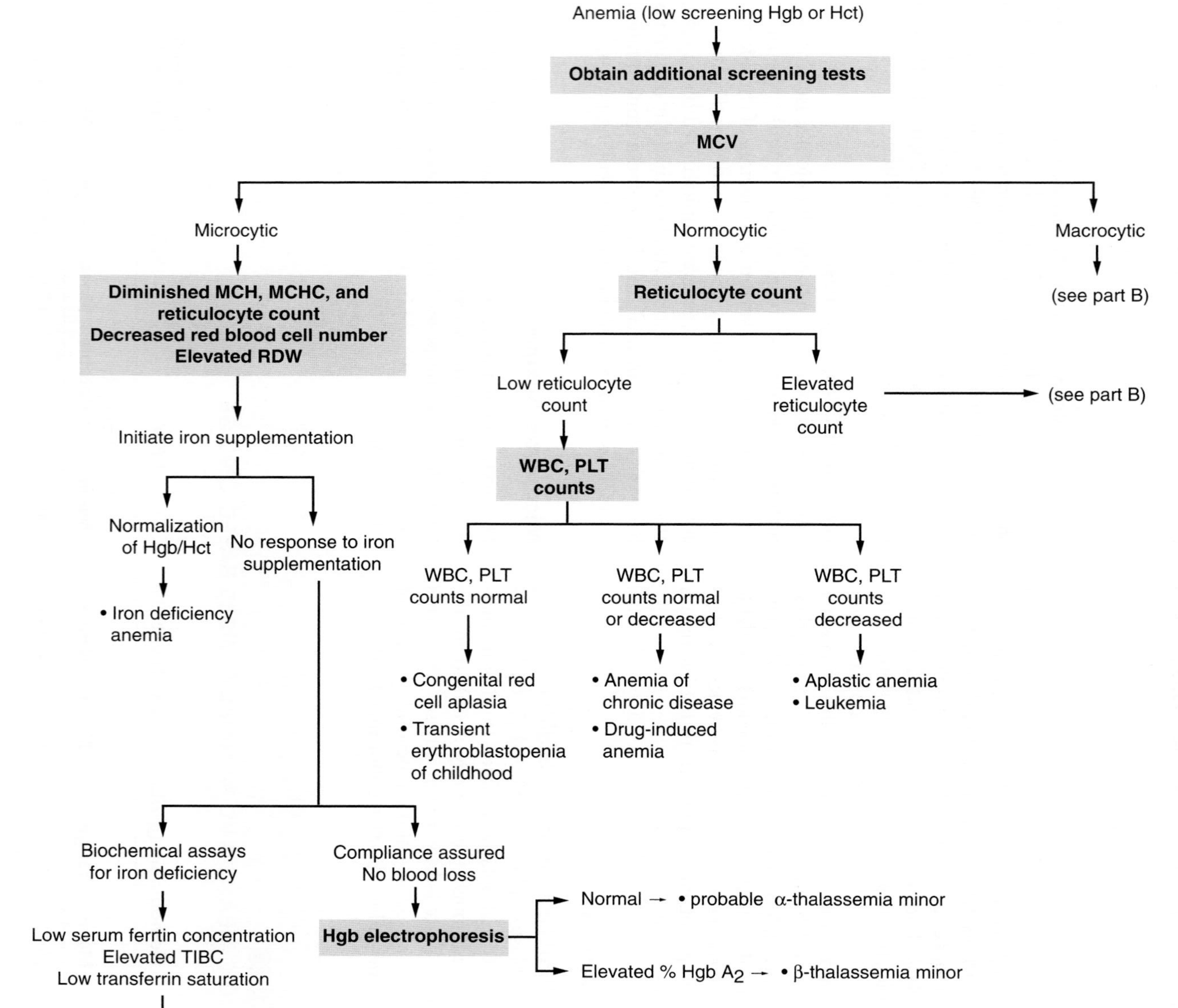

Figure 15-1 Evaluation of anemia beyond the neonatal period.

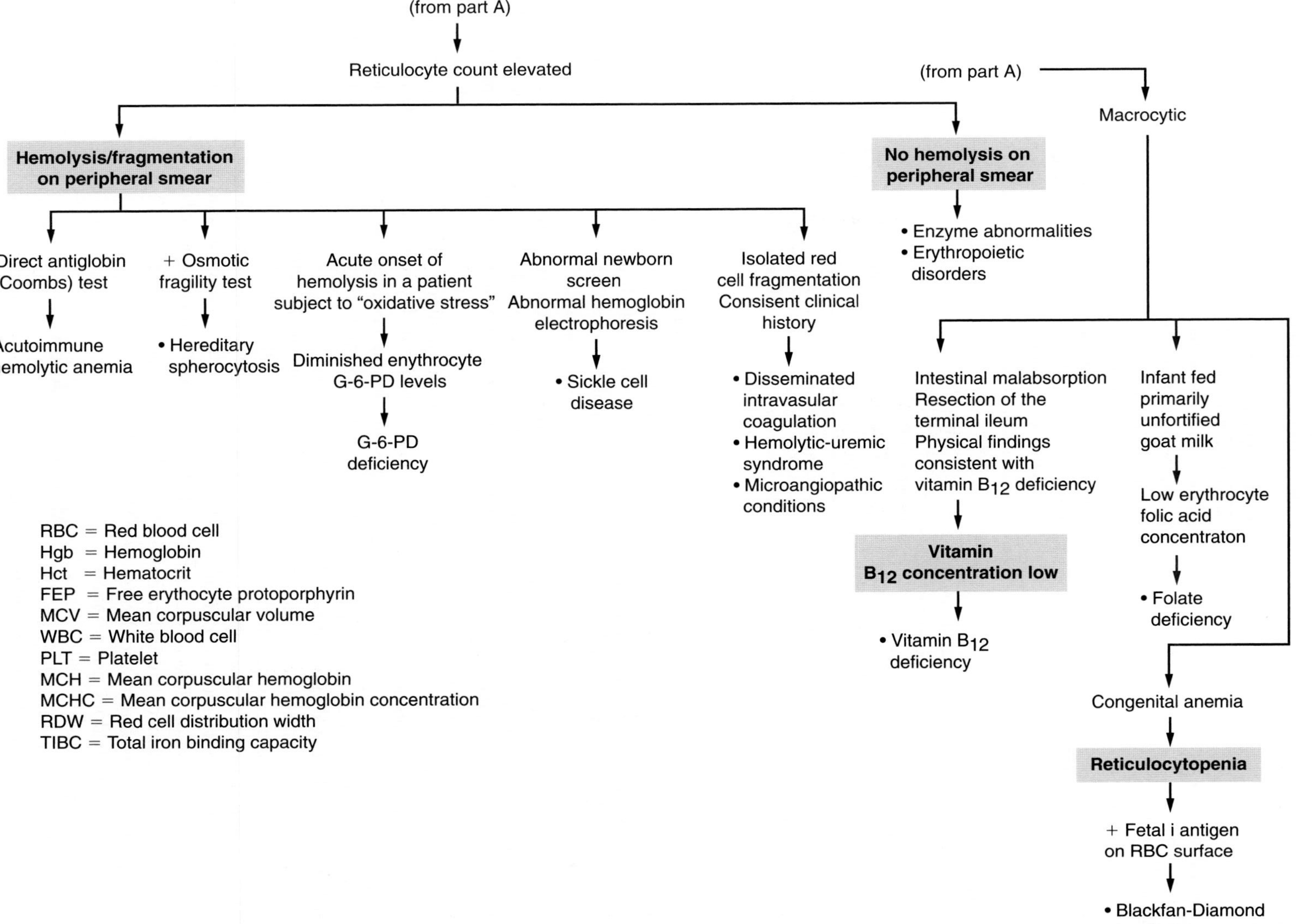

Figure 15-1 *(continued)*

TABLE 15-2
ANEMIA: SCREENING TESTS

Complete blood count (CBC) and differential
Red blood cell indices
- Mean corpuscular volume (MCV)
- Mean corpuscular hemoglobin (MCH)
- Mean corpuscular hemoglobin concentration (MCHC)
- Red cell distribution width (RDW)

Reticulocyte count
Peripheral blood smear

Iron-Deficiency Anemia

As noted in Chapter 2, the timely diagnosis and management of iron deficiency anemia is of great importance in growing children. Iron deficiency is associated with cognitive impairment, poor school performance, and behavior problems, even prior to the onset of anemia. The most common cause of iron deficiency is poor diet; iron deficiency is the major nutritional deficit of American youths. Chronic blood loss (e.g., gastrointestinal bleeding or heavy menses) can result in decreased iron stores and anemia; ongoing bleeding should be suspected in the patient with iron deficiency anemia who is consuming a normal diet or does not respond to iron supplementation. Infants and toddlers who consume large amounts of cow milk are prone to anemia for several reasons: cow milk is low in iron, and the iron in cow milk is poorly absorbed; excessive cow milk is filling and discourages the intake of other, iron-rich foods; the calcium in milk interferes with iron absorption; and intake in an individual with cow protein allergy results in gastrointestinal blood loss.

Laboratory changes consistent with iron deficiency anemia are provided in Table 15-3.

Once the diagnosis has been made, oral iron replacement therapy is initiated at 6 mg/kg/day divided into two or three doses. Intravenous and intramuscular routes are not appropriate. Adverse effects of iron therapy include nausea, stomach cramping, and diarrhea or constipation. Supplements should be taken with fruit or juices containing vitamin C, which increases absorption. Repeat studies 10 to 14 days after initiation of treatment are indicated to document increasing reticulocyte count and hemoglobin concentrations. Anemia which does not respond following a month of iron therapy warrants further investigation. Non-compliance and continued bleeding are the most common causes of treatment failure. Improvement is temporary unless predisposing conditions are addressed (bleeding, excessive milk intake, poor diet). Oral iron supplements should be continued at least two months beyond normalization of the hemoglobin concentration in order to replete body iron stores.

TABLE 15-3
LABORATORY EVIDENCE OF IRON DEFICIENCY ANEMIA

Hematologic screening results
- ↓ mean corpuscular volume
- ↓ mean corpuscular hemoglobin
- ↑ red cell distribution width
- ↓ reticulocyte count
- ↓ red blood cell number
- ↓ mean cell hemoglobin

In the case of a questionable history or insufficient response to iron therapy, consider:

Biochemical studies (can detect iron deficiency prior to the onset of anemia)

Serum ferritin concentration (↓)*
Total iron binding capacity (↑)
Transferrin saturation (↓)
Free erythrocyte protoporphyrin (↑, but also elevated in lead poisoning)

*Serum ferritin is an acute phase reactant. It is the first laboratory value to become abnormal when iron deficiency is present; however, it also becomes elevated in the setting of infection and inflammation, even when iron stores are low.

Thalassemia minor is an inherited defect of globin chain synthesis, which is most common in people of Southeast Asian, Mediterranean, and African ancestry. Although technically a hemolytic disease, α-thalassemia minor is touched on here because it is similar in presentation to iron deficiency anemia. The presence of two defective α-globin chains (out of four) results in a mild hypochromic microcytic anemia, which does not respond to iron supplementation. Affected patients are asymptomatic, and most maintain hemoglobin concentrations within or just below the low-normal range. Alpha-thalassemia trait is primarily a diagnosis of exclusion, although genetic testing is available to confirm the defect. Hemoglobin electrophoresis is normal in these patients.

Beta-thalassemia minor produces a mild hemolytic anemia. The presentation is virtually identical to that of α-thalassemia minor, although evidence of hemolysis may be impressive on the peripheral smear. Hemoglobin electrophoresis demonstrates an elevated percentage (5% to 7%) of hemoglobin A_2, composed of two α-chains and two delta-chains.

Macrocytic Anemia

Macrocytic anemia is uncommon in children. The development of megaloblastic anemia is related to deficiency of vitamin B_{12} or folic acid (inadequate intake or impaired absorption).

Deficiency in vitamin B_{12} can result from several different mechanisms:

- Dietary deficiency, as may occur in an infant who is exclusively breastfed by a strictly vegan mother
- Impaired gastric or small bowel absorption, due to surgical resection or malabsorption that affects the terminal ileum
- Bacterial overgrowth of the terminal ileum
- Insufficient intrinsic factor (pernicious anemia)

A deficiency due to pernicious anemia can be congenital or autoimmune.Vitamin B_{12}-deficient individuals may initially present with glossitis, paresthesias, and/or peripheral neuropathies. Hypersegmented neutrophils are present in the peripheral blood. The criteria for diagnosis include a consistent dietary, surgical, or disease history; sub-normal serum B_{12} concentration; and positive response to treatment. Intramuscular vitamin B_{12} results in rapid resolution of the megaloblastic bone marrow and normalization of the hemoglobin concentration within 1 to 2 months.

Megaloblastic anemia resulting from folate deficiency is less common that that from inadequate vitamin B_{12}. Infants fed primarily unfortified goat milk are at risk for folate deficiency resulting in anemia. The primary laboratory tests available for the confirmation of folate deficiency are the serum and (preferably) erythrocyte folic acid concentrations. In considering treatment for folate deficiency, it is important to document adequate vitamin B_{12} levels, because the longer vitamin B_{12} deficient-anemia persists without treatment, the higher the risk of neurologic complications (ataxia, posterior spinal column degeneration).

Diamond-Blackfan syndrome (congenital hypoplastic anemia) is a rare inherited insensitivity to erythropoietin which presents in infancy with macrocytic anemia and reticulocytopenia. One in four patients also has associated anomalies of the facial features (micrognathia), thumbs, and/or heart. The diagnosis is confirmed through hemoglobin electrophoresis (elevated hemoglobin F) and detection of fetal i antigen on the red blood cells. Diamond-Blackfan syndrome is managed with long-term corticosteroid therapy and/or chronic transfusions; bone marrow transplantation is curative.

Hemolytic Anemia

Autoimmune Hemolytic Anemia

Autoimmune hemolytic anemia (AIHA) should be considered part of the differential diagnosis in any child presenting with the characteristic signs and symptoms of hemolytic anemia [pallor, scleral icterus/jaundice, splenomegaly, fatigue, abdominal pain, and (occasionally) dark urine]. The condition often follows a nonspecific viral illness. In AIHA, the red blood cells become coated with antibody (usually IgG) and/or complement, and are then destroyed in the spleen. Screening studies reveal a normochromic, normocytic anemia, reticulocytosis, and normal white blood cell and platelet numbers. Microspherocytes, polychromasia, and nucleated red blood cells are noted on the peripheral smear. AIHA is the only hemolytic condition resulting in a positive direct antiglobin (Coombs) test. Patients with mild disease recover spontaneously and require no treatment. Corticosteroids are indicated for patients with moderate anemia who are hemodynamically stable. Transfusion is problematic in these patients and should only be undertaken in consultation with a hematologic specialist.

Hereditary Spherocytosis

Hereditary spherocytosis is the most common inherited disorder of the red cell membrane. Multiple variations of the gene are recognized, accounting for substantial variation in presentation. Defective red cells cannot maintain the natural shape, instead becoming spherical and less deformable. Abnormal cells are destroyed in the spleen, leading to the classic presentation of anemia, jaundice, splenomegaly, and chronic hemolysis.

Most patients with mild-to-moderate disease remain asymptomatic and require no specific treatment. Severe disease is defined by a hemoglobin concentration ≤8g per dL. Hereditary spherocytosis should be considered part of the differential in any of the following clinical scenarios:

- A neonate with jaundice appearing in the first 24 hours of life
- A neonate with persistent jaundice
- A child with exercise intolerance, poor growth, and/or academic difficulties
- An older child with cholecystitis and bilirubin stones
- Any patient with laboratory evidence of hemolytic anemia (elevated unconjugated bilirubin, elevated lactate dehydrogenase, depressed haptoglobin)

Results of initial screening tests include low hemoglobin levels, elevated reticulocyte counts, and increased mean cell hemoglobin concentrations. The peripheral smear is significant for the presence of small, spherical red blood cells with no central pallor. The osmotic fragility test is useful in patients older than 1 year of age; increased fragility is consistent with hereditary spherocytosis.

Children with hereditary spherocytosis require regular visits to monitor growth, development, spleen size, complete blood count, and reticulocyte count. A reticulocyte count which is suppressed in the presence of anemia may be due to iron or folic acid deficiency. Parents should be instructed to seek medical attention at the first sign of increasing pallor or jaundice. Pallor may precede the development of severe anemia due to aplastic crisis, most commonly resulting from infection with parvovirus B19, which suppresses red cell production. Progressive jaundice is a sign of increased hemolysis.

Red cell transfusions and splenectomy may be indicated in patients with severe disease or complications. Transfusions can benefit patients with acute exacerbation of their anemia due to traumatic bleeding or hypersplenism. Splenectomy should be considered for patients with severe anemia, extramedullary hematopoisis, poor growth, and fatigue which significantly interferes with activities of daily living. The procedure results in significant improvement in anemia and jaundice but increases the risk of serious infection with encapsulated bacteria. If possible, removal is delayed until children are at least 5 years old. Patients scheduled for surgery should be vaccinated against *Streptococcus pneumoniae*, *Haemophilus influenzae*, and *Neisseria meningitidis* at least several weeks prior to splenectomy, if possible.

Glucose-6-Phosphate Dehydrogenase Deficiency

Glucose-6-phosphate dehydrogenase (G-6-PD) deficiency is an X-linked red cell enzyme defect with an increased prevalence in black (A^-), Asian, and Mediterranean (Med) populations. The half-life of G-6-PD is decreased to weeks in A^--variant disease and hours in Med-variant deficiency. G-6-PD is instrumental in protecting the red cell against oxidative stress, which may accompany infection or the ingestion of certain medications (sulfonamides, nitrofurantoin, some anti-malarials, aspirin, chloramphenicol, dimercaprol), toxins (naphthalene in mothballs), and foods (fava beans).

G-6-PD deficiency should be considered in neonates (particularly those of the ethnicities listed above) under the following circumstances:

- Jaundice in the first 24 hours of life
- Jaundice despite exclusive ingestion of formula
- Jaundice associated with a fall in hematocrit
- Jaundice which is poorly responsive to phototherapy

Older infants and children remain asymptomatic until placed under oxidative stress, whereupon they develop jaundice, hyperbilirubinemia, pallor, and anemia, which may be severe enough to result in heart failure. During an acute hemolytic event, red cell G-6-PD results may be normal (false negative) in patients with A^- disease, given that older cells with lower levels of the enzyme are destroyed before newer cells and reticulocytes. The diagnosis is confirmed through laboratory demonstration of low erythrocyte G-6-PD levels at least 2 months after an episode of hemolysis. Patients should avoid exposures that prompt hemolysis whenever possible.

Sickle Cell Disease

Sickle cell disease (SCD) is an autosomal recessive disorder of beta-chain synthesis. Black and Hispanic populations have the highest prevalence of disease. Beta-chain hemoglobinopathies are detected on newborn screens in most states. Children usually become symptomatic in the latter half of the first year of life. The major clinical manifestations of SCD (Table 15-4) are related to:

- occlusion of the microvasculature by sickled cells
- chronic anemia due to ongoing hemolysis
- increased susceptibility to infections

TABLE 15-4
CLINICAL MANIFESTATIONS OF SICKLE CELL DISEASE

Infants Older than 6 Months of Age and Toddlers

- Splenomegaly (resolves with time as spleen becomes progressively fibrotic)
- Dactylitis (painful swelling of the hands and/or feet)
- Overwhelming infection with encapsulated bacteria (*Streptococcus pneumoniae*, *Haemophilus influenzae*, *Neisseria meningitidis*) or *Salmonella* sp.
- Vaso-occlusive crises
- Scleral icterus, pallor

Children and Adolescents

- Vaso-occlusive ("pain") crises :most common in the bones, joints, and muscles of the limbs and back
  :also occur in the abdomen (mesenteric sickling) and lungs
  :may be triggered by dehydration, cold weather, or infection, but usually no identifiable precipitating event
  :patient is in obvious pain, with tenderness at the involved site on physical examination
- Acute chest syndrome :infarction or infection of the lung preceded by sickling
  :presents with acute onset of severe chest pain, cough, hypoxemia, and chest infiltrates
  :characterized by focal signs on lung auscultation
- Stroke :vaso-occlusion of tributaries of the internal carotid, anterior cerebral, or middle cerebral arteries
  :transient ischemic events and strokes present with neurologic signs
  :periodic transcranial Doppler imaging is indicated in all patients with SCD
- Priapism :intermittent or prolonged
- Sequestration crisis :red cell trapping within the spleen associated with impressive splenic enlargement
  :presents with rapid onset of severe anemia, often accompanied by cardiovascular instability
  :anemia requires emergent treatment with intravascular fluids and/or blood transfusion
- Aplastic crisis :temporary failure of erythropoiesis following infection with parvovirus B19 (or, less commonly, other viruses)
  :presents with increasing pallor; progressive, severe anemia with no associated reticulocytosis
  :may be accompanied by cardiovascular instability, necessitating emergent treatment with intravascular fluids and/or blood transfusion
- Cholelithiasis :chronic hemolysis and hyperbilirubinemia lead to formation of biliary stones
  :presents with right upper quadrant pain and clinical and laboratory manifestations of biliary colic or acute cholecystitis
  :abdominal ultrasonography detects biliary sludge and stone formation

Hemoglobin electrophoresis is the most definitive laboratory study for diagnosing SCD. Most patients with SCD have hemoglobin concentrations in the 6 to 10 g per dL range, with slightly elevated MCV (>80) and elevated reticulocyte counts. Irreversibly sickled cells are evident on the peripheral blood smear; red blood cell sizes and shapes are quite varied, and nucleated erythrocytes are not uncommon.

Patients with SCD are at increased risk of death due to overwhelming bacterial sepsis, which may present suddenly and be rapidly progressive. In fact, infection is the most common cause of death in children with SCD. Oral penicillin prophylaxis is initiated at diagnosis, consisting of 125 mg twice a day until age 3 years, when the dosage is increased to 250 mg twice a day. Vaccination of patients with sickle cell disease is covered in Chapter 3. Individuals with SCD are counseled to seek immediate medical attention if they become febrile. Minimum assessment includes the history and physical examination, complete blood count, and blood cultures. Broad-spectrum antibiotics are administered for two days until culture results become known. Medical intervention is also strongly advised in the event of chest pain or respiratory symptoms, neurologic signs, splenomegaly, pallor, priapism, or severe pain. Pain crises and most vaso-occlusive events are managed with hydration, analgesics, and, if appropriate, admission to the hospital for pain management, supportive care, and possibly transfusion. Chronic transfusion therapy with iron chelation is indicated for patients who have a history of a stroke, high risk for a stroke, recurrent chest syndrome, or frequent and debilitating pain crises. Hydroxyurea has been shown to decrease the incidence of vaso-occlusive events in adults with SCD; it should be initiated only in consultation with an experienced hematologist.

LEUKOCYTE DISORDERS

The hallmark of leukocyte disorders, whether of number or function, is recurrent bacterial infection. Neutropenia is defined below according to the severity of the suppression of the absolute neutrophil count. Abnormal neutrophil function may instead be to blame in children with recurrent significant bacterial illnesses who have normal neutrophil counts.

Quantitative Disorders

Absolute neutrophil counts vary by age. Neutrophils account for about 35% of leukocytes in infancy; this number increases to about 50% at age 2 years and 60% in the adult. The absolute neutrophil count (ANC) is calculated by multiplying the total white blood cell count by the sum of the percentages of segmented cells and bands in the differential. Severity of neutropenia is classified by ANC result:

- ANC of 1,000 to 1,500 per mm^3 constitutes mild neutropenia.
- ANC of 500 to 1,000 per mm^3 constitutes moderate neutropenia.
- aANC <500 per mm^3 constitutes severe neutropenia, which is associated with a significant risk of life-threatening infection.

Infections that are more common in patients with neutropenia include cutaneous and soft tissue infections (cellulitis, abscesses, or furuncles); mucosal lesions (stomatitis, perirectal infections); otitis media; pneumonia; and sepsis. Patients with neutropenia may become infected with their own skin, respiratory tract, and bowel flora, particularly *Staphylococcus aureus* and gram-negative organisms. They are also more likely to become colonized with nosocomial pathogens. Infected patients who are neutropenic often have blunting of the inflammatory response, with diminished evidence of fever, erythema, purulence, or exudate; this can make localization of disease difficult. Neutropenia does not appear to disproportionately predispose children to viral, fungal, or parasitic disease. Isolated, mild neutropenia may present with persistent gingivitis or mucosal ulcerations rather than overwhelming infection.

Neutropenia may be congenital or acquired, chronic or acute and self-limited (Table 15-5). Patients with acquired neutropenia due to malignancy or chemotherapy are especially susceptible to bacterial sepsis, which is the most common cause of death in these patients. Overwhelming bacterial sepsis may precipitate neutropenia (and/or thrombocytopenia) in an otherwise competent neonate or young infant; in fact, one or both of these laboratory abnormalities may be the presenting sign(s) of infection.

Recombinant human granulocyte colony-stimulating factor (rhG-CSF) is successful in raising neutrophil counts in patients with myelosuppression secondary to chemotherapy; drug-induced neutropenia which does not resolve upon discontinuation of the drug; autoimmune neutropenia of infancy; and disorders of proliferation and maturation of myeloid stem cells (cyclic neutropenia, severe congenital neutropenia, common variable immune deficiencies, Shwachman-Diamond syndrome). Disorders of neutrophil function (e.g., chronic granulomatous disease) do not respond to rhG-CSF administration.

Qualitative Disorders

Chronic granulomatous disease is discussed in Chapter 9.

PLATELET DISORDERS

Petechiae, purpura, and abnormal bleeding are the presenting features of both quantitative and qualitative platelet disorders. Excessive, persistent, or spontaneous bleeding, discussed in detail below (see "Coagulation Disorders"), is usually related to platelet or clotting factor abnormalities. Platelets, clotting factors, and characteristics of the vasculature prevent extravasation of blood from the vessel; disorders of any of these three may result in petechiae and/or purpura. However, petechiae and particularly purpura may

TABLE 15-5
CAUSES OF NEUTROPENIA

Chronic Idiopathic Neutropenia of Childhood
- Persistence of absolute neutrophil counts <1,000 mm^3 (often <500 mm^3)
- Severity of infections varies; many patients do not appear to have increased susceptibility
- Diagnosed through serial neutrophil counts, bone marrow examination (adequate numbers of erythroid, myeloid, and platelet precursors)

Cyclic Neutropenia
- Rare autosomal dominant disorder of regular episodic periods of neutropenia
- Cycles average 21 days in length, with a 3 to 10 day period of symptomatic neutropenia
- Diagnosed through serial neutrophil counts, bone marrow examination (arrest of maturation of granulocytes during neutropenic phase)
- Treated with recombinant human granulocyte colony-stimulating factor

Severe Congenital Neutropenia
- Rare sporadic disorder of severe persistent neutropenia (<300/mm^3)
- High incidence of severe infections beginning in the first month of life
- Bone marrow biopsy demonstrates arrested terminal differentiation of myeloid precursors
- Treated with recombinant human granulocyte colony-stimulating factor and/or bone marrow transplantation
- May convert to acute myelogenous leukemia

Immune Neutropenia
- Neonatal alloimmune neutropenia occurs when maternally-derived antibody interacts with paternally-derived antigens on the neutrophil; the ANC normalizes over several weeks
- Neonatal autoimmune neutropenia is secondary to granulocyte-specific antibodies generated by the infant; resolves over the first few years of life
- Diagnosis rests on antibody detection

Drug-Induced Neutropenia
- Many medications may have isolated neutropenia as a possible adverse reaction
- Examples include carbamazepine and other anticonvulsants, sulfonamides, chloramphenicol, and phenothiazine
- Identified medications should be discontinued if possible, which usually results in resolution of the neutropenia

Neutropenia Associated with Viral Suppression
- Most common cause of transient neutropenia in children
- More commonly associated with Epstein-Barr virus, influenza, hepatitis a and b, measles, rubella, varicella, and respiratory syncytial virus
- Onset in the first 1 to 2 days of illness; duration 3 to 7 days
- Resolves spontaneously with no significant complications; however, repeat complete blood count and differential two weeks later advised to document recovery

Neutropenia Associated with Malignancy
- Invasion of the bone marrow
- Myelosuppressive chemotherapy

be caused by disease primarily involving other systems. Petechiae or purpura in the setting of normal or elevated platelet counts indicates one of the following:

- Trauma
- Viral infection
- Prolonged crying or vigorous coughing (petechiae on face only)
- Defective platelet aggregation (inherited, drug-induced)
- Vasculitis (leukocytoclastic vasculitis; acute hemorrhagic edema of infancy; polyarteritis nodosa)

Leukocytoclastic vasculitis (acute hemorrhagic edema of infancy) is an inflammatory vasculitis of the small vessels. Antibodies deposited in the vascular walls incite an inflammatory cascade which increases permeability, resulting in localized areas of petechiae and purpura. Acute hemorrhagic edema of infancy is rare; when it occurs, it is typically seen in patients younger than 3 years of age.

Polyarteritis nodosa is a rare disorder characterized by necrotizing inflammation of small- and medium-sized arteries of the skin, muscles, organs, and central nervous system. The diagnosis is based on clinical presentation and supportive biopsy results.

Thrombocytopenia is defined as a platelet count less than the normal range of 150 to 400 × 10^3/mcL. A partial differential diagnosis of thrombocytopenia is provided in Table 15-6. When an ill-appearing child presents with thrombocytopenia and petechiae/purpura, conditions to consider include:

- infection—*Neisseria meningitidis, Neisseria gonorrhoeae* (and various other bacteria); Rocky Mountain spotted fever
- disseminated intravascular coagulation/purpura fulminans
- hemolytic-uremic syndrome
- malignancy
- aplasia

TABLE 15-6
DIFFERENTIAL DIAGNOSIS OF THROMBOCYTOPENIA

Neonatal Thrombocytopenia

Bacterial sepsis (infection-induced thrombocytopenia)

Congenital viral infection (most notably cytomegalovirus)

Neonatal alloimmune thrombocytopenia

- Platelets are destroyed after being coated by maternally-derived antibody specific for antigens on the infant's platelets.
- Resolves slowly over several weeks

Thrombocytopenia-absent radius syndrome (congenital amegakaryocytic thrombocytopenia)

- May be autosomal recessive
- Associated with abnormalities of the carpal bones and phalanges, clubbed hands, and/or phocomelia
- Thumbs are usually *present.*
- Thrombocytopenia is severe ($<$10 to 15 $\times$ 10^3/mcL), resulting in spontaneous hemorrhage, which, when intracranial, is the most serious complication of the disease.
- Platelet levels typically normalize by 2 years of age.
- Management consists of platelet transfusions to maintain level in excess of 10 to 15 $\times$ 10^3/mcL, and avoidance of trauma and elective surgery.

Fanconi anemia

- Persistent aplastic anemia
- Most patients exhibit congenital anomalies of the distal upper extremity or genitourinary system.
- Physical features include hyperpigmentation of the skin; short stature; upper limb anomalies (absent, hypoplastic, supernumerary, or bifid thumbs and aplasia of the first metacarpal or the radius); hypogonadism; and microcephaly.
- Bone marrow transplantation is curative.
- Prenatal diagnosis should be offered to parents.

Maternal drug exposure

- Medications include quinine, thiazide, hydralazine, tolbutamide, heparin, vancomycin.

Venous thrombosis due to long-term indwelling vascular catheter

Childhood Thrombocytopenia

Immune thrombocytopenic purpura

- Most common in children ages 2 to 10 years
- Presents in an otherwise healthy child with bruises, purpura, petechiae
- Clinical diagnosis; thrombocytopenia is isolated and usually not terribly low
- Patient should avoid medication known to suppress platelet function (sulfonamides, valproic acid, aspirin).
- Patient should limit physical activity (no contact sports until platelet count exceeds 50 $\times$ 10^3/mcL).
- Patient must promptly seek medical attention for fever, bleeding (mucous membranes), or head or abdominal trauma.
- Most cases resolve within 6 months with no serious complications.
- Thrombocytopenia that lasts longer than 6 months requires referral to a hematologist for further evaluation/management.
- If the platelet count falls to less than 20 $\times$ 10^3/mcL, or there is extended cutaneous bleeding, mucous membrane bleeding, or surgery, treat with corticosteroids, intravenous immunoglobulin, or anti-d immunoglobulin.

Henoch-Schönlein purpura

- IgA-mediated systemic vasculitis of small vessels of the skin, gastrointestinal tract, joints, and kidneys
- Cutaneous lesions (purpura) concentrated in the dependent areas
- Begins as erythematous macules/papules, progressing to palpable purpura on the lower extremities and buttocks (dependent areas) within days
- Abdominal and/or joint pain
- Patient has low-grade or no fever; does not appear systemically ill.

Wiskott-Aldrich syndrome

- X-linked recessive disorder
- Classic presentation includes thrombocytopenia, eczema, and immunodeficiency.

Kasabach-Merritt syndrome

- Rare disorder which typically presents in early infancy
- Consumptive thrombocytopenia due to an enlarging vascular tumor

Medications

- Chemotherapeutic agents, chloramphenicol, phenylbutazone, gold, and valproic acid may all cause isolated thrombocytopenia.

Broad-spectrum antibiotic coverage (i.e., vancomycin plus ceftriaxone) is indicated in patients older than three months of age with petechiae, palpable purpura, and fever due to the possibility of life-threatening infection. Once the pathogenic organism has been isolated and susceptibilities identified, coverage can be narrowed.

PANCYTOPENIA

Pancytopenia, defined as a shortage of red blood cells, white blood cells, and platelets, is due to bone marrow suppression or failure. Clinically, pancytopenia is suggested by physical signs and symptoms associated with disruption of least two of the following:

- Erythroid cell lines (anemia)—pallor, general fatigue, easy fatigability, weakness
- Myeloid cell lines (neutropenia)—increased susceptibility to infection
- Megakaryocytic cell lines (thrombocytopenia)—easy bruising, purpura, epistaxis

Bone marrow suppression may be associated with any of the following conditions:

- Viral infection
- Aplastic anemia (autoimmune or drug-induced)
- Myelofibrosis
- Leukemia
- Malignancies which metastasize to the bone marrow
- Exposure to various drugs, chemicals, and irradiation

Acute Lymphoblastic Leukemia

Acute lymphoblastic leukemia (ALL) is the most common malignancy of childhood. Incidence peaks in children ages 2 to 5 years, although affected patients may be any age. Signs and symptoms may include any combination of the following: fever, malaise, bone and/or joint pain, easy bruising, abdominal pain, lymphadenopathy, and organomegaly (spleen, liver). Half of patients with ALL have a white blood count $<10 \times 10^3$/mcL at diagnosis; only 20% have a white blood count $>50 \times 10^3$/mcL. While depression in at least two cell lines is usually noted, affected children may present with isolated disruption of a single cell line. Bone marrow biopsy is required for diagnosis; lymphoblasts are usually noted on the peripheral smear, but absence of blasts in the peripheral blood of a patient with pancytopenia does not rule out the diagnosis of leukemia. This is in stark contrast to the bone marrow results of the patient with aplastic anemia, which may have a very similar presentation to ALL.

Greater than 95% of patients with standard-risk acute lymphoblastic leukemia will enter remission with initial treatment. Children at high risk for relapse (Table 15-7) are treated more aggressively, improving their survival. The relapse rate in ALL is about 20%. While relapse is most frequent in the marrow, the central nervous system and testicles are also common sites of relapse, necessitating regular self-examination of the testicles and periodic CNS imaging.

TABLE 15-7
POOR PROGNOSTIC FACTORS IN ALL

Age older than 10 years or younger than 1 year at diagnosis
White blood count >50,000 per mcL at diagnosis
Mature B-cell leukemia
Cell hypodiploidy
Poor response to induction therapy or early relapse (within 18 months of diagnosis)

Survivors of childhood cancer, including ALL, are at least ten times more likely than their peers to develop a second malignant neoplasm over their lifetimes (beginning about five years after primary therapy). Common associations between initial treatment and subsequent malignancy are provided below:

- Chemotherapy—acute myelogenous leukemia
- Radiation therapy—solid tumors located at the site of irradiation

Cranial irradiation for ALL increases the lifetime risk of solid central nervous system tumors, the most common secondary malignant neoplasm of ALL therapy. The association is stronger in children treated when they are younger than five years, and the risk increases in direct proportion to the amount of radiation received.

Acute myelogenous leukemia (AML) is less common than ALL but has a similar presentation. Exposure to radiation or chemotherapy increases an individual's risk of AML. The incidence of AML peaks in adolescence. AML has a higher relapse rate and lower cure rate than ALL. It is treated with intensive chemotherapy followed by bone marrow transplantation (if available) from an antigen-identical sibling.

COAGULATION DISORDERS

The severity of bleeding or thrombosis among hereditary coagulation disorders is extremely varied due to the myriad of genetic mutations which may occur and, in some cases, variable disease penetrance. Signs of severe congenital factor deficiency in the neonate include excessive or persistent bleeding following circumcision, oozing with umbilical cord separation, and significant scalp or intraventricular hemorrhage. In the older child and adolescent, easy bruising, severe menorrhagia, and severe/persistent/recurrent epistaxis suggest coagulation abnormalities. Bleeding disorders should be suspected in patients with positive family histories, bleeding which requires medical intervention (iron supplementation, transfusion), bleeding from more than one site, persistent bleeding following venipuncture, and spontaneous hemorrhage. Initial screening studies include a complete blood count, prothrombin time, partial thromboplastin time, and bleeding time (Fig. 15-2).

Patients with a strong family history of deep vein thrombosis or pulmonary embolism may be similarly affected with heritable thrombophilia.

Hemophilia

Hemophilia is an X-linked deficiency of factor VIII (*hemophilia A*) or factor IX (*hemophilia B*). Hemophilia A is by far the more common disorder. One third of all cases occurs in patients with no affected family members and represents new mutations. As is true for all X-linked disorders, females born to affected males are obligate carriers; 50% of the male offspring of female carriers will have hemophilia, and 50% of the female offspring will be carriers. Prenatal diagnosis is available. Factor levels are usually abnormal at birth; males with known hemophilia routinely receive factor replacement shortly after delivery to prevent intracranial hemorrhage.

Hemophilia is characterized by recurrent bleeding into soft tissue and joints. Hemorrhaging into the brain, spinal cord, abdomen, or throat is obviously life-threatening, and signs and symptoms which are at all consistent with such should be aggressively managed with factor replacement prior to further evaluation. Significant bleeding into the soft tissue of the limbs may result in compartment syndrome. Repetitive bleeding limited to a specific joint is associated with chronic changes, decreased range of motion, and arthritis.

Factor replacement is indicated for prophylaxis and in the setting of acute bleeding. Viral transmission is no longer a concern with current products, but patients may develop IgG antibodies to the factor for which they are deficient. The goal is to keep patients with moderate disease at 50% or more of normal factor levels. Severe trauma or spontaneous hemorrhage as described above necessitates replacement to 100% of normal factor levels, even (in the case of trauma) in the absence of overt signs of bleeding. Surgery and femoral/jugular venipuncture are contraindicated in patients with hemophilia until factor levels are normalized.

von Willebrand Disease

von Willebrand disease (vWD) is the most common congenital bleeding disorder. Inheritance is autosomal dominant, and severity of bleeding is extremely varied. Most patients develop only mild symptoms. Heavy menstrual bleeding may be the initial presenting feature in adolescent girls. The diagnosis is made through documentation of a positive family and/or clinical history and consistent laboratory results (prolonged bleeding time, normal PT, normal or slightly prolonged PTT, and reduced ristocetin co-factor or von Willebrand factor activity). Studies which are initially normal do not rule out vWD; repetitive testing may be necessary as von Willebrand factor levels fluctuate over time.

Management depends on severity. The administration of intravenous or intranasal desmopressin acetate (DDAVP) results in release of von Willebrand factor and factor VIII from platelet and endothelial cells. DDAVP has been proven to increase circulating levels of von Willebrand factor (and factor VIII) in the acute setting and often controls active bleeding. Adverse effects (tachyphylaxis) limit the amount that can be administered. Factor replacement is indicated for patients with continued bleeding. DDAVP is often prescribed monthly to adolescent girls with vWD-associated menorrhagia; oral contraceptives are also beneficial in limiting bleeding in these patients.

Acquired Coagulation Disorders

Acquired coagulopathies are usually related to liver disease or renal failure. Thrombin time is consistently prolonged in patients with disordered bleeding related to these disorders.

Disseminated intravascular coagulation consists of fibrin deposition within the walls of small vessels, with widespread consumption of platelets and clotting factors. Petechiae and palpable purpura are almost universally present, along with oozing from multiple sites (venipuncture sites, mucous membranes). PT, PTT, and prothrombin times are prolonged; fibrinogen is typically low, with a corresponding increase in the level of fibrin degradation products. Emergent treatment of DIC involves blood product replacement in the form of fresh frozen plasma, platelets, and red blood cells if needed. DIC-related thromboembolysis does not resolve until the underlying condition is addressed. Disorders predisposing to the development of DIC include sepsis, malignancy, burns, and transfusion or hemolytic reactions.

Thromboembolic Disorders

Thrombosis is generally rare in the pediatric population. The prolonged presence of a central venous catheter is the predominant risk factor for thrombus formation in this age group, so most deep vein thromboses (DVTs) are located in the subclavian or jugular veins. DVTs may also develop in the setting of sepsis, malignancy, congenital heart disease, or nephrotic syndrome. Most symptomatic DVTs present with local pain/swelling or pulmonary embolism.

ERYTHROCYTE TRANSFUSION REACTIONS

The majority of erythrocyte transfusions take place without incident and are of invaluable benefit to the patient; however, transfusion reactions due occur. Early recognition and timely treatment of complications limit mortality.

Febrile reactions typically result from the presence of host cell antibodies against human leukocyte antigens

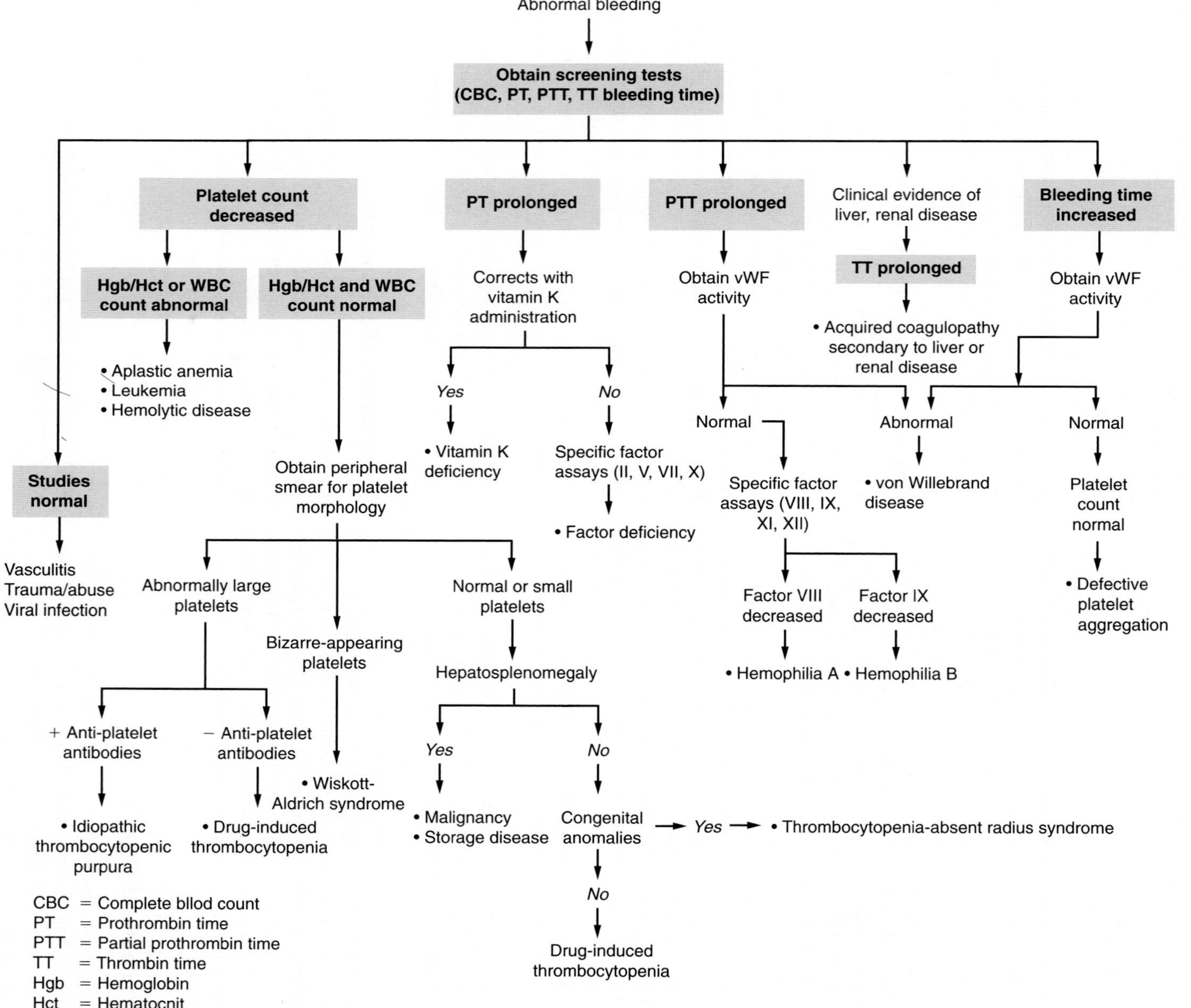

Figure 15-2 Simplified algorithm for the evaluation of abnormal bruising, bleeding in a nontoxic-appearing child.

(HLA) in the blood product. Pregnancy and previous transfusion can result in sensitization. The reactions consist of chills, fever, and, in severe cases, pulmonary infiltrates. Leukoreduction of blood products decreases the risk of both febrile reactions and intracellular viral transmission (e.g., cytomegalovirus, Epstein-Barr virus).

Allergic reactions, such as urticaria, itching, or frank anaphylaxis, occur in patients who have hypersensitivity to donor plasma proteins. The plasma is removed from "washed" red blood cells, reducing the risk of this reaction.

Hemolytic transfusion reactions are the rarest but most often fatal response to administration of blood. Overwhelming intravascular hemolysis follows the inadvertent transfusion of ABO incompatible blood products, with the potential for massive internal hemorrhage, renal failure, and death. Early signs and symptoms include fever, chills, abdominal pain, chest tightness, hypotension, and a sense of impending doom. The presence of any of these mandates immediate cessation of transfusion.

Hemosiderosis is the progressive accumulation of iron that results from prolonged transfusion therapy for conditions such as sickle cell disease and thalassemia. Manifestations of hemosiderosis include:

- heart failure secondary to cardiomyopathy
- arrhythmias resulting from deposition of iron in the conductive tissues of the heart
- liver failure
- endocrine failure (diabetes, hypothyroidism)
- delayed puberty
- short stature

Chelation with subcutaneous desferoxime is used to reduce the excessive iron load.

NEOPLASTIC DISORDERS

Lymphoma

Lymphoma is the third most common malignancy in the pediatric population. These cancers are highly malignant but have relatively high cure rates. Hodgkin lymphoma (HL) is slightly more prevalent than non-Hodgkin lymphoma (NHL) in young children; the ratio is reversed in adolescents. Features of HL and NHL are compared in Table 15-8. NHL, and to a lesser degree HL, occur with higher frequency in patients with genetic (e.g., Wiskott-Aldrich, severe combined immunodeficiency) or acquired (HIV) immunodeficiency syndromes.

Painless lymphadenopathy is a common initial presentation of lymphoma in the pediatric population. Characteristics of lymphadenopathy which should prompt consideration of lymphoma include location of the enlargement (posterior auricular, supraclavicular areas); painless enlargement; rubbery or firm nodes; and discrete or matted nodes. Lymph node biopsy and chest radiograph (to assess for mediastinal adenopathy and tumors) are indicated for patients with any of the above features. Anterior mediastinal tumors may be asymptomatic or present with symptoms related to compression of adjacent structures:

- Dysphagia (esophagus)
- Dyspnea (airway)
- Pain or swelling of face, neck, upper extremities (superior vena cava syndrome)

Specific management of lymphomas depends on the type (HL vs. NHL), histology, and stage of the tumor. Given its rapid growth, diagnosis and staging of NHL is considered a medical emergency. NHL has metastasized to the central nervous system and/or bone marrow in the majority of patients

TABLE 15-8
COMPARISON OF HODGKIN, NON-HODGKIN LYMPHOMA

Feature	Hodgkin Lymphoma	Non-Hodgkin Lymphoma
Onset of symptoms	Insidious	Rapid/acute
Characteristic location of adenopathy	Cervical, supraclavicular, mediastinal locations	Supraclavicular, abdominal, mesenteric locations
Constitutional symptoms	Fever, malaise, night sweats, weight loss (in up to one third of cases)	Uncommon
Abdominal involvement	Rare	Abdominal pain, intermittent obstruction, intussusception*
Mediastinal symptoms	Less common	Airway compression/obstruction; superior vena cava syndrome
Histology	Reed-Sternberg cell is diagnostic; divided into four histologic subtypes	Most common form is small cell lymphoma (Burkitt and non-Burkitt)

*NHL is the most common cause of intussusception in children 6 years of age and older, with mesenteric lymphadenopathy forming the lead point of the intussusception.

at diagnosis. Poor prognostic features associated with HL include any of the following systemic symptoms at diagnosis:

- Fever >38°C for 3 consecutive days
- Night sweats
- Weight loss

Long-term sequelae of lymphoma are related to the chemotherapeutic agents used and whether the spleen has been laproscopically removed or irradiated. Patients with functional or anatomic asplenia are at risk for overwhelming bacterial sepsis. Prophylactic antibiotic therapy is indicated for these patients, and their caretakers must be instructed to seek medical attention at the first sign of fever or illness.

Neuroblastoma

Neuroblastoma is an embryonal cancer of sympathetic nervous system tissue derived from neural crest cells. It is the fourth most common childhood malignancy, with the highest incidence in young children under the age of 5 years. Clinical manifestations of neuroblastoma may include any of the following:

- An intra-abdominal tumor arising from the adrenal gland or a paravertebral sympathetic ganglion; the mass presents as a fixed, typically painless, irregularly-shaped enlargement which may cross the midline
- An intrathoracic mass arising from a thoracic sympathetic ganglion; the growth is localized to the posterior mediastinum
- A cervical mass diagnosed as part of the evaluation of Horner syndrome
- A paraspinal tumor which compresses the cord, resulting in back pain or lower extremity paresis, paralysis, and bowel/bladder dysfunction.
- Widespread lymphadenopathy in disseminated disease
- Purplish discoloration of the periorbital area resulting from mass effects of enlarged lymphoid tissue
- Fever, weight loss, flushing, sweating, and irritability due to excess catecholamine production
- Watery, explosive diarrhea secondary to excess secretion of vasoactive intestinal peptide
- Opsoclonus or "dancing eyes"
- Stage 4S neuroblastoma, a unique presentation in children younger than a year of age, consisting of subcutaneous nodules, hepatomegaly, and a small primary tumor without bony involvement

Homovanillic acid (HVA) and vanillylmandelic acid (VMA) are catecholamine metabolites; urinary levels are usually elevated in patients with neuroblastoma and can serve as non-invasive screening tests. Various imaging studies assist in evaluation of the primary tumor. Bone scan and marrow biopsies are indicated to assess for marrow metastases, which are present in the majority of patients at diagnosis. Staging is based on extent of primary and metastatic disease; prognosis is closely tied to the disease stage. Stages 1 and 2 disease in low-risk patients is curable in the vast majority of cases. High-risk patients with Stages 2, 3, and 4 disease have significantly lower survival rates. The presence of N-myc amplification confers a poor prognosis.

Wilms Tumor

Wilms tumor is the most common renal neoplasm of childhood. It usually presents as an asymptomatic abdominal mass noted in a young child by the parents or physician. Symptoms, when present, may include abdominal pain, vomiting, and constipation due to partial obstruction. Palpation of a large flank mass which neither moves with respiration nor crosses the midline is consistent with Wilms tumor. Tumors which compress the renal artery result in hypertension. Microscopic hematuria may be present as well. Constitutional symptoms are uncommon. Abdominal ultrasonography is indicated in patients with suspected abdominal tumors; this study can demonstrate whether the lesion is intrarenal or extrarenal (neuroblastoma) and can also be used to assess the extent of vascular extension. Chest radiographs are indicated for patients with suspected Wilms tumor due to the high rate of lung metastasis. Treatment consists of surgical removal of the affected kidney. Histologic evidence of anaplasia results in a poorer prognosis. Stages 1 and 2 tumors can be completely excised. Stage III disease is defined by local spread. Stage IV disease involves metastasis to the lung, liver, brain, or bone. Bilateral renal involvement defines Stage V. Greater than 95% of patients with Stage 1 disease survive >4 years. Relapse is most common in the lungs and in the first 2 years after diagnosis.

Wilms tumor usually develops in isolation but may occur in conjunction with congenital anomalies, particularly aniridia and anatomic abnormalities of the genitourinary system. *WAGR syndrome* is the rare constellation of Wilms tumor, aniridia, genitourinary abnormalities, and mental retardation. Children with hemihypertrophy or syndromes of somatic overgrowth (e.g., Beckwith-Wiedemann syndrome) are at increased risk for Wilms tumor and hepatoblastomas; surveillance consists of serum alpha-fetoprotein, urinalysis, and abdominal ultrasound every 3 months from birth until the age of 5 years.

Central Nervous System Tumors

As a group, central nervous system tumors comprise almost a quarter of pediatric malignancies. The medical practitioner must maintain a high degree of suspicion in order to recognize the clinical presentation of a brain tumor, which may be quite subtle. Early diagnosis often results in fewer complications by limiting the amount and/or duration of treatment. Signs and symptoms are typically related to one of the following:

- Increased intracranial pressure—Headaches are often the earliest indicator of increased intracranial pressure. Intermittent nonspecific headaches evolve over time into morning or near-constant pain over the occipital or frontal region, which may be accompanied by vomiting and, eventually, lethargy. Horizontal diplopia and papilledema are ophthalmologic findings of severe or long-standing pressure increases. Affected infants present with irritability, poor feeding/growth, developmental regression, macrocephaly and/or splitting of the cranial sutures, a bulging anterior fontanelle, and occasionally the "setting sun" sign.

- Localizing signs—Lesions of the cerebrum, basal ganglia, thalamus, hypothalamus, and optic chiasm (supratentorial lesions) are more likely to cause hemiparesis or hemisensory loss, hyperreflexia, seizures, or visual changes. Infratentorial tumors may also present with hemiparesis and/or hyperreflexia; however, ataxia and cranial nerve deficits (diplopia, nystagmus) are more common than seizures.
- Global signs—Changes in affect, memory, energy level, behavior, or weight; sexual precocity or delayed puberty; growth failure; declining school performance.

Craniopharyngioma is a tumor that arises from the remnants of the Rathke pouch in the hypothalamic-pituitary region. Most early signs and symptoms are related to disordered endocrine function or compression of the optic chiasm, including: short stature (growth hormone deficiency); central diabetes insipidus; central hypothyroidism; precocious puberty; and visual field defects. Tumors which enlarge beyond the sella turcica may obstruct the third ventricle, leading to hydrocephalus and signs of increased intracranial pressure. Resection is associated with a high rate of survival. Recurrences and incomplete resections are treated with cranial irradiation.

Bone Lesions

Fibrous cortical defect is a benign, asymptomatic bone lesion which is often an incidental radiographic finding. These defects are extremely common, occurring in a significant minority of children older than 2 years of age. Plain radiographs demonstrate a sharply demarcated lucent area in the metaphyseal cortex, with the long axis of the lesion oriented along the long axis of the bone. In questionable cases, biopsy is diagnostic. Fibrous cortical defects regress spontaneously when skeletal maturity is attained. Treatment is unnecessary unless the lesion occupies more than half the diameter of the bone, in which case orthopedic surgery and bone grafting may be required.

Osteoid osteoma is a benign but painful bony lesion most commonly found in older children and adolescents. The sharp, focal pain may be constant; it is often worse at night and does not vary with changes in activity. In some cases, the pain is severe enough to result in disuse atrophy, scoliosis, or apparent limb-length discrepancy. It is consistently relieved with aspirin, naproxen, or other nonsteroidal anti-inflammatory medications. Palpation of the area over the lesion (usually the metaphyseal region of the femur or tibia) elicits tenderness. Plain films may be negative early in the course of development despite the presence of pain; bone scan or computed tomography confirms the presence of the lesion. When positive, radiographs demonstrate a small radiolucent center surrounded by sclerotic bone. Osteoid osteomas regress with skeletal maturation, but surgical removal may be indicated for pain relief.

Osteosarcoma is a malignant tumor often localized to the metaphyseal area of the long bones, particularly around the knee. It may be painful but usually presents as a painless bony mass or pathologic fracture. The radiologic hallmark of the disease is the "sunburst" pattern of calcified spikes surrounding an irregular sclerotic lesion. Chemotherapy is variably successful; amputation may be necessary. The cure rate is relatively low; about one third of affected patients die of their disease.

Ewing sarcoma is a rare and highly malignant bone tumor which presents as acute pain and possibly swelling, occasionally accompanied by constitutional symptoms. Males and older children/adolescents are disproportionately affected. Pathologic fractures are common. Any bone may be involved. The characteristic radiographic "onionskin" lesion represents a lytic area surrounded by ongoing periosteal reaction. Metastatic disease at diagnosis confers a poor prognosis.

Histiocytosis

Histiocytosis syndromes of childhood are alike in that they all involve proliferation of monocyte/macrophage cell lines. They are categorized according to physical and histologic findings:

- Class I (Langerhans cell) histiocytosis includes eosinophilic granuloma and Hand-Schüller-Christian disease. The Langerhans cell is the antigen-presenting cell of the skin. The diagnosis is confirmed on skin biopsy through detection of the characteristic Birbeck granule on histology or demonstration of CD1a cell surface markers.
- Class II histiocytosis includes juvenile xanthogranuloma and familial hemophagocytic lymphohistiocytosis syndromes. These diseases are characterized by widely disseminated lesions of many organ systems.
- Class III histiocytosis consists of disorders involving malignant proliferation of monocytes, macrophages, or immature dendritic cells. Malignant histiocytosis and a variant of AML are included in this category.

Therapeutic Considerations

Tumor lysis syndrome results when intracellular components are released into the bloodstream, resulting in hyperkalemia, hyperphosphatemia, and elevated lactate dehydrogenase levels. It can complicate the initial stage of chemotherapeutic treatment, when a cancerous tumor or cell line is undergoing rapid cell lysis. Eventually, renal function is compromised by the shear magnitude of the solute load and obstruction of the tubules with uric acid and phosphate precipitants. Tumor lysis syndrome should be anticipated during induction therapy in patients with ALL whose presenting leukocyte counts exceed 50×10^3/mcL. Aggressive hydration is indicated for at-risk patients, along with alkalinization of the urine, diuretic therapy, and allopurinol.

Children undergoing chemotherapy should receive all routine inactivated bacterial and viral vaccines, polysaccharide-protein conjugate vaccines, and toxoid vaccines. Immunosuppressed patients may be incapable of mounting optimal or even adequate responses to these vaccinations. The risk-benefit of delaying an inoculation in order to generate a stronger response should be weighed against the need for additional protection against these pathogens. Patients can also be re-vaccinated following the end of their chemotherapy. The annual influenza vaccine should be administered to all patients undergoing chemotherapy as well as their household contacts. Live virus vaccines (MMR) should not be given to patients undergoing chemotherapy until at least 3 to 6 months after the completion of the course. They can be administered to household contacts, however, as they are not transmitted person-to-person. The varicella vaccine is thought to be safe and protective in patients receiving chemotherapy.

TABLE 15-9
LONG-TERM COMPLICATIONS OF CANCER THERAPY

Alkylating Agents
- Examples: cyclophosphamide, cisplatin, busulfan
- Gonadal toxicity, which is affected by the agent, the regimen (multi-agent), the total dosage, and the gender and stage of sexual development of the patient
- Subsequent infertility in males; pubertal development and sexual function remain normal
- Ovaries are more resistant to toxic effects than testes; premature menopause is a long-term possibility.

Cranial Irradiation
- Panhypopituitarism (younger children are most susceptible; growth hormone is often affected first)
- Poor academic achievement
- Behavior changes
- Secondary neoplasms

Chemotherapy-induced neutropenia is managed with rhG-CSF and prompt evaluation and treatment of fevers.

Alkylating agents and radiation are associated with the most significant long-term complications of cancer treatment (Table 15-9). Normal pubertal development does not assure fertility. Total body irradiation in conjunction with myeloablative doses of alkylating agents, the typical preparations for bone marrow transplantation, result in total and irreversible testicular or ovarian failure.

SOURCES

Allen GA, Glader B. Approach to the bleeding child. *Pediatr Clin North Am.* 2002;49:1239–1256.

Boxer LA. Neutrophil abnormalities. *Pediatr Rev.* 2003;24:52–61.

Di Paola JA, Buchanan GR. Immune thrombocytopenic purpura. *Pediatr Clin North Am.* 2002;49:911–928.

Fixler J, Styles L. Sickle cell disease. *Pediatr Clin North Am.* 2002;49:1193–1210.

Friedman Dl, Meadows AT. Late effects of childhood cancer therapy. *Pediatr Clin North Am.* 2002;49:1083–1106.

Hermiston ML, Mentzer WC. A practical approach to the evaluation of the anemic child. *Pediatr Clin North Am.* 2002;49:877–891.

Journeycake JM, Buchanan GR. Coagulation disorders. *Pediatr Rev.* 2003;24:83–91.

Kaplan RN. Differential diagnosis and management of thrombocytopenia in childhood. *Pediatr Clin North Am.* 2004;51:1109–1140.

Kyono W, Coates TD. A practical approach to neutrophil disorders. *Pediatr Clin North Am.* 2002;49:929–971.

Mortimor W. Focus on diagnosis: Screening for von Willebrand factor disease. *Pediatr Rev.* 2005;26:302–303.

Pierce JM, Sills RH. Consultation with the specialist: Childhood leukemia. *Pediatr Rev.* 2005;26:96–104.

Piomelli S. Childhood lead poisoning. *Pediatr Clin North Am.* 2002;49:1285–1304.

Reaman GH. Pediatric oncology: Current views and outcomes. *Pediatr Clin North Am.* 2002;49:1305–1318.

Richardson M. Microcytic anemia. *Pediatr Rev.* 2007;28:5–14.

Segal GB, Hirsh MG, Feig SA. Managing anemia in pediatric office practice (Part 1). *Pediatr Rev.* 2002;23:75–84.

Segal GB, Hirsh MG, Feig SA. Managing anemia in pediatric office practice (Part 2). *Pediatr Rev.* 2002;23:111–122.

Shah S, Vega R. Hereditary spherocytosis. *Pediatr Rev.* 2004;25:166–171.

Velez MC. Consultation with the specialist: Lymphomas. *Pediatr Rev.* 2003;24:380–386.

QUESTIONS

1. Infants and children who consume large amounts of cow milk are prone to iron deficiency anemia due to all of the following reasons EXCEPT:

A) Excessive cow milk ingestion is associated with menorrhagia in adolescent females.
B) The iron in cow milk is poorly absorbed.
C) The calcium in cow milk interferes with absorption of iron.
D) Cow milk slows gastric emptying and may decrease the intake of iron-rich foods.
E) Cow milk ingestion in a patient with protein allergy results in gastrointestinal blood loss.

2. A 3-year-old boy presents with his second episode of culture-positive staphylococcal skin infection. There is minimal warmth, erythema, and tenderness at the site. The discharge is non-purulent. Which of the following laboratory studies is most likely to be abnormal in this patient?

A) White blood cell count
B) Absolute neutrophil count
C) CD4+ lymphocyte count
D) Total hemolytic complement assay
E) Serum immunoglobulin levels

3. An 18-month-old boy with sickle cell disease is brought to the emergency department in the middle of the night by his grandmother for a fever of 39°C. He is fussy but not toxic-appearing, and his affect brightens as the acetaminophen begins to take effect. The physical examination is significant for a well-nourished, well-developed male in no acute distress. Mild scleral icterus is noted; otherwise the physical examination is within normal limits. A complete blood count (CBC) and culture are obtained; the results of his CBC are similar to his baseline counts. Which of the following is the most appropriate management of this patient?

A) Continue penicillin prophylaxis and follow-up with the family in the pediatric hematology clinic the following day.
B) Observe the patient for 4 to 6 hours (or until morning) in the emergency department.
C) Admit the patient to the hospital and repeat the complete blood count in the morning.
D) Admit the patient to the hospital and administer broad-spectrum antibiotics until culture results are available.
E) Admit the patient to the hospital and obtain chest radiographs and a bone scan.

4. A 6-year-old girl with no significant past medical history presents with a chief complaint of fever for the last three days. The temperature is 38.6°C; other vital signs are stable. The examination is significant for a well-nourished, well-developed, alert and well-appearing child. The anterior cervical lymph nodes are mildly enlarged and minimally tender; no other lymphadenopathy is noted. Results of a complete blood count are as follows:

white blood count 3.1×10^3/mcL
20% neutrophils
hemoglobin 13.0 g per dL
platelet count 225,000 per mm^3

Which of the following is the most appropriate next step in the evaluation of this patient's neutropenia?

A) Ask the laboratory to re-run the sample.
B) Obtain a new sample for laboratory analysis.
C) Obtain a peripheral blood smear to look for blasts.
D) Repeat a complete blood count in 10 to 14 days.
E) Obtain complete blood counts every 21 days for the next 3 months.

5. A 5-year-old girl is brought to the emergency department by her mother complaining of abdominal pain. The mother tells you that the girl's urine is darker than normal. Vital signs reveal moderate tachycardia, and the physical examination is significant for pallor, scleral icterus, diffuse abdominal tenderness, and a palpable spleen tip. Laboratory results are obtained as follows:

white blood count 11.0×10^3/mcL
hemoglobin 5.5 g per dL
platelet count 175,000 per mm^3
reticulocyte count 6.0%
blood urea nitrogen 10 mg per dL
serum creatinine 0.5 mg per dL

Which of the following tests is most likely to provide a definitive diagnosis in this child?

A) Red blood cell fetal i antigen testing
B) Hemoglobin electrophoresis
C) Bone marrow biopsy
D) Peripheral blood smear
E) Direct antiglobin (Coombs) test

6.A 12-month-old boy is found to have a screening hematocrit of 29%. Results of a venous complete blood count include a hemoglobin of 9.7 g per dL; reticulocyte count 1.5%; mean corpuscular volume 65 fL; mean cell hemoglobin 22 picograms per cell. The hemoglobin level is unchanged following a 4-week course of iron supplementation. Which of the following is the most likely cause of failure of iron therapy in this patient?

A) Thalassemia minor
B) Noncompliance
C) Continued bleeding
D) Inactive or insufficient iron-binding globulin
E) Lead poisoning

7. A mother brings her 24-month-old daughter to your office because the child appears pale and is less able to keep up with her peers at preschool. The patient has no significant history, and screening questions suggest a low risk for iron deficiency anemia. The physical examination is significant for marked pallor and moderate tachycardia at rest. Screening laboratory results include the following:

white blood count 10.0×10^3/mcL
hemoglobin 4.2 g per dL
mean cell volume 72 fL
platelet count 250,000 per mm^3
reticulocyte count 0.2%

Which of the following is the most likely cause of this patient's anemia?

A) Iron deficiency anemia
B) Transient erythroblastopenia of childhood
C) Acute lymphoblastic anemia
D) Hereditary spherocytosis
E) Histiocytosis syndrome of childhood

8. A 5-year-old boy presents for evaluation of his recurrent nosebleeds over the past week. He also has a 3-week history of increasing pain in his arms and legs which does not respond to acetaminophen. Scattered petechiae are noted on physical examination. The following laboratory results are obtained:

white blood count 3.0×10^3/mcL
9% neutrophils
85% lymphocytes
5% monocytes
1% eosinophils
hemoglobin 8.7 g per dL

platelet count 21 × 10^3/mcL
peripheral blood smear negative for blasts
Which of the following is the most likely cause of this child's hematologic abnormalities?

A) Kasabach-Merritt syndrome
B) Fanconi anemia
C) Acute lymphoblastic leukemia
D) Acute myeloblastic leukemia
E) Aplastic anemia

9. You are lecturing a group of medical residents about von Willebrand disease. You would be correct in telling them each of the following EXCEPT:

A) Heavy menstrual bleeding may be the first manifestation of von Willebrand disease in girls.
B) von Willebrand disease is the most common congenital bleeding disorder.
C) The inheritance pattern of von Willebrand disease is autosomal dominant.
D) Desmopressin acetate may be used in the acute setting to limit active bleeding.
E) Screening results consistent with a diagnosis of von Willebrand disease include prolonged bleeding time, prolonged prothrombin time, and normal or slightly prolonged activated partial thromboplastin time.

10. A 10-year-old boy with known hemophilia A is brought to the emergency department via ambulance for closed head trauma (vehicular collision). The patient did not loose consciousness, has no headache, and has not vomited. Vital signs are stable, and a rapid neurologic assessment, including mental status testing, is normal. Which of the following is the most appropriate next course of action in this patient?

A) Discharge with reliable caretaker, who is instructed to call immediately with any vomiting, confusion, or headache
B) Observation in the emergency department for 6 to 8 hours, with immediate factor VIII replacement if any neurologic signs develop
C) Computed tomography of the head; factor VIII replacement if intracranial bleeding is documented
D) Replacement of factor VIII to 100% of normal levels following documentation of a prolonged activated partial thromboplastin time
E) Immediate replacement of factor VIII levels to 100% of normal

11. Which of the following percentages indicates the likelihood that a male born to a woman whose father has hemophilia A will have the disorder?

A) 25%
B) 50%
C) 66%
D) 75%
E) 90%

12. Recombinant human granulocyte colony-stimulating factor may be indicated for patients with all of the following immunodeficiency syndromes EXCEPT:

A) Autoimmune neutropenia of infancy
B) Chronic granulomatous disease
C) Cyclic neutropenia
D) Severe congenital neutropenia
E) Shwachman-Diamond syndrome

13. A 10-year-old boy presents to the emergency department with regular, episodic, progressive abdominal pain of a few hours duration. He denies fever, vomiting, or diarrhea. He feels fine between the episodes of pain but becomes anxious as the pain develops again. The physical examination is remarkable for stable vital signs between the episodes of pain; a tender, indistinct mass in the right upper quadrant; and generalized non-tender lymphadenopathy, including rubbery enlargement of the supraclavicular nodes. Intussusception is diagnosed and successfully reduced on air contrast enema. Which of the following diagnostic test(s) is (are) most likely to yield a positive result in this patient?

A) Chest radiographs
B) Lymph node biopsy
C) A and B
D) Platelet count
E) Serum IgA concentration

14. A 2-year-old girl with a month-long history of weight loss, watery diarrhea, and irritability presents with a fixed, non-tender, irregular abdominal mass which crosses the midline. Which of the following screening studies is most likely to be abnormal in this patient?

A) Serum creatinine concentration
B) Random urine calcium-creatinine level
C) Urinalysis (red blood cells)
D) Urinary homovanillic acid (HVA) and vanillylmandelic acid (VMA) levels
E) Urinalysis (protein)

15. Abdominal ultrasonography obtained to evaluate a left-sided flank mass in a hypertensive 3-year-old child demonstrates an intrarenal tumor compressing the renal artery. Which of the following radiographic studies is indicated in this patient prior to initiation of treatment for the tumor?

A) Echocardiography
B) Magnetic resonance imaging of the brain
C) Computed tomography of the brain
D) Radiographs of the abdomen
E) Radiographs of the chest

16. A mother brings her 3-year-old son to your office because she noted a "large swollen place" in his abdomen while she was bathing him. You note a large mass in the left upper abdominal/flank area, which does not move with respiration or cross the midline. His vital signs are normal. Urinalysis reveals microscopic hematuria. Abdominal ultrasonography is most likely to demonstrate which of the following?

A) An intrarenal mass
B) An extrarenal mass
C) A paravertebral mass
D) Splenomegaly
E) Gastric outlet obstruction

17. A 2-week-old infant is noted to have aniridia. There is no history of the condition in his family. This infant should undergo regular monitoring consisting of which of the following for the next several years?

A) Random urine calcium/creatinine ratio
B) Renal ultrasonography
C) Thyroid stimulating hormone levels
D) Growth hormone levels
E) Echocardiography

18. The physical examination of a 17-year-old adolescent demonstrates Stage V genital and pubic hair development. His height is at the 25th percentile, and his weight is at the 50th percentile. The patient's past medical history is significant for successful treatment of acute lymphoblastic leukemia at the age of 4 years. He is still in remission. Which of the following statements regarding this patient's reproductive potential is TRUE?

A) This patient is not at an increased risk of infertility since he was younger than 5 years of age during initial treatment.
B) Successful progression through puberty predicts normal fertility.
C) Successful progression through puberty predicts normal sexual function.
D) This patient has a high risk of passing his underlying leukocyte abnormality to his offspring.
E) If this patient was found to have abnormal Leydig cell function, he would not need to use barrier contraception with his sexual partners.

19. A 4-year-old girl diagnosed with acute lymphoblastic leukemia has a peripheral leukocyte count of 70,000 per mcL at diagnosis. Which of the following courses of treatment is most likely to prevent significant acute electrolyte abnormalities in this patient during the first 12 to 24 hours of chemotherapy?

A) Pretreatment with acetaminophen and prochlorperazine
B) 0.45 normal saline with 20 mEq per L KCL at ¼ maintenance
C) Maintenance plus replacement fluids; allopurinol
D) Aggressive intravenous hydration; diuretic therapy; alkalinization of the urine
E) Use of a single alkylating agent rather than a multidrug regimen

20. A mother brings her 11-year-old son to your office for evaluation of his leg pain. The pain started several weeks ago in his left lower leg; it is focal, sharp, and progressive. The pain is worse at night and does not improve with rest; however, naproxen generally relieves his symptoms. Palpation of the metaphyseal area of the left tibia reveals an isolated area of tenderness. Plain radiographs of the area demonstrate a small radiolucent lesion surrounded by sclerotic bone. Which of the following conditions is the most likely cause of this patient's pain?

A) Osteosarcoma
B) Pathologic fracture
C) Ewing sarcoma
D) Fibrous cortical defect
E) Osteoid osteoma

21. A previously well 16-year-old adolescent is brought to the emergency department for evaluation of his high fever and rash. The patient's temperature is 40°C on arrival, with heart rate 130 beats per minute, respiratory rate 30 breaths per minute, and blood pressure 90/60 mm Hg. Petechiae and purpura are visible on the patient's distal upper and lower extremities; more petechiae are scattered over the trunk and proximal extremities. Which of the following is indicated prior to further evaluation of this patient?

A) Intravenous vancomycin plus ceftriaxone
B) Intravenous doxycycline plus ceftriaxone
C) Intravenous vancomycin plus tetracycline
D) Intravenous vancomycin alone
E) Intravenous ceftriaxone alone

ANSWERS

1. A	8. C	15. E
2. B	9. E	16. A
3. D	10. E	17. B
4. D	11. B	18. C
5. E	12. B	19. D
6. A	13. C	20. E
7. B	14. D	21. A

Renal Disorders

16

RENAL FUNCTION: AGE-RELATED NORMS

Although renal architecture at gross and microscopic levels is virtually identical in neonates and adults, age-related changes in renal function occur over the first 2 years of life as tubules continue to grow and develop. Nephrogenesis is not complete until 36 weeks of gestation. Immature kidneys are relatively poor at concentrating urine; thus, premature infants are more susceptible to fluid, pH, and electrolyte shifts. Fractional excretion of sodium, a measure of the adequacy of the renal response to solute load, is higher in premature infants, placing them at increased risk of fluid overload and (dilutional) hyponatremia.

Glomerular filtration rate (GFR) is defined as the quantity of filtrate generated by all the nephrons in both kidneys per minute. The GFR can be approximated if the serum creatinine is known, factoring in the patient's age, weight, and gender. It is not surprising, then, that both GFR and serum creatinine, a product of muscle breakdown which undergoes renal clearance, rise toward adult levels as the child ages (Table 16-1). The relatively low GFR in infants during the first few months of life results in diminished renal clearance of certain drugs; this dilemma presents most frequently in relation to antimicrobials. When a neonate requires treatment with a medication which undergoes renal clearance, it is important to ascertain whether changes in the recommended dosage or intervals are required for this age group. For example, aminoglycosides can accumulate and result in short-term nephrotoxicity and often irreversible ototoxicity in neonates when standard dosing intervals are not appropriately increased. It is also imperative to maintain good hydration in the young infant when administering a drug which undergoes renal clearance. The risk of drug toxicity is even greater in infants who are dehydrated, septic, or in acute or chronic renal failure.

Urea nitrogen is a product of protein metabolism. Serum blood urea nitrogen levels are an indirect but useful indicator of hydration status; the serum creatinine concentration is more reflective of renal function.

TABLE 16-1

GLOMERULAR FILTRATION RATE AND SERUM CREATININE: AGE-RELATED NORMS

The *glomerular filtration rate* at birth is relatively low, due primarily to reduced effective renal blood flow.

GFR in the premature infant—less than 10% of normal adult GFR; directly proportional to gestational age

GFR at birth—10% of normal adult GFR

GFR at age 3 months—50% of normal adult GFR

GFR at age 12 months—80% of normal adult GFR

GFR at age 24 months—essentially equal to normal adult GFR

At birth, the *serum creatinine* concentration is reflective of maternal values. Serum creatinine rises more slowly in relation to adult values because levels are related to overall muscle mass, which increases with age.

Serum creatinine in the premature infant—0.7 mg per dL

Serum creatinine at age 3 months—0.3 mg per dL

Serum creatinine at age 24 months—0.4 mg per dL

Serum creatinine at age 6 years—0.6 mg per dL

Serum creatinine at age 18 years—0.9 mg per dL

Urinalysis

Proteinuria

Protein in the urine may be factitious, transient, benign, or pathologic (Table 16-2). A dipstick reading of 2+ or greater usually represents a true positive test. Samples which are positive for both protein and blood suggest underlying glomerular pathology, especially in the setting of hypertension or edema. Additional investigative testing is based on the history and physical examination but may include a complete blood count, serum electrolytes, serum creatinine, blood urea nitrogen, serum complement levels, and an antinuclear antibody test. Orthostatic proteinuria presents as isolated proteinuria in an asymptomatic patient with normal blood pressure, physical examination, and serum electrolyte results. Protein is excreted into the urine when the patient is erect, but not when the patient is supine. The benign nature of the condition is confirmed if the ratio of urinary protein/urinary creatinine is <0.2 on a first-morning-void specimen.

TABLE 16-2
CAUSES OF PROTEINURIA

Factitious Proteinuria (dipstick result)
Urine is overly concentrated
Urine pH is alkaline
Dipstick is immersed in the urine for too long
Dipstick is placed in the urinary stream rather than dipped into the sample
Mucoproteins are present in the urine
Transient Proteinuria
Fever
Vigorous exercise
Dehydration
Cold exposure
Seizures
Stress
Chronic Benign Proteinuria
Orthostatic proteinuria
Pathologic Proteinuria
Nephrotic syndrome
Glomerulonephritis (acute and chronic)
Acute tubular necrosis
Toxin exposure
Adverse effect of medication

TABLE 16-3
CAUSES OF HEMATURIA

Factitious Hematuria
Dipstick positive
Myoglobin secondary to muscle breakdown (exercise, crush injury, malignant hyperthermia, inherited myopathy)
Hemoglobin (usually occurs in the setting of hemolysis)
Porphyrins
Discolored urine without red blood cells
Foods (beets)
Medications
Additives (red dye)
Vaginal bleeding
Transient Hematuria
Hemorrhagic cystitis (adenovirus)
Chronic Benign Hematuria
Benign familial hematuria
Hypercalciuria (idiopathic or due to hypercalcemia)
Pathologic Hematuria
Glomerular disease
Interstitial renal disease
Tubular renal disease
Urinary tract infection
Nephrocalcinosis
Renal tumor
Papillary necrosis secondary to sickle cell disease or trait

Hematuria

Hematuria is defined as discolored (red, brown) or normal-appearing urine which contains red blood cells. Like proteinuria, hematuria can be factitious, transient, benign, or pathologic (Table 16-3). Many conditions may cause either gross or microscopic hematuria, but overall gross hematuria is more likely to result from an underlying pathologic renal condition. Brown urine typically signifies bleeding in the kidney, whereas bleeding in the lower tract results in bright red urine or clots. Urine may appear red/brown or test positive for blood in the absence of hematuria; for example, urinary presence of myoglobin, a heme-containing protein present in muscle, will produce a positive dipstick result. Microscopic urinalysis is indicated in these cases to confirm whether red blood cells or casts are indeed present (normal: zero to two red blood cells/hpf). Significant myoglobinuria can precipitate acute renal failure and is managed with intravenous hydration and alkalinization of the urine.

Information gathered from the history and physical examination often assists in the diagnosis of hematuria:

- Family history—renal disease, benign familial hematuria, renal failure, stones, hypertension, sickle cell disease
- History of current illness—duration of hematuria; history of skin rash, cellulitic infection, or pharyngitis; history of hemolytic disease; current and recent medications
- Symptoms—fever, weight gain, pain (abdominal, flank, cystitis), arthritis, bruising
- Signs—hypertension, edema, jaundice, splenomegaly

The evaluation and management of hematuria is provided in Table 16-4.

Benign familial hematuria is a common cause of asymptomatic microscopic and occasionally gross hematuria. Renal function and architecture are normal. Because transmission is autosomal dominant, asymptomatic microscopic hematuria is usually found in other family members. No treatment is necessary for this benign condition.

Urinary Symptoms

Dysuria

Dysuria is a relatively common complaint in pediatrics. Urinary tract infections usually cause dysuria, but so do multiple other conditions:

- Pinworm infestation, nonspecific vulvitis, and dysfunctional voiding patterns in young children
- Adolescent females with sexually transmitted infections, vulvovaginitis, urethritis, and chemical irritation
- Urethritis in males resulting from a sexually transmitted infection
- Trauma to the urinary and/or genital tract

TABLE 16-4
EVALUATION AND MANAGEMENT OF HEMATURIA

Repeat the urinalysis in 1 to 2 weeks if all of the following are present:

- Isolated, microscopic hematuria
- Urine dipstick ≤2+ blood
- No family history of renal disease
- No history of trauma
- No history of easy bleeding
- Patient is asymptomatic
- No evidence of hypertension or edema

If the patient does not fit the criteria listed above, or if hematuria is persistent, immediate laboratory investigation is warranted:

- Complete microscopic urinalysis (red cells, white cells, bacteria)
- Urine culture
- Complete blood count
- Serum electrolyte, creatinine, and blood urea nitrogen
- Serum complement levels (C3, C4)
- Spot urine calcium/creatinine ratio (normal <25)

Radiologic evaluation is guided by results of the clinical and laboratory phases, but usually begins with ultrasonography of the kidneys and urinary tract.

Microscopic or gross hematuria in the patient with sickle cell disease or trait

Given the increased incidence of glomerular and particularly tubular disease in patients with sickle cell disease or trait, patients in these populations who develop hematuria warrant:

- a renal sonogram to assess the architecture of the renal medulla
- intravenous pyelography to evaluate for *papillary necrosis*, which is usually insidious in onset but occasionally presents with the sudden onset of gross hematuria and flank pain

Urinary tract infection may occur at any age but is more common in infants, toddlers, and adolescent females. The presentation and family history are often helpful in cases of nephrolithiasis. Dysuria may be the only clinical manifestation of hypercalciuria.

The adolescent female with dysuria can be presumptively treated for a urinary tract infection once the urine culture has been obtained if the dipstick is positive for leukocyte esterase and nitrites; there are no abnormalities of the external genitalia; and she is not sexually active. Pelvic examinations and testing for sexually transmitted diseases is indicated for the female adolescent with dysuria who does not fit the criteria above. *Staphylococcus saprophyticus* infection should be considered in patients with dysuria who test negative for nitrites. Dysuria in the adolescent male requires identification of the pathogen. Males diagnosed with sexually transmitted infections should be adequately screened and treated. Because infection of the urinary tract is so uncommon in adolescent males, further investigation is warranted in patients found to have a typical urinary pathogen.

Frequency/Incontinence

Successful bladder control is usually achieved between the ages of 24 and 36 months, although many developmentally normal children take significantly longer (up to 48 months). Enuresis is the involuntary loss of urine in a child older than 5 years of age:

- Primary enuresis is diagnosed in patients who have never successfully maintained a dry period. Primary enuresis is much more common in boys. Postulated benign causes of primary enuresis include maturational delay and small functional bladder capacity.
- Secondary enuresis is diagnosed in patients who remain dry for six months or more before regular wetting recurs. Secondary enuresis is more likely to be pathologic in origin (e.g., constipation, infection, diabetes, psychosocial stress, and rarely child abuse). Enuresis which persists for >2 weeks in a previously continent child requires evaluation. Urinalysis is the most appropriate initial screening test; other studies to consider based on results of urinalysis include urine culture, renal sonogram, and serum electrolytes, creatinine, and blood urea nitrogen. Patients with normal physical examinations and negative urinalysis results are unlikely to have underlying systemic disease; behavioral therapy may be more appropriate for these children.

Enuresis is also classified as *diurnal* (day and night) or exclusively nocturnal. Occasional daytime wetting is rare beyond the age of 5 to 6 years. When the history, physical examination, and urinalysis results are all normal, management of diurnal enuresis consists of increasing fluid intake to counteract urinary "holding" behavior in a resistant child; establishment of a regular voiding schedule; and treatment of constipation, if present.

Primary nocturnal enuresis is very common in children. About 20% of 5-year-olds and 10% of 6-year-olds continue to wet the bed at night, with 15% achieving nighttime dryness per year thereafter. Nocturnal enuresis usually results from a small bladder and/or depressed arousal. No further evaluation is necessary beyond urinalysis to rule out diabetes and infection. Compliance is a problem with alarms, which nevertheless have good long-term success rates. Intranasal or oral desmopressin acetate (DDAVP) decreases the volume of urine produced overnight and may be effective for sporadic use, but it is not appropriate for daily administration due to the incidence of adverse effects (headache, flushing, nausea, diarrhea).

Conditions which should be considered part of the differential diagnosis of enuresis in the child are discussed below.

Inappropriate parental expectations are an important cause of "incontinence" in the young child. Parents should be questioned regarding expectations as well as methods of toilet training. Early anticipatory counseling may prevent parental and childhood anxiety and promote successful, non-stressful toilet training.

Bladder instability is a cause of frequent urination and incontinence in the young child. Peripheral nervous system dyssynergy coupled with a small bladder capacity results in urinary frequency, enuresis, and occasionally dysuria; urine cultures remain negative. Oxybutynin, an antispasmodic agent, is indicated for patients with wetting which does not resolve with conservative behavioral intervention or that which interferes with placement in school. Imipramine is an alternative. Adverse effects of oxybutynin include urinary retention and gastrointestinal upset; imipramine can cause dry mouth, constipation, and rarely hypotension and cardiac arrhythmias. Neither medication is effective in the management of primary nocturnal enuresis which is not due to bladder dyssynergy.

Overflow incontinence is suggested when enuresis is associated with unusually frequent or infrequent voiding. Enuresis due to infrequent voiding is less common and usually results from voluntary withholding in the younger child. Overflow incontinence in the setting of frequent voiding occurs primarily in elementary school-age girls. It is a secondary form of enuresis, which may be related to bladder instability. Chronic constipation causes secondary diurnal enuresis in a minority of patients; the diagnosis is suggested by the stooling history and can be confirmed on an abdominal plain radiograph.

Diabetes insipidus (DI) is a condition in which the kidneys do not concentrate the urine, either because the pituitary gland does not secrete sufficient antidiuretic hormone (central DI) or because there is a defective receptor on the renal collecting duct (nephrogenic DI). Affected individuals are unable to achieve urinary specific gravities in excess of 1.005. Obstructive uropathy can cause sufficient renal damage to impair concentration of the urine, but enuresis is rarely the sole presenting feature of this abnormality.

Patients with *spina bifida occulta* may present with urinary incontinence or dribbling as the only manifestation of their condition. These children often develop frequent urinary tract infections due to urinary stasis. A sacral dimple may be noted superior to the gluteal cleft; magnetic resonance imaging demonstrates distal spinal dysraphism. Spinal cord tumors are a rare cause of secondary urinary incontinence; back pain and lower extremity weakness usually accompany the tumor.

An abnormally weak urinary stream can contribute to urinary frequency. Males may have posterior urethral valves. Ureteroceles and ectopic urethra are rarer conditions in females with can affect the strength of urination. Ultrasonography of the renal/urinary systems and voiding cystourethrogram are indicated for patients with voiding abnormalities.

Diabetes mellitus and Fanconi syndrome both cause glucosuria/polyuria and may present with enuresis in the young child. Urinary tract infection should also be considered part of the differential diagnosis in the incontinent child.

Evaluation of enuresis begins with assessment of growth parameters, blood pressure, history and physical examination, urinalysis, and urine specific gravity. Further assessment is guided by results of the above. Withholding of urine associated with toilet training is discussed in Chapter 28.

Renal Studies

Prenatal ultrasonography beyond 12 to 14 weeks gestation is the diagnostic procedure of choice for the in utero assessment of renal architecture and size. Hydronephrosis, renal agenesis, and fluid in the bladder are evident if present. Evaluation of the quantity of amniotic fluid is important; oligohydramnios suggests possible urinary tract obstruction and/or Potter syndrome. Although kidney damage may already be irreversible by the time ultrasonographic changes become apparent, postnatal interventions can be set in place to prevent further degeneration of renal function in the postnatal period.

Hydronephrosis (distension of the renal pelvis) is a relatively common prenatal finding. Physiologic hydronephrosis is transient and resolves without treatment. Pathologic hydronephrosis is usually secondary to an obstructive uropathy such as ureteropelvic junction obstruction (UPJO) or posterior urethral valves (PUV). Most cases of prenatal pathologic hydronephrosis are addressed once the infant is delivered. However, when the obstruction and resultant distension become so severe that there is a risk of irreversible loss of kidney or lung function, endoscopic placement of a stent may be attempted to shunt fluid from the renal pelvis to the amniotic fluid space. This procedure is technically complex, variably successful, and fraught with complications (subsequent obstruction or displacement of the shunt; preterm labor; introduction of infection).

Ultrasonography (US) is the most appropriate initial method of evaluating the urinary tract in children. This study permits assessment of: the size of the kidneys, bladder, and ureters (if enlarged); renal architecture, including corticomedullary differentiation; renal echogenicity; and, when coupled with Doppler flow analysis, renal venous and arterial vascularization.

The voiding cystourethrogram (VCUG) is primarily used to detect and classify vesicoureteral reflux (VUR), although ureteral abnormalities (e.g., megaureter, duplicated ureter) and posterior urethral valves are also clearly visible on VCUG if present. Sterility of the urine should be documented prior to the procedure.

Intravenous pyelography used to be the radiographic study of choice for the diagnosis of obstructive hydronephrosis; however, nuclear medicine scans (renal scintigraphy) are now preferred. The scans are used to evaluate renal function and assess for obstructive uropathy. Renal angiography is obtained when there is suspicion of renal artery stenosis or other vascular abnormalities. Renal biopsy is reserved for cases in which the diagnosis is in doubt and a specific diagnosis is required for therapeutic or prognostic indications.

The 24-hour urine collection, which provides a wealth of information in adults, is usually unnecessary and frequently impossible to collect in children. Young patients often do not excrete the requisite 15 to 20 mg per kg of creatinine needed to standardize the sample against reference rates. Instead, a single random sample is used to generate a ratio of the urinary concentration of a particular substance to that of creatinine.

Congenital Renal Disorders

Obstructive Uropathy in the Infant

In congenital obstructive uropathy, the blockage can occur anywhere along the urinary system, including the infundibulum, renal pelvis, ureteropelvic junction, kidney, ureter, uretovesicular junction, bladder, and urethra. Obstructive uropathy may present with prenatal hydronephrosis, urinary tract infection, or an abdominal mass; in fact, hydronephrosis is the second most commonly palpated abdominal mass in infancy. The differential diagnosis of congenital urinary tract obstruction is provided in Table 16-5. Once identified, the obstruction must be relieved to preserve renal function. Chronic obstruction predisposes to recurrent urinary tract infection, kidney scarring, decreased renal function, and renal failure.

Lax abdominal musculature, cryptorchidism, and urinary tract anomalies are the defining features of *prune belly (Eagle-Barrett) syndrome.* Most patients exhibit some degree of hydronephrosis, which is usually obstructive (e.g., ureteropelvic junction obstruction, posterior urethral valves) but may be nonobstructive in some cases. Abdominal US and VCUG are indicated in any neonate suspected of having prune belly syndrome due to the high incidence of associated vesicoureteral reflux. Most patients eventually develop renal failure despite antibiotic prophylaxis, urinary diversion, and/or surgical repair.

TABLE 16-5
DIFFERENTIAL DIAGNOSIS OF CONGENITAL OBSTRUCTIVE NEUROPATHY

Unilateral Hydronephrosis **(proximal or upper tract obstruction)**

Uretopelvic junction obstruction*

Mid-ureteral obstruction

Unilateral megaureter

Ureterocele (more common in females; may present with visible prolapse through the urethral meatus)

Bilateral Hydronephrosis **(distal/lower tract obstruction or abnormal retrograde flow)**

Posterior urethral valves (males)—hydronephrosis and oligohydramnios

Vesicoureteral reflux

Bladder neck obstruction

Prune belly syndrome (rare)

Enlarged Kidneys Without Obstruction

Polycystic kidney disease

Multicystic dysplastic kidney

Renal tumor (rare)

Renal vein thrombosis

*Most common congenital cause of urinary tract obstruction

Renal Dysplasia and Multicystic Dysplastic Kidney

Congenital renal dysplasia is severe, widespread malformation of renal glomeruli and tubules during early development, which results in a nonfunctional kidney. US reveals marked thinning of the renal parenchyma with increased echogenicity throughout. When renal cysts are noted in the setting of the aforementioned signs, the condition is referred to as multicystic dysplastic kidney (MDK), the most common cause of abdominal mass in infancy.

In the neonate, MDK presents as an abdominal or flank mass (the enlarged, palpable kidney). Hydronephrosis is due to communicating cysts within the organ. Both kidneys should be assessed by US given the high rate of anomalies in the contralateral organ (ureteropelvic junction obstruction; vesicoureteral reflux; hydronephrosis secondary to posterior urethral valves). VCUG is indicated in patients with bilateral renal abnormalities. Finally, renal scintigraphy is necessary to confirm nonfunctionality of the dysplastic kidney.

Renal concentrating ability is suboptimal in most patients with significant renal dysplasia, including those with MDK. Once the affected infant begins voiding, fluids should be liberalized to prevent dehydration and salt depletion. Most dysplastic kidneys involute over time. However, a minority undergo progressive enlargement due to cystic growth, resulting in pain. Although there is no demonstrated risk of malignant transformation of the dysplastic kidney, surgical removal may be indicated for relief of pain.

MDK can arise in isolation or be part of a known sequence or syndrome. VATER (or VACTERL) is the association of the following anomalies (at least two must be present for diagnosis):

- Vertebral anomalies (*example: hemivertebrae*)
- Anal atresia
- Cardiac defects (*example: ventricular septal defect*)
- Tracheoesophageal fistula
- Renal anomalies (*examples: renal dysplasia; renal agenesis*)
- Radial limb defects (*examples: club hand; absence of thumb*)

Chromosomal analysis is indicated for all patients with VATER association in order to rule out rare underlying structural defects. MDK also occurs with increased frequency in patients with CHARGE association, Beckwith-Wiedemann syndrome, and multiple trisomy syndromes.

Potter syndrome is characterized by neonatal pulmonary hypoplasia in the setting of severe bilateral renal dysplasia/aplasia and oligohydramnios. Low amniotic fluid levels result in anomalies consistent with fetal constraint, including growth restriction, flattened facies, low-set ears, micrognathia, and joint contractures. Neonatal pulmonary hypoplasia has a high mortality rate, even when optimal treatment is rendered.

Polycystic Kidney Disease

Although bilateral cystic disease is a feature of both infantile (autosomal recessive; ARPKD) and adult (autosomal dominant; ADPKD) polycystic kidney disease, these two disorders are distinct in their presentations. ARPKD presents in early infancy with bilateral flank masses and renal dysfunction of variable severity. Cysts are not usually visualized on US in the neonatal period, but both kidneys are enlarged and abnormally echogenic. The diagnosis may be confirmed by computed tomography or magnetic resonance imaging. Up to half of affected patients die before the age of one year due to pulmonary hypoplasia or end-stage renal disease. Disease of mild severity may result in only minimal renal insufficiency with or without hypertension. However, the other major element of ARPKD, congenital hepatic fibrosis, eventually leads to portal hypertension, hepatomegaly or hepatosplenomegaly, bleeding esophageal varices, and hepatic failure. Transplantation is a viable option in some patients.

ADPKD usually does not present until after 30 years of age, but severe cases may become symptomatic in late childhood or adolescence. Younger patients present with some combination of the following: abdominal and/or flank pain, hypertension, and hematuria. Flank masses (hydronephrosis) are detectable in some cases. Abdominal US demonstrates large cysts in both kidneys and possibly the spleen, pancreas, and liver. Involvement of the vasculature is not uncommon; at least one in ten affected individuals develops intracranial aneurysms. ADPKD which manifests in children and adolescents is typically extremely severe, with progression to end-stage renal disease in early adulthood. Changes in the renal architecture may be noted long before the disease becomes symptomatic, and genetic testing is available. However, there is general agreement within the medical community that US and molecular screening studies are not indicated for asymptomatic children with an affected parent; treatment in the presymptomatic stage does not affect progression, and individuals should be allowed to decide whether testing is in their best interests once they have reached adulthood.

Ureteropelvic Junction Obstruction

Ureteropelvic junction obstruction (UPJO) is the most common congenital cause of urinary tract obstruction. Intrinsic fibrosis at the junction of the renal pelvis and ureter, kinking of the ureter, and a crossing renal vessel may all obstruct the urinary tract. The obstruction is bilateral in 20% of cases. Hydronephrosis is occasionally detected in the infant with UPJO. The older child presents with abdominal or flank pain and an abdominal mass on deep palpation. Infection due to urinary stasis is not uncommon. Abdominal US demonstrates enlargement of the involved kidney(s), thinning of the renal parenchyma, and dilation of the pelvis. Radioisotope renography is used to localize the site of obstruction. Dilatation is noted proximal to the lesion, and excretion below the obstruction is delayed. Administration of furosemide results in rapid clearance of the isotope below the obstruction, but the signal is increased proximal to the obstructed area. This increase in signal intensity following administration of a diuretic corresponds clinically with pain these patients experience when they are given diuretics. Pyeloplasty (surgical correction) reestablishes transport of urine from the pelvis to the ureter and relieves the obstruction.

Vesicoureteral Reflux

Vesicoureteral reflux (VUR) results from incompetence of the functional valve preventing backflow of urine into the ureter during bladder contraction. VUR is usually bilateral but may be more severe on one side than the other. The most frequent presentation is recurrent urinary tract infection (including pyelonephritis). Severe congenital reflux causes hydronephrosis in utero.

VCUG detects abnormalities at ureteral insertion sites and allows grading of the reflux based on extent of retrograde flow and associated dilatation of the ureter and renal pelvis. Low grades (I-II) of reflux often resolve spontaneously within a few years of diagnosis; VCUG should be repeated every year until resolution is demonstrated. Antibiotic prophylaxis is unnecessary in patients with grade I reflux; patients with grade II reflux do not require prophylaxis unless they are in diapers, have recurrent urinary tract infections, or experience dysfunctional voiding.

High grades of reflux produce large, tortuous ureters and marked distortion of the renal pelvis and calyces. Recurrent pyelonephritis results in progressive scarring and loss of renal function. Antibiotic prophylaxis is recommended for all patients with grades III-V reflux (amoxicillin in the infant; trimethoprim-sulfamethoxazole or nitrofurantoin in the older child). Deflux surgery (i.e., injection of polymer material into the region of insertion) is indicated for grades III-V reflux which does not resolve within 12 months of diagnosis. Ureteral reimplantation surgery may be preferable in some patients.

Bladder Outlet Obstruction

Occurring only in males, posterior urethral valves (PUV) consist of posteriorly-situated leaflets within the prostatic urethra which result in partial bladder outlet obstruction. The increased pressure causes urethral dilation followed by bladder neck hypertrophy, mucosal trabeculation, and (not infrequently) vesicoureteral reflux and renal dysgenesis. PUV is the most common cause of end-stage renal disease in childhood.

Prenatal detection of hydronephrosis or palpation of a distended bladder during the newborn examination should prompt consideration of PUV. In older infants, parents may note a weak or dribbling urinary stream or unexplained daytime wetting; however, a strong urinary stream does not rule out PUV. Occasionally, the condition is diagnosed during radiologic evaluation related to a urinary tract infection. The leaflets are clearly visible on VCUG, with proximal urethral dilatation and distal narrowing forming a "spinning top" appearance. Transurethral ablation is the treatment of choice. Temporary placement of a vesicostomy is an option for neonates who are too small for the procedure. Prognosis depends on the degree of renal and bladder impairment at the time of repair; patients with reduced renal function and significantly involvement of the renal parenchyma are likely to progress to end-stage renal disease within several years, despite ablation of the valves and repair of associated urinary tract defects. Long-term monitoring via renal US, serum electrolytes, and urine output is indicated for patients at high risk for ESRD.

Bladder outlet obstruction is uncommon in female children. If it is suspected, VCUG is the diagnostic study of choice. Narrowing of the female urethra in the setting of a normal urinary stream does not increase a patient's risk of UTI and requires no treatment. The narrowing is benign and resolves as the patient grows.

Alport Syndrome

Alport syndrome (also called hereditary or familial nephritis) is an inherited defect of type IV collagen, part of the makeup of the glomerular basement membrane. Multiple forms of inheritance are possible; X-linked dominant is the most common form. The essential features of the condition are progressive renal failure, sensorineural hearing loss (up to half of patients), and abnormalities of the ocular lens, all of which are variable in severity within and between different people. Relatives of patients with Alport syndrome are screened for the presence of blood in the urine, which is present even in early infancy in affected individuals. The diagnosis is confirmed through renal biopsy or genetic testing.

Males are affected earlier and more severely than females, who may remain asymptomatic carriers or have microscopic hematuria and mild disease. Males develop end-stage renal disease in early adulthood and are more likely to experience cochlear and ocular manifestations.

Congenital Nephrotic Syndrome

Congenital nephrotic syndrome, a rare condition (except in the Finnish population), is caused by a genetic defect in nephrin, a basement membrane protein which provides a barrier to leakage of proteins into the urine. Not surprisingly, patients present in the neonatal period with marked edema and proteinuria. Renal abnormalities may be noted on prenatal US; in some cases, fetal demise occurs due to hydrops. The protein loss accounts for many features of the disease, including:

- edema (secondary to loss of albumin and the subsequent decrease in vascular oncotic pressure)
- failure to thrive/malnutrition
- hypothyroidism (resulting from the loss of thyroid-binding globulin in the urine)
- bleeding diathesis (loss of clotting factors)
- increased susceptibility to infection (excessive excretion of serum immunoglobulins)

Hydronephrosis is noted in all affected infants by 2 months of age, if not in utero. US demonstrates increased echogenicity of the renal cortex and progressive blurring of corticomedullary borders. Eventually, the kidneys become small, fibrotic, and nonfunctional.

The primary goals of management are protein replacement (through enteral, parenteral routes and/or via albumin infusions); administration of low-dose aspirin, thyroxine, and antibiotic prophylaxis to prevent specific complications as noted above; angiotensin-converting enzyme inhibitors to staunch protein loss; dialysis; and (eventually) renal transplantation. As opposed to minimal change nephrotic syndrome, corticosteroids and cyclophosphamide have not been found to be beneficial in the treatment of congenital nephrotic syndrome.

Urinary Tract Infection

Bacterial urinary tract infection (UTI) is a frequent cause of pediatric morbidity. Infection may be limited to the bladder (*cystitis*) *or* may also involve the kidney (pyelonephritis). The genders are equally affected in the first year of life; thereafter, girls have almost a ten-fold risk over boys. The most significant risk factor is the presence of a urinary tract abnormality that causes urinary stasis, obstruction, reflux, or dysfunctional voiding. Children with pyelonephritis usually sustain damage to the infected area of the renal parenchyma, resulting in localized scarring and decreased function.

In febrile infants, the urinary tract is the most common site of bacterial infection. The source is almost always hematogenous seeding of the kidneys, which correlates with the high rate of renal scarring seen in this group of patients. UTI in the infant warrants special consideration because:

- Fever may be the only manifestation of UTI in this age group. Absence of pyuria does not rule out UTI in febrile infants.
- UTI is often the first suggestion of an obstructive anomaly or vesicoureteral reflux. Ideally, urine should be collected, analyzed, and cultured in all febrile patients under the age of 2 years. Urine may be obtained by suprapubic tap (in neonates) or sterile catheterization of the bladder.

UTI in patients beyond infancy more often results from ascent of exterior fecal flora into the urinary tract. Common pathogens include *Escherichia coli* (80%) and *Proteus* and *Klebsiella* species. In older children, the signs and symptoms of cystitis are similar to those in adults and include low-grade fever, frequency, urgency, dysuria, incontinence, abdominal pain, and hematuria. In contrast, pyelonephritis presents with high fever, chills, nausea, vomiting, and flank pain. Elevation of the peripheral white blood count, erythrocyte sedimentation rate, and C-reactive protein are more consistent with upper tract involvement.

Although pyuria, hematuria, and bacteriuria on urinalysis suggest a UTI, a positive urine culture is the gold standard for diagnosis. The absence of white or red blood cells in the urine does not rule out a urinary tract infection; however, urine which is negative for nitrites is unlikely to be infected. Bagged specimens are adequate for assessment of cellular material but are not appropriate for culture. Patients with positive leukocyte esterase dipstick results should be treated for a presumed urinary tract infection until culture results are available. Appropriate oral antibiotics include amoxicillin, ampicillin, nitrofurantoin, or trimethoprim-sulfamethoxazole. If the culture is negative, antibiotics may be discontinued. Patients with positive urine cultures should complete a 5- to 10-day course with an appropriate oral antibiotic based on sensitivity results. Three days of trimethoprim-sulfamethoxazole may be sufficient in the adolescent.

Nontoxic-appearing children with suspected pyelonephritis are treated with oral cefixime or intravenous ampicillin plus gentamicin or cefotaxime until culture results are available. Patients who are unstable, unable to tolerate oral medications, septic, or under 2 months of age warrant admission to the hospital for intravenous antibiotics and observation.

Recommendations regarding assessment for underlying pathology following an initial UTI in the pediatric patient are controversial and depend on the patient's age, severity of infection, and response to treatment. A diagnostic algorithm for children with urinary tract infections is provided in Figure 16-1. Current American Academy of Pediatrics guidelines recommend that all children under the age of 24 months undergo renal US to rule out hydronephrosis or structural lesions that predispose to infection. Those who do not respond to appropriate antibiotic therapy within 48 hours should also be evaluated with VCUG. In prompt responders, the VCUG is optional. Other experts argue that all children under a certain age (6 to 12 months; 5 years) should receive a VCUG regardless of response to treatment. It is likely that further studies will clarify the diagnostic picture.

The prognosis for patients with isolated cases of cystitis is excellent; morbidity increases with recurrent infection. Most UTI-related complications accompany pyelonephritis, including perinephric abscess, renal scarring, and renal failure.

Glomerulonephritis

Glomerulonephritis is inflammation within the glomerulus. Antigen-antibody complexes are formed or deposited in subepithelial or subendothelial areas; immune mediators

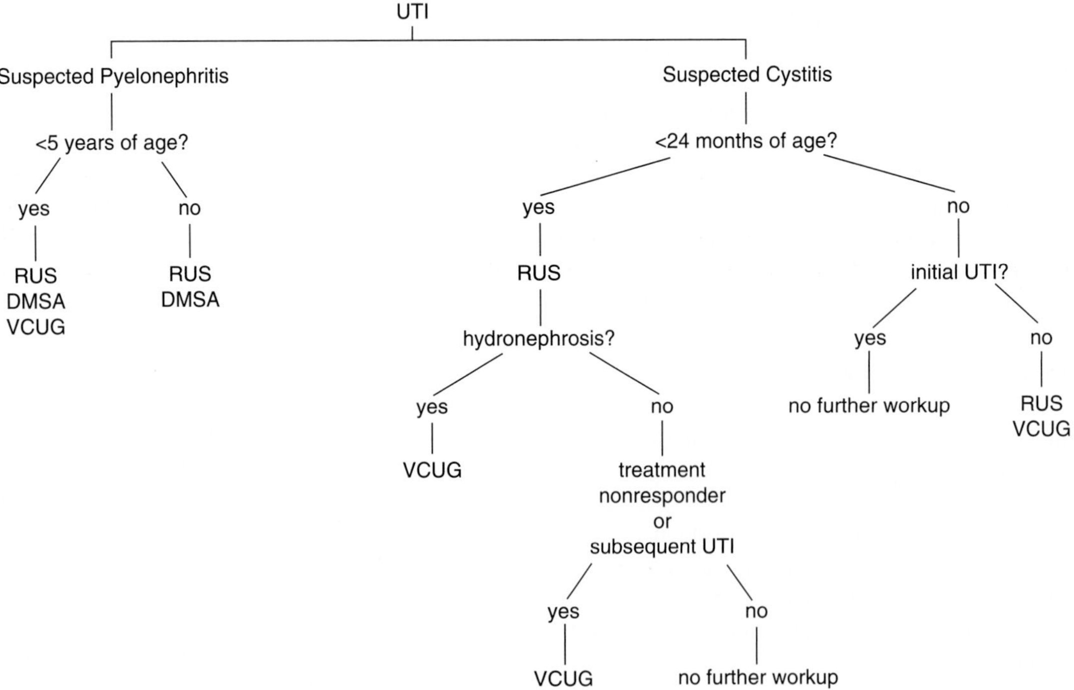

Figure 16-1 Diagnostic algorithm for pediatric urinary tract infection. (From Marino BS and Fine KS. *Blueprints Pediatrics.* 4th ed. Philadelphia: Lippincott Williams & Wilkins; 2006 with permission.)

follow, resulting in inflammatory injury. Hematuria with red cell casts is the hallmark of the disease; other presenting features include oliguria, malaise, abdominal pain, edema, hypertension, and azotemia (evidenced by elevated serum creatinine and blood urea nitrogen concentrations). Proteinuria is less prominent than in nephrotic syndrome. A decrease in GFR precipitates circulatory overload and temporary disruption of sodium and potassium regulation. Laboratory studies to consider in the patient with suspected glomerulonephritis include urinalysis, urine culture, complete blood count, coagulation studies, serum electrolyte levels, blood urea nitrogen and creatinine, streptococcal antibody titers, and complement levels.

Acute Glomerulonephritis

Postinfectious acute glomerulonephritis (PIAGN) is the term used to describe generalized glomerular inflammation that follows an infection not directly involving the renal or genitourinary systems. It is the most common pediatric glomerulonephritis and is typically benign and self-limited. PIAGN is usually associated with group A beta-hemolytic streptococcal (GAS) infection of the throat or skin, but other bacterial and viral infections can be associated with this condition. Appropriate treatment of the causative pathogen does not prevent renal inflammation. Infection precedes the onset of glomerular disease by 1 to 3 weeks. Clinical manifestations include microscopic (or occasionally gross) hematuria, edema, and hypertension due to retention of salt and water caused by the diminished GFR. Management consists of antibiotic therapy to eradicate GAS from the oropharynx and, in hypertensive, oliguric, or edematous patients, loop diuretics and fluid restriction. The prognosis is excellent; PIAGN rarely progresses to chronic renal failure. However, patients with rapidly progressive disease and acute renal failure are less likely to regain normal renal function; such children may require dialysis.

Laboratory evaluation is indicated for determining whether a GAS infection has occurred and for differentiating PIAGN from other causes of glomerulonephritis. Elevated antistreptolysin-O or anti-DNAase B titers are consistent with recent streptococcal infection. Total hemolytic complement levels are low, and the C3 component of the complement pathway is diminished, but C4 values are typically normal. The C4 is low in membranoproliferative glomerulonephritis and lupus nephritis, whereas serum complement levels remain normal in IgA nephropathy and focal segmental glomerulonephritis. Renal biopsy is unnecessary in cases of PIAGN, but if the diagnosis is in doubt, histologic examination demonstrates mesangial and capillary cell proliferation, inflammatory cell infiltration, and granular "humps" of IgG and C3 below the glomerular basement membrane.

Normalization of renal function and serum complement levels is complete within 6 months. Hypertension, hematuria, and proteinuria may rarely persist several months longer.

Chronic Glomerulonephritis

Rapidly progressive glomerulonephritis is the description given to a number of glomerulopathies that, for unknown reasons, deteriorate over a few weeks or months to renal failure, uremia, encephalopathy, and even death. All forms produce generalized crescent formation in the glomeruli, thought to represent cellular destruction by macrophages with subsequent necrosis and fibrin deposition. Many chronic glomerulonephritic syndromes eventually recur in a transplanted kidney.

Rapidly progressive glomerulonephritis is rare in children.

Nephrotic Syndrome

Nephrotic syndrome (NS) is a glomerular disorder characterized by proteinuria, hypoalbuminemia, hyperlipidemia, and edema. Minimal change disease (MCD) is by far the most common cause of primary nephrotic syndrome in the pediatric population; focal segmental glomerulosclerosis (FSGS) and membranoproliferative glomerulonephritis (MPGN) account for the remainder of pediatric cases. Patients typically present between the ages of 2 to 10 years, and boys outnumber girls. The criteria for diagnosis of NS include:

- generalized edema
- hypoproteinemia (≤2 g/dL), with proportionately lower serum albumin in relation to serum globulin (serum albumin/globulin ratio <1.0)
- urinary protein/creatinine ratio >2 on first morning void (normally <0.2), OR documented protein loss >50 mg/kg/day
- hypercholesterolemia (>200 mg/dL; often >500 mg/dL) and elevated triglyceride levels

Patients with nephrotic syndrome initially appear quite well, usually manifesting only periorbital or facial edema. Generalized edema and ascites occur later in the course of the disease, often accompanied by anorexia, diarrhea, and abdominal pain. Pulmonary effusions may develop in severe cases.

Electrolyte abnormalities are not uncommon in patients with NS. Hyperkalemia and hyponatremia can reach symptomatic levels, whereas hypocalcemia is generally mild. Hypertension and hematuria are less common in MCD when compared with other causes of nephrotic syndrome. Patients with NS who are found to have low C3 and C4 levels are more likely to have MPGN than MCD. Serum complement levels are typically normal in MCD and FSGS.

Treatment of an initial episode of NS consists of salt restriction and oral corticosteroid therapy, which is begun immediately following a documented negative tuberculin skin test. Prednisone is prescribed daily for 4 to 6 weeks, or until remission, followed by every other day dosing. Progress is initially measured by daily weights; protein levels in the urine should begin to fall in the second week of therapy and clear within 3 to 4 weeks. The stable patient with a good diuretic response may be discharged from the hospital after a short stay. Cyclophosphamide and chlorambucil are alkylating agents are beneficial for inducing remission in subsequent episodes of proteinuria. Administration of one of these medications in combination with corticosteroids may increase the responsiveness of steroid-resistant disease.

Patients who are markedly edematous, oliguric, or unstable at diagnosis are managed with infusion of albumin over 8 to 12 hours coupled with a loop diuretic. Diuretic therapy alone removes fluid from the intravascular space only and may precipitate hypovolemic collapse. Adverse effects associated with use of loop diuretics include electrolyte imbalances (hypokalemia is the most common, but hyponatremia, hypochloremia, hypercalciuria, and hypomagnesemia can also occur), alkalosis, hyperglycemia, hyperuricemia, and ototoxicity. Loop diuretics are bound to albumin for transport, so they may be less effective in patients with severe hypoalbuminemia. Thiazide diuretics may be more appropriate in some cases.

Renal biopsy is indicated for patients outside the typical age range for MCD, frequent relapsers, and those who do not respond to standard corticosteroid treatment within 8 weeks. Biopsy is unnecessary at initial presentation because results do not effect first-line treatment. True to the name, gross sections in MCD show few if any abnormalities; the only consistent finding is effacement of epithelial cell foot processes demonstrated by electron microscopy. FSGS is characterized by focal sections of distorted glomeruli, with mesangial hypertrophy and segmental capillary loop fibrosis. Increased mesangial cellularity and glomerular basement membrane thickening are found in diffuse MPGN.

Prognosis is closely linked to response to initial therapy. Rapid resolution with steroid treatment is associated with a better long-term prognosis and fewer relapses. Though MCD recurs in most patients at least once, the majority of affected individuals eventually remain disease-free, with normal renal function and life expectancy. In general, the prognosis is less favorable for NS due to MPGN or FSGS; progression to end-stage renal disease is not uncommon, and both conditions recur in a transplanted kidney.

Bacterial infection is the most frequent complication of NS. Patients lose IgG and other immune proteins in their urine, and susceptibility is further increased by immunosuppressant medications. Spontaneous bacterial peritonitis (infection of ascites fluid) presents with abdominal pain, nausea, vomiting, and fever. Culture typically grows *Streptococcus pneumoniae* or *Escherichia coli*. Definitive diagnosis requires paracentesis. A fluid sample which yields the following results is consistent with peritonitis:

- White blood count >2.5 X 10^3/mcL
- pH <7.35
- Glucose <50 mg per dL
- LDH >225 U per L
- Total protein level >10 g per dL
- Organisms present on Gram stain

Patients with NS and spontaneous bacterial peritonitis are managed with 10 to 14 days of intravenous antibiotics (ceftriaxone, cefotaxime, or cefotetan).

Other complications of NS include thromboembolism (hypercoagulability) and impaired growth due to protein loss and chronic steroid therapy.

Hemolytic-Uremic Syndrome

Hemolytic-uremic syndrome (HUS), the triad of renal insufficiency, microangiopathic hemolytic anemia, and thrombocytopenia, is the most common cause of acute renal failure in the pediatric population. "Typical" HUS follows a bacterial diarrheal infection with a verotoxin-producing pathogen, most commonly *E. coli* 0157:H7. Patients are usually between the ages of 6 months and 5 years. As the diarrhea begins to resolve 10 to 14 days into the illness, the patient suddenly develops irritability, pallor, petechiae, abdominal pain, and oliguria. Hypertension is common. The white blood count may be normal or elevated but usually has a left shift. Hemoglobin levels are typically below 8.0 g per dL, and platelet counts rarely exceed 60,000 per mcL. Emergency treatment of HUS involves judicious fluid and/or blood product replacement, bowel rest, and dialysis if the patient becomes anuric or has a serum potassium >6.5 mEq per L. Plasma exchange is reserved for severe cases. HUS resolves without sequelae in the majority of patients who are appropriately managed. "Atypical" HUS does not follow a diarrheal illness and has a poorer prognosis. Older patients and those who develop bowel necrosis, seizures, or altered mental status also tend to fair less well.

IgA Nephropathy

IgA nephropathy (Berger disease), once thought to be a benign condition, is now known to progress to end-stage renal disease in over half of affected individuals. It is rarely diagnosed in children younger than 10 years of age. Although the etiology remains unclear, IgA nephropathy is more common in family members of patients with the condition. Affected individuals present with asymptomatic gross hematuria and a history of recent upper respiratory infection. Some patients complain of mild abdominal discomfort; hypertension is notably absent. Many red blood cells are noted on urinalysis, but samples are negative for protein, and renal function is initially normal. The serum IgA concentration may or may not be elevated; C3 levels are normal. Renal biopsy is required for diagnosis, demonstrating mesangial deposits of IgA-containing immune complexes in the glomeruli. Recurrent episodes of hematuria are the norm and frequently follow infectious illnesses. One third of cases progress to end-stage renal disease within 10 years of diagnosis (more common in males), with another one third over the second decade. Progression is signaled by increasing serum creatinine concentration, proteinuria, and/or hypertension. IgA nephropathy which presents in childhood tends to be more severe. Immunosuppressive therapy with corticosteroids does not appear to slow progression of the disease. Patients with IgA are followed quarterly with urinalysis and random urinary protein/creatinine ratios, serum electrolytes, serum creatinine concentrations, and blood pressure checks.

Henoch-Schönlein Purpura

Henoch-Schönlein purpura (HSP), a systemic vasculitis characterized by lower extremity purpura, cramping abdominal pain, and arthralgia/arthritis, may progress to a glomerulonephritis-type syndrome that is indistinguishable from IgA nephropathy. Up to half of patients with HSP manifest renal involvement (usually isolated microscopic hematuria). Biopsy is rarely necessary; results are very similar to those for IgA nephropathy. Long-term renal impairment related to HSP is rare; renal failure is more common in patients who present with proteinuria, hypertension, and reduced GFR. Corticosteroids are often given to patients with HSP but do not appear to affect renal involvement. HSP is discussed in further detail in Chapter 21.

Renal Failure

Acute Renal Failure

Renal failure is an uncommon but potentially life-threatening condition in children. Acute renal failure (ARF) involves the abrupt reduction in renal function (occurring over hours-to-days), retention of nitrogenous waste products (azotemia), and fluid and electrolyte imbalances. The mechanism of ARF may be prerenal, intrarenal (intrinsic), or postrenal. Prerenal failure results when a normal kidney experiences significant hypoperfusion due to hypovolemia and/or hypotension. Dehydration, sepsis (in the neonate), and congestive heart failure can all lead to prerenal failure. The substantial decrease in glomerular filtration rate is evidenced by oliguria or even anuria. Prerenal failure is completely reversible unless it remains unrecognized or is inappropriately treated.

Intrinsic renal failure results from an abnormality of the kidney itself, such as glomerulonephritis, interstitial nephritis, renal vasculitis, or acute tubular necrosis, a condition in which damaged tubules become obstructed with cellular debris. Intrinsic renal failure may follow administration of certain drugs known to be nephrotoxic (ACE inhibitors, indomethacin, amphotericin). Intrarenal conditions typically present with oliguria, although the urine output may remain normal (nonoliguric renal failure).

In postrenal failure, obstructive lesions at or below the collecting ducts produce increased intrarenal pressure, hydronephrosis, and compromised glomerular filtration. Obstructive uropathy, vesicoureteral reflux, and nephrolithiasis may all result in postrenal failure. Patients with complete obstruction will be anuric; urine output is generally preserved in the setting of partial obstruction.

ARF presents with edema, oliguria, and hypertension. Hyperkalemia, azotemia, and metabolic acidosis develop as the GFR falls, and increases in the serum creatinine concentration parallel diminishing renal function. Anemia is variably present. Urine and plasma sodium, urea nitrogen, creatinine, and osmolality are useful for differentiating prerenal and intrinsic failure (Table 16-6).

The management of ARF is individualized based on the underlying cause, volume status of the patient, and concurrent electrolyte abnormalities. Optimal fluid management is essential. Volume depletion, if present, should be corrected. Ins, outs, and insensible losses are calculated and replaced. Diuretics such as furosemide that help preserve renal blood flow may be indicated in the early stages of ARF. Hyperkalemia and other electrolyte imbalances are reversed with appropriate therapy, and pH is normalized. Protein is restricted to replacement needs only. Short-term hemodialysis is necessary in some patients. The prognosis of ARF depends on the underlying etiology, length of impairment, and severity of functional disturbance. Medications that undergo renal clearance may require dosing adjustments in acute (and chronic) renal failure to avoid toxicity.

Chronic Renal Failure

Chronic renal failure (CRF) implies that renal function has dropped below 30% of normal; function at 10% or less defines end-stage renal disease. The most common cause of CRF in the pediatric population is obstructive uropathy, followed by renal dysplasia, glomerulonephropathies (particularly FSGS), and hereditary renal conditions (e.g., cystic kidney disease).

Patients with CRF may be largely asymptomatic or experience any combination of the following: anorexia, nausea, malaise, lethargy, polyuria, recurrent dehydration, salt craving, and decreased exercise tolerance. Hypertension and pallor are usually noted on examination. Long-standing CRF

TABLE 16-6
TYPICAL FINDINGS IN PRERENAL VERSUS INTRINSIC ACUTE RENAL FAILURE IN CHILDREN

Diagnostic Index	Prerenal	Intrinsic
Fractional excretion of sodium (%) = $[(U_{Na} \times P_{Cr})/(P_{Na} \times U_{Cr})] \times 100$	<1	>1
Urine creatinine/Plasma creatinine	>40	<20
Urine urea nitrogen/Plasma urea nitrogen	>8	<3
Urine osmolality (mOsm/L)	>500	<350
Urine osmolality/Plasma osmolality	>1.5	<1.5
Urine specific gravity	>1.020	<1.020
Plasma urea nitrogen/Plasma creatinine	>20	<15

P_{Cr}, plasma creatinine concentration; P_{Na}, plasma sodium concentration; U_{Cr}, urine creatinine concentration; U_{Na}, urine sodium concentration.

produces rickets or other forms of disordered bone growth which may be visually evident. Patients with CRF develop many of the same laboratory abnormalities seen in ARF, including azotemia, acidosis, sodium imbalance, and hyperkalemia. Anemia is virtually always present to some degree.

The major sequelae of CRF include growth failure, anemia, renal osteodystrophy, and developmental/social delay:

- Growth retardation affects nearly all children with CRF and is thought to be primarily due to end-organ resistance to growth hormone (due to uremia), inhibition of pulsatile growth hormone secretion (metabolic acidosis), and increased protein catabolism. Caloric intake should be maintained despite protein restriction, particularly in patients younger than 2 years of age, in whom catch-up growth remains suboptimal even after renal transplantation. Recombinant human growth hormone has been proven to augment height growth in patients with CRF but must be administered daily (parenteral route) until the child reaches the expected height for age or receives a transplanted kidney.
- Anemia is more closely associated with CRF than with acute renal failure. It is typically normocytic and normochromic. Folate supplementation is routine; oral iron is added for patients with low serum ferritin levels (as may occur with the institution of erythropoietin). Recombinant human erythropoietin is usually required to maintain adequate hemoglobin concentrations in patients undergoing hemodialysis; overcorrection increases the risk of thrombosis.
- Renal osteodystrophy is a form of delayed and disordered bone growth associated with CRF. Long-standing CRF predisposes to skeletal deformities, rickets, osteopenia, and bone pain. The underlying abnormality is secondary hyperparathyroidism resulting from parathyroid hormone resistance and hypocalcemia. Alterations in calcium and phosphate metabolism in chronic renal failure are presented in Figure 16-2. Children with CRF require calcium carbonate and activated vitamin D supplements for prevention or reversal of bony changes.
- CRF management is complex and time-consuming. Pediatric patients with CRF often experience a diminished quality of life and are predisposed to developmental and social delays.

Treatment for CRF includes optimization of nutritional intake (in spite of protein and salt restriction); pharmacologic intervention (diuretics, recombinant erythropoietin); and dialysis therapy. Children with <10% of normal renal function evidenced by a serum creatinine concentration >10 mg per dL require either dialysis or renal transplantation. Peritoneal dialysis, which can be performed at home, is the preferred method for most children undergoing long-term dialysis. Peritonitis, the most frequent complication of peritoneal dialysis, is usually due to gram-positive organisms. Hernias may occur at the catheter insertion site in the groin.

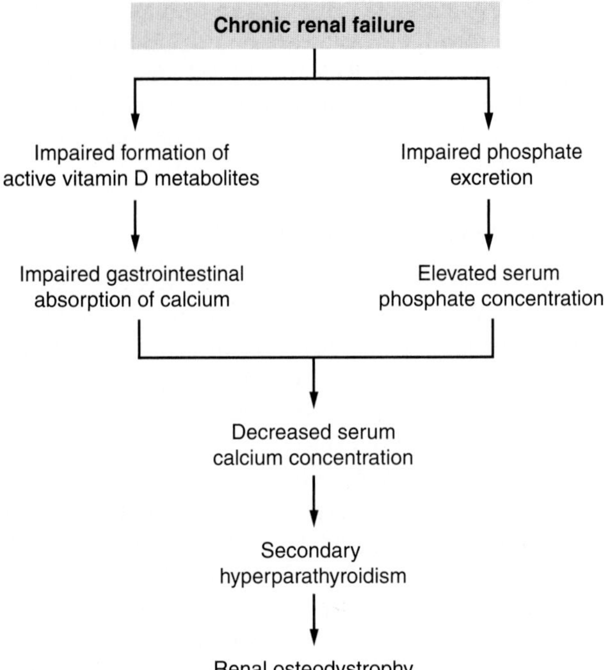

Figure 16-2 Alterations in calcium and phosphate metabolism in chronic renal failure.

Other potential complications include pain, cellulitis, tunnel infections, and peritoneal membrane failure. Hemodialysis provides close to 10% of normal renal function but is time-consuming. Disequilibrium syndrome, a form of cerebral edema that results when the serum urea nitrogen level drops too rapidly, is a known complication of hemodialysis which presents with headache, nausea, vomiting, abdominal pain, muscle cramps, and seizures progressing to coma. Other complications include bleeding, thrombosis, and infection. Hemodialysis-associated mortality is low at specialized pediatric centers, but availability is limited, and complications can occur despite appropriate care.

Renal transplantation is the definitive therapy for all children with end-stage renal disease, and there are few absolute contraindications. The donated organ may come from a living-related or deceased donor; living-related donor transplants have better host and graft survival rates. Improvements in the surgical and intensive care of infants has led to transplantation at earlier ages, substantially increasing both the quality and duration of life in infants with CRF due to congenital disorders.

Renal Trauma

The most common cause of blunt abdominal trauma is motor vehicle collision. Computed tomography of the abdomen with intravenous contrast is the preferred initial diagnostic study in the stable pediatric trauma victim. Abdominal US can be performed in children who are too unstable to be transferred to the radiology department, but it is not as sensitive as computed tomography. Diagnostic peritoneal lavage is reserved for patients who are already in the operating room for surgical care of their injuries.

Renal injury should be suspected in the trauma patient who presents with flank pain, gross or microscopic hematuria, abdominal or flank tenderness, or a palpable flank mass. Computed tomography of the abdomen with intravenous contrast is the diagnostic modality of choice for evaluation of patients with renal trauma and injury. Renal contusion, the most common injury of the kidney, responds to bed rest and symptomatic care. Significant lacerations of the kidney should be surgically repaired. Traumatic fragmentation of the parenchyma or disruption of a major vessel usually necessitates nephrectomy.

Placement of a Foley catheter is contraindicated in patients with visible blood at the urethral meatus due to the possibility of urethral trauma. Trauma is the most common cause of urethral stricture in the pediatric population. Urethral stricture is much more common in males.

Renal Toxins

A list of medications known to cause renal toxicity is presented in Table 16-7.

TABLE 16-7

RENAL TOXICITY AND MEDICATIONS

Aminoglycosides

- Aminoglycosides are the most likely class of antibiotics to result in nephrotoxicity.
- The mechanism of action is related to concentrated uptake of the drug within the proximal renal tubular cells.
- Nephrotoxicity is more likely to occur in the setting of extended or high-dose therapy and dehydration.
- The classic presentation involves gradual increases in serum blood urea nitrogen and creatinine concentrations, which may be accompanied by hypertension.
- Nephrotoxicity associated with aminoglycoside administration is reversible once the drug is discontinued.
- Examples of commonly used aminoglycosides in children include gentamicin, tobramycin, amikacin, streptomycin, and kanamycin.

Tacrolimus (oral)

- Nephrotoxicity is uncommon but does occur, especially when the drug is used post-renal transplantation.
- Presentation consists of gradual compromise in the glomerular filtration rate, which is reversible if the drug is discontinued in the early stages.
- Peak and trough levels should be monitored frequently.

Cyclosporine

- Nephrotoxicity is rare in the acute setting, but chronic use invariably leads to morphologic changes (interstitial fibrosis, glomerular sclerosis).

Renal Stones

The formation of stones within the urinary system (also called renal calculi, nephrolithiasis, or urolithiasis) involves the interplay of multiple factors, including genetic predisposition, concurrent systemic disorders, local anatomy, and biochemical environment. Stones are more likely to occur in the setting of low urinary volume, high concentration, acidic pH, low mobility, and bacterial infection. Conditions associated with stone formation in children are provided in Table 16-8.

Adolescents with renal stones present similarly to adults, with the sudden onset of severe colicky flank pain. Children may have nonspecific abdominal cramping, or flank or inguinal pain. Hematuria, gross or microscopic, is virtually always noted. Asymptomatic renal stones may be found during the work-up of a urinary tract infection, especially if the stone is obstructive or otherwise results in renal stasis.

The initial evaluation of a patient with suspected nephrolithiasis consists of plain abdominal radiographs. With the exception of xanthine stones, most renal calculi are radiopaque. US or preferably spiral computed tomography provides additional information regarding associated lesions (obstructive uropathy/hydronephrosis) or multiple stones. Immediate urologic referral is indicated for stones associated with obstruction and hydronephrosis. Metabolic studies identify predisposing conditions, if present. Although 24-hour urine collections are preferred, spot analysis of random specimens for calcium, oxalate, cystine, citrate, and uric acid concentrations may be sufficient. Excretion of these substances may be "standardized" through comparison of their ratios to urinary creatinine concentration. The composition of any stones which are recovered should be analyzed.

Hydration and pain control form the foundation of nephrolithiasis therapy in the acute setting. Specific therapies are listed in Table 16-8. Extracorporeal shock wave lithotripsy has been used in children with good results. Endoscopic and percutaneous removal may be appropriate in some cases.

Renal Tubular Acidosis

All forms of renal tubular acidosis (RTA) are characterized by hyperchloremic metabolic acidosis (Fig. 16-3) resulting from insufficient renal transport of bicarbonate or acids. Most bicarbonate filtered from the plasma is reabsorbed in the proximal tubule, along with amino acids, glucose, sodium, potassium, calcium, phosphate, and water. In the distal tubule, the remainder of the bicarbonate is reabsorbed in exchange for hydrogen ions. Defects involving either transport site compromise pH homeostasis. RTA may be hereditary or sporadic, acute or chronic, isolated or part of a disease complex.

TABLE 16-8
CONDITIONS ASSOCIATED WITH URINARY STONE FORMATION IN THE PEDIATRIC POPULATION

Calcium Oxalate Stones (hypercalciuria)

- Calcium oxalate stones are one of the more common types of renal calculi.
- Hypercalciuria usually occurs in the setting of normal serum calcium.
- Conditions known to cause hypercalciuria include familial idiopathic hypercalciuria and distal (type 1) renal tubular acidosis.
- Loop diuretics enhance calcium excretion, resulting in hypercalciuria.
- Nephrocalcinosis is the generalized deposition of calcium within the renal parenchyma, which may be overt or microscopic. The condition is most common in ill term or preterm infants with protracted NICU courses. Other disorders which predispose to the development of nephrocalcinosis include the use of a loop diuretic in a patient with undiagnosed hypercalciuria; hypercalciuria in the setting of hypercalcemia; and chronic metabolic acidosis.
- Specific treatment of urinary stones associated with hypercalciuria consists of increasing fluid intake, limiting dietary salt, and administration of a thiazide diuretic. Supplementation with vitamin C or D should be avoided, but restriction of dietary calcium intake is not recommended.

Struvite (magnesium-ammonium-phosphate) Stones

- Struvite stones develop in the setting of chronic infection with urease-producing bacteria (e.g., *Proteus* sp.; some *Klebsiella* sp. and enterococci).
- The stones are more common in females.
- Struvite stones may take on a "staghorn" appearance due to branching into the renal calyces.

Oxalate Stones

- Hyperoxaluria is due to oxalosis, which may be primary (congenital) or acquired (bowel resection; inflammatory bowel disease).
- Calcium oxalate is deposited in multiple tissues including the kidneys (nephrocalcinosis and/or nephrolithiasis), with progression to renal insufficiency/failure.
- Other manifestations include osteoporosis and destructive arthritis, failure to thrive, and uremia.
- Patients require specialized management. Foods which are high in oxalate (spinach, nuts, tea, wheat bran) should be avoided. Dialysis is not effective.

Cystinuria

- Cystinuria is an autosomal recessive defect in renal tubular transport, resulting in excessive excretion of cystine, arginine, lysine, and ornithine.
- The renal stones may be composed of any of the above but most commonly contain cystine.
- Management consists of aggressive hydration and alkalinization of the urine.
- Cysteine stones may require surgical removal as they are relatively refractory to extracorporeal shock wave lithotripsy.

Figure 16-3 Diagnostic evaluation of hyperchloremic metabolic acidosis in a patient with suspected renal tubular acidosis (RTA).

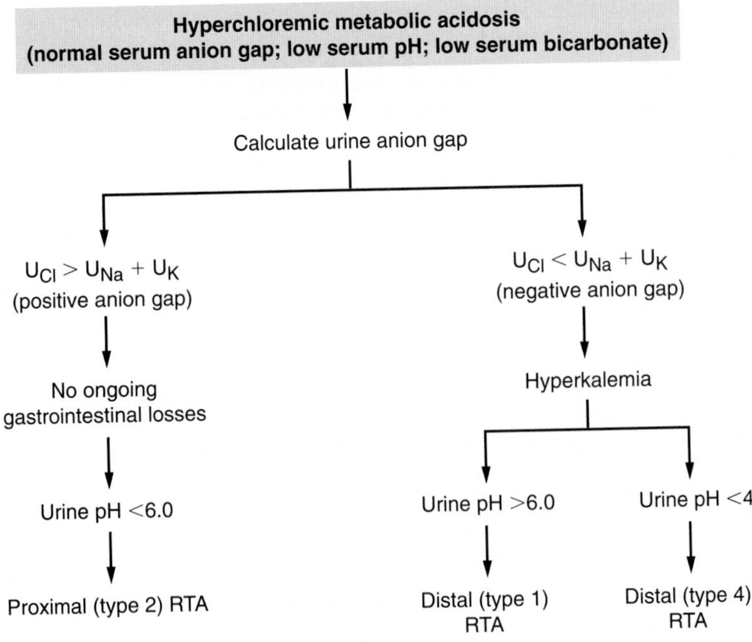

In proximal RTA (type 2), the proximal tubule fails to reabsorb bicarbonate from the ultrafiltrate. Proximal RTA type 2 is usually noted in the setting of Fanconi syndrome, a generalized disorder of proximal tubule transport resulting in excessive urinary losses of bicarbonate, amino acids, small proteins, glucose, electrolytes, and water. Patients who manifest proximal RTA type 2 as part of Fanconi syndrome present with polyuria and polydipsia, anorexia, failure to thrive, chronic acidosis, hypokalemia, volume contraction, and hypophosphatemic rickets.

Distal RTA results from either deficient hydrogen secretion (type 1) or impaired ammonia production in the face of hyperkalemia from hypoaldosteronism or pseudohypoaldosteronism (type 4):

- Distal RTA type 1 presents with metabolic acidosis and failure to thrive. Hypokalemia, hypercalciuria, and kidney stones are common. Distal RTA may occur in conjunction with related proximal tubule dysfunction.
- Type 4 is the most common RTA in adults but is rather rare in childhood. The acidosis in distal RTA type 4 occurs in the setting of hyperkalemia related to primary or secondary hypoaldosteronism or end-organ resistance.

Treatment consists of providing children with sufficient amounts of an alkalinizing agent (either bicarbonate or citrate) to completely correct the acidosis and restore normal growth. Thiazide diuretics are administered in proximal RTA to increase reabsorption of bicarbonate. Hypokalemia is treated concurrently when the alkali is coupled with potassium as a salt. Hyperkalemia is more difficult to correct; furosemide is prescribed unless the defect results in salt wasting. If RTA is associated with an underlying condition, the primary disorder must be addressed.

Nephrogenic Diabetes Insipidus

Diabetes insipidus (DI) results in an inability to produce concentrated urine. Affected individuals produce up to 400mL/kg/day of very dilute urine regardless of hydration status. DI may be central or nephrogenic in origin:

- *Central DI* results when the production or release of antidiuretic hormone (ADH; also known as arginine vasopressin) is insufficient. Usually, the condition is related to an identifiable central nervous system abnormality such as infection, tumor, or trauma.
- Congenital nephrogenic DI arises from end-organ resistance to ADH. The hormone is appropriately released from the posterior pituitary gland, but a receptor defect prevents binding and transport of water within the renal cortical tubules. The majority of cases follow an X-linked inheritance pattern, although autosomal inheritance is described as well.
- Acquired nephrogenic DI usually results from primary or secondary renal disease (polycystic kidney disease, pyelonephritis, sickle cell disease) but may be an adverse effect of certain medications (e.g., lithium).

Congenital nephrogenic DI (CNDI) presents in the first few years of life with overwhelming polyuria and compensatory polydipsia. Other features may include intermittent fever, irritability, vomiting, and failure to thrive. Most patients have histories of recurrent hypernatremic dehydration. Developmental delay is less common unless frequent hypernatremic seizures have occurred. Some patients manifest no symptoms until they are stressed with illness. Others remain completely unable to keep themselves in fluid balance without continual therapy.

Figure 16-4 provides a suggested evaluation of a patient with suspected diabetes insipidus. Other conditions that may present in a similar manner include diabetes mellitus, RTA, renal failure, and compulsive water drinking.

Patients with congenital nephrogenic DI are maintained on a diet restricted in salt and protein. Thiazide or potassium-sparing diuretics decrease urinary sodium reabsorption; nonsteroidal anti-inflammatory medications reduce water excretion and may have an additive effect when combined with diuretics.

Cystinosis

Nephropathic cystinosis is an autosomal recessive lysosomal storage disease. The accumulation of cysteine in the cells of the proximal tubule results in tubule destruction. Large amounts of sodium, bicarbonate, phosphate, and glucose are then lost in the urine, giving rise to the characteristic features of the disease: polyuria and polydipsia; failure to thrive; hypophosphatemic rickets (bowing of the legs); and (normal anion gap) hyperchloremic metabolic acidosis. This constellation of clinical findings is termed "Fanconi syndrome." Most patients progress to end-stage

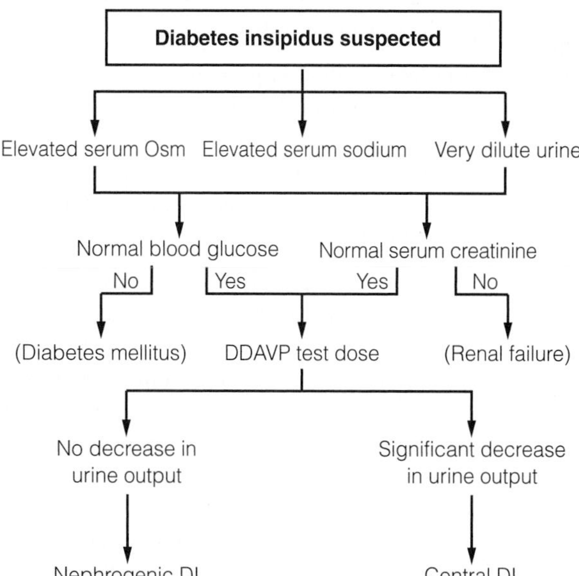

Figure 16-4 Diagnosing nephrogenic diabetes insipidus. (From Marino BS and Fine KS. *Blueprints Pediatrics*. 4th ed. Philadelphia: Lippincott Williams & Wilkins; 2006 with permission.)

renal disease by ten years of age. Kidney transplantation resolves the renal manifestations of the disease; however, accumulation of cysteine in other organs remains unchecked. Affected individuals suffer from blindness, hepatic failure, and central nervous system lesions beginning in early-to-middle adulthood.

Hypertension

Blood pressure rises as a child grows, reaching adult values during adolescence. Hypertension in the pediatric population is defined as blood pressure greater than the 95th percentile for age, gender, and height on three separate occasions. If both diastolic and systolic are less than the 90th percentile, blood pressure is considered normal. Patients with pressures which average between the 90th to 95th percentiles are prehypertensive; these patients are at increased risk of becoming hypertensive as time progresses. A single measurement is sufficient in symptomatic patients and patients with extremely high blood pressures. Essential (primary) hypertension is the most common form in adults and adolescents; unfortunately, the prevalence of essential hypertension is rising among older children as well, paralleling the rise in obesity rates. Despite this increase, children are more likely to manifest secondary hypertension. The younger the patient at diagnosis, the more likely the hypertension is due to an underlying condition. Essential hypertension does not occur in infants and is extremely rare in young children. Endocrine, vascular, and neurologic conditions may be associated with increased blood pressure (Table 16-9). However, a renal or renovascular condition is diagnosed in up to 80% of preadolescent children with secondary hypertension.

Renal disease causes hypertension through its effects on the renin-angiotensin-aldosterone system. Renin secretion is affected by each of the following:

- Afferent arteriolar perfusion pressure
- Sodium concentration in the plasma
- Sodium concentration in the tubular urine
- Sympathetic nervous system activation
- Other factors (prostaglandins, potassium uptake, atrial natriuretic peptide)

Renovascular hypertension may be due to stenosis of the renal artery or any of its tributaries. Vasculitis, renal trauma, abdominal aortic malformations (which decrease renal artery perfusion), William syndrome, radiation exposure, and surgical repair of the vessel are all associated with an increased incidence of renal artery stenosis. Ill neonates who undergo umbilical artery catheterization are at risk for embolization in the renal artery or one of its segments, which presents as the sudden onset of hypertension. The most common cause of renovascular stenosis in the pediatric population is fibromuscular dysplasia, which usually occurs in isolation but is also associated with neurofibromatosis. Compression of the renal artery by a

TABLE 16-9
DIFFERENTIAL DIAGNOSIS OF HYPERTENSION

Factitious
Anxiety
Inappropriate cuff size

Primary (essential) Hypertension

Renal*
Glomerulonephritis
Recurrent pyelonephritis with renal scarring
Parenchymal (cystic) disease
Obstructive uropathy
Reflux nephropathy
Hemolytic-uremic syndrome
Renal tumor
Renal trauma
Acute renal failure

Neurologic
Pain
Increased intracranial pressure
Hemorrhage
Familial dysautonomia

Drugs and Toxins
Oral contraceptives
Corticosteroids
Decongestants
Beta-agonist bronchodilators
Cyclosporine
Nicotine
Cocaine/amphetamines/phencyclidine

Endocrine
Congenital adrenal hyperplasia
Cushing syndrome
Hyper- or hypothyroidism
Pheochromocytoma
Hyperparathyroidism
Hyperaldosteronism
Hypercalcemia

Vascular
Coarctation of the aorta*
Renal vein thrombosis
Renal artery thrombosis/embolism*
Fibromuscular dysplasia
Large arteriovenous fistula
Vasculitis
William syndrome (multiple vascular stenoses)

Other
Immobilization in traction#
Chronic upper airway obstruction
Malignant hyperthermia
Acute intermittent porphyria

*Coarctation of the aorta, renovascular abnormalities (particularly embolism secondary to umbilical artery catheter), and side effects of medication comprise the majority of neonatal hypertension.
#Most cases occur within 3 weeks of surgery in young children in traction for femoral, pelvic, or humeral fractures. Hypertension related to immobilization is asymptomatic, does not require treatment, and resolves within a week of removal of traction.

TABLE 16-10
CLASSES OF ANTIHYPERTENSIVE MEDICATIONS

Angiotensin Converting Enzyme Inhibitors
- Examples—captopril (the initial drug in this class), enalapril and lisinopril (longer-acting forms)
- Primary mechanism of action is blocking the conversion of angiotensin I to angiotensin II
- Should not be used when GFR is low
- Does not affect cardiovascular performance, so good for hypertensive athletes
- Contraindicated during pregnancy

Angiotensin Receptor Blockers
- Examples—losartan, candesartan
- Mechanism of action—prevent action of angiotensin II by blocking cell membrane receptors
- Similar to ACE inhibitors; most useful in cases of renin-mediated hypertension
- Fewer adverse effects than ACE inhibitors

Calcium Channel Blockers
- Extended-release nifedipine, nicardipine
- Mechanism of action—inhibit vasoconstriction by blocking movement of calcium into smooth muscle; most agents used are selective for arteriolar smooth muscle
- Safe, effective, few adverse side effects

Beta-Adrenergic Antagonists
- Examples—propranolol, atenolol, labetalol (which also has alpha-adrenergic blocking potential and a synergistic effect (vasodilation))
- Mechanism of action—block beta-receptors, thereby decreasing cardiac output, peripheral vascular resistance, renin secretion, and CNS sympathetic activity
- Many adverse side effects, including some that limit compliance in athletes (decreased exercise capacity) and adolescents (decreased sexual function)

Diuretics
- Examples—furosemide, hydrochlorothiazide
- Mechanism of action—promote water and salt excretion
- Most effective in hypertension due to fluid retention
- Generally a second-line therapy, but therapeutic intervention of choice in cases of postinfectious acute glomerulonephritis
- Should not be used in athletes
- Adverse dose-related effects of furosemide include mild-to-moderate hypokalemia, dehydration, and contraction alkalosis; nephrotoxicity and ototoxicity are potential long-term dose-related sequelae of furosemide therapy

Central Alpha-Adrenergic Blockers
- Examples—clonidine, alpha methyldopa
- Mechanism of action—activation of central nervous system alpha-2-adrenergic receptors
- Minimal adverse effects
- Should never be suddenly stopped due to risk of rebound hypertension
- Methyldopa is treatment choice in pregnancy

Peripheral Alpha-Adrenergic Blockers
- Example—prazosin
- Mechanism of action—blocks alpha-1-receptors on the vasculature, resulting in peripheral vasodilatation

Direct Vasodilators
- Examples—hydralazine, minoxidil
- Mechanism of action—smooth muscle relaxation
- Sodium nitroprusside is used for hypertensive emergencies due to ability to titrate continuous intravenous infusion based on blood pressure changes

mass results in effective renal artery stenosis. The elevated blood pressure may require antihypertensive medication until surgical or medical correction of the underlying condition can be achieved. Calcium channel blockers are first-line therapy in patients with renovascular hypertension. ACE inhibitors should not be used in patients with a single kidney or bilateral renal artery stenosis (due to risk of ARF and hypotension), but they are beneficial in cases of unilateral renal artery stenosis. The definitive treatment is percutaneous transluminal angioplasty or surgical revascularization.

Essential (primary) hypertension is elevated blood pressure which is not found to result from any identifiable underlying cause; thus, it is a diagnosis of exclusion. The condition is more common in patients with a positive family history and patients of certain ethnic backgrounds (African-American). Half of patients with essential hypertension are obese, and half have hypertension which is salt-sensitive. Nonpharmacologic treatments include weight management, regular exercise, and a salt-restricted diet.

Adrenal hypertension arises in the presence of catecholamine-secreting tumors (e.g., pheochromocytoma). The classic presentation of pheochromocytoma includes paroxysmal flushing, tachycardia, and headaches, which result from sudden and severe spikes in blood pressure. The hypertension is more often what is described as "paroxysmal" in adults, whereas children may be harder to diagnose because their blood pressures typically remain consistently elevated. Increased levels of urinary catecholamines (epinephrine, norepinephrine, VMA, and HVA) are consistent with the condition, but definitive diagnosis rests on detection of the tumor with a meta-iodobenzylguanidine (MIBG) radionucleotide scan. Other pathologic conditions which may cause acute increases in blood pressure include cocaine abuse and thyroid storm.

Most children with hypertension are asymptomatic at presentation. Stable or slowly progressive hypertension is particularly unlikely to cause symptoms. Family history is often positive for hypertension, stroke, or premature heart attack. Patients with secondary hypertension may seek medical attention for complaints related to their underlying disease (e.g., growth failure, edema). Severe hypertension or hypertension that has developed over a short period of time can cause headache, dizziness, and vision changes. Hypertensive encephalopathy is characterized by vomiting, ataxia, mental status changes (stupor), seizures, and coma.

Since most patients are asymptomatic and the examination is usually normal, laboratory evaluation is of paramount importance. The initial evaluation should include a complete blood count, serum electrolytes, blood urea nitrogen, creatinine, renin level, and urinalysis with culture. A lipid profile is indicated in adolescents and patients who are obese and/or have positive family histories. Doppler US of the kidneys allows assessment of anatomy as well as renal vasculature. Chest radiograph, electrocardiogram, and echocardiogram evaluate heart size and function, whether cardiac deficits are the cause or effect of the hypertension. Other tests to consider, depending on information gathered during the history and physical examination, include thyroid function tests, measurement of urinary catecholamines, serum aldosterone, drug screens, and adrenal function studies.

Pharmacologic intervention is indicated for patients with persistent or refractory hypertension or abnormalities on electrocardiogram. Diuretics, beta-blockers, and occasionally calcium channel blockers are used in younger children; angiotensin converting enzyme inhibitors (ACEI) are second-line treatment in this age group but are effective first-line agents in adolescents and adults because of fewer side effects. Table 16-10 describes the different mechanisms of action of different classes of antihypertensive drugs. Essential hypertension is often treated with long-acting calcium channel blockers or ACEIs. Athletes cannot use diuretics because they are banned (considered performance-enhancing drugs), and medications which compromise cardiovascular function are obviously undesirable; ACEIs and calcium-channel blockers are the preferred medications in these patients.

In patients with severe hypertension, rapid decreases in blood pressure compromise organ perfusion. Hypertensive crisis is treated with oral or sublingual nifedipine (in the absence of an intravenous line), intravenous nitroprusside, or labetalol. The blood pressure should be dropped to normal over at least 24 hours. Continuous infusion of sodium nitroprusside, nicardipine, or labetalol is best because it allows minute-to-minute titration in response to alterations in blood pressure. Stroke, heart attack, and irreversible renal disease are the most devastating complications of severe hypertension. Prognosis depends on the underlying disorder and degree of control.

SOURCES

Bergstein J, Leiser J, Andreoli S. The clinical significant of asymptomatic gross and microscopic hematuria in children. *Arch Pediatr Adolesc Med.* 2005;159:353–355.

Chan JC, Williams DM, Roth KS. Kidney failure in infants and children. *Pediatr Rev.* 2002;23:47–60.

Gillespie RS, Stapleton FB. Nephrolithiasis in children. *Pediatr Rev.* 2004;25:131–139.

Kennedy WA. Assessment and management of fetal hydronephrosis. *Neoreviews.* 2002;3:214–219.

Li SC. Risk factors for the development of Nephritis in Henoch--Schonlein purpura. *AAP Grand Rounds.* 2006;16:14–15.

Marino BS, Fine KS. Nephrology and Urology. In: Marino BS, Fine KS, eds. *Pediatric Blueprints.* 4th ed. Philadelphia: Lippincott Williams & Wilkins; 2007:226–241.

Norwood VF. Hypertension. *Pediatr Rev.* 2002;23:197–208.

Roberts KB. Urinary tract infection treatment and evaluation: Update. *Pediatr Infect Dis J.* 2004;23:1163–1164.

Roth KS, Amaker BH, Chan JC. Nephrotic syndrome: Pathogenesis and management. *Pediatr Rev.* 2002;23:237–248.

QUESTIONS

1. Upon examining a newborn on the first day of life, you note an imperforate anus and a holosystolic murmur loudest at the left lower sternal border accompanied by increased intensity of the second heart sound. Echocardiography confirms a moderate-to-large ventricular septal defect. Which of the following radiographic studies is the most appropriate next step in the evaluation of this patient?

A) Renal sonogram
B) Plain radiographs of the distal lower extremities
C) Magnetic resonance imaging of the lower spine

D) Fluoroscopy of the chest
E) Plain radiographs of the radius

2. A neonate with a history of mild bilateral hydronephrosis on prenatal ultrasound is diagnosed with infantile polycystic kidney disease. She is most at risk for which of the following complications in late childhood/adolescence?
A) Intracranial aneurysm
B) Bleeding esophageal varices
C) Sensorineural hearing loss
D) Anterior lenticonus
E) Giant-cell thrombocytopenia

3. You are called to the delivery room to evaluate a newborn infant with respiratory distress. The infant is eventually intubated and transferred to the neonatal intensive care unit. Multiple congenital anomalies include a flattened face, low-set ears, micrognathia, and bilateral club feet. Review of the maternal chart reveals a history of oligohydramnios and a gestational age of 37 weeks by dates. This infant's respiratory distress is most likely due to which of the following?
A) Respiratory distress syndrome
B) Transient tachypnea of the newborn
C) Pulmonary hypoplasia
D) Bacterial pneumonia
E) Choanal atresia

4. A normally-voiding neonate with a palpable abdominal mass undergoes abdominal ultrasonography, which reveals left-sided multicystic dysplastic kidney. The organ is found to be nonfunctional on nuclear medicine scanning. In addition to liberalizing fluids to prevent dehydration, which of the following is the most important next step in the management of this patient?
A) Replacement of excessive potassium losses
B) Replacement of excessive bicarbonate losses
C) Replacement of excessive sodium losses
D) Assessment of the contralateral kidney, collecting system, and urethra
E) Echocardiography

5. You are discussing familial nephritis (Alport syndrome) with a group of medical interns during morning rounds on the specialty floor. You are correct in telling them each of the following EXCEPT:
A) Patients with Alport syndrome are at risk for the development of ocular lens abnormalities.
B) Patients with Alport syndrome are at risk for the development of sensorineural hearing loss.
C) Patients with familial nephritis have microscopic hematuria in infancy.
D) Males with Alport syndrome are more severely affected than females.
E) The majority of cases of Alport syndrome are autosomal recessive in inheritance.

6. A 1-day-old infant with a history of several voids appears edematous. Crackles are noted throughout all lung fields. During the evaluation, the patient becomes progressively hypotensive. Urinalysis obtained as part of a sepsis work-up is negative for blood and white cells but documents 4+ protein. A prenatal ultrasound was positive for "nonspecific renal abnormalities." Which of the following statements regarding this patient's condition is TRUE?
A) This patient will require renal transplantation early in childhood.
B) This patient is at risk for sensorineural hearing loss.
C) This patient is at risk for intracranial hemorrhages later in life.
D) This patient should be assessed for radial limb abnormalities.
E) This patient probably also has congenital hepatic fibrosis.

7. Mild bilateral hydronephrosis is noted on a prenatal sonogram at 16 weeks of gestation. On a repeat ultrasound at 20 weeks of gestation, labia are visible, and the hydronephrosis is now judged to be "moderate." Which of the following conditions is least likely to be the cause of hydronephrosis in this patient?
A) Vesicoureteral reflux
B) Posterior urethral valves
C) Bilateral ureteropelvic junction obstruction
D) Multicystic dysplastic kidneys
E) Infantile polycystic kidney disease

8. Prenatal ultrasonography is useful for detecting all of the following conditions EXCEPT:
A) Renal agenesis
B) Hydronephrosis
C) Renal size prior to 12 weeks of gestation
D) Oligohydramnios
E) Renal architecture

9. You are performing a newborn examination on a 12-hour-old infant who has not yet voided. You note lax abdominal musculature, wrinkled skin over the abdomen, and bilateral undescended testes. Further evaluation of this patient should include which of the following studies?
A) Computed tomography of the chest
B) Plain films of the distal upper extremities
C) Head ultrasound
D) Abdominal sonogram and voiding cystourethrogram
E) Upper gastrointestinal series with small bowel follow-through

10. A 5-year-old girl is brought to the emergency department with a chief complaint of abdominal pain. The pain started about 12 hours ago and is not associated with fever, vomiting, or diarrhea. Vital signs include a

temperature of 37°C, respiratory rate 23 breaths per minute, heart rate 96 beats per minute, and blood pressure 110/60 mm Hg. The pain is localized to the left side of the abdomen on physical examination, and a left-sided mass is noted on deep palpation. Abdominal ultrasonography reveals unilateral hydronephrosis. Which of the following studies is most specific for confirming the diagnosis of ureteropelvic junction obstruction?

A) Renal sonogram
B) Doppler color flow study
C) Voiding cystourethrography
D) Computed tomography with oral contrast
E) Diuretic nuclear scintigraphy

11. A newborn infant has a history of severe bilateral hydronephrosis on prenatal sonogram and failed placement of a vesicoamniotic shunt. Posterior urethral valves are confirmed. Which of the following studies is indicated for all patients with posterior urethral valves in order to rule out the most common associated abnormality?

A) Voiding cystourethrogram
B) Diuretic nuclear renogram
C) Intravenous pyelogram
D) Computed tomography with intravenous contrast
E) Technetium 99m-DMSA scan

12. Which of the following conditions is the most common cause of end-stage renal disease in childhood?

A) Ureteropelvic junction obstruction
B) Posterior urethral valves
C) Multicystic dysplastic kidney
D) Infantile polycystic kidney disease
E) Congenital nephrotic syndrome

13. A 15-month-old boy with failure to thrive has a history of polyuria and polydipsia. A screening urinalysis is negative for ketones and glucose; the urine specific gravity is 1.005 g per mL, with an osmolality of 50 mOsm per L. The serum osmolality is 300 mOsm per L. Which of the following is the most likely cause of this child's polyuria?

A) Renal tubular acidosis
B) Water intoxication
C) Diabetes insipidus
D) Infantile polycystic kidney disease
E) Diabetes mellitus

14. A 12-month-old girl with hypophosphatemic rickets is diagnosed with Fanconi syndrome. Which of the following conditions is consistent with this patient's clinical presentation?

A) Vitamin D deficiency
B) Acute renal failure
C) Distal renal tubular acidosis
D) Nephropathic cystinosis
E) Parathyroid malignancy

15. A 3-month-old infant with failure to thrive undergoes a screening serum electrolyte panel, the results of which are provided below. His urine pH is 5.5. Which of the following is the most likely cause of this child's failure to thrive?

Sodium 138 mEq per L
Potassium 4.7 mEq per L
Chloride 115 mEq per L
Bicarbonate 12 mEq per L
Blood urea nitrogen 9 mg per dL
Creatinine 0.3 mg per dL

A) Nephrogenic diabetes insipidus
B) Acute renal failure
C) Distal (type 4) renal tubular acidosis
D) Distal (type 1) renal tubular acidosis
E) Proximal (type 2) renal tubular acidosis

16. Which of the following radiologic tests is most sensitive and specific for the presence of a renal stone?

A) Spiral computed tomography
B) Abdominal ultrasonography
C) Plain radiographs of the abdomen
D) Extracorporeal shock wave lithotripsy
E) Intravenous pyelography

17. A 13-year-old girl with a fever to 39°C presents to the emergency department complaining of severe, colicky left flank pain radiating to her left groin area. Results of the urinalysis include TNTC ("too numerous to count") red blood cells, TNTC white blood cells, and bacteria. You suspect pyelonephritis. An abdominal film reveals a radiopaque stone in the left renal pelvis. Which of the following pathogens is most likely to be the cause of this patient's urinary tract infection?

A) Enterococci
B) *Proteus* species
C) *Klebsiella* species
D) *Neisseria gonorrhoeae*
E) *Chlamydia trachomatis*

18. Which of the following adjustments is not beneficial for decreasing the risk of nephrotoxicity due to aminoglycoside administration?

A) Prevent dehydration during treatment.
B) Limit the dose.
C) Administer gentamicin rather than kanamycin.
D) Limit the duration of therapy.
E) Discontinue the drug as soon as the glomerular filtration rate begins to fall.

19. A 10-year-old boy has sustained abdominal trauma in a motor vehicle accident. He is complaining of unremitting abdominal pain and has gross hematuria. His spine has been cleared and his Glascow coma score is 15. Which of the following studies is the most

appropriate initial radiographic test for the evaluation of this patient's abdominal pain?
A) Nuclear medicine renogram
B) Abdominal sonogram
C) Intravenous pyelography
D) Abdominal computed tomography with intravenous contrast
E) Supine and upright plain films of the abdomen

20. You are asked to prepare a lecture for Grand Rounds about changes in renal function with regard to patient age. You are correct in including all of the following facts EXCEPT:
A) Nephrogenesis is generally complete by 36 weeks of gestation.
B) The serum creatinine concentration is higher in premature infants that in term infants.
C) The glomerular filtration rate is lower in premature infants than in term infants.
D) The glomerular filtration rate in children reaches that of adults at about 24 months of age.
E) The serum creatinine concentration in children reaches that of adults at about 24 months of age.

21. A 12-year-old boy with no significant past medical history and a normal physical examination is found to have 2+ proteinuria. His parent denies a family history of renal disease. Both systolic and diastolic measurements are at the 50th percentile for age, weight, and gender. Serum electrolytes, creatinine, blood urea nitrogen, and a complete blood count are within normal limits. The urinalysis demonstrates zero to two white blood cells and zero to two red blood cells per hpf. Which of the following is the most appropriate next step in the management of this patient?
A) Obtain a first morning void specimen for urinary protein/creatinine ratio.
B) Reassure the parent that the boy's condition is benign.
C) Refer the patient to a pediatric nephrologist.
D) Obtain a renal sonogram.
E) Obtain a renal biopsy.

22. A 30-month-old girl has a one week history of grabbing herself and complaining of pain when she urinates. She has no significant past medical history. She provides a urine sample in your office, which is negative for nitrites, red blood cells, and white blood cells. Examination of her perineum reveals multiple excoriations on the labia minora and majora and around the anus. Which of the following is the most appropriate next step in the management of this patient?
A) Contact Child Protective Services.
B) Instruct the parent in the correct procedure for the "tape" test for pinworms.
C) Repeat the urine sample in 7 days.
D) Order microanalysis of the urine sample to look for parasitic eggs.
E) Instruct the parent to use only all-cotton underwear.

23. A previously well 8-year-old girl is brought to your office complaining of persistent dysuria for the past 3 months. Her vital signs and physical examination are normal, with no evidence of growth failure, hypertension, or edema. The urinalysis is positive for 10 to 20 red blood cells/hpf but negative for glucose, protein, leukocyte esterase, or nitrites. A urine culture is obtained. Serum electrolytes, including a serum calcium concentration and serum creatinine and blood urea nitrogen are all within normal limits. The urine culture is negative, and a repeat urinalysis 2 weeks later yields similar results. Which of the following laboratory studies are indicated in this patient at this time?
A) Serum complement levels (C3, C4)
B) Complete blood count
C) Spot urinary calcium/creatinine ratio
D) A and B
E) A, B, and C

24. You are lecturing a group of medical students about renal manifestations of sickle trait and sickle cell disease. You are correct in reporting which of the following?
A) Glomerular disease is not more common in patients with sickle cell disease.
B) Tubular disease is not more common in patients with sickle cell disease.
C) Patients with sickle trait do not have an increased incidence of papillary necrosis when compared with the general population.
D) Renal ultrasonography and intravenous pyelography are indicated in individuals with sickle cell trait or disease who develop hematuria.
E) Papillary necrosis is always an asymptomatic condition.

25. A 5-year-old boy is in your office for his pre-kindergarten health maintenance visit. His mother is concerned that the boy has never been able to sleep overnight without a diaper because he does not wake to urinate. He achieved daytime dryness at 30 months of age. You are correct in telling her all of the following EXCEPT:
A) This child's primary nocturnal enuresis is unlikely to be due to an underlying pathologic condition.
B) Nighttime wetting which persists beyond the age of 5 years is unlikely to resolve.
C) Long-term nightly use of intranasal desmopressin is appropriate for her son.
D) Alarms have not been proven to achieve any measure of long-term success.
E) About 15% to 20% of 5-year-old children still wet the bed at night.

26. Which of the following renal conditions is not paired with the diagnostic study of choice for detecting it?
A) Vesicoureteral reflux—voiding cystourethrogram
B) Hydronephrosis—renal sonogram
C) Oligohydramnios—prenatal ultrasound
D) Intravenous pyelography—corticomedullary differentiation
E) Nephrolithiasis—spiral computed tomography

27. Multicystic dysplastic kidney occurs with increased frequency in patients with which of the following conditions?
A) VATER association
B) CHARGE association
C) Beckwith-Wiedemann syndrome
D) Trisomy 21
E) All of the above

28. An infant with a history of moderate hydronephrosis noted on prenatal ultrasound is found to have posterior urethral valves. Renal function is moderately compromised, with some reduction in typical renal parenchyma noted on a postnatal renal sonogram. Successful transurethral ablation is performed in the first week of life without complication. The parents are concerned about the child's long-term prognosis. You are correct in telling them all of the following EXCEPT:
A) Posterior urethral valves are the most common cause of pediatric end-stage renal disease.
B) Patients with moderate obstructive hydronephrosis who remain undiagnosed experience progressive renal insufficiency.
C) Patients with moderate hydronephrosis who undergo repair early in infancy do not experience progressive renal insufficiency.
D) Prognosis depends on the degree of renal and bladder impairment at the time of repair.
E) Long-term monitoring via renal sonogram, serum electrolytes, and urine output is indicated in this patient.

29. A 5-year-old girl with recurrent urinary tract infections is found to have grade IV vesicoureteral reflux on voiding cystourethrogram. Renal scintigraphy is consistent with minimal bilateral renal scarring. Which of the following is the most appropriate management of the girl's reflux at this time?
A) Due to the patient's young age, no intervention is necessary at this time.
B) Immediate ureteral reimplantation
C) Immediate deflux surgery
D) Antibiotic prophylaxis with trimethoprim-sulfamethoxazole
E) Weekly urine cultures

30. A 9-year-old girl with a history of recent group A *Streptococcus* pharyngitis presents to the emergency department with tea-colored urine and lower extremity edema. Her blood pressure is found to be 150/94 mm Hg. Faint crackles are noted in both lung bases. The patient is admitted to the hospital with a diagnosis of postinfectious acute glomerulonephritis. Fluids are restricted, and she is placed on a loop diuretic. Which of the following electrolyte imbalances is most likely to occur in this patient?
A) Hyponatremia
B) Hypokalemia
C) Hypocalcemia
D) Hypochloremia
E) Hypomagnesemia

31. A 4-year-old boy who was diagnosed 12 days ago with nephrotic syndrome presents to the emergency department with nausea, vomiting, and abdominal pain. His current temperature is 38.5°C; other vital signs are stable. An abdominal sonogram demonstrates excess peritoneal fluid; a sample is collected for analysis. Which of the following results is most consistent with the diagnosis of spontaneous bacterial peritonitis?
A) white blood count $>2.5 \times 10^3$/mcL
B) pH >7.35
C) LDH <225 U per L
D) glucose >50 mg per dL
E) total protein level <10 g per dL

32. Which of the following patients with HUS has the poorest prognosis for return of normal renal function?
A) A 3-year-old boy with typical HUS
B) A 15-year-old boy with atypical HUS
C) A 3-year-old girl with typical HUS
D) An 18-month-old boy with a hemoglobin level of 7.6 g per dL at presentation
E) A 24-month-old girl with abdominal pain at presentation

33. A 24-month-old girl presents with a 2-day history of vomiting and diarrhea. Her parents are unable to tell you whether she has urinated in the past 12 hours because she is still in diapers. Which of the following laboratory values is most consistent with a diagnosis of "prerenal" acute renal failure?
A) Fractional excretion of sodium >1
B) Urine urea nitrogen/blood urea nitrogen ratio <3
C) Urine creatinine/serum creatinine ratio >40
D) Urine osmolality <350 mOsm per L
E) Blood urea nitrogen/serum creatinine ratio <15

34. Which of the following supplements is not indicated for patients with chronic renal failure?
A) Oral folate
B) Oral iron

C) Oral calcium carbonate
D) Oral potassium salts
E) Oral vitamin D

35. You have decided to treat a septic full-term neonate with ampicillin and gentamicin. The medical student working with you wants to prepare sample orders for you to evaluate. You would be correct in reminding him of all of the following EXCEPT:
A) Infants with severe infections are at increased risk of drug toxicity.
B) The glomerular filtration rate in neonates is lower than that in children and adults.
C) Excessive accumulation of an aminoglycoside can result in ototoxicity.
D) The dosing interval should be increased in the neonate.
E) The dosage of gentamicin should be decreased in the neonate.

36. Which of the following is a long-term dose-related complication of furosemide therapy?
A) Otoxicity
B) Hepatotoxicity
C) Behavior changes
D) Persistent acidosis
E) Hyperkalemia

37. Which of the following results computed from laboratory data is most consistent with a diagnosis of intrinsic renal failure?
A) Urine creatinine to plasma creatinine ratio >40
B) Fractional excretion of sodium >1
C) Urine osmolality >500 mOsm per L
D) Urine specific gravity >1.020
E) Urine osmolality to plasma osmolality ratio >1.5

38. Which of the following results computed from laboratory data is most consistent with a diagnosis of prerenal failure?
A) Urine creatinine to plasma creatinine ratio <20
B) Fractional excretion of sodium >1
C) Urine osmolality >500 mOsm per L
D) Urine specific gravity >1.020
E) Urine osmolality to plasma osmolality ratio <1.5

39. A 9-year-old girl who was a restrained back seat passenger in a car involved in a motor vehicle collision presents with right-sided flank pain and tenderness and gross hematuria. Vital signs are stable, the patient is awake and alert, and there is no history or evidence of head trauma. Which of the following is the diagnostic study of choice for the evaluation of this patient's suspected renal injury?
A) Renal sonogram
B) Intravenous pyelography
C) Voiding cystourethrogram
D) Computed tomography of the abdomen with intravenous contrast
E) Computed tomography of the abdomen without contrast

40. A mother brings her 30-month-old son to you because she is "having trouble toilet training him." She began toilet training at age 24 months by having the child sit on the toilet twice a day after meals. She has progressively lengthened the amount of time the child must sit on the toilet before he can get up and play. His sister was trained the same way by age 27 months without difficulty. Although the boy was initially willing, he has become very resistant to sitting on the toilet in the past 4 weeks. He generally has a single soft bowel movement without straining every day. The child's growth is consistent with pre-established normal curves. Which of the following represents the best management of the boy's wetting at this time?
A) Advise the mother to stop toilet training for a few months until the child expresses interest on his own.
B) Advise the mother to institute a reward program for sitting on the toilet.
C) Advise the mother to institute a reward program for producing urine and/or stool in the toilet.
D) Refer the child for a renal sonogram.
E) Obtain a urine sample for screening urinalysis.

41. The mother of a 6-year-old girl brings her daughter to your office for evaluation because the girl has begun wetting her pants over the past 2 weeks. The child was successfully toilet trained at 30 months of age and has not wet her bed or her clothing since then. The mother has noticed no change in appetite or bowel habits, and the child does not complain of pain when she urinates. About a month ago, the child was moved from her first grade class back into a kindergarten class. The child's growth continues along pre-established normal growth curves. Which of the following represents the best next step in the management of this patient?
A) Reassure the mother that her daughter's wetting is a reaction to the stress of a change in classrooms.
B) Obtain a urine sample for urinalysis.
C) Refer the child for cognitive testing to ensure correct school placement.
D) Refer the child to a pediatric urologist for further evaluation and management.
E) Obtain a renal sonogram.

42. The mother of a 7-year-old boy with primary nocturnal enuresis is interested in hearing about treatment options. You would be correct in telling her all of the following EXCEPT:
A) Treatment is not required for his condition.
B) About 15% of patients 6 years of age and above with primary nocturnal enuresis will experience resolution of bed wetting each year thereafter.

C) Oxybutynin will have little effect on nocturnal bed wetting, which is not due to bladder dyssynergy.
D) Compliance is a problem with alarms, which never-the-less have good long-term success rates.
E) Intranasal or oral desmopressin acetate is appropriate for daily use in patients with primary nocturnal enuresis.

ANSWERS

1. A
2. B
3. C
4. D
5. E
6. A
7. B
8. C
9. D
10. E
11. A
12. B
13. C
14. D
15. E
16. A
17. B
18. C
19. D
20. E
21. A
22. B
23. E
24. D
25. C
26. A
27. E
28. C
29. D
30. B
31. A
32. B
33. C
34. D
35. E
36. A
37. B
38. C
39. D
40. A
41. B
42. E

Disorders of the Genital System

17

INGUINAL/SCROTAL MASSES

As the testes descend from the abdominal cavity into the scrotum, they bring with them a portion of the peritoneum called the processus vaginalis. Patency is normally lost early in infancy as the tunica vaginalis surrounds the testis and the processus vaginalis becomes obliterated. Hydroceles are fluid-filled sacs in the scrotal cavity consisting of remnants of the processus vaginalis. They are usually diagnosed in infancy. Hydroceles are painless and often bilateral. When a light source is placed behind the scrotum, the light is transmitted through the clear fluid of the hydrocele (transillumination). When the processus vaginalis remains fully patent, the resultant "communicating hydrocele" may noticeably enlarge when the patient is crying or straining due to increased intra-abdominal pressure. A hydrocele that communicates with the peritoneal cavity places the patient at risk for herniation of bowel into the scrotum. Surgical repair is indicated for communicating hydroceles, scrotal hernias, and hydroceles that persist beyond 18 months of age. Most noncommunicating hydroceles involute by 12 months of age.

An indirect inguinal hernia consists of herniation of intra-abdominal contents into the proximal processus vaginalis, which remains patent despite distal obliteration. Peak incidence occurs at 3 months of age, and the condition is more common in premature infants. Ten percent are bilateral. A bulge which increases in size with crying is noted in the groin at the external inguinal ring. The hernia should be reducible; those which are not may be incarcerated, representing a surgical emergency. Patients with incarcerated inguinal hernias are irritable and in pain; vomiting is not uncommon. Reducible inguinal hernias should be differentiated from retractile testes, which are benign and resolve without intervention.

A varicocele is made up of the dilated testicular vein and enlarged pampiniform plexus resulting from the absence of the venous valves responsible for advancing the blood toward the heart. Varicoceles typically become detectable in boys during adolescence and occur more commonly on the left. The classic presentation consists of a painless scrotal mass superior to the testis which resembles a "bag of worms;" it is not visible when the patient is supine but become evident upon standing when the veins distend. Indications for surgical repair include pain, interference with testicular hormone function, and ipsilateral testicular atrophy. Painless lesions are managed with frequent monitoring of testicular size. As a group, patients with unrepaired varicoceles have a slightly higher rate of infertility.

Trauma is an unlikely cause of a scrotal mass in the infant but is occasionally encountered in children and adolescents. A specific history consistent with the injury is virtually always present. Testicular hematomas are painful; the affected scrotum is edematous and discolored. Testicular tumors are rare in the pediatric population, but should be suspected upon palpation of a firm intratesticular mass.

The differential diagnosis of the painful scrotal mass includes the conditions noted above as well as testicular torsion, torsion of the testicular appendix, epididymitis, and orchitis (see "Acquired Abnormalities of the Male Genital Tract").

Vaginal Discharge and/or Bleeding in the Preadolescent Girl

Vaginal discharge in the prepubescent female patient often occurs in the setting of vulvovaginitis (inflammation of the lining of the vagina and the external genital region). The differential diagnosis of vaginal discharge in this age group is provided in Table 17-1. A detailed history should be followed by inspection of the external genitalia (perineum and anus) with the patient in the knee-chest position, which may allow visualization of the vaginal canal and identification/removal of a foreign body, if present. Vaginal fluid specimens are easily obtained in this position as well.

Thin, milky-white vaginal discharge is common in newborn females. This physiologic leukorrhea is due to maternal estrogen stimulation and is usually accompanied by visible swelling of the external genitalia. Scant vaginal bleeding may also be noted in the first few weeks of life; this blood is uterine in origin and represents withdrawal bleeding as maternal estrogen levels decline in the infant.

Male Congenital Abnormalities

Hypospadias

Hypospadias is the most common congenital anomaly of the penis. Incomplete development of the distal urethra leads to malpositioning of the urethral meatus along the ventral shaft of the glans (first-degree), penis (second-degree), scrotum, or perineum (third-degree). Proximal hypospadias may cause curving of the penis *(chordee)*. Since

TABLE 17-1
VAGINAL DISCHARGE IN THE PREPUBESCENT FEMALE

Primary Symptoms are Vaginal Discharge and/or Vulvovaginal Irritation

Sexually-transmitted infection (sexual abuse; see Chapter 24 for discussion of specific pathogens)

- Normal findings on physical examination do not rule out sexual abuse.

Candidal vulvovaginitis

- History of recent oral broad-spectrum antibiotic use, diabetes mellitus; otherwise unusual in immunocompetent prepubescent child (excepting toddlers still in diapers)

Group A beta-streptococcal infection

- Most common infectious cause of vulvovaginitis in this age group
- Vaginal discharge may be green or bloody
- Often accompanied by a well-demarcated area of intense erythema around the external genitalia or anus
- Other causative infectious agents include respiratory and enteric bacterial pathogens

Pinworm infection

- Usually accompanied by pruritus and visible excoriations

Vaginal foreign body

- Presents with malodorous, possibly bloody discharge
- Toilet paper is the most frequently retained substance
- Removal, followed by sitz baths, is generally adequate treatment

Nonspecific/irritant vulvovaginitis

- Most common cause in children
- Poor hygiene often a factor
- Irritants include soaps, detergents, bubble bath solution, shampoos
- Maceration may result from tight-fitting clothing such as tights, bathing suits, nylon underwear, and leotards
- Managed with sitz baths, avoidance of irritants, looser clothing

Dermatitis

- Specific conditions include severe diaper rash, psoriasis, seborrhea

Primary Symptom is Vaginal Bleeding

Urethral prolapse

- Typically presents as blood in the diaper or underwear of an asymptomatic child
- Bleeding more likely urethral in origin
- "Donut-shaped" extrusion of highly-vascularized tissue at the introitus of the urethra
- Treated with topical estrogen cream

Lichen sclerosus et atrophicus

- Typically presents as blood in the underwear of child with vulvar pruritus
- Atrophy of the superficial skin in a "figure 8" pattern around the vulva and anus
- Exacerbations managed with topical corticosteroids

Vaginal trauma

- Bloody discharge
- May be secondary to sexual abuse or masturbation

the critical period for phallic development occurs later than that for the kidneys, radiologic studies to look for related anomalies of the genitourinary tract are unnecessary. A karyotype is indicated in infants with hypospadias and bilateral cryptorchidism in order to rule out female virilization. Circumcision is contraindicated before surgical reconstruction, although many cases are now repaired without the use of preputial tissue. Surgical repair should be performed within the first year of life it at all possible, preferably at about 6 months of age. Prognosis is excellent for distal lesions; proximal lesions may require multiple revisions before an acceptable result is achieved.

Cryptorchidism

Cryptorchidism is defined as testes that have not fully descended into the scrotum and, unlike retracted testes, cannot be manipulated into the scrotum with gentle pressure. Term infants have a 3% to 4% incidence at birth; the rate is much higher (30%) in premature infants. Cryptorchidism may occur as part of a genetic syndrome or be an isolated anomaly. Ninety percent of affected patients have associated inguinal hernias. Undescended testes may be found in the abdomen or along the inguinal canal; most are palpable. More than 99% of males have bilateral descended testicles at 12 months of age. Testes that remain outside the scrotum develop progressive ultrastructural changes, have impaired sperm production, and confer an increased risk of malignancy for *both* testes, even if one is normally descended. Surgical repair takes place at 12 to 18 months of age and has a high success rate. Orchiopexy does not appear to alter the incidence of malignant degeneration (2% to 3%), but it does render the testis accessible for regular self-examination and improves fertility. Bilateral cryptorchidism results in oligospermia and infertility.

Micropenis

Congenital micropenis is an uncommon condition, which usually occurs in association with an endocrine, hormonal, or chromosomal abnormality. Proper measurement consists of gently stretching the penis to its full length and measuring from the tip to the symphysis pubis, which negates apparent shortening in the patient with a large pubic fat pad. Available tables record the range of normal penile lengths based on age. A penis which measures <2.5 cm in length during the first several months of life in a full-term infant is consistent with the diagnosis of micropenis.

Acquired Abnormalities of the Male Genital Tract

Testicular Torsion

Torsion is a surgical emergency; prompt recognition and intervention may prevent loss of the torsed testicle. Most patients with testicular torsion lack the posterior attachment to the tunica vaginalis that keeps the testis from rotating around the spermatic cord. This condition is more common in preadolescent males but may occur at any age.

Clinical manifestations include the acute onset of unilateral scrotal pain; nausea; vomiting; a firm or edematous, exquisitely tender testis; scrotal edema and erythema; and absent cremasteric reflex. Occasionally, the torsion is limited to the testicular or epididymal appendix, localized tenderness, a "blue dot" sign on the upper aspect of the scrotum, and a normal cremasteric reflex suggest limited involvement. Doppler ultrasonography allows differentiation of the two conditions based on blood flow to the testis (restricted/absent vs. normal/increased), but should not delay appropriate treatment. Symptomatic pain relief is all that is required for a torsed appendix.

Early surgical intervention is critical; 90% of gonads survive when detorsion and fixation take place within 6 hours of symptom onset. Necrotic testes must be removed. The contralateral testis is fixed to the posterior scrotal envelope during surgery to avoid subsequent torsion. Torsion of the testicular or epididymal appendix resolves spontaneously.

Epididymitis

Epididymitis, a common cause of acute hemiscrotal pain in sexually active adolescents, results from an ascending infection through the vas deferens. The pain is often less severe than that from testicular torsion and develops more gradually. Patients frequently complain of urinary frequency and dysuria as well. On examination of the genitals, the pain is usually most severe posterior and superior to the testis, in the area of the epididymis. The cremasteric reflex remains intact. Urethral discharge may be present. Adolescent patients with epididymitis should be screened for sexually transmitted diseases and treated with antimicrobials effective against *Neisseria gonorrhoeae* and *Chlamydia trachomatis*.

Orchitis

Orchitis, or inflammation of the testes, frequently follows the spread of pathogenic organisms from an infected epididymis. Orchitis which occurs in isolation is usually viral, and a large number of viruses are capable of causing this condition. Mumps orchitis develops in up to a third of adolescent males who contract the infection. One or both testes become swollen and tender. When fever and parotid swelling are present as well, the diagnosis may be straightforward. However, because the cremasteric reflex is a less reliable indicator in these patients, Doppler ultrasonography is usually indicated; increased blood flow to the affected testicle rules out torsion. Males with concurrent epididymitis are treated as above. Viral orchitis resolves without specific treatment; atrophy is later noted in some involved testes but does not appear to significantly affect fertility.

Urethritis

Urethritis often occurs in association with epididymitis in adolescent males and is usually due to a sexually transmitted infection, particularly *C. trachomatis*. In contrast, urethritis secondary to a bacterial urinary infection is rare in males beyond the age of 12 months. Dysuria, urinary frequency, and urethral discharge are virtually always present. Examination of a first-voided urinary sample or urethral discharge is positive for white blood cells. The inflammation may not be infectious in origin; instrumentation of the urethra frequently results in mild, transient urethritis. Antibiotics are not indicated for the patient with a negative urine culture and history of urethral foreign body or instrumentation; treatment is symptomatic. Patients with positive urine cultures should be treated appropriately.

Testicular Cancer

Testicular carcinoma is rare in prepubertal boys but occurs with some frequency in adolescent and adult males. A firm testicular mass is usually noted by the patient or physician. A history of cryptorchidism places the individual at high risk for the development of this tumor, especially if the testis remains in the abdomen. All postpubertal males should be instructed in the proper method of testicular self-examination and encouraged to check themselves monthly. Children with a history of cryptorchidism should be examined monthly by their parents until they are old enough to do so themselves. Disease which is localized to the testicle at diagnosis is associated with an excellent prognosis.

Female Congenital Abnormalities

Imperforate Hymen

Imperforate hymen results when the hymenal opening does not develop and there is no communication between the uterus and the outside of the body. It is the most common obstructive abnormality of the female genital tract. The anomaly is often diagnosed on the newborn examination when a fluid-filled bulge is noted at the vaginal outlet. The mass results from hydrometrocolpos, or fluid trapped in the uterine and vaginal cavities; maternal estrogens stimulate vaginal secretions that cannot escape from the body and eventually are absorbed. When the condition is not identified in infancy, it may instead present during puberty with the onset of menstruation. The typical presentation involves an adolescent female with Stage 4 breast and pubic hair who experiences cyclic (monthly) lower abdominal pain, often associated with nausea and back pain. A bluish, bulging mass is noted at the vaginal introitus on examination of the external genitalia, and the distended vagina may be palpable on the digital rectal examination. Imperforate hymen is surgically correctable.

Labial Adhesions

Labial adhesions are not actually a congenital lesion; they are acquired in infancy or early childhood. Fusion of the labia minora may result from irritation due to poor hygiene, diaper dermatitis, or low-normal estrogen levels. The fusion typically originates at the posterior introitus and may be insignificantly small or involve virtually the entire length of the minora. Most labial fusions resolve spontaneously; those which do not are likely to recur regardless of treatment. Daily application of a mild ointment often halts progression of the fusion. Topical estrogen cream applied daily for up to 3 weeks is indicated if there is partial obstruction of vaginal secretions or urine output. Surgical separation is inappropriate.

Acquired Abnormalities of the Female Genital Tract

Ovarian Torsion

Ovarian torsion is a surgical emergency. Although torsion can occur in a normal ovary, this is uncommon. Most cases involve an organ which is enlarged due to a cyst or mass; the ovary twists on its vascular stalk, which impairs perfusion of the ovary and distal Fallopian tube. Adnexal torsion can occur in any age group but is more common in late puberty. The classic presentation consists of the sudden onset of severe colicky pain localized to a lower quadrant of the abdomen. The pain may be referred to the flank, thigh, or lower back as well. It is usually accompanied by nausea and vomiting. About half of patients with ovarian torsion have a history of a similar painful episode that resolved spontaneously. Fever and urinary symptoms are notably absent, and the white blood count is generally normal. An ovarian mass may be palpable during bimanual or rectal examination.

Pelvic ultrasonography with Doppler flow is the diagnostic method of choice for differentiating ovarian torsion from other painful abdominal conditions. Unilateral ovarian enlargement, the presence of multiple peripheral follicles, and diminished or absent blood flow to the organ support the diagnosis of torsion. Even with early laparoscopic evaluation and intervention, the majority of torsed adnexa are nonsalvagable at surgery.

The differential diagnosis of lower abdominal pain in the adolescent female in particular is extensive. Right-sided ovarian torsion often cannot be distinguished clinically from appendicitis or ectopic pregnancy. Any female of reproductive age who presents with abdominal or pelvic pain must have a pregnancy test completed early in the diagnostic process due to management implications and the relatively high rate of morbidity and mortality associated with ectopic pregnancy.

Ovarian Masses in the Adolescent

When an ovarian mass is discovered in the adolescent, the differential diagnosis includes ovarian cysts, benign growths, and malignancy. Ovarian cysts are very common; they usually represent persistence of follicles or, less commonly, the corpus luteum. Ovarian cysts are often asymptomatic but may present with pain, irregular menses, urinary frequency, or a sensation of pelvic fullness. Ultrasonography permits sizing and characterization of ovarian masses, including cysts. When a simple fluid-filled cyst <6 cm in size is present, resolution is expected within 4 to 8 weeks and can be documented by a repeat study. Corpus luteum cysts take longer to regress (up to three months) and have a higher rate of complications (e.g., ovarian torsion). Oral contraceptive pills which contain both estrogen and progestin have been shown to prohibit future cyst formation, but they have no effect on existing cysts. Laparoscopic aspiration or removal is indicated for cysts which are symptomatic or larger than 6 to 8 cm. Aspiration alone is associated with a high rate of recurrence; however, since no ovarian tissue is removed with this procedure, it is often preferred for initial intervention.

Solid masses and cysts with septations, calcifications, or multiloculated areas are suspicious for malignancy. Initial screening consists of measurement of serum tumor markers. Further assessment with computed tomography or magnetic resonance imaging is indicated, followed by studies of the liver and/or lungs to look for metastatic disease. Surgical intervention is based on radiologic findings and serum tumor markers. Affected patients need specialized counseling regarding the risk/benefit ratio of proposed treatment options with regard to cure rates and preservation of reproductive potential.

SOURCES

Adelman WP, Joffe A. Testicular masses/cancer. *Pediatr Rev.* 2005;26:341–344.

Bundy DG, Serwint J. Vesicoureteral reflux. *Pediatr Rev.* 2007;28:e6–e8.

Ein S, Njere I, Ein A. Six thousand three hundred sixty-one pediatric inguinal hernias: A 35-year review. *J Pediatr Surg.* 2006;41:980–986.

Emans SJ. Vulvovaginal problems in the prepubertal child. In: Emans SJ, Laufer MR, Goldstein DP, eds. *Pediatric and Adolescent Gynecology.* 5th ed. Philadelphia: Lippincott, Williams, & Wilkins; 2005:83–119.

Kokotos F, Adam HM. Vulvovaginitis. *Pediatr Rev.* 2006;27:116–117.

LeeL, Homme J, Henrichsen T, et al. Monstrous surprise at a female adolescent's routine visit. *Contemp Pediatr.* 2006;23:17–24.

Maisonet L. Inguinal hernia. *Pediatr Rev.* 2003;24:34–35.

Posner JC, Spandorfer PR. Early detection of imperforate hymen prevents morbidity from delays in diagnosis. *Pediatrics.* 2005;115:1008–1012.

Powell JK. Benign adnexal masses in the adolescent. *Adolesc Med Clin.* 2004;15:535–547.

Raj GV, Wiener JS. Varicoceles in adolescents: When to observe, when to intervene. *Contemp Pediatr.* 2004;21:39–54.

Snodgrass WT. Hypospadias. *Pediatr Rev.* 2004;25:62–66.

Sugar NF, Graham EA. Common gynecologic problems in prepubertal girls. *Pediatr Rev.* 2006;27:213–223.

QUESTIONS

1. A mother brings her 6-year-old daughter to the clinic because the child has developed a greenish, slightly bloody vaginal discharge. She also has a painful rash which the mother is treating with topical petroleum jelly. The child is otherwise asymptomatic. She lives in an intact family and attends her neighborhood school. The physical examination reveals a well-nourished, well-developed child with visible thin, green, slightly bloody discharge accumulated in the posterior fourchette. The hymenal ring is intact, with no evidence of trauma. A dramatic, well-demarcated scarlet rash is noted in the perineal region. The anus appears normal. Which of the following is the most appropriate next step in the management of this patient?

A) Culture of the inner labia for group A beta-hemolytic *Streptococcus*
B) Sitz baths twice a day for 2 weeks, followed by re-evaluation
C) Topical estrogen cream
D) Pinworm tape test
E) Involvement of the local Child Protection Services agency

2. A 2-month-old infant is brought to your clinic by her parents because they have noticed blood in her diaper intermittently for the past week. There is no history of fever, irritability, or change in bowel or bladder habits. They care for their daughter at home and have not left her with a sitter. Examination of the external genitalia and anus reveals a vascular ring of congested, reddened, edematous tissue at the introitus of the urethra. Which of the following is the most appropriate next step in the management of this patient?

A) Daily sitz baths and avoidance of perfumed soaps
B) Daily application of estrogen cream to the lesion for 1 week, with a scheduled follow-up visit at that time
C) Reassurance that the condition is physiologic and does not require treatment
D) Obtain vaginal fluid for cultures of *Neisseria gonorrhoeae* and *Chlamydia trachomatis*
E) Referral to a pediatric gynecologist

3. Parents of a 2-week-old infant bring her to your office because they saw blood in the diaper this morning. She is feeding, urinating, and stooling normally. A small amount of bloody spotting is noted on the diaper lining, which is also saturated with urine. The patient is afebrile and alert; no irritability is noted. The physical examination, including visualization of the external genitalia and anus, is normal except for a minute amount of blood noted in the posterior fourchette. The child's vaginal bleeding is most likely secondary to which of the following?

A) Vaginal trauma
B) Presence of maternal estrogens
C) Withdrawal of maternal estrogens
D) Perinatally-acquired sexually-transmitted infection
E) Vaginal foreign body

4. A 16-year-old male in your office for his routine health maintenance visit is noted to have an ill-defined nontender mass located in the left scrotum superior to the testicle. The mass has the consistency of a "bag of worms" and disappears when the patient is in the supine position. The testicles are symmetric in size, and the genital examination is otherwise normal. Which of the following statements regarding this patient's condition is TRUE?

A) This patient's condition is probably bilateral.
B) This patient's condition requires immediate referral to a urologist.
C) This patient's lesion would be expected to fully transilluminate.
D) The sizes of the testes should be monitored and compared every 3 to 6 months.
E) This patient's lesion places him at increased risk for fertility problems.

5. A mother brings her 3-month-old infant to your office because he has developed scrotal swelling. There is no history of fever, and the patient is feeding normally and otherwise appears well. The physical examination is significant for nontender bilateral scrotal swelling. Both testes are palpable and without abnormality. Bilateral transillumination is present. When the patient cries, the swelling does not change in size or become more tense than before. This patient's scrotal enlargement is most likely due to which of the following?

A) Communicating hydroceles
B) Bilateral varicoceles
C) Bilateral scrotal hernias
D) Bilateral inguinal hernias
E) Noncommunicating hydroceles

6. A 3-month-old infant is brought to the emergency department by his mother because he has been crying for the past hour and has vomited twice. When the diaper is removed, an impressive bulge is noted in the right groin. There is no discoloration. A firm mass is palpated at the external inguinal ring. You are unsuccessful in reducing the contents of the mass into the abdomen. Which of the following is the most appropriate next step in the management of this patient?

A) Emergent surgical consultation
B) Administration of a narcotic for pain control, followed by another attempt at reduction
C) Abdominal sonogram with Doppler flow studies
D) Abdominal computed tomography with intravenous and oral contrast
E) Needle aspiration of the mass

7. A 17-year-old girl is brought to your office by her mother for a complaint of persistent, nonspecific pelvic discomfort for the past 2 months. The patient denies sexual activity, and a pregnancy test is negative. Her last menstrual period was 3 weeks ago, and her periods have remained regular. A right-sided ovarian mass is palpated on the bimanual examination. Which of the following is the most appropriate next step in the evaluation of this patient?

A) Pelvic computed tomography with intravenous contrast
B) Pelvic sonogram
C) Measurement of serum tumor markers
D) Referral to a gynecologist
E) Referral to a general surgeon for aspiration of the mass

8. An 11-year-old girl is brought to the emergency department complaining of abdominal pain. The severe, colicky pain began abruptly about 90 minutes ago. She has had two previous episodes of similar pain; each resolved spontaneously within an hour. She is afebrile, and vital signs are stable. Bowel sounds are normal, and the abdomen is soft. Tenderness is noted on deep palpation of the left lower quadrant. A complete blood count and urinalysis are within normal limits. Pelvic ultrasonography reveals an enlarged, complex ovarian mass with multiple follicles in the cortical region. The contralateral ovary appears normal. Which of the following statements regarding this patient's condition is TRUE?

A) This patient does not require a pregnancy test prior to treatment.
B) This patient will probably retain her left ovary.
C) This patient will probably have abnormal Doppler flow study results on pelvic ultrasonography.
D) This patient probably has an elevated white blood count.
E) This patient probably has appendicitis.

9. You are providing a lecture to medical interns on the topic of gynecologic problems in prepubertal girls. Which of the following statements concerning imperforate hymen is FALSE?

A) Imperforate hymen is the most common obstructive abnormality of the female genital tract.
B) The typical presentation involves an adolescent female with Stage 4 breast and pubic hair development who experiences cyclic (monthly) lower abdominal pain.
C) On examination of the external genitalia of an adolescent female with symptomatic imperforate hymen, a bluish, bulging mass is noted at the vaginal introitus.
D) Imperforate hymen cannot be diagnosed prior to the onset of menses.
E) Imperforate hymen is usually fully surgically correctable.

10. While performing a routine health maintenance examination on a 24-month-old girl, you note labial

fusion involving 60% of the labia minora, with visible pooling of urine at the opening. Which of the following is the most appropriate management of this patient?
A) No treatment is indicated at this time.
B) Referral to a general surgeon
C) Intravenous pyelogram
D) Application of a hypoallergenic ointment twice a day until the fusion resolves
E) Application of an estrogen-containing cream once a day until the fusion resolves, but no longer than 2 to 3 weeks

11. While examining a full-term, 1-week-old infant who was circumcised in the newborn nursery, you note what appears to be the opening of the urethra along the ventral portion of the glans of the penis. Which of the following is the most appropriate next step in the management of this patient?
A) Referral to a pediatric urologist
B) Renal ultrasonography
C) Catheterization of the opening for urine to confirm the diagnosis
D) Inform the infant's parents that surgical repair is not possible since the boy has already been circumcised.
E) Question the parents regarding the force of the child's stream, with no further intervention if flow is unobstructed.

12. The newborn examination of an infant born at 35 weeks of gestation is significant for bilateral undescended testicles. The left testicle is palpable high along the inguinal canal. The parents are concerned about the child's prognosis for normal testicular development. You are correct in telling them all of the following EXCEPT:
A) If the testes have not fully descended by 12 months of age, they are unlikely to spontaneously descend thereafter.
B) Orchiopexy is associated with a decreased risk of malignant transformation.
C) Infertility is a complication of bilateral cryptorchidism.
D) The incidence of cryptorchidism is higher in premature infants than in term infants.
E) About 99% of males have bilateral descended testes by 12 months of age.

13. A full-term newborn whose weight is appropriate for gestational age has a penile length of 3.9 cm. Which of the following is the most appropriate initial management of this patient's condition?
A) Measurement of serum concentration of growth hormone
B) Measurement of serum concentration of thyroid-stimulating hormone
C) The patient's penile length is within normal limits.
D) Renal ultrasonography
E) Karyotype

14. A 13-month-old patient with bilateral intra-abdominal cryptorchidism is undergoing surgical orchiopexy. Which of the following statements regarding long-term sequelae of his condition is TRUE?
A) Adolescent males without a history of cryptorchidism do not appear to develop testicular cancer.
B) Monthly testicular examinations are not indicated for this child until he reaches puberty.
C) Orchiopexy decreases this patient's future risk of testicular cancer.
D) Orchiopexy allows better detection of testicular masses in the future.
E) Orchiopexy does not affect fertility in patients with cryptorchidism.

15. A 3-year-old boy who had a fever without a source was catheterized for urine 48 hours ago in the emergency department. He now becomes anxious when he has to urinate and says that "it hurts." The first-void urine sample contains 10 to 20 white blood cells per hpf; however, the mid-void sample contains zero to two white blood cells per hpf, and no bacteria are noted on Gram stain. Which of the following is the most appropriate next step in the management of this patient?
A) Schedule the patient for renal ultrasonography.
B) Reassure the parents that the dysuria will resolve.
C) Obtain urine culture; administer parenteral antibiotics.
D) Obtain urine culture; begin oral antibiotics.
E) Obtain urine culture; no antibiotics at this time.

16. A 16-year-old adolescent presents with a swollen, tender right testicle. He denies sexual activity. There is no history of fever, parotid swelling, nausea, or vomiting. The testis is diffusely tender, with scrotal edema but no overlying erythema. The cremasteric reflex is absent on the right side. Color Doppler ultrasonography reveals increased blood flow to the right testicle. Which of the following is the most likely cause of testicular pain in this patient?
A) Viral orchitis
B) Bacterial orchitis
C) Epididymitis
D) Testicular torsion
E) Testicular carcinoma

17. A 17-year-old sexually active adolescent presents to your clinic complaining of right scrotal pain, dysuria, and urinary frequency. The pain has developed over the past 72 hours and is described as "intense." The physical examination is significant for bilateral intact cremasteric reflexes and tenderness localized to an area of tissue just posterior and superior to the right testis.

Which of the following conditions is the most likely cause of testicular pain in this patient?
A) Testicular torsion
B) Epididymitis
C) Testicular carcinoma
D) Orchitis
E) Urethritis

18. An 11-year-old boy presents to the emergency department with a 4-hour history of severe left scrotal pain. The pain was acute in onset. He has vomited twice since the pain started. The physical examination is significant for left-sided scrotal edema and overlying erythema; a firm, exquisitely tender left testicle, and the absence of a cremasteric reflex on the left side. Which of the following the most appropriate next step in the management of this patient?
A) Intravenous antibiotics
B) Doppler ultrasonography
C) Immediate surgery
D) Nuclear medicine scan
E) Urinalysis

19. An 8-year-old boy presents to the emergency department with a 4-hour history of severe left scrotal pain. The pain was acute in onset. He has vomited twice since the pain started. The physical examination is significant for tenderness localized to the superior aspect of the left testicle with an overlying "blue spot." The cremasteric reflex is intact on the left side. Doppler ultrasonography confirms increased blood flow to the left testis. Which of the following the most appropriate next step in the management of this patient?
A) Immediate surgery
B) Nuclear medicine scan
C) Urinalysis
D) Adequate pain control
E) Intravenous antibiotics

ANSWERS

1. A	8. C	15. E
2. B	9. D	16. A
3. C	10. E	17. B
4. D	11. A	18. C
5. E	12. B	19. D
6. A	13. C	
7. B	14. D	

Neurologic Disorders

18

CLINICAL MANIFESTATIONS OF NEUROLOGIC DISORDERS

Headache

When presented with a complaint of headache, it is most important to determine early in the evaluation whether the condition is primary or secondary:

- *Primary (benign) headaches* are not associated with underlying neuropathology. Tension headaches and migraine headaches fall into this category.
- *Secondary (pathologic) headaches* originate from an underlying neurologic process, usually through the mechanism of increased intracranial pressure (ICP) (Table 18-1).

Neither computed tomography (CT) nor magnetic resonance imaging (MRI) of the head is necessary in the patient with recurring headaches and a normal neurologic examination. *Neuroimaging* is indicated in the setting of any of the following: recent onset of severe headaches; headaches that are changing in severity, frequency, or character; and headaches accompanied by neurologic signs such as papilledema, strabismus, unilateral weakness or sensory loss, dysarthria, ataxia, and changes in mental status, personality, behavior, and arousability. Such signs typically develop within 6 months of the onset of headaches in patients with underlying neuropathology. Neuroimaging should also be strongly considered in the patient with headaches and a history of neurodevelopmental impairment or seizures. Structural lesions large enough to produce increased ICP are almost always visible on head CT. The additional detail provided by MRI may be beneficial in patients with abnormal CT scans or suspected posterior fossa lesions.

Benign tension headaches are often associated with psychological stress or fatigue. They are described as generalized, nonthrobbing, and bandlike in distribution. Most respond to over-the-counter analgesics, removal of the inciting stressor, and rest. *Chronic headaches* occur more than five times a week or average >15 a month over 3 to 6 months. Chronic primary headaches may be due to benign tension headaches, analgesic overuse headaches, and/or depression. Analgesic use should be restricted to no more than two to three times per week; chronic use resets pain centers within the brain, precipitating rebound headaches when the medication is discontinued. Although aspirin, nonsteroidal anti-inflammatory agents, and acetaminophen are most frequently associated with analgesic overuse headaches, chronic administration of ergotamines, sedatives, and narcotics can also produce rebound headaches. Resolution of the headaches follows discontinuation of all analgesic medications. Headaches that accompany *depression* typically occur daily over several weeks or months; alternatively, chronic headaches of any etiology may precipitate depression. Daily prophylaxis should be considered in headache patients requiring medication more than two to three times a week. Referral to a mental health professional prior to the initiation of prophylactic treatment for chronic headaches may be beneficial in patients with suspected social or emotional stressors.

Migraine headaches are hypothesized to result from sudden progressive depolarization of a hyperexcitable cerebral cortex ("spreading cortical depression"). They are characterized by recurrent attacks of severe, throbbing, frontal or frontotemporal pain that lasts for several hours and resolves with sleep. Patients who suffer from migraine headaches remain asymptomatic and have normal neurologic examinations between episodes of pain. Migraine headaches run in families, and approximately half of affected individuals have a prior history of sleep disorder or motion sickness. Other childhood syndromes believed to

TABLE 18-1
FEATURES SUSPICIOUS FOR PATHOLOGIC HEADACHES

Headaches that are:
- Focal
- Frontal or occipital
- Incapacitating
- Increasing in frequency and/or severity
- Worse in the morning (or waken the patient from sleep)
- Associated with persistent vomiting that is not accompanied by abdominal pain or diarrhea
- Accompanied by neurologic signs
- Occurring in a patient without a family history of migraine headaches

be precursors of migraine complexes include *abdominal migraine, benign paroxysmal vertigo of childhood,* and *cyclical vomiting.* Migraine headaches may be categorized as classic or common:

- Approximately one third of patients experience *classic migraines,* headaches heralded by *auras* that are typically visual (scotomas, monocular vision impairment) but may also be sensory (vertigo), motor (hemiparesis), or verbal (aphasia).
- *Common migraines* are not associated with auras, although they may be preceded by nonspecific symptoms such as malaise, anorexia, irritability, or pallor.

Both classic and common migraines are commonly accompanied by nausea, vomiting, photophobia, phonophobia, and a preference for sleep. A few migraine complex variants may initially present with neurologic impairment (Table 18-2).

Migraine headaches are highly responsive to therapy; in fact, as many as one third of patients report remission of the headache following administration of a placebo. Treatment begins with reassurance that the headache is not due to underlying neuropathology. A headache diary assists in identification of triggers, if present, which can include fatigue, sleep deprivation, fasting, caffeine, menstruation, and stress. Nonpharmacologic interventions (e.g., biofeedback, relaxation techniques, cognitive therapy, acupuncture, aromatherapy) are often very beneficial for controlling migraine headaches. Patients should be instructed to eat regular meals, exercise, remain well-hydrated, and avoid fatigue and sleep deprivation. Over-the-counter medications (e.g., acetaminophen, ibuprofen) work well as abortive medications in children; intranasal or oral *sumatriptan* is reserved for children ≥12 years of age with headaches that are severe or unresponsive to over-the-counter medications. Subcutaneous sumatriptan is inappropriate for children. If abortive medication is necessary more than three to six times a month, prophylaxis should be considered; anticonvulsants, antidepressants, and beta-blockers have been prescribed with variable success.

TABLE 18-2
MIGRAINE VARIANTS

Basilar Migraine

- Pain is typically occipital rather than frontal or frontotemporal.
- Headache is preceded by some combination of the following: changes in vision (diplopia, visual field defects); dysarthria; vertigo; tinnitus or auditory sensitivity or impairment; mental status changes, altered level of consciousness; and bilateral paresthesias.

Familial Hemiplegic Migraine

- Focal headache preceded by contralateral hemiparesis
- Positive family history

Altered Level of Consciousness

The differential diagnosis of pediatric *encephalopathy,* or deterioration in mental status due to generalized cerebral dysfunction, is extensive (Table 18-3). Fortunately, the age of the patient, past medical history, history of present illness, and physical examination often suggest the cause. Encephalopathy secondary to a systemic process such as electrolyte imbalance, infection, or liver failure is characterized by fluctuating mental status and nonlocalizing neurologic manifestations (myoclonus, tremors, temperature instability). In contrast, levels of consciousness are abnormal but fairly stable when encephalopathy results from structural lesions in the brain (tumor, abscess, hemorrhage), and focal neurologic signs are more common. Specific identification of the underlying disorder is critical to resolving the encephalopathy and preserving brain function. Signs and symptoms suggesting an intracranial process warrant immediate neuroimaging (CT in the child and sonogram or CT in the infant).

Somnolence, lethargy, and particularly coma correspond with encephalopathy in the neonate, especially if alterations in consciousness are preceded by refractory seizures. *Hypoxic-ischemic encephalopathy,* discussed in Chapter 5, is always accompanied by a history of perinatal asphyxia and resuscitation; other confirmatory findings include multiorgan system dysfunction and seizures on the first day of life. Ultrasonography of the head is indicated for infants with suspected *intraventricular hemorrhage* or *congenital structural lesions* of the brain. *Septic* infants may become comatose whether or not they have concurrent *meningitis. Drug intoxication or withdrawal* is identified through maternal history of drug use or positive maternal and infant drug screens. Laboratory evaluation for *inborn errors of metabolism,* including serum ammonia, amino acids, glucose, electrolytes, lactate concentrations, and urine organic acid levels, should take place early in the workup of neonatal coma.

Ataxia

Ataxia refers to incoordination of purposeful movement or unsteadiness of posture that is not due to weakness. Although relatively uncommon in children, ataxia can arise from a large number of underlying processes (Table 18-4). Most causes of acute ataxia in childhood are self-limited and require no treatment beyond supportive care. Chronic ataxia generally has a poorer prognosis. Evaluation is aided by a basic understanding of the structures responsible for coordination of voluntary movement. A thorough neurologic examination may help pinpoint the origin of the abnormality. For example, horizontal nystagmus is often noted in cases of acute labyrinthitis; vertical nystagmus is more commonly associated with hydrocephalus. Phenytoin toxicity results in both vertical and horizontal nystagmus.

Toxicology screens should be considered in ambulatory patients or patients with suspected abuse. Neuroimaging permits assessment for cerebellar masses (tumor, abscess,

TABLE 18-3
DIFFERENTIAL DIAGNOSIS OF ENCEPHALOPATHY IN CHILDREN

Infection
- Infection of the central nervous system is by far the most common cause of acute encephalopathy in children.
- Infections that may present with altered level of consciousness include meningitis, encephalitis, postinfectious encephalomyelitis, brain abscess, and subdural empyema.
- Sepsis can produce generalized cerebral depression in the absence of central nervous system involvement.
- Infection with *Shigella* species occasionally presents with isolated encephalopathy.

Trauma/Abuse
- Hemorrhage (epidural, subdural, subarachnoid, intraparenchymal, intraventricular)
- Concussion/cerebral contusion
- Cerebral edema/increased intracranial pressure

Central Nervous System Disorders
- Increased intracranial pressure/hydrocephalus/shunt malfunction
- Acute disseminated encephalomyelitis—follows viral or *Mycoplasma* upper respiratory infection by a few days to a few weeks; characterized by multifocal neurologic signs, lethargy, coma due to widespread neuritis in the brain, spinal cord, and optic nerves; specific MRI findings confirm the diagnosis; treatment with high-dose corticosteroids
- Seizures, postictal phase
- Neoplastic infiltration or brain tumor
- Arteriovenous malformation, embolism, stroke

Ingestions (see Chapter 4)

Electrolyte Imbalances
- Hyponatremia
- Hypernatremia
- Hypocalcemia
- Hypercalcemia
- Hypomagnesemia

Metabolic Disorders
- Aminoacidopathies
- Organicacidopathies
- Disorders of carbohydrate metabolism
- Disorders of fatty acid oxidation

Mitochondrial Disorders
- Reye syndrome—acute-onset encephalopathy and degenerative liver disease that most commonly follows a childhood viral illness treated with aspirin

Disorders of the Liver
- Hepatic encephalopathy

Renal Disease
- Hypertensive encephalopathy
- Kidney failure/uremia

Pulmonary Disease
- Acute, chronic hypoxia

Cardiovascular Disease
- Cardiovascular failure/shock/compromised perfusion

Endocrinopathy
- Hypoglycemia
- Diabetic ketoacidosis
- Adrenal insufficiency
- Hashimoto encephalopathy

Gastrointestinal Disorders
- Intussusception

TABLE 18-4
CAUSES OF ACUTE, EPISODIC, AND CHRONIC ATAXIA IN CHILDREN

Acute Ataxia

Infectious disease
- Labyrinthitis
- Meningitis
- Encephalitis
- Cerebellar abscess

Acute cerebellar ataxia

Head trauma
- Cerebellar hemorrhage
- Subdural hematoma in the posterior fossa
- Brain contusion

Brain tumor
- Cerebellar tumor
- Posterior fossa tumor

Cerebrovascular thrombosis, embolism, stroke

Proprioceptive disorders
- Posterior spinal column disease
- Neuropathy

Hydrocephalus

Drug or toxin exposure
- Anticonvulsants
- Thallium
- Ethanol (and others)

Episodic Ataxia

Basilar migraine

Inborn errors of metabolism

Malingering

Conversion disorder

Chronic (progressive) Ataxia

Friedreich ataxia—autosomal recessive disorder presenting in late childhood with progressive ataxia, weakness, and muscle wasting; long-term sequelae include kyphoscoliosis and hypertrophic cardiomyopathy

Ataxia telangiectasia—autosomal recessive neurodegenerative disorder that presents in the second year of life with progressive ataxia, extensive telangiectasias (evident on the bulbar conjunctiva and ears), and immunodeficiency (chronic sinopulmonary infections); patients invariably have elevated serum alpha-fetoprotein concentrations

Congenital anomalies of the posterior fossa
- ***Dandy-Walker malformation***—a cystic malformation of the fourth ventricle presenting early in life with hydrocephalus followed by ataxia
- ***Joubert syndrome***—presents in early infancy with nystagmus, periodic hyperpnea/apnea; ataxia in early childhood

Abetalipoproteinemia—inherited inability to absorb fat (and thus fat-soluble vitamins) that presents in infancy with failure to thrive, steatorrhea, and developmental delay; ataxia, peripheral neuropathy, and retinitis pigmentosa develop by late childhood

Hartnup disease—inherited metabolic disorder characterized by aminoaciduria, skin rash, and cerebellar ataxia that usually presents in early childhood

Biotinidase deficiency—an inherited enzyme deficiency presenting in infancy or early childhood with seizures, ataxia, and developmental delay; cutaneous manifestations include eczematous rash and alopecia

hemorrhage). CT of the head should always precede lumbar puncture (LP) in patients with ataxia unless deep tendon reflexes (DTRs) are absent on examination; intracranial processes do not interfere with DTRs. LP permits analysis for abnormalities noted in meningitis, acute disseminated encephalomyelitis, and Guillain-Barré syndrome.

The incoordination resulting from *acute cerebellar ataxia* may be relatively minor; alternatively, the child may be unable to walk or stand. The condition is most common between the ages of 2 and 7 years and often follows a viral illness. The patient appears otherwise well, with no changes in level of consciousness or mental status. The prognosis of acute cerebellar ataxia that involves only the trunk, limbs, and mild nystagmus is quite good, with return of normal coordination within a few weeks. Cases associated with opsoclonus or tremors of the head and neck may require treatment with systemic corticosteroids or intravenous immunoglobulin and can result in permanent neurologic impairment.

Vertigo

Vertigo is the false sensation of rotational movement that is present even if the patient is still. In young patients, differentiation between ataxia and vertigo may be difficult, if not impossible. The age of the patient, duration of the episodes, and associated hearing deficits and neurologic findings provide clues to the diagnosis (Table 18-5). The most common cause of vertigo in pediatric patients is eustachian tube dysfunction/middle ear disease (e.g., otitis media with effusion, acute or chronic suppurative otitis media).

Involuntary Movements

Movement disorders are manifested by involuntary or disordered movement that is not related to ataxia, weakness, or abnormalities in muscle tone such as spasticity (although these may coexist with the movement disorder). Most movement disorders in children are categorized as *dyskinesias*, which are characterized by repetitive abnormal, involuntary movements. Dyskinesias (tics, chorea, myoclonus, tremors, and dystonia, among others) are caused by local or systemic disorders that affect neurologic functioning of the basal ganglia or frontal cortex.

Tics are sudden, involuntary behaviors that serve no functional purpose and recur in frequent bouts throughout the day. Tic disorders run in families and are more common in males. They usually begin prior to the age of 10 years. Transient tic disorders last <1 year. Tics that occur daily for >1 year are chronic. *Motor tics* involve skeletal muscle, usually of the head and/or neck (e.g., facial grimacing). *Vocal tics* result from abnormal stimulation of the diaphragmatic, laryngeal, or pharyngeal muscle (e.g., throat clearing). Isolated vocal tic disorders are not known to persist longer than a year in children. Tics can also be classified as *simple* (a single behavior such as eye blinking) or *complex* (such as a consistent sequence of motor tics that occurs without variation). Patients experience more tics when they are stressed or feeling self-conscious about the disorder; tics decrease in frequency during sleep and periods of intense concentration. Although most patients can voluntarily suppress their tics with some difficulty, they are often unable to concentrate on anything else during this time, and eventually the behaviors occur with increased amplitude. The frequency and severity of tics vary over time; in more than half of patients, the behaviors eventually resolve. The diagnosis of "tic disorder" is a clinical one, arrived at via consistent history and normal neurologic examination. In classic cases, no further evaluation is needed. Behavioral therapy can be beneficial in some patients. Pharmacologic intervention is reserved for patients with significant impairment. The α-2-agonists clonidine and guanfacine are first-line agents in the management of tic disorder. A transient exacerbation of tics is known to occur in affected patients who are placed on methylphenidate; this is not a contraindication to the use of the drug in this population.

Patients with *Tourette syndrome* suffer from motor *and* vocal tics (although not necessarily simultaneously) that persist almost daily for over a year. Common comorbid conditions include obsessive-compulsive behaviors (50%), attention-deficit/hyperactivity disorder (50%), mood disorders (20%), and anxiety disorders (20%). The goal of pharmacologic management of Tourette syndrome consists of identifying a single agent that addresses both the tic disorder and any comorbid conditions.

Chorea is difficult to describe but remarkably easy to identify. The term refers to the recurrence of unexpected, chaotic, purposeless movements that flow from body part to body part. Chorea that involves large-amplitude movements is termed *ballismus*. Primary chorea is rare in children. The two most common causes of secondary chorea in the pediatric population are acute renal failure and rheumatic fever. *Sydenham (rheumatic) chorea* is a major criterion for the diagnosis of acute rheumatic fever after group A beta-hemolytic *Streptococcus* infection, but it may not become evident for weeks or even months after the initial infection. It is more common in girls, usually between the ages of 5 and 15 years. The onset of chorea is often preceded by progressive clumsiness, erratic behavior, and mood swings, followed about a week later by hypotonia, dysarthria, and generalized (although often asymmetric) chorea. The emotional lability and hypotonia are consistent and quite marked; affected patients without these characteristic manifestations are unlikely to have Sydenham chorea. Cultures and titers may be noncontributory by the time the abnormal movements begin. Sydenham chorea follows a waxing and waning course; it eventually resolves but may recur with subsequent streptococcal infections. Carbamazepine and valproic acid are appropriate for symptomatic treatment in patients with significant impairment, but this is rarely necessary. Any child with chorea should be assessed for rheumatic heart disease.

Chorea may be the sole presenting feature of *systemic lupus erythematosus*, but this is uncommon. Marked elevation of serum antiphospholipid antibodies is consistent with lupus chorea. Other causes of secondary chorea in childhood include neurodegenerative disorders, genetic diseases, kernicterus, thyrotoxicosis, trauma, brain tumors, and exposure to various toxins and medications (e.g., carbon monoxide, metoclopramide, phenytoin, amitriptyline).

Acute dystonic reactions and *tardive dyskinesia* are drug-induced movement disorders most frequently associated with neuroleptic use (e.g., haloperidol, metoclopramide, promethazine, prochlorperazine). Acute dystonic reactions can occur following a single dose of any of the above medications but more commonly develop 2 to 3 days after the start of treatment. The patient presents with sustained,

TABLE 18-5
COMMON CAUSES OF VERTIGO IN THE PEDIATRIC POPULATION

Acute Vertigo without Hearing Loss

Benign paroxysmal vertigo

- Most common between the ages of 1 and 3 years
- Typical presentation involves an anxious-appearing child with pallor and obvious unsteadiness/dizziness
- Often associated with nystagmus or rapid eye movements
- Episodes last minutes to hours
- Thought to be a migraine precursor

Benign paroxysmal positional vertigo

- Episodes of vertigo last 20 seconds or less
- Onset of episodes associated with changes in head position
- Can be elicited during physical examination by the Hallpike-Dix maneuver

Vestibular neuronitis

- Most common in adolescents
- Typically follow a viral illness
- Recurrent episodes of vertigo, nausea, and vomiting that occur with decreasing frequency and eventually resolve

Labyrinthine concussion

- Recurrent episodes of severe vertigo following head trauma to the temporal area
- May be associated with temporal bone fracture
- Vertigo accompanied by falling to the affected side
- Episodes resolve over several weeks

Acute Vertigo with Hearing Loss

Eustachian tube dysfunction/middle ear disease

- Most common cause of imbalance in children
- Vertigo due to otitis media with effusion and acute or chronic suppurative otitis media is associated with conductive hearing loss

Labyrinthitis

- Vertigo occurs with the onset of movement and subsides when the patient is still
- Symptoms resolve within several days

Perilymphatic fistula

- Acute onset of hearing loss and vertigo following minor head trauma or abrupt changes in barometric pressure, such as occurs in decompression syndrome
- Hearing loss is sensorineural rather than conductive
- Results when a tear in the round window allows fluid to flow from the inner ear to the middle ear, which is usually filled with air
- Associated symptoms include dizziness, nausea, and vomiting
- May be complicated by recurrent episodes of meningitis when it remains undiagnosed
- Diagnosis and treatment aided by consultation with an experienced pediatric otolaryngologist

Ménière disease

- This condition is rare in the pediatric population, usually occurring in adult patients
- A recurrent disorder that involves tinnitus, vertigo, and progressive hearing loss related to changes in fluid levels within the membranous labyrinth

Persistent (continuous) Vertigo

Vertigo that persists for weeks is uncommon in children. The differential diagnosis includes vestibular schwannoma (neurofibromatosis type II), cholesteatoma, drug toxicity (e.g., aminoglycosides, furosemide), and demyelination disorders. Persistent vertigo is best evaluated and managed by referral to a specialist (otolaryngologist, neurologist).

often painful muscle contractions that may produce an abnormally twisted posture. This reaction is also (less commonly) linked with some anticonvulsants. The dystonia resolves within 24 hours of discontinuing the offending agent. Diphenhydramine or benztropine (in children older than 3 years of age) is indicated to ameliorate the spasms.

Tardive dyskinesia is an extrapyramidal syndrome characterized by involuntary chorealike movements of the face, mouth and tongue, and/or extremities. The abnormal movements develop after months or years of daily neuroleptic treatment. Tardive dyskinesia is rare and may be irreversible despite discontinuation of the drug. *Neuroleptic malignant syndrome* is a potentially fatal adverse reaction consisting of high fever, delirium, and severe rigidity that presents a few days after initiation of a neuroleptic drug and may last as long as 2 to 4 weeks. Care is supportive; no specific therapy is proven to alter the course or duration of the disorder.

Increased Intracranial Pressure

Gradually increasing ICP may initially be difficult to diagnose given the nonspecific nature of early signs and symptoms (Table 18-6). Acute elevations are less subtle. Regardless of the underlying cause, increased ICP is an emergency. Immediate neuroimaging is indicated for patients with suspected increased ICP, which is evident on both CT and MRI.

Management of increased ICP involves the following strategies:

- Achieve modest fluid restriction (if possible) in order to minimize cerebral edema without compromising systemic or cerebral tissue perfusion.
- Administer oxygen to limit cerebral vasodilatation.
- Place the patient's head in the midline at 30 degrees of elevation.
- If hypertension is present, achieve measurable but minimal reduction in blood pressure so as not to compromise cerebral blood flow.
- Administer furosemide (if indicated) to decrease production of cerebrospinal fluid (CSF) and address fluid overload.
- Begin intravenous dexamethasone in the setting of a suspected mass lesion to counteract anticipated *vasogenic edema* (resulting increased permeability of the cerebral capillaries).

Increased ICP with impending brainstem herniation may respond to mannitol and hyperventilation in the acute setting. Although these therapies do not address the underlying condition, they are often successful in delaying herniation of the brainstem until more definitive surgical amelioration can be achieved. Transtentorial herniation (displacement of the uncus of the temporal lobe into the posterior fossa through the tentorial notch) presents with unilateral dilation of the pupil followed by ipsilateral hemiparesis; immediate intervention is necessary to prevent loss of brainstem function and subsequent death.

Pseudotumor cerebri is a benign form of increased ICP that is not associated with underlying neurologic pathology. Idiopathic pseudotumor cerebri is most common in obese adolescent girls. Secondary causes of pseudotumor cerebri are listed in Table 18-7; most can be ruled out through careful history and physical examination. *Headache* and *papilledema* are present in virtually all patients with pseudotumor cerebri; some also complain of diplopia. The LP serves as both a diagnostic tool and treatment; obviously, CT of the head is indicated prior to this procedure in affected individuals. An opening pressure of 20 to 25 cm H_2O with the patient in the decubitus position is consistent with the diagnosis. CSF cell counts and glucose are normal; protein levels may be normal or slightly low. The headache and papilledema usually improve or resolve following LP. Persistent or recurrent headaches are treated with serial LP or pharmacologic therapy (oral acetazolamide and furosemide). The condition is self-limited, and long-term sequelae are rare; persistent papilledema may eventually result in partial vision loss.

TABLE 18-6
CLINICAL MANIFESTATIONS OF INCREASED INTRACRANIAL PRESSURE

Clinical Manifestations	Infants	Children/Adolescents
Nonspecific signs and symptoms	Irritability Shrill cry Anorexia Poor growth Persistent projectile vomiting Somnolence	Persistent vomiting Changes in behavior Changes in mental status Decreasing academic performance Fatigue Vague intermittent headaches Persistent vomiting without abdominal pain or diarrhea
Neurologic signs and symptoms	Macrocephaly Separation of cranial sutures Increasing head circumference Developmental regression Lethargy "Setting sun" sign Asymmetric pupils (anisocoria) Head tilt (abducens nerve palsy)	Headaches in the occipital or frontal region that are increasing in frequency and severity; that occur upon wakening or wake the child; that worsen with lying flat, coughing, or Valsalva Horizontal diplopia (inability to abduct the eye due to abducens nerve palsy) Other cranial nerve palsies Papilledema (if long-standing; initially absent) Lethargy Ataxia (posterior fossa tumor) Cushing triad (hypertension, bradycardia, variable respirations)

TABLE 18-7

POTENTIAL CAUSES OF SECONDARY PSEUDOTUMOR CEREBRI

Medications
- Retinoids (including isotretinoin)
- Tetracycline, minocycline
- Corticosteroids (chronic use)
- Oral contraceptives (chronic use)
- Nitrofurantoin

Hyper- or hypovitaminosis A

Endocrine disorders
- Addison disease
- Hypoparathyroidism or pseudohypoparathyroidism

Systemic lupus erythematosus

Pregnancy

Iron deficiency

Polycythemia

TABLE 18-8

COMMON CAUSES OF PATHOLOGIC WEAKNESS IN THE PEDIATRIC POPULATION

Acute Weakness

Electrolyte disturbances
- Hypercalcemia
- Hypocalcemia
- Hypomagnesemia

Brainstem or cerebellar stroke

Infection
- Poliomyelitis
- Diphtheria
- West Nile virus
- Botulism

Tick paralysis

Toxicities
- Organophosphates
- Lead

Acute intermittent porphyria

Chronic Weakness

Muscular dystrophy
- Duchenne muscular dystrophy
- Becker-type muscular dystrophy

Polymyositis/dermatomyositis

Tumor or abscess of the brain or spine

Transverse myelitis

Myasthenia gravis

Guillain-Barré syndrome

Weakness

Weakness may be acute or insidious in onset and static or progressive (Table 18-8). Acute weakness is typically vascular, infectious, toxin-mediated, or traumatic. Subacute or chronic onset is more likely due to myositis or degenerative disease. Episodic weakness may result from periodic paralysis or myasthenia gravis (MG). Weakness originates at the level of the muscle fiber, neuromuscular junction, peripheral motor nerve or its axon, spine, brainstem, or cerebellum. Muscle disorders produce symmetric weakness that is greater in the proximal extremities (shoulders, hips); the serum creatinine kinase level is invariably elevated. Symmetric weakness is also a feature of neuropathies, which may be accompanied by diminished DTRs and sensory loss. Nerve conduction studies demonstrate diminished impulse velocity or amplitude. Neuromuscular junction disorders cause weakness that becomes more pronounced throughout the day. Weakness originating from a spinal cord process may be accompanied by sensory deficits below the lesion or limited to a specific dermatome. Asymmetric weakness and cranial neuropathies are consistent with a brainstem disorder. When a cerebral abnormality is the source of the weakness, the characteristic hemiparesis and ipsilateral hyperreflexia may occur in the setting of visual disturbances and/or dysarthria.

Neonatal hypotonia, a form of weakness, bears special consideration. Central hypotonia is typically generalized; reflexes are normal or increased, and there may be associated developmental delay and/or microcephaly. Causes include meningitis/encephalitis, hypoxic-ischemic encephalopathy, genetic syndromes, cerebral palsy (CP), and congenital malformations of the brain. Oropharyngeal manifestations (tongue fasciculations, disordered suck and/or swallow) and diminished or absent reflexes are more likely in the setting of peripheral hypotonia (congenital MG, botulism, congenital myopathies).

NEURODIAGNOSTIC TESTING/PROCEDURES

Neurodiagnostic testing is best guided by results of the history and physical examination. *Neuroimaging* is indicated for any patient with focal neurologic signs, including focal seizures.

Lumbar Puncture

LP provides invaluable information in the evaluation of the patient with suspected neurologic disease. The LP permits measurement of the opening pressure and provides CSF samples for analysis of cells counts/differentials/histology and protein and glucose levels. Normal results are listed in Table 18-9. CSF is normally clear; CSF that is cloudy or bloody contains cells. If blood in the CSF is due to a traumatic tap, red cell counts of successive samples will fall; counts remain steady in the setting of herpes

TABLE 18-9
NORMAL RESULTS OF LUMBAR PUNCTURE AND CEREBROSPINAL FLUID ANALYSIS

	Term Infant	Child	Adolescent
Opening pressure (lateral recumbent positioning)	8 to 10 cm H_2O	12 to 16 cm H_2O	8 to 18 cm H_2O
White blood cell (WBC) count	0 to 15 WBC/μL (up to 7 PMNs)	0 to 5 WBC/μL (0 PMNs)	0 to 5 WBC/μL (0 PMNs)
Protein	<120 mg/dL	10 to 40 mg/dL	10 to 40 mg/dL
Glucose	60% to 100% blood glucose	60% blood glucose (generally 40 to 80 mg/dL)	50% to 60% blood glucose

PMNs, polymophonuclear cells.

simplex virus (HSV) encephalitis or subarachnoid hemorrhage. A contrast-enhanced CT should be obtained prior to LP in any patient with signs or symptoms consistent with increased ICP; focal seizures or focal neurologic findings; or altered level of consciousness (i.e., comatose patients, in whom the neurologic examination is often unreliable). LP is contraindicated if the patient is unstable, if there is a skin infection at the LP site, or if the patient has evidence or a history of a bleeding diathesis.

Electroencephalography

Electroencephalography (EEG) records cerebral brain wave electrical activity. As such, it is indicated in patients with transient neurologic symptoms (seizures, paroxysmal disorders) and cases of unexplained encephalopathy or coma. Level of consciousness can also be determined through EEG, which is often performed for prognostic purposes or to document brain death. Focal EEG findings, such as sharp waves and periodic lateralizing epileptiform discharges, are common findings in HSV encephalitis. EEG is of no benefit in the evaluation of structural lesions of the brain.

Electromyography

Electromyography measures the rate, amplitude, and shape of motor unit discharge in response to voluntary movement. Results are most informative in the setting of lower motor neuron disease. Nonspecific changes seen with upper motor neuron or extrapyramidal disease are rarely informative.

Nerve Conduction Studies

Nerve conduction studies record the amount of time it takes for a nerve stimulus to travel between two points. They are most beneficial in confirming peripheral nerve demyelination (e.g., Guillain-Barré syndrome). Conduction times increase in the setting of demyelination but remain normal when weakness results from axonal degeneration or myopathy.

Evoked Potentials

Evoked potentials measure the response of the brain to a standard visual, auditory [brainstem auditory evoked response (BAER)] or somatosensory [somatosensory evoked potential (SSEP)] stimulus. BAERs are discussed in Chapters 5 and 23. SSEPs are used to diagnose central demyelination of the brain or posterior columns of the spinal cord (e.g., multiple sclerosis).

Head Ultrasonography

Ultrasonography through an open anterior fontanelle is a useful screen for ventriculomegaly, hemorrhage, intracranial malformations, or periventricular leukomalacia. Serial sonograms provide a method of monitoring changes against an initial study. Finally, ultrasonography does not expose the patient to radiation. Subsequent CT or MRI provides additional anatomic detail if needed; these studies are usually indicated to provide a more specific prognosis or accurately delineate a surgical lesion.

Computed Tomography

CT is the modality of choice for emergent imaging of the ill child when there is suspicion of hemorrhage, tumor, or abscess. CT is quicker to obtain and, in children older than 5 years, requires no sedation. It is the preferred study for evaluation of head trauma victims. Intracranial calcifications are better identified on CT than MRI. A drawback of the procedure is the amount of radiation to which the patient is subjected (up to 100 times that of a single plain radiograph). Contrast should be included if abscess or tumor is suspected.

Magnetic Resonance Imaging

MRI provides more detailed images than CT, making it superior for the detection and analysis of small intracranial malformations, contusions, and tumors. MRI is also more sensitive for demyelinating or subtle epileptogenic brain lesions. Length of time needed to obtain the study means that sedation is usually required in children, making the procedure unsuitable for patients who are unstable or at high risk for complications from conscious sedation. MRI is the preferred diagnostic modality for nonurgent imaging of the brain in patients with partial seizures and those with suspected HSV encephalitis. MRI is the only appropriate study for assessment of spinal cord trauma, compression, and tumor. Like ultrasonography, MRI does not expose the patient to radiation.

Cerebral Angiography

Cerebral angiography provides highly detailed pictures of the intracranial vasculature [arteriovenous malformations (AVMs)] but is of no benefit in the evaluation of other forms of intracranial pathology.

CENTRAL NERVOUS SYSTEM INFECTIOUS DISEASE

Meningitis

Meningitis is inflammation of the leptomeninges, which may be bacterial, aseptic, or noninfectious. *Bacterial meningitis* occurs most commonly in children younger than 5 years of age, with peak incidence in the first year of life. It is more prevalent in the winter months. Fever, headache, and stiff neck are the most common manifestations in children and adults, although nuchal rigidity and other clinical evidence of meningeal irritation (positive Kernig and Brudzinski signs) are often absent in patients younger than 2 years of age. Nausea, vomiting, and photophobia are frequently present; lethargy, somnolence, and altered consciousness are worrisome signs. Inflammation of the subarachnoid space and increased ICP may rarely be sufficient to produce cranial neuropathies, particularly abducens palsy. The combination of vancomycin and a broad-spectrum third-generation cephalosporin is required empiric therapy for suspected bacterial meningitis in children beyond the neonatal period due to high rates of *Streptococcus pneumoniae* resistance. Rifampin is substituted for the cephalosporin in penicillin-allergic patients. Once the pathogen is identified and sensitivities are known, antibiotic coverage is narrowed, and vancomycin is discontinued if possible. Dexamethasone is indicated for all patients >6 weeks of age with suspected *Haemophilus influenzae* meningitis; its use in infection due to *S. pneumoniae* is controversial. Fluid restriction is no longer recommended for uncomplicated cases of bacterial meningitis. Fever often takes as much as a week or more to resolve; it may normalize following administration of dexamethasone but recurs when the medication is discontinued. If the causative organism and sensitivities have been determined, persistent fever is unlikely to be due to inadequately treated disease; drug fever, suppurative complications, or acquisition of a nosocomial infection is more probable.

Every febrile neonate (temperature >100.4°F) should be evaluated for meningitis. The most common neonatal pathogens are noted in Table 18-10. Infants may not manifest fever due to immaturity of the brain and disruption of intracranial thermoregulatory processes. Initial signs of meningitis are nonspecific in neonates (irritability, somnolence, vomiting, and lethargy). Bulging of the anterior fontanelle indicates increased ICP; in febrile infants with asymmetric findings on neurologic examination, meningitis is the most likely cause. Empiric therapy for suspected neonatal meningitis consists of ampicillin in conjunction with gentamicin or cefotaxime. If the infant is older than 1 month of age and *S. pneumoniae* is a concern, vancomycin and cefotaxime are most appropriate.

Aseptic meningitis occurs when there is evidence of meningeal inflammation without the presence of bacteria. It should be suspected in the patient with a poor response to initial antibiotic therapy and negative bacterial cultures. Most cases of aseptic meningitis are due to viruses, particularly enteroviruses, but also arbovirus, echovirus, and coxsackievirus group B. Viral meningitis peaks in incidence in

TABLE 18-10
PEDIATRIC MENINGITIS: BACTERIAL PATHOGENS

Neonatal Meningitis (birth to 3 months)

Group B *Streptococcus* (early or late onset)
Escherichia coli
Listeria monocytogenes (older than 7 days of age)
Streptococcus pneumoniae (older than 30 days of age)
Enterococci
Gram-negative enteric bacilli (often nosocomial)

Meningitis (3 months to 12 years of age)

Streptococcus pneumoniae (more common in younger children)
Neisseria meningitidis (more common in older children and adolescents; may present with petechial/purpuric rash and/or septic shock)
Haemophilus influenzae (rare in the immunized population)
Consider *Cryptococcus neoformans* in **immunocompromised patients**, particularly those with human immunodeficiency virus (HIV).

the summer and fall months. Affected individuals typically complain of headaches, low-grade fever, and photophobia, but they appear less ill than patients with bacterial meningitis. Nausea, vomiting, abdominal pain, and diarrhea may also be present and suggest a viral etiology. The headache generally improves or resolves following LP. Human immunodeficiency virus (HIV) meningitis should be considered in high-risk patients with aseptic meningitis. Other nonbacterial causes of meningitis are detailed in Table 18-11.

LP should be performed in any patient with suspected meningitis. CT of the brain is not indicated for patients with uncomplicated meningitis but should be obtained prior to LP in patients with papilledema or other evidence of increased ICP, patients with focal neurologic signs, comatose patients, and patients with suspected masses (including abscesses). Normal LP results do not exclude the diagnosis of meningitis; a repeat study several hours later may be markedly abnormal despite partial treatment. Analysis of CSF allows preliminary diagnosis based on results:

- In *bacterial meningitis*, organisms are often noted on Gram stain, and the CSF may appear cloudy. The white blood cell count is quite elevated, occasionally >1,000 per μL, with a predominance of neutrophils. The glucose is typically <50% of serum glucose (<30 mg/dL), and the protein is elevated (>100 mg/dL). The causative organism is recovered through culture of the peripheral blood approximately 80% of the time.
- The CSF glucose level is normal in cases of *viral meningitis*, with protein levels normal or slightly increased. The CSF is sterile, and the white blood count, although increased, is less so than with bacterial meningitis.

TABLE 18-11
CAUSES OF ASEPTIC MENINGITIS

Infectious Aseptic Meningitis

Viruses (most common)

Herpes simplex virus
- Peak incidence of HSV meningitis in the neonatal period; secondary peak in adolescence (sexually active)
- Patients usually toxic appearing
- Suggested by the presence of red blood cells (up to 500/μL) in the cerebrospinal fluid (CSF) or CSF red blood cell counts that do not decrease between first and final sample tubes

Treponema palladium
- Neurosyphilis detailed in Chapters 5 and 24

Borrelia burgdorferi
- Lyme disease is more common in the summer and in certain geographic locations but has been documented throughout the country
- May be history of travel to an endemic area, tick bite, or erythema migrans
- CSF significant for increased white blood count, normal glucose and protein, negative CSF cultures

Rickettsia rickettsii
- Rocky Mountain spotted fever

Mycobacterium tuberculosis
- Insidious in onset, with nonspecific symptoms preceding neurologic signs by 1 to 2 weeks
- Most common in children 6 months to 4 years of age
- CSF white blood count lower than that for bacterial meningitis, with a lymphocytic predominance

Noninfectious Aseptic Meningitis

Parameningeal inflammation
- May accompany cases of sinusitis
- Typical CSF findings include normal glucose, mildly increased protein, and increased WBC count with predominance of neutrophils

Medications
- Nonsteroidal anti-inflammatory agents, allopurinol
- Intrathecal chemotherapeutic drugs

Systemic illnesses
- Systemic lupus erythematosus
- Wegener granulomatosis
- Sarcoidosis

Postinfectious inflammation

Neoplastic disease

Identification of a specific viral pathogen can be achieved in the majority of cases by polymerase chain reaction (PCR) studies.

The most common acute complication of bacterial meningitis is *syndrome of inappropriate antidiuretic hormone* (SIADH). Careful monitoring of serum electrolytes, osmolality, and urine specific gravity permits early detection of SIADH (hyponatremia, low serum osmolality, high urine specific gravity). The condition usually develops 2 to 4 days after the onset of therapy. Increased ICP associated with SIADH presents with irritability and altered consciousness. SIADH in the setting of central nervous system (CNS) pathology is managed with fluid restriction, normalization of serum sodium and osmolality, and administration of mannitol to promote diuresis and decrease ICP to <30 mm H_2O. SIADH resolves spontaneously as the CNS pathology normalizes.

Subdural effusions are another acute complication of meningitis; they occur in up to a third of patients and are most common in young children Subdural effusions are generally of no consequence but require drainage if they become infected or result in increased ICP or focal seizures. *Subdural empyemas* are differentiated from noninfected effusions by contrast-enhanced CT. Other acute complications of bacterial meningitis are listed in Table 18-12.

TABLE 18-12
COMPLICATIONS OF BACTERIAL MENINGITIS

Acute Complications

Syndrome of inappropriate antidiuretic hormone (SIADH)
Subdural effusions
Seizures (including hyponatremic seizures due to SIADH)
Increased intracranial pressure
Cranial neuropathies
Stroke
Cerebral or cerebellar herniation
Sagittal or venous sinus thrombosis
Brain abscess
Systemic thrombosis
Disseminated intravascular coagulation

Long-Term Sequelae (may develop months later)

Sensorineural hearing loss
Hydrocephalus
Seizures
Cranial neuropathies
Motor deficits
Learning disorder
Developmental delay
Behavior problems
Cerebral palsy

Sensorineural hearing loss is the most frequent long-term neurologic consequence of bacterial meningitis, although conductive, mixed, and central hearing loss have also been associated with this infection. The hearing impairment is irreversible and typically presents early in the course of illness. The likelihood of acquiring hearing loss and the degree of resulting impairment appear unrelated to the severity of the meningeal infection. Infection with certain pathogens (e.g., *S. pneumoniae*) is associated with a higher likelihood of hearing loss. Administration of intravenous dexamethasone prior to infusion of antibiotics has shown some success in limiting hearing loss in children with *H. influenzae* meningitis; its role in meningitis due to other pathogens has not been elucidated. Early administration of an appropriate antibiotic does not appear to prevent subsequent hearing loss. Patients with low CSF glucose levels, seizures prior to pharmacologic intervention, longer durations of fever following initiation of therapy, treatment with oral antibiotics prior to diagnosis, and ataxia on initial presentation are at higher risk for sensorineural hearing loss. Hearing assessment is indicated for any patient with a history of bacterial meningitis and should be performed before or soon after discharge.

Encephalitis

Encephalitis in children is typically viral in origin. Important pathogens are listed in Table 18-13.

In *acute disseminated encephalomyelitis*, the onset of widespread CNS demyelination is heralded by irritability, lethargy, mental status changes, mood swings, ataxia, and occasionally seizures. The condition almost always follows a nonspecific respiratory or gastrointestinal illness and is most common in children under the age of 10 years. MRI of the brain demonstrates disseminated CNS lesions. LP is beneficial for distinguishing acute disseminated encephalomyelitis from multiple sclerosis, which may present in a similar manner. The disorder is typically responsive to high-dose systemic corticosteroids and rarely recurs.

HSV encephalitis is an uncommon but potentially devastating infection. In perinatally infected neonates, abnormalities become evident in the second or third week of life. Skin and oral lesions, when present, are virtually diagnostic. HSV encephalitis should be suspected in any infant with seizures, whether focal or generalized, or other signs of encephalitis. Due to the high incidence of permanent neurologic impairment following CNS HSV, intravenous acyclovir should be initiated prior to confirmation of the diagnosis when the disease is suspected.

HSV encephalitis beyond the newborn period may be equally destructive. The infection should be suspected in toxic-appearing patients with high fevers who present with focal seizures and/or other asymmetric neurologic signs. Mental status is frequently altered; meningismus is uncommon. EEG reveals abnormal brain wave activity in the temporal region. Changes are noted in the temporal lobe

TABLE 18-13
VIRAL ENCEPHALITIS

Arboviruses (mosquito-borne pathogens)
- Eastern equine encephalitis
- Western equine encephalitis
- St. Louis encephalitis
- California encephalitis
- West Nile encephalitis

Enterovirus
- Encephalitis typically follows a viral prodrome (fever, upper respiratory symptoms), with the subsequent acute onset of irritability and mental status changes.
- Neurologic signs are usually generalized and symmetric.

Herpes simplex virus

Mumps Meningoencephalitis
- Usually a mild form of encephalitis
- Seasonal (late winter, early spring)
- More common in nonimmunized patients
- Parotid swelling may be present

Rabies (discussed at length in Chapter 10)

on CT. CSF results may be nonspecific or positive for increased protein, pleocytosis, and increased red cell counts that do not clear between sample tubes. Gram stains are negative, and bacterial cultures remain so as well. CSF viral cultures are usually negative; PCR testing for HSV DNA in the CSF is the most reliable diagnostic study and, when positive, is diagnostic of HSV encephalitis. As with neonatal herpes encephalitis, treatment with acyclovir should be initiated when the infection is suspected, even before neurodiagnostic testing if possible.

Brain Abscess

Brain abscesses are less common in children than meningitis and encephalitis. As is true for abscesses in other parts of the body, brain abscesses are usually polymicrobial, containing both Gram-positive and Gram-negative aerobes and anaerobes (*Staphylococcus aureus, Streptococcus viridans, S. pneumoniae, H. influenzae, Pseudomonas aeruginosa, Bacteroides fragilis, Escherichia coli, Klebsiella* species, enterococci, and *Proteus* species). Organisms reach the brain via hematogenous spread (patients with right-to-left shunting and congenital heart disease; emboli from endocarditis) or spread from contiguous structures (sinusitis, trauma). Patients with chronic lung disease are also at increased risk for CNS abscesses. Symptoms are insidious in onset and often nonspecific early in infection. Patients may or may not have low-grade fever; pyrexia is rarely marked. Headache, vomiting, irritability, failure to thrive, generalized seizures, and signs of increased ICP may all be present. Focal neurologic signs are common and depend on the region of the brain primarily affected. When a brain abscess is suspected, neuroimaging with contrast should be obtained prior to LP. Contrast delineates the characteristic ring-enhancing lesion. LP is nondiagnostic.

Empiric treatment should include coverage for the organisms mentioned earlier (e.g., metronidazole, a broad-spectrum third-generation cephalosporin, and nafcillin or vancomycin). Penicillin and metronidazole alone may be sufficient in a patient with known congenital heart disease. Optimal management consists of long-term antibiotic therapy coupled with drainage of the abscess, which both aids in diagnosis and alleviates increased ICP and/or mass effect. Corticosteroids have demonstrable benefit for patients with brain abscess. Affected individuals who do not have a history of trauma or sinusitis should be evaluated for congenital heart disease and endocarditis by echocardiography.

Citrobacter species are a recognized cause of brain abscess in the neonate. Exposure to this Gram-negative organism at birth results in asymptomatic late-onset meningeal seeding and subsequent development of a multiloculated brain abscess. These abscesses are managed with drainage of the loculated areas, if possible, and intravenous therapy with an aminoglycoside and third- or fourth-generation cephalosporin. Due to the extensive nature of the lesions, significant cognitive impairment and developmental delay are the rule.

Myelitis

In children, *transverse myelitis* (inflammation of the spinal cord) is usually postinfectious in origin. Viruses that have been associated with the development of postinfectious myelitis include Epstein-Barr virus, HSV, influenza, mumps, rubella, and varicella, among others. Fever and malaise typically precede the onset of neurologic signs by 24 to 48 hours; patients may also complain of back pain. Lower extremity weakness, sensory changes, and diminishing reflexes progress over several days and plateau before the evolution of spasticity, hyperreflexia, and bowel/bladder dysfunction. MRI of the spine demonstrates fusiform swelling at the involved area of the cord; it is the diagnostic study of choice in patients with these symptoms because it is also sensitive for tumor and cord compression. LP may be necessary if the MRI is unremarkable; moderate elevation of the white blood count with a lymphocytic predominance and a normal or slightly elevated protein concentration are consistent with transverse myelitis and differentiate this condition from Guillain-Barré syndrome. Treatment with corticosteroids is controversial. Most patients recover completely; up to a third are left with residual weakness.

CONGENITAL MALFORMATIONS

Spina Bifida

Spina bifida, or *myelomeningocele*, results from failed closure of the embryonic neural tube, which surrounds and protects the spinal cord. The spinal cord and associated meninges protrude through a defect in the vertebral column and skin, with sensory and motor paraplegia caudal to the lesion. Inheritance is multifactorial. Parents with one affected child have a 1 in 25 chance of having another child with myelomeningocele. Routine maternal folate supplementation has decreased the number of affected newborns. Evaluation for associated orthopedic and urologic anomalies should be conducted early in the neonatal period. Chromosomal analysis is indicated for infants with dysmorphic features or other anomalies. Spina bifida is a static lesion; an underlying cause should be sought in the patient with progressive neurologic dysfunction (*herniation of the brainstem, shunt malfunction, tethered cord*).

The development of *hydrocephalus* due to a Chiari II malformation occurs in virtually all patients with spina bifida, with the great majority requiring permanent placement of a shunt (usually ventriculoperitoneal). Manifestations of hydrocephalus in the neonate consist of increasing head circumference, bulging fontanelle, widely split sutures, irritability, poor feeding, vomiting, and apnea/bradycardia. Hydrocephalus is evident on ultrasonography. Ventricular shunts are fraught with complications. *Extracranial shunt malfunction*, suggested by headache, nausea, vomiting, poor feeding, and lethargy or somnolence, mimics more benign conditions that frequently affect children (e.g., viral infections), resulting in frequent shunt studies early in life. Shunt malfunction in older children may be more insidious and nonspecific, with behavior changes, declining school performance, new-onset seizures or increasing seizure frequency, or changes in ambulation, postural control, or bowel/bladder function. Alternatively, papilledema may be an isolated indicator of a malfunctioning shunt. *Shunt infections* are usually due to *Staphylococcus epidermis* and are most common in the first 3 months after placement.

Tethering of the cord is universal in patients with myelomeningocele; growth of the vertebral column stretches and stresses the cord, leading to back or leg pain, decreased strength and sensation, impairment of bowel/bladder function, and orthopedic deformities of the back or lower extremities. These complications are severe enough to require surgical untethering in about half of cases. Tethering is best evaluated with MRI of the spine.

A renal sonogram and voiding cystourethrogram are performed in the neonatal period to assess for the presence of urinary retention in the bladder (*neurogenic bladder*), associated hydronephrosis, and renal failure. Infants with residual voiding function are closely monitored with serial studies and serum creatinine concentrations as they grow, given their high risk of progressive bladder dysfunction. Neurogenic bladder can usually be managed with urethral dilatation, clean intermittent catheterization, or vesicostomy. Impaction associated with *neurogenic bowel* may be avoided with stool softening and/or scheduled assisted emptying of the bowels.

Orthopedic anomalies noted with increased frequency in patients with myelomeningocele include spinal/vertebral malformations, developmental hip dysplasia, and congenital anomalies of the foot. Scoliosis, kyphosis, and joint contractures are not uncommon as the child grows. Early management of associated orthopedic conditions may permit ambulation and preserve function.

Patients with myelomeningocele may have average or low-normal intelligence, learning disabilities, and/or mental retardation. Performance skills are typically lower than verbal skills.

Spina Bifida Occulta

Spina bifida occulta is a posterior vertebral column defect in the lumbosacral region. The lesion is not associated with protrusion of the cord or meninges, and the skin is intact over the defect. This condition should be suspected in patients with hair, a cleft, or a birthmark over the lumbosacral area. Spina bifida occulta is often an asymptomatic, incidental radiographic finding. Alternatively, patients with this anomaly can experience one or more of the following: bowel/bladder incontinence, abnormal gait, lower extremity sensory/motor deficits, back pain, hip dislocation, tethered cord, and Chiari malformation with hydrocephalus. Neurologic impairment may be absent at birth, only to develop later in life as the child grows.

Abnormal Head Shape

Craniosynostosis is the premature fusion of one or more cranial sutures. It may be idiopathic or occur as part of a syndrome. Bony growth continues along open sutures, resulting in an abnormally shaped head. If early obliteration of the sagittal suture occurs (most common), the child will have a long head and a narrow face (scaphocephaly). In contrast, premature closure of the coronal sutures results in a very wide face with a short, almost boxlike, skull. Lambdoidal synostosis is rare. Most synostosis is evident on plain radiographs of the skull; CT may be required in questionable cases. The need for and timing of surgical intervention, which consists of reopening the sutures and retarding their subsequent fusion, are controversial. Most defects are repaired before age 2 years for cosmetic reasons. Craniosynostosis with associated hydrocephalus, subnormal brain growth, or developmental delay is addressed sooner.

Positional plagiocephaly is the benign flattening of the back of the head often seen in infants placed to sleep exclusively on their backs. A variant results when an infant preferentially lies with the head turned toward one side; flattening of the parieto-occipital area is accompanied by prominence of the forehead on the same side. Most cases require no intervention beyond counseling the parents to encourage the child to lie with the head tilted to the opposite side (by moving a mobile or colorful object to that side). If there is a cosmetic concern, a soft plastic helmet fitted by a plastic surgeon may be successful in gently molding the back of the head into a more acceptable shape when instituted prior to 9 months of age.

Isolated macrocephaly is discussed in Chapter 1.

Cerebral Palsy

Cerebral palsy (CP) is a nonprogressive disorder of movement and posture that results from a fixed lesion of the immature brain. Most cases occur in the absence of identifiable risk factors:

- *Antenatal* conditions that increase the risk of CP include prematurity, intrauterine growth retardation, congenital infection, chromosomal abnormalities, multiple gestation, and congenital malformations of the brain.
- Birth asphyxia and perinatal hypoxia are recognized *perinatal* risk factors. These are present in <10% of children with CP.
- *Postnatal* risk factors include cerebral hemorrhage with resultant periventricular leukomalacia, CNS infection, and traumatic brain injury.

The most common form of CP is *spastic (pyramidal) CP*, which is the consequence of injury to motor tracts in the brain. It is characterized by increased muscle tone in the affected limbs. The disorder is further classified by which limbs are involved (Table 18-14). Patients with CP are generally hypotonic throughout the first few months of life, only later developing the characteristic spasticity. It is usually very difficult to diagnosis CP until an infant fails to meet motor developmental milestones or the spasticity becomes apparent on examination.

Extrapyramidal CP is a rare disorder resulting from damage to the basal ganglia, which is involved in the regulation of muscle tone and coordination. Affected patients exhibit involuntary choreoathetoid movements and postural ataxia, in addition to some spasticity. In contrast to spastic CP, most patients with extrapyramidal CP have an identifiable brain insult (e.g., perinatal asphyxia, placental infarction, maternal toxemia, kernicterus).

Some children with CP are otherwise cognitively normal, but this is the exception. The majority have cognitive deficits ranging from learning disabilities to mental retardation. One third of patients suffer from seizure disorders. Many have hearing and vision impairments. Other frequently encountered conditions include oral-motor dysfunction, constipation, poor growth, gastroesophageal reflux, joint contractures and other skeletal malformations, language disorders, and behavior problems. A multidisciplinary care team, consisting of the primary pediatrician, physical and occupational therapists, nutritionist, speech-language therapist, and social support services, results in optimal therapy and maximization of function. Benzodiazepines, dantrolene, or baclofen may be helpful in addressing spasticity in the acute setting. Recently, however, significant improvements in motor function have been achieved with botulinum toxin motor point blocks.

TABLE 18-14
TOPOGRAPHIC CLASSIFICATION OF SPASTIC (PYRAMIDAL) CEREBRAL PALSY

Diplegia—bilateral lower extremity spasticity

Quadriplegia—all limbs involved, with spasticity greater in lower limbs

Hemiplegia—one side involved, upper extremity more than lower

Double hemiplegia—all limbs involved, with spasticity greater in upper limbs

DEGENERATIVE DISORDERS

Rett syndrome is an X-linked dominant neurodegenerative disorder characterized by developmental regression in social, language, gross, and fine motor skills. It is thought that spontaneous mutation occurs during spermatogenesis. Affected boys die in utero or shortly after birth. In girls, impairment is noted in the second year of life in a child who heretofore had normal achievement of developmental milestones. Decelerated head growth velocity results in acquired microcephaly. *Repetitive hand-wringing* is the most characteristic behavior in these patients. Other manifestations of disease include generalized tonic-clonic seizures, mental retardation, progressive gait disturbances, poor feeding, constipation, sleep disorders, breath-holding spells, scoliosis, muscle wasting, and cardiac arrhythmias. Most affected girls die in late adolescence. Genetic testing is available; presence of an abnormal MECP2 gene confers the diagnosis.

SEIZURE DISORDERS

A *seizure* is a temporary disruption of brain function resulting from abnormal, excessive, synchronous cerebral neuron discharge. A patient is diagnosed with seizure disorder (epilepsy) when unprovoked (idiopathic) seizures become recurrent. The majority of children who have a first seizure will not experience another. Factors associated with an increased risk of recurrence include:

- first seizure beyond age 12 years
- history of severe head trauma
- CP or other major motor handicap
- mental retardation
- abnormal findings on EEG

"Transient slowing" is frequently noted on EEG within the first 48 hours after a seizure; this is an expected finding that does not indicate any underlying disorder. MRI assessment for a structural focus is indicated for the child with focal findings on EEG.

Patients with a second seizure within 6 months and those whose seizures require multiple medications are also at higher risk for recurrences. Initiation of anticonvulsant therapy is not indicated after a first seizure; such treatment does not affect the likelihood that the child will eventually be diagnosed with a seizure disorder, and most anticonvulsants are associated with significant adverse effects. Antiseizure medication should be considered in children who experience a second or third seizure within 6 to 12 months. The decision to start anticonvulsant medication is guided by the risk of seizure recurrence balanced against the anticipated adverse effects of the medications.

Patients with seizure disorder should be allowed to resume their normal activities with as few restrictions as possible. Swimming and bathing are permitted with strict supervision; for adolescents, baths are replaced with showering. Patients of driving age may drive unaccompanied when they have been seizure-free for a period of 3 to 12 months (depending of the state), regardless of whether they are taking anticonvulsants. Birth control is mandatory for sexually active girls with seizure disorder due to the high incidence of birth defects associated with anticonvulsant use. Concurrent use of oral contraceptive pills is known to decrease serum levels of many anticonvulsants, and the efficacy of oral contraceptive pills is diminished when administered with anticonvulsants such as phenobarbital, phenytoin, carbamazepine, and oxcarbamazepine. Strategies for negating these effects include the use of newer anticonvulsant medications (gabapentin or lamotrigine) that do not interfere with oral contraceptive use, switching to high-dose estrogen oral contraceptive pills, or discontinuing estrogen birth control in favor of medroxyprogesterone acetate, which does not affect serum levels of anticonvulsants and is thought to raise the seizure threshold.

A trial off anticonvulsant medication is typically attempted when the patient has remained seizure-free for at least 2 years, especially when the risk of recurrence is low based on the factors listed earlier. EEG has no established role of providing helpful information on which to base this decision.

Many diseases, derangements, and disorders are known to cause seizures (Table 18-15); most of these also lower the seizure threshold in patients with idiopathic epilepsy. Seizures that result from underlying systemic metabolic abnormalities are typically refractory to anticonvulsant therapy.

Seizures should be differentiated from other conditions of altered consciousness and/or abnormal movements, including:

- breath-holding spells
- tics
- self-stimulation
- syncope
- gastroesophageal reflux
- pseudoseizures
- sleep disturbances

TABLE 18-15
RECOGNIZED CAUSES OF CHILDHOOD SECONDARY SEIZURES

Fever
Meningoencephalitis
Trauma (parenchymal contusion)
Structural lesions of the brain
- Congenital
- Neoplastic
- Abscess
- Hemorrhage

Electrolyte imbalances
- Hyponatremia
- Hypocalcemia
- Hypomagnesemia

Hypoglycemia
Uremia
Inborn errors of metabolism
Hypertensive crisis
Medications
- Meperidine
- Bupropion
- Isoniazid
- Ephedra

Medication toxicity
- Methotrexate
- Cyclosporin
- Imipenem
- Lidocaine

Illicit drug ingestion/overdose
- Amphetamines
- Sympathomimetics
- Phencyclidine
- Inhalants
- Cocaine

Neonatal seizures (i.e., those that occur in the first month of life) are considered a separate entity from epilepsy. Most seizures in the neonatal period result from an underlying structural or metabolic abnormality. The differential diagnosis of neonatal seizures is relatively small (Table 18-16). Identifying underlying pathology is particularly important because many neonatal seizures are refractory to anticonvulsant therapy unless the causative condition is addressed. Neonatal seizures may present as any of the following: generalized tonic seizures (stiffening of the body, arms, and legs for up to 20 seconds); focal or multifocal clonic seizures (rhythmic shaking of one or more extremities); myoclonic seizures (brief, isolated jerks); or subtle seizures (eye deviation, apnea, lip smacking, cycling of the extremities), which may not be identified as such. Although neonatal seizures can be an indicator of underlying brain damage, most affected infants remain neurologically

TABLE 18-16
DIFFERENTIAL DIAGNOSIS OF NEONATAL SEIZURES

Hypoxic-ischemic encephalopathy
Trauma
Intracranial hemorrhage
Meningitis
Herpes simplex virus encephalitis
Congenital infection (toxoplasmosis, cytomegalovirus)
Hypoglycemia
Hypocalcemia (e.g., DiGeorge syndrome)
Structural malformations
Benign familial neonatal convulsions
Inborn errors of metabolism
Inherited pyridoxine dependency

intact, and less than half develop an ongoing seizure disorder. Hypoxic-ischemic encephalopathy, intracranial hemorrhage, and structural malformations have the poorest prognoses. Abnormalities on neurologic examination and EEG are also associated with poor outcomes.

Aicardi syndrome is a congenital constellation of abnormalities consisting of cerebral dysgenesis, agenesis of the corpus callosum, and coloboma of the iris. The condition occurs exclusively in females. Infantile spasms begin at 3 to 5 months of age. Patients develop complex seizure disorders and mental retardation early in life, with most dying in the first decade. *Benign familial neonatal convulsions* are an autosomal condition in which seizures (often 10 to 20 per day) begin on or after the third day of life, with spontaneous resolution within weeks or months. Seizures due to *inborn errors of metabolism* typically present beyond the first 48 hours of life; affected infants are usually obtunded as well. In inherited pyridoxine dependency, seizures begin in utero and are often mistaken for fetal hiccups; generalized clonic seizures that develop soon after birth are refractory to anticonvulsant therapy but resolve with administration of intravenous pyridoxine. This condition requires lifelong pyridoxine supplementation.

Febrile seizures do not represent true epilepsy. They are most common in children 6 months to 5 years old with fevers >39°C. The rapid rise in temperature, rather than the height of the fever, seems to be the important determinant. A *simple febrile seizure* is generalized, lasts <10 to 15 minutes, and does not recur for the duration of the precipitating illness. Simple febrile seizures do not require evaluation beyond determining the source of the fever. *Complex febrile seizures* last >10 to 15 minutes, recur within 24 hours, or have focal features. Such children should receive additional studies (e.g., CT of the head, LP) and close follow-up or hospitalization for observation. Children who are toxic-appearing or have meningismus, abnormal neurologic signs, or an underlying brain abnormality should not be presumed to have had a febrile seizure without ruling out more serious etiologies. Persistent neurologic deficits resulting from febrile seizures are exceedingly rare. Only a third of affected children will have a second seizure with a subsequent febrile episode; risk factors for recurrence include decreasing age, family history of febrile seizures, short duration of fever, and relatively low fever with initial seizure. Although antipyretics do not prevent future febrile seizures, caretakers should be counseled concerning fever avoidance and seizure precautions. Children with a history of febrile seizures are at a minimally increased risk of epilepsy later in life; the risk is greatest in those with a family history of epilepsy, but complex febrile seizure and recognized neurodevelopmental abnormality are also associated with a higher incidence of subsequent epilepsy.

Infantile spasms, a particularly devastating seizure syndrome, usually presents between 3 and 12 months of age. The characteristic recurrent, mixed flexor-extensor spasms (involving all four extremities) last only a few seconds but may repeat >100 times in a row. The condition may occur in isolation but is frequently associated with certain neurologic disorders (e.g., congenital malformations, chromosomal abnormalities, inborn errors of metabolism, tuberous sclerosis). An EEG demonstrating hypsarrhythmia is diagnostic of infantile spasms. Approximately 90% of affected infants develop mental retardation and mixed seizure disorders such as Lennox-Gastaut, which is characterized by the frequent occurrence of generalized seizures that are notoriously refractory to pharmacologic treatment.

High-dose adrenocorticotropin (ACTH) controls the seizures in many patients with infantile spasms but does not seem to prevent developmental delay. Prednisone, valproic acid, and clonazepam have also been shown to be beneficial as second-line agents.

Absence (petit mal) seizures typically present between 5 and 7 years of age. These are sudden staring or blinking episodes associated with alteration of consciousness. The child is unaware of the event and immediately returns to the task at hand, with no postictal phase. Although very brief, petit mal seizures can occur hundreds of times a day and may interfere with learning and socialization. Hyperventilation or photic stimulation can precipitate an absence episode in susceptible individuals. An EEG demonstrates the characteristic generalized, symmetric, three-per-second spike and wave pattern. Ethosuximide is the preferred agent for the treatment of these seizures. Most children experience resolution of their seizures within several years, after which medication can be discontinued. Atypical absence seizures may occasionally be mistaken for complex partial seizures but are shorter (<30 seconds in duration) and occur more frequently (multiple times a day).

The abnormal brainwave activity associated with *simple partial seizures* involves only a small focus in one hemisphere. The child remains conscious, and there is no postictal phase. Partial seizures may involve very specific movements or sensations that remain stable with recurrent episodes. The symptoms are specific to the area of the brain involved and may be motor, cognitive, affective, or somatosensory. *Complex partial seizures* result in alteration or impairment of consciousness. Semipurposeful movement continues without direction, or the child may begin lip-pursing or picking at clothes. The episodes may be preceded by an aura and typically last <2 minutes. Both carbamazepine and valproic acid are appropriate first-line agents for patients with recurrent simple or complex partial seizures. Complex partial seizures may rarely progress to generalized convulsions.

Rolandic epilepsy is a benign, self-limited seizure disorder of childhood characterized by unilateral somatosensory or tonic-clonic seizures involving the facial structures or muscles. The condition may remain undiagnosed because seizures frequently occur at night. The presence of characteristic centrotemporal spikes on EEG confirms the diagnosis. Treatment is generally unnecessary, with the seizures remitting in the majority of patients by adulthood. Rarely, these seizures may progress to generalized tonic-clonic convulsions.

Juvenile myoclonic epilepsy (also called myoclonic epilepsy of Janz) is a syndrome of sudden involuntary jerking contractions of the extremities. Onset is between 8 and 12 years of age, and patients may have a history of absence seizures. The condition does not remit, requiring lifelong therapy with valproic acid. Sleep deprivation potentiates the episodes; hyperventilation may provoke a seizure during evaluation. EEG demonstrates bilateral three to six cycle per second spike and wave discharges. More than half of affected individuals develop recurrent generalized tonic-clonic seizures later in life.

With medication, approximately 50% of patients with seizures will become seizure-free. Another 30% will have significant reductions in seizure frequency, intensity, or both. There has been a dramatic increase in the number of medications available for the management of seizures. The newer medications have better toxicity profiles. Their names, indications, and side effects are listed in Table 18-17.

Anticonvulsants have significant adverse effects, many of which involve changes in blood counts or liver transaminases. Most undergo hepatic metabolism. Carbamazepine, phenytoin, and phenobarbital result in enzyme induction and, if used together, lower plasma levels of each other by increasing metabolism. Enzyme inhibition by other medications, most notably macrolide antibiotics, increases circulating levels of these anticonvulsants. Valproic acid displaces phenytoin and phenobarbital from plasma-binding proteins, increasing their serum concentrations into the toxic range.

Serum anticonvulsant levels should be viewed as guidelines or starting points rather than inviolate parameters. A drug level is considered "therapeutic" when seizures are

TABLE 18-17
INDICATIONS AND SIDE EFFECTS OF ANTICONVULSANTS

Medication	Indications	Side Effects/Toxicity
Conventional Drugs		
Carbamazepine (Tegretol)	Partial, tonic-clonic	Diplopia, nausea and vomiting, ataxia, leukopenia,[a] thrombocytopenia
Ethosuximide (Zarontin)	Absence	Rash, anorexia, leukopenia, aplastic anemia
Phenobarbital (Luminal)	Tonic-clonic, partial, neonatal	Hyperactivity, sedation, nystagmus, ataxia
Phenytoin (Dilantin)	Tonic-clonic, partial, neonatal	Rash, nystagmus, ataxia, drug-induced lupus, gingival hyperplasia, anemia, leukopenia, polyneuropathy
Valproic acid (Depakote)	Tonic-clonic, absence, partial	Hepatotoxicity, nausea and vomiting, abdominal pain, weight loss, weight gain, anemia, leukopenia, thrombocytopenia, neural tube and other birth defects
Newer Drugs		
Gabapentin (Neurontin)[b]	Partial	Somnolence, dizziness, ataxia, and fatigue
Lamotrigine (Lamictal)	Tonic-clonic, partial, absence, and Lennox-Gastaut	Dizziness, ataxia, blurred or double vision, nausea, vomiting, rash (including Stevens-Johnson syndrome)
Oxcarbazepine (Trileptal)	Parital, tonic-clonic	Somnolence, hyponatremia, rash
Topiramate (Topamax)	Tonic-clonic, partial, Lennox-Gastaut, infantile spasms	Somnolence, fatigue, confusion, headache, ataxia, weight loss
Zonisamide (Zonegran)	Partial, generalized, infantile spasms, myoclonic seizures	Somnolence, ataxia, confusion, irritability, renal stones

[a]Leukopenia does not cause immunodeficiency and is not an indication for stopping the drug.
[b]Undergoes renal excretion without metabolism, avoiding drug interactions.

controlled and adverse effects are minimal. Levels are most helpful in the following settings:

- At initiation of therapy or when a new drug is added to an established regimen
- During periods of accelerated patient growth
- When the patient is on a multidrug regimen
- When there is a change in the formulation of the drug (generic vs. brand name)
- When there is a change in seizure type, persistence of seizures, or increased frequency of seizures
- When there are concerns about compliance

Status epilepticus is defined as a prolonged episode of seizure activity (>30 minutes) or an extended period of recurrent seizures between which the patient does not regain consciousness. Status epilepticus has the potential for significant morbidity (hypoxic-ischemic injury, brain damage) and death, although any residual neurologic impairment is more likely to be related to the underlying cause rather than the episode of status itself. Airway, breathing, and circulation are evaluated and supported as necessary; oxygen is routinely administered. STAT labs should include measurements of glucose, electrolytes (including calcium, phosphorus, and magnesium), blood urea nitrogen, and liver transaminases; complete blood count with differential; toxicology screens; and anticonvulsant levels, if applicable. Short-acting benzodiazepines (intravenous lorazepam, intravenous or rectal diazepam) often "break" the seizure and should be administered if seizure activity persists for >5 minutes, with one to two repeat doses thereafter at 5- to 10-minute intervals unless the seizure abates. Fosphenytoin, phenytoin, or phenobarbital loading doses are usually administered concurrently to prevent recurrence (Table 18-18). Patients in refractory status may require thiopental induction of anesthesia.

TABLE 18-18

DOSAGES AND ROUTES OF ADMINISTRATION OF DRUGS FOR THE MANAGEMENT OF STATUS EPILEPTICUS

Diazepam
- Intravenous: 0.1 to 0.3 mg/kg dose over 2 to 5 minutes
- Rectal: 0.2 to 0.5 mg/kg/dose

Lorazepam
- Intravenous: 0.05 to 0.1 mg/kg/dose over 2 to 5 minutes
- Injectable form may be given rectally

Phenobarbital
- Intravenous loading dose: 15 to 20 mg/kg administered at a rate of 1 mg/kg/min
- May also be administered via intraosseous line

Phenytoin
- Intravenous loading dose: 15 to 20 mg/kg administered at a rate of 1 mg/kg/min

Fosphenytoin
- Intravenous loading dose: phenytoin equivalent dose of 15 to 20 mg/kg administered at a rate of up to 3 mg/kg/min
- May also be administered via intramuscular route (multiple sites)

CEREBROVASCULAR DISEASE

Stroke consists of the sudden onset of focal neurologic impairment caused by an interruption of cerebral blood flow, which may be transient or permanent. In children, stroke is rare and is usually precipitated by one of the following:

- Cardiac disease (congenital heart disease, endocarditis)
- Vascular disease (arteriovenous malformation, aneurysm)
- Hematologic disorders (sickle cell disease and diseases that predispose to the formation of thrombi or bleeding)
- Metabolic disease (most commonly homocystinuria)

Most strokes in children occur in the cerebral hemispheres, presenting with hemiparesis, visual field defects, and/or aphasia. Brainstem and cerebellar strokes are less common. The neurologic manifestations correlate with the location of the ischemia.

Arteriovenous malformations (AVMs) may present with the sudden or insidious onset of headache, vomiting, nuchal rigidity, progressive hemiparesis, diplopia, ataxia, and focal or generalized seizures. At least half of AVMs are asymptomatic until rupture. Surgical removal, embolization, or radiotherapy is necessary to prevent recurrent stroke or hemorrhage.

SPINAL CORD DISEASE

Spinal cord impairment can result from extrinsic compression, abscess, trauma, and transverse myelitis. Signs and symptoms may include any of the following, combined or in isolation: motor deficits, sensory deficits, and autonomic dysregulation. Immediate MRI of the spinal cord with gadolinium contrast is indicated for any patient with a suspected spinal cord lesion.

Patients with Down syndrome are at increased risk for atlantoaxial dislocation, presenting with neck pain, limitation of neck mobility, head tilt, incoordination, gait abnormalities, hyperreflexia, clonus, and/or bowel/bladder dysfunction. Symptomatic children should be evaluated with an MRI of the spine. Dislocation with cord compression necessitates emergent referral to a neurosurgeon or orthopedist.

Spinal cord compression from an extramedullary tumor has a similar presentation, although the pain is typically more severe and specific to the area of involvement. Back pain in the setting of motor, sensory, or bowel/bladder control changes should prompt suspicion of an extrinsic spinal cord tumor. Intravenous dexamethasone is administered to patients with suspected cord compression immediately in order to reduce edema and preserve function. Surgical removal of the mass is indicated within 24 to 48 hours.

PERIPHERAL NERVE AND MUSCLE DISORDERS

Guillain-Barré syndrome (GBS) is characterized by the acute onset of rapidly progressive ascending weakness, diminished or absent DTRs, and a history of recent respiratory or gastrointestinal viral illness. GBS results from autoimmune-mediated demyelination of the peripheral nerves. Weakness may be minimal or progress to total flaccid paralysis. Truncal ataxia and cranial nerve palsies are not uncommon. If present, respiratory muscle weakness necessitates mechanical ventilation. Back pain and paresthesias occur in some patients. Although rarely prominent, autonomic impairment may occasionally precipitate life-threatening fluctuations in heart rate and blood pressure. Bowel and bladder function are generally preserved. The CSF protein concentration is quite elevated; cell count is typically <10 per μL, glucose remains normal, and red cells are absent ("albuminocytologic dissociation"). Motor nerve conduction studies are particularly helpful in the first 1 to 2 weeks of disease, during which CSF results may be normal. Characteristic abnormalities include reduced or absent F waves and sensory nerve action potentials and prolonged latencies consistent with demyelination. Symptoms progress for up to 4 weeks, and resolution beginning about 4 weeks thereafter. Recovery is usually complete in children, although the rare patient will experience permanent lingering disability. Intravenous immunoglobulin administered on 5 consecutive days shortens the duration and severity of GBS and should be administered as soon as the diagnosis is made. Plasmapheresis is equally effective but has more potential adverse effects.

NEUROPATHY

Peripheral neuropathy is rare in children. As opposed to adults, who typically complain of numbness and paresthesias, children present with weakness and diminished or absent DTRs. Isolated ataxia is not uncommon early in the course. The differential diagnosis includes:

- GBS
- diphtheria (in unimmunized patients and underdeveloped countries; diagnosed by throat culture demonstrating *Corynebacterium diphtheriae*)
- botulism (descending paralysis with cranial neuropathies, hyporeflexia; diagnosed through demonstration of toxin in the serum or presence of *Clostridium botulinum* in the stool)
- Charcot-Marie-Tooth disease (an inherited disorder of peripheral sensory and motor nerves; it is slowly progressive and usually does not produce weakness until late adolescence or adulthood)
- leukodystrophies (including Refsum disease)
- tick paralysis
- toxin-mediated neuropathy (organophosphates, lead, cisplatin, vincristine)
- spinal muscle atrophy (infantile/Werdnig-Hoffmann, juvenile-onset)

Bell palsy is the most common cause of facial weakness/paralysis in the pediatric population. Swelling of the facial nerve within the canal may be idiopathic or follow a viral infection. Usually, an entire side of the face is affected, although the forehead is spared. When the intermediate branch of the facial nerve is also affected, patients may experience inability to close the ipsilateral eye, hyperacusis, and loss of taste over the anterior region of the tongue. Recovery is spontaneous and complete in nine out of ten cases. Prednisone reduces swelling of the nerve within the canal and decreases the risk of permanent facial sequelae. An ocular lubricant is prescribed for nighttime use in patients who are unable to close an eye. Further assessment with MRI is indicated if there is a concern for a brainstem abnormality, a proximal facial nerve process, loss of hearing, or cranial neuropathies, or if the existing palsy does not improve.

Neonatal brachial plexus injuries are more common in difficult extractions or breech deliveries. Most occur on the right side; a small minority are bilateral. *Erb-Duchenne palsy* results from injury to cervical nerves 5 to 7. The infant is unable to abduct the affected arm at the shoulder, externally rotate the arm, or supinate the forearm. *Klumpke paralysis* develops following injury to cervical nerves 7 and 8 and the first thoracic nerve; the ability to grasp the hand on the involved side is impaired. A physical therapist should be consulted for any infant with a brachial plexus injury to promote return of function and prevent contractures.

Myasthenia gravis (MG) is a chronic autoimmune disorder involving the neuromuscular junction. Autoantibodies bind to postsynaptic acetylcholine receptors, blocking their interaction with acetylcholine. The rate of receptor breakdown also increases, resulting in fewer functional receptors. Predominant symptoms include rapid fatigability and weakness of skeletal muscles that is exacerbated by sustained activity and improves with rest. *Juvenile MG* typically presents in late childhood or adolescence; the onset may be rapid or, more typically, insidious. Weakness is initially worse in the afternoons and evenings, and symptoms wax and wane over time. Ptosis and double vision develop early in the course of the disease in 50% of patients. Weakness of bulbar musculature follows, resulting in difficulty with speech and feeding. The diagnosis is confirmed through administration of an intravenous anticholinesterase (edrophonium chloride), which produces a transient increase in muscle strength by blocking the breakdown of acetylcholine in the synaptic cleft. Nerve stimulation studies demonstrate a significant decrease in strength over several rapid-fire trials. Serum acetylcholine receptor antibodies are measurable in the majority of cases. Anticholinesterase therapy (neostigmine or pyridostigmine bromide) often relieves symptoms in patients with mild involvement. Corticosteroids and other immune suppressants help curb the autoimmune response. Finally, thymectomy results in substantial improvement in many patients with juvenile MG. The disorder may go into complete or partial remission after several years; however, most patients continue to experience periodic exacerbations throughout adulthood. Mechanical ventilation is required in the setting of severe respiratory muscle fatigue, hypoventilation, or apnea. Plasmapheresis may also be indicated in this setting.

MUSCULAR DYSTROPHIES

Muscular dystrophies are inherited disorders of skeletal muscle without evidence of central or peripheral nervous system involvement. Individual disorders are categorized as congenital muscle dystrophies or limb girdle muscle dystrophies. *Duchenne muscular dystrophy* results from an X-linked mutation in the gene encoding for dystrophin, an integral component of the sarcolemma (the extensible membrane covering the contractile substance of the muscle fiber). Instability of the sarcolemma leads to muscle damage and initiation of the inflammatory cascade; further muscle damage progresses to necrosis and fibrosis of both skeletal and cardiac muscle. Although the disease is present from birth (as evidence by elevated creatinine kinase levels), clinical signs become evident between 3 and 5 years of age. Affected individuals are usually late walkers and tend to walk primarily on their toes. Their inability to conclusively hop, jump, or run places them in sharp contrast to their peers. They often fall and have difficulty rising, essentially needing to climb up their legs (*Gower maneuver*). Proximal extremity weakness precedes distal weakness, and the lower extremities are affected before the upper extremities. As pelvic muscles weaken, affected boys develop lumbar lordosis and a Trendelenburg (rocking) gait. Many also have delayed motor and/or language development and poor attention spans but benefit from academic intervention. Most patients are wheelchair bound by the age of 10 years and lose the upper extremity strength needed to feed and care for themselves several years thereafter. Orthopedic procedures are required to correct spinal curvature within 3 to 4 years of wheelchair dependence; surgical care is also indicated for lower extremity contractures. Pulmonary function begins to decline in late childhood; as the cough weakens, the patient is unable to effectively clear respiratory secretions, predisposing to recurrent pneumonias. Most patients die in their late teens or early twenties from respiratory disease or heart failure.

Creatinine kinase levels are markedly elevated (up to 100-fold over normal levels); in fact, Duchenne muscular dystrophy is the only known cause of such high levels. Creatinine kinase levels are elevated at birth, despite normal muscle strength and tone. EMG demonstrates only nonspecific changes and is not helpful in the diagnosis of Duchenne muscular dystrophy. Genetic identification is available for diagnosis of 80% to 90% of cases; histologic examination of muscle tissue obtained through biopsy is required in the remaining 10% to 20%. Corticosteroids can slow but not halt the progressive muscle injury and destruction, but they have significant adverse effects, including obesity, which is already problematic in these patients when they become wheelchair bound. Newer formulations such as deflazacort, an oxazolone derivative of prednisone, are better tolerated and equally effective.

CENTRAL NERVOUS SYSTEM TRAUMA

CNS trauma in children most often results from motor vehicle accidents, bicycle mishaps, falls, or child abuse. Prognosis depends on the severity of the initial insult and factors contributing to secondary neuronal injury such as hypotension and hypoxia. In cases of minor head trauma with no alteration in or loss of consciousness and normal findings on physical examination, the risk of intracranial injury is extraordinarily low; neither extended observation nor imaging studies are indicated under these circumstances. Approximately 10% of children hospitalized for a *traumatic brain injury* will experience at least one seizure. Long-term sequelae can include behavioral changes, motor impairment, memory problems, and seizure disorder.

A *concussion* is a brief (usually <1 minute) alteration in or loss of consciousness following mild head trauma. CT of the head without contrast may be appropriate in select patients with concussion, although observation alone is equally acceptable. Brain injury is typically undetectable, and the neurologic examination returns to normal within hours. In contrast, *cerebral contusions* represent direct injury to brain parenchyma that can be appreciated on noncontrast head CT. Concussion in the athlete is discussed in detail in Chapter 25.

Traumatic brain hemorrhages may be epidural, subdural, and/or subarachnoid:

- An *epidural hematoma* should be suspected in the patient with significant head trauma who experiences a brief loss of consciousness, followed by a lucid period, with subsequent rapid neurologic deterioration ("waxing and waning" consciousness). Bleeding from a damaged artery produces an acute increase in ICP, evidenced by the rapid alteration in consciousness.
- Bleeding from injured bridging veins traversing the subdural space results in a *subdural hematoma*. Increased ICP can also develop during subdural bleeding, but deterioration is typically slower and delayed several hours or even days after the initial injury. Altered consciousness may be preceded by headache, irritability, lethargy, and vomiting (or poor feeding in the infant). Alternatively, patients may not regain consciousness following the injury, presenting instead with coma. Subdural bleeding

should be suspected when the injury mechanism involves acceleration-deceleration forces, such as may occur with motor vehicle collision or shaken baby syndrome.

- Severe brain injury usually results in some degree of *subarachnoid hemorrhage*, manifested by blood in the CSF.

Severe brain injury may occur in absence of external signs of trauma. The preferred method of detecting epidural, subdural, and subarachnoid hemorrhage in the trauma patient is noncontrast CT of the head. This study should be obtained in patients with altered mental status or altered levels of consciousness, a history of loss of consciousness lasting >1 minute, amnesia for the event, recurrent vomiting, severe or progressive headache, focal neurologic findings, or findings consistent with underlying skull fracture.

Blunt injury, vertebral fracture dislocations, and whiplash forces are all capable of resulting in significant *spinal cord injury* (contusion, laceration). The C1-2 and C5-6 joints are the most common sites of cervical cord injury. Spinal immobilization should be secured prior to transport in any patient who has sustained significant body trauma; removal is delayed until the possibility of spinal damage has been safely eliminated. Many patients can be "cleared" following clinical evaluation and plain radiographs of the neck; spinal CT and MRI are reserved for patients with questionable films or neurologic findings. Manifestations of spinal injury include midline focal back pain and weakness or sensory loss in the extremities. *Spinal shock syndrome* describes the temporary loss of all sensorimotor and reflex function inferior to the cord injury. Urinary retention and constipation are typical. The symptoms gradually resolve over hours to days.

Intravenous methylprednisolone is indicated for any patient with history and physical examination suggestive of spinal cord injury. The administration of an initial bolus followed by drip infusion during the first 24 hours after injury has been demonstrated to reduce neuronal edema and subsequent ischemic injury.

The characteristics of head injuries suspicious for physical abuse are discussed in Chapter 28.

SOURCES

Biggar WD. Duchenne muscular dystrophy. *Pediatr Rev.* 2006;27:83–88.

Chavez-Bueno S, McCracken GH. Bacterial meningitis in children. *Pediatr Clin North Am.* 2005;52:795–810.

Dias MS. Neurosurgical management of myelomeningocele (spina bifida). *Pediatr Rev.* 2005;26:50–60.

Forghani N, Cohen RA. Radiation risks of CT scans. *Pediatr Rev.* 2006; 27:79.

Friedman MJ, Sharieff GQ. Seizures in children. *Pediatr Clin North Am.* 2006;53:257–278.

Gladstein J, Mack KJ. Chronic daily headache in adolescents. *Pediatr Ann.* 2005;34:472–485.

Lewis DW. Pediatric migraine. *Pediatr Rev.* 2007;28:43–53.

Lewis DW, Pearlman E. The migraine variants. *Pediatr Ann.* 2005; 34:486–497.

Lewis DW, Yonker M, Winner DO, et al. The treatment of pediatric migraine. *Pediatr Ann.* 2005;34:448–460.

MacGregor DL. Vertigo. *Pediatr Rev.* 2002;23:10–16.

McVicar K. Seizure-like states. *Pediatr Rev.* 2006;27:e42–e44.

Oleson J. The international classification of headache disorders. *Cephalalgia.* 2004;24(suppl 1):1–160.

Rubin DH, Suecoff SA, Knupp KG. Headaches in children. *Pediatr Ann.* 2006;35:345–353.

Schlaggar BL, Mink JW. Movement disorders in children. *Pediatr Rev.* 2003;24:39–51.

Thiessen ML, Woolridge DP. Pediatric minor closed head injury. *Pediatr Clin North Am.* 2006;53:1–26.

Wolf SM, McGoldrick PE. Recognition and management of pediatric seizures. *Pediatr Ann.* 2006;35:332–344.

Zinner SH. Tourette syndrome: much more than tics. *Contemp Pediatr.* 2004;21:22–49.

Zupanc ML. Neonatal seizures. *Pediatr Clin North Am.* 2004;51:961–978.

QUESTIONS

1. A 14-year-old girl presents to your office for evaluation of her headaches. She has had four headaches over the past 3 months, which she describes as sudden in onset, pounding, severe, and located in the bifrontal region. The headaches are not present upon wakening, but otherwise occur at variable times of day. She often feels nauseous during the headaches, which are made worse by exposure to light but resolve with sleep. The pain does not respond to acetaminophen or ibuprofen. The vital signs and physical examination, including a complete neurologic assessment, are normal. Which of the following is the most appropriate management of the patient's headaches at this time?

A) Oral sumatriptan at the first sign of headache
B) Intravenous sumatriptan at the first sign of headache
C) Subcutaneous sumatriptan at the first sign of headache
D) CT of the head with intravenous contrast
E) Discontinue all over-the-counter and prescription analgesics

2. A 12-year-old boy presents with a history of morning headaches for the past several weeks. The headaches are located at the back of his head and are occasionally accompanied by vomiting. The child has normal vital signs and a normal physical examination except for mild asymmetry in upper and lower extremity strength (5/5 on the left, 4/5 on the right). Which of the following is the most appropriate management for the patient at this time?

A) Prescription for intranasal sumatriptan, to be given at the first sign of headache
B) Computed tomography scan of the head
C) EEG
D) Prescription for oral metoclopramide, to be given at the first sign of headache
E) Prescription for daily amitriptyline

3. A 15-year-old girl presents to your office for evaluation of her daily headaches. The headaches started about 3 months ago. She describes them as "like a rubber band" around her head. They usually occur in the late afternoon or evening and are worse on the weekends when she stays with her father (her parents are recently divorced). Her vital signs and physical examination, including the neurologic assessment, are completely normal. This patient's pain is most likely a result of which of the following?
A) CNS mass effect
B) Increased intracranical pressure
C) Benign tension headaches
D) Basilar migraine headaches
E) Common migraine headaches

4. A full-term neonate delivered without complication following an uneventful pregnancy develops multifocal seizures at 16 hours of age. A screening head sonogram is negative for structural abnormality or hemorrhage. Initial serum electrolyte, calcium, magnesium, and glucose levels are normal. The infant continues to seize intermittently despite the administration of lorazepam, phenobarbital, and fosphenytoin. The boy's mother denies illicit drug and alcohol use during the pregnancy. The clinical presentation of this patient's seizures is most consistent with which of the following?
A) Narcotic withdrawal
B) Group B streptococcal sepsis
C) *Listeria monocytogenes* meningitis
D) Inborn error of metabolism
E) Reye syndrome

5. A 7-year-old boy developed intermittent, repetitive, nonrhythmic sniffing and throat clearing 2 months ago. The child has now started back to school after summer vacation. He attends a private school with small class sizes. His parents report that the teacher says his tics are near-continuous at school and are interfering with the other children's educations. In addition, he is now being teased about his behavior. The boy continues to do well in school despite his tic disorder and has no history of compulsive behavior. Which of the following agents is recommended as an initial treatment for tics in this child?
A) Risperidone
B) Haloperidol
C) Methylphenidate
D) Dextromethorphan
E) Clonidine

6. An 8-year-old boy has an 18-month history of daily tics, including chirping and facial grimacing (although not necessarily concurrently). His physical examination, including the neurologic assessment, is normal. This child meets the diagnostic criteria for which of the following conditions?
A) Tourette syndrome
B) Chronic motor tic disorder
C) Chronic vocal tic disorder
D) Sydenham chorea
E) Motor rhythmias

7. Which of the following comorbid conditions is most frequently associated with Tourette syndrome?
A) Pervasive developmental disorder
B) Attention-deficit/hyperactivity disorder
C) Oppositional-defiant disorder
D) Conduct disorder
E) Learning disorder

8. An 11-year-old girl is brought to your office by her mother because she is making unusual movements. Upon questioning, she describes the movements as frequent, brief, unpredictable, involuntary twitching movements that resemble fidgeting. The girl has also been clumsier than normal, occasionally has difficulty speaking, and has wide mood swings. The physical examination is remarkable for mild hypotonia throughout. This child should be evaluated for which of the following conditions?
A) Myotonic dystrophy
B) Tourette syndrome
C) Acute rheumatic fever
D) Generalized torsion dystonia
E) Benign paroxysmal vertigo

9. A mother brings her previously well 2-year-old daughter to you because the girl seemed "off-balance" when she got out of bed this morning and now falls whenever she tries to ambulate. There is no antecedent history of a viral infection, but there is a family history of migraine headaches. The physical examination reveals a well-nourished, well-developed girl who appears nontoxic but unsteady when asked to sit unsupported or stand. Her gait is unsteady, and she falls after taking a few steps. Strength and sensation are intact throughout, and no cranial nerve palsies are noted. Which of the following is the most likely cause of this child's unsteadiness?
A) Postinfectious cerebellar ataxia
B) Basilar artery migraine
C) Labyrinthine concussion
D) Benign paroxysmal vertigo
E) Benign paroxysmal positional vertigo

10. A previously well, 6-month-old infant develops recurrent seizures that are difficult to control with anticonvulsant monotherapy. At 9 months of age, the child is unable to sit unsupported, which is thought to be due to unsteadiness since his tone and strength are grossly normal. He develops an eczematous rash and, by age 12 months, is globally delayed and has no hair

on his head. This patient's clinical presentation is most consistent with which of the following conditions?
A) Abetalipoproteinemia
B) Hartnup disease
C) Ataxia-telangiectasia
D) Friedreich ataxia
E) Biotinidase deficiency

11. A 16-year-old obese female presents to the emergency department with a headache of 3 days in duration that is increasing in intensity. The headache is generalized and constant; lying down, coughing, or defecating makes the pain worse. She denies fever, vomiting, recent infection, weakness, or dizziness. Her only medication is daily oral contraceptives. Vital signs are normal in the emergency room. The physical examination is within normal limits except for bilateral papilledema. Contrast-enhanced CT of the head is negative. The LP opening pressure is 25 cm H_2O. Which of the following is the most appropriate management of this patient's ICP?
A) Counsel the patient to substitute another form of birth control for the oral contraceptive use.
B) Reassure the patient that she has a self-limited condition that is not associated with underlying neuropathology.
C) Schedule the patient for serial LPs.
D) Refer the patient for a lumboperitoneal shunt.
E) Prescribe daily acetazolamide and furosemide, with follow-up in the neurology clinic in 3 months.

12. A 3-week-old former full-term infant is referred to the emergency department by his primary care physician for fever of 38.5°C, irritability, and poor feeding for 24 hours. Pregnancy and delivery were uncomplicated, and the infant has been gaining weight appropriately. Results of a LP are consistent with bacterial meningitis. Which of the following pathogens is the most likely cause of meningitis in this patient?
A) *Listeria monocytogenes*
B) Group B *Streptococcus*
C) *Streptococcus pneumoniae*
D) HSV
E) *Cryptococcus neoformans*

13. A 7-month-old girl who is in the hospital receiving intravenous antibiotics for bacterial meningitis due to *Streptococcus pneumoniae* becomes increasingly irritable on the third day of treatment. Serum sodium concentration measures 126 mEq per L. This patient's hyponatremia is most likely due to which of the following?
A) End-organ insensitivity
B) Administration of hypotonic fluids
C) Syndrome of inappropriate antidiuretic hormone secretion
D) Acute renal failure
E) Diabetes insipidus

14. A 10-day-old former full-term infant develops irritability and poor feeding. As part of his evaluation, a LP is performed, which yields cloudy fluid and elevation of the CSF white blood count with a predominance of neutrophils. Which of the following treatments should be instituted in this patient without delay?
A) Securing of the airway
B) Intravenous dexamethasone
C) Intravenous vancomycin and cefotaxime
D) Intravenous ampicillin and cefotaxime
E) Intravenous ampicillin and vancomycin

15. You suspect postinfectious transverse myelitis in a patient with lower extremity spasticity, hyperreflexia, and sensory deficits. No abnormalities are noted on MRI of the spine. Which of the following sets of LP results is consistent with the diagnosis of transverse myelitis?
A) Cloudy fluid with a white blood count in excess of 1,000 per μL; predominance of monocytes; low glucose; normal protein
B) Cloudy fluid with a white blood count in excess of 1,000 per μL; predominance of neutrophils; low glucose; normal protein
C) Normal white blood count, differential; normal glucose and protein; increased red cell counts that clear between sample tubes
D) Marked elevation of the white blood count; predominance of lymphocytes; normal glucose; increased protein; increased red cell counts that do not clear between sample tubes
E) Moderate elevation of the white blood count; predominance of lymphocytes; normal glucose; normal or slightly elevated protein

16. While rounding with a group of medical students, you decide to elaborate on HSV encephalitis, which has been diagnosed in a 6-year-old girl on the unit. You are correct in telling the students all of the following EXCEPT:
A) Viral cultures of the CSF are typically positive for HSV.
B) Meningismus is uncommon in HSV encephalitis.
C) Acyclovir should be started prior to obtaining neurodiagnostic studies when HSV infection of the CNS is suspected.
D) Abnormal brain wave activity in the temporal lobe is consistent with the diagnosis of HSV encephalitis.
E) HSV encephalitis has a high incidence of permanent neurologic sequelae.

17. A previously well, 30-month-old girl develops a low-grade fever, lethargy, and focal seizures. Neuroimaging reveals a single brain abscess in the right frontal lobe. The sinuses appear normal for age, and there is no history of trauma. Which of the following

studies should be performed first, once the patient has been stabilized and begun effective treatment?
A) MRI of the spine
B) Echocardiography
C) Cognitive testing
D) Hearing assessment
E) Radionuclide bone scan

18. A 14-day-old infant presents to the pediatric emergency department with poor feeding and irritability. His temperature upon arrival is 38.0°C. He experiences a focal seizure and becomes comatose. CT of the head is obtained with contrast and demonstrates multiloculated ring-enhanced lesions in both frontal lobes. Which of the following is the most likely cause of this patient's condition?
A) Group B *Streptococcus*
B) *Listeria monocytogenes*
C) *Citrobacter* species
D) *Bacteroides fragilis*
E) *Staphylococcus aureus*

19. Parents of a full-term 2-month-old infant bring the child to you for evaluation of the shape of the girl's head. Weight, height, and head circumference continue to tract along established curves. The physical examination is significant for a patent anterior fontanelle, normal neurologic assessment, and subtle flattening of the right parieto-occipital region with mild prominence of the right forehead. No cranial ridges are noted along suture lines. Which of the following is the most appropriate next step in the management of this patient?
A) Refer the patient to a neurosurgeon.
B) Refer the patient to a plastic surgeon.
C) Obtain plain radiographs of the skull.
D) Counsel the parents to encourage the infant to turn her head toward the left when she is lying on her back.
E) Obtain CT of the head.

20. Which of the following is not considered part of the differential diagnosis of acute neurologic deterioration in a child with myelomeningocele?
A) Herniation of the brainstem
B) Shunt malfunction
C) Tethered cord
D) Normal progression of the condition
E) All of the above are part of the differential.

21. A previously well, 3-year-old boy is brought to your clinic by his mother because he is "walking funny." She also notes that he has been intermittently constipated for the past few months and has begun to wet his pants several times a day. His physical examination is significant for a midline hairy tuft above the gluteal cleft. This patient's clinical presentation is most consistent with which of the following?
A) Spina bifida occulta
B) Myelomeningocele
C) Cerebral palsy
D) Syringomyelia
E) Atlantoaxial dislocation

22. You are giving a lecture about cerebral palsy (CP) to a group of residents. You are correct in telling them all of the following EXCEPT:
A) CP is a nonprogressive disorder of movement and posture that results from a fixed lesion of the immature brain.
B) A history of birth asphyxia or perinatal hypoxia is present in at least 50% of patients with CP.
C) The most common form of CP is spastic (pyramidal) CP.
D) Infants with CP are hypotonic early on, with spasticity developing later.
E) Traumatic brain injury is a recognized postnatal risk factor for the development of CP.

23. You are called about a newborn patient belonging to your practice who has just been transferred to the neonatal intensive care unit with multifocal clonic seizure activity. A student working with you asks you about neonatal seizures. You are correct in telling him all of the following EXCEPT:
A) Neonatal seizures are not a form of epilepsy.
B) Most seizures in the neonatal period result from an underlying structural or metabolic abnormality.
C) The majority of patients who experience a seizure in the neonatal period develop an ongoing seizure disorder.
D) Infants with neonatal seizures associated with hypoxic-ischemic encephalopathy are likely to manifest significant neurologic impairment.
E) Generalized tonic-clonic seizures are uncommon in the neonatal period.

24. A previously well, 20-month-old girl in your practice experienced a generalized tonic-clonic seizure last night that lasted between 5 and 10 minutes. She was transported to the emergency department. Her temperature on presentation was 39.7°C. Following a complete history, physical examination, and laboratory evaluation, she was diagnosed with a simple febrile seizure and an upper respiratory infection. She is now in your office for a follow-up visit, and her parents are concerned about her prognosis. You are correct in telling them each of the following EXCEPT:
A) Approximately one third of children with an initial febrile seizure will have at least one recurrence with a subsequent febrile illness.
B) Children with a history of febrile seizures are at a minimally increased risk of epilepsy later in life.

C) Significant neurologic deficits resulting from febrile seizures are exceedingly rare.
D) Administration of anticonvulsant medication following an initial febrile seizure does not affect the risk of subsequent epilepsy.
E) The judicious use of antipyretics can prevent further febrile seizures.

25. A mother brings her 4-month-old son to your office because she believes he is suffering from "acid reflux." Weight and length are at the 25th percentile; head circumference is at the 10th percentile. During the physical examination, you observe recurrent flexor-extensor spasms involving all four extremities that last only a few seconds but are repeated several times in a row. Which of the following interventions is most likely to decrease the frequency of this patient's episodes?
A) Ranitidine
B) Carbamazepine
C) Felbamate
D) Clonazepam
E) High-dose adrenocorticotropic hormone

26. A 6-year-old previously well kindergarten student is referred to you with a working diagnosis of attention deficit disorder. Her teacher comments that the child seems to be daydreaming off and on during the day, and her schoolwork is suffering. The child's mother has also noticed frequent brief spells of blank staring. The child's physical examination is normal in your office. Hyperventilation produces a brief episode of altered consciousness and cessation of activity. Which of the following results is most consistent with this child's condition?
A) Three-per-second generalized spike and wave discharges on EEG
B) Hypsarrhythmia on EEG
C) Focal slowing in the left temporal lobe on EEG
D) Agenesis of the corpus callosum on CT of the head
E) Periventricular leukomalacia on MRI of the brain

27. An 8-year-old girl is brought to your office following her fourth complex partial seizure within the past 6 months. Which of the following anticonvulsant agents is most appropriate for initial treatment of this patient's seizure disorder?
A) Ethosuximide
B) Carbamazepine
C) Phenobarbital
D) Phenytoin
E) Vigabatrin

28. A 9-month-old boy is brought to the emergency department via ambulance in status epilepticus. He was well until 2 days ago, when he began vomiting. The emesis lasted for 8 hours and was followed by watery diarrhea, which has persisted. For the past 48 hours, his mother has withheld all oral supplementation except for apple juice cut in half with water. This child's seizure is most likely due to which of the following metabolic imbalances?
A) Hypocalcemia
B) Hypernatremia
C) Hyponatremia
D) Hypophosphatemia
E) Hypomagnesemia

29. A mother brings her 8-year-old boy to the emergency department for evaluation of his dizziness and vomiting. The child was well until 2 days ago, when he developed a mild upper respiratory infection. This morning, he began complaining that the room was spinning whenever he tried to sit up in his bed. He has vomited twice. He is most comfortable lying on his left side and resists efforts to turn or move him. The patient's physical examination, including neurologic and funduscopic evaluation, is normal except for diminished hearing in the right ear. Which of the following conditions is most consistent with this patient's clinical picture?
A) Labyrinthine concussion
B) Ménière disease
C) Benign positional vertigo
D) Acute labyrinthitis
E) Benign paroxysmal vertigo

30. Acute dystonic reactions are a recognized adverse effect of all of the following medications EXCEPT:
A) Promethazine
B) Metoclopramide
C) Haloperidol
D) Phenytoin
E) Diphenhydramine

31. Which of the following sets of symptoms is paired with a lesion that may result in this pattern of weakness?
A) Hemiparesis and ipsilateral hyperreflexia—cerebral abnormality
B) Symmetric weakness, dysarthria, sensory defects—brainstem lesion
C) Symmetric weakness that is greater in the distal extremities than proximally—myopathy
D) Weakness that is most pronounced upon rising in the morning—neuromuscular junction disorder
E) Increased deep tendon reflexes and asymmetric weakness—peripheral neuropathy

32. A 4-year-old Caucasian girl is brought to the emergency department by ambulance with her preschool teacher. Her parents are out of the country, and you are unable to contact them. The teacher noticed that the girl was limping and occasionally falling to her left side. She also tells you that the child has had problems with her eyes and wears glasses because she cannot see things well unless they are very close to her. The neurologic examination is significant for left-sided weakness that is more pronounced in the upper extremity than the lower one. Which of the following studies is most likely to be abnormal in this girl?

A) Hemoglobin electrophoresis
B) Urinary homocysteine level
C) MRI of the spine
D) Serum antiphospholipid antibody concentration
E) Serum hepatitis B surface antigen

33. An 8-year-old boy with Down syndrome suddenly develops an abnormal gait, excessive clumsiness, and recurrent enuresis. His physical examination is significant for hyperreflexia and a head tilt to the left. Which of the following is the most appropriate next step in the management of this patient?

A) Plain radiographs of the cervical spine
B) Plain radiographs of the lumbar spine
C) MRI of the spine with gadolinium
D) MRI of the spine without gadolinium
E) CT of the spine with nonionic contrast

34. A 10-year-old boy is brought to the emergency department following a motor vehicle collision. He was a front-seat passenger in one of the cars. He was unconscious when he was pulled from the wreck but regained consciousness in the ambulance and has been alert and able to appropriately answer questions since arrival in the emergency department. Vital signs are within normal limits, and the physical examination, including the neurologic assessment, is normal except for a gaping laceration over the left parietal region and some initial bruising. While the physician's assistant is cleaning the cut and preparing to suture, the patient becomes progressively confused and then difficult to arouse. This patient has most likely sustained which of the following injuries?

A) Subarachnoid injury
B) Simple concussion
C) Subdural hematoma
D) Epidural hematoma
E) Cerebellar hemorrhage

35. A mother brings her 4-year-old son to you for evaluation of his gait. She is concerned because he seems to have difficulty jumping and running and walks with a waddling gait. He often falls and has to balance his arms on his thighs to push himself up. The history is significant for independent walking at age 16 months. His mother also describes him as easily frustrated, with a short attention span. On physical examination, proximal muscle weakness exceeds distal muscle weakness; the weakness is most pronounced in the patient's lower extremities. Which of the following studies is most appropriate for the initial screening of this patient?

A) SSEPs
B) Nerve conduction studies
C) Electromyography
D) Serum immunoglobulin G concentration
E) Serum creatinine kinase concentration

36. A 3-year-old boy develops drooping of his left upper eyelid and seems less active than usual to his mother, particularly in the afternoons, when he prefers to lie on the couch. Which of the following studies is most specific for the diagnosis of juvenile myasthenia gravis?

A) Nerve stimulation studies before and after administration of edrophonium chloride
B) MRI of the brain with gadolinium
C) MRI of the spine with gadolinium
D) EEG
E) LP and CSF analysis

37. A previously well, 8-year-old boy presents with "sagging" of his face on the left side. He recovered from an upper respiratory infection approximately 10 days ago. He denies any alteration in his hearing, taste, or vision. He is unable to fully close his left eye. The physical examination is significant for normal neurologic findings except for left-sided facial weakness; the forehead is spared. Which of the following is indicated in the management of this patient?

A) Intravenous immunoglobulin
B) Systemic corticosteroids
C) Plasmapheresis
D) Exchange transfusion
E) No treatment is indicated for this patient.

38. A 3-year-old boy develops progressive lower extremity weakness over several days and is now barely able to stand. He was well until a week ago, when he started complaining that his back hurt in the middle. Vital signs are normal; neurologic assessment reveals 2/5 strength in the lower extremities (symmetric) and 4/5 strength in the upper extremities. You are unable to elicit lower extremity deep tendon reflexes. CT of the head is normal. Analysis of CSF obtained by LP yields the following results:

White blood cells: 3 per μL
Differential: 0 neutrophils
Red blood cells: 0 per μL
Glucose: 55 mg per dL
Protein: 130 mg per dL

This patient's weakness is most likely due to which of the following conditions?

A) Myasthenia gravis
B) Multiple sclerosis
C) Guillain-Barré syndrome
D) Tick paralysis
E) Polymyositis

39. A 4-year-old boy who has recently arrived from Papua New Guinea develops ascending weakness over 48 hours.

You are unable to elicit deep tendon reflexes. This child's weakness is most likely due to which of the following?
A) Hypervitaminosis A
B) Hypovitaminosis A
C) Brucellosis
D) Diphtheria
E) Myasthenia gravis

40. Which of the following conditions is paired with the neurodiagnostic procedure most appropriate for detecting it?
A) SSEPs—Guillain-Barré syndrome
B) MRI—intracranial calcifications
C) CT—CNS demyelination
D) Head sonogram—traumatic epidural hematoma
E) Electromyography—lower motor neuron disease

41. Which of the following does not increase the risk of developing sensorineural hearing loss in the child with bacterial meningitis?
A) Administration of systemic corticosteroids prior to the administration of the initial antibiotic dose
B) Infection with *Streptococcus pneumoniae*
C) Seizures at presentation
D) Ataxia at presentation
E) Prior treatment with oral antibiotics

42. You are attending morning rounds with a team of pediatric residents. A 4-year-old boy was admitted to the floor overnight with a diagnosis of *Streptococcus pneumoniae* meningitis. Which of the following statements regarding sensorineural hearing loss after bacterial meningitis is TRUE?
A) This patient is likely to show progressive hearing loss necessitating regular monitoring of his hearing ability.
B) This patient should be evaluated for hearing impairment prior to or soon after discharge.
C) Patients with viral meningitis have approximately the same risk of developing sensorineural hearing loss as patients with bacterial meningitis.
D) Bacterial meningitis is not associated with conductive or mixed hearing loss.
E) Patients with meningitis due to *Streptococcus pneumoniae* are less likely to develop hearing loss than patients with *Haemophilus influenzae* meningitis.

43. A 16-year-old girl is in your office complaining of dizziness. Her imbalance developed shortly after participating in a scuba diving expedition with her parents while on vacation last week. She has also noted clear but persistent drainage from her right ear and a change in her ability to hear with that ear. Her dizziness was worst during airplane take-off and landing on her return trip; the abrupt changes in altitude resulted in nausea and vomiting. The physical examination is significant for a small amount of clear drainage through a perforation in the left tympanic membrane. This patient's symptoms are most likely due to which of the following conditions?
A) Labyrinthitis
B) Temporal bone fracture
C) Perilymph fistula
D) Ménière disease
E) Labyrinthine concussion

44. A 6-year-old girl is brought to the emergency department in status epilepticus. She appeared well this morning when her mother dropped her off at the daycare center. About 3 hours later, the lead teacher in the room noticed that the girl's eyes were glazed over; then the child lost consciousness and began to have generalized tonic-clonic movements. One dose of rectal diazepam was given en route to the emergency department by ambulance technicians in communication with an emergency department physician. Following initial assessment of airway, breathing, circulation, and dextrose-stick, which of the following is the most appropriate initial pharmacologic management of this child's seizure?
A) A dose of ketamine following pretreatment with fentanyl
B) Thiopental induction of anesthesia
C) A dose of a short-acting benzodiazepine
D) A dose of a short-acting benzodiazepine in conjunction with a loading dose of fosphenytoin
E) A loading dose of fosphenytoin

45. You are unsuccessful in obtaining intravenous or intraosseous access in a child in status epilepticus. You have already administered two doses of rectal diazepam. Which of the following medications can be given via the intramuscular route?
A) Lamotrigine
B) Valproic acid
C) Phenobarbital
D) Phenytoin
E) Fosphenytoin

46. A 6-year-old girl fell off the back of a see-saw onto her head. She cried immediately. She is now in the emergency department for repair of a 2-cm laceration over the right occipital area. While in the waiting area, she vomits once and falls asleep. She is easily rousable. Vital signs are stable, and neurologic findings are normal. Moderate swelling is noted in the immediate vicinity of the laceration; no bony "step-off" is appreciated. Following repair of the laceration, the most appropriate management of this child consists of which of the following?
A) Discharge to home with appropriate instructions for observation
B) Discharge to home following a 4- to 6-hour observation period
C) Discharge to home following an overnight observation period
D) Plain radiographs of the skull
E) CT of the head with intravenous contrast

47. An 18-month-old toddler is brought into the emergency department by ambulance after falling from a second story window of his house. He has not regained consciousness. Rapid assessment following placement of an endotracheal tube and intravenous access reveals a large hematoma over the mid-forehead/frontal region without other obvious facial or skull deformities. The right pupil is fixed and dilated. This patient's clinical manifestations are most consistent with which of the following?

A) Blowout fracture of the orbital floor
B) Uncal herniation
C) Basilar skull facture
D) Longitudinal temporal bone fracture
E) Transverse temporal bone fracture

ANSWERS

1. A
2. B
3. C
4. D
5. E
6. A
7. B
8. C
9. D
10. E
11. A
12. B
13. C
14. D
15. E
16. A
17. B
18. C
19. D
20. D
21. A
22. B
23. C
24. E
25. E
26. A
27. B
28. C
29. D
30. E
31. A
32. B
33. C
34. D
35. E
36. A
37. B
38. C
39. D
40. E
41. A
42. B
43. C
44. D
45. E
46. A
47. B

Musculoskeletal Disorders

19

CONGENITAL MUSCULOSKELETAL DISORDERS

Osteogenesis Imperfecta

Osteogenesis imperfecta (OI) consists of a group of closely related genetic disorders resulting in fragile, brittle bones. The common denominator in all variants is the abnormal synthesis of type I collagen, which normally constitutes approximately 90% of the bone matrix but is also dispersed in the teeth, ligaments, skin, ears, and sclerae.

Clinical severity depends on the subclass of OI (Table 19-1). Treatment involves standard fracture care, pneumatic bracing, physical therapy, and careful avoidance of even minor trauma. Patients with severe disease may benefit from pamidronate or other bisphosphonate medications.

Achondroplasia

Achondroplasia is a disorder of cartilage calcification and remodeling. Inheritance of the defective gene, which is responsible for encoding fibroblast growth factor receptor 3, is autosomal dominant; however, 80% of cases result from a spontaneous gene mutation of paternal origin. Parents who do not themselves have achondroplasia have a recurrence risk in subsequent pregnancies of <1%. The physical appearance of patients with achondroplasia is strikingly characteristic (Table 19-2). Heterozygote patients have fairly normal intelligence, sexual function, and life expectancy, although early speech and motor skills are typically delayed. Hydrocephalus and restrictive pulmonary disease are known complications of achondroplasia but are amenable to treatment. Infants younger than 1 year of age are at risk for sudden death due to brainstem compression; early signs include apnea, hypotonia, weakness, hyperreflexia or asymmetric reflexes, and clonus. Homozygous achondroplasia is fatal in the neonatal period.

Arthrogryposis Multiplex Congenita

Arthrogryposis is a congenital syndrome of multiple joint contractures thought to result from decreased fetal movement. The condition can be idiopathic, but often there is

TABLE 19-1
CLASSIFICATION OF OSTEOGENESIS IMPERFECTA

Syndrome	Mode of Inheritance	Orthopedic Manifestations	Nonorthopedic Manifestations	Life Expectancy
Type I	Autosomal dominant	Frequent fractures from the neonatal period through adolescence;[a] severe bone fragility; bow legs; joint laxity; short stature	Blue/gray sclerae; adult-onset sensorineural hearing loss (deafness); abnormal dentition	Generally shortened
Type II	Autosomal recessive	Short, deformed limbs; multiple in utero and neonatal fractures; severe bone fragility	Intrauterine growth retardation; stillbirth; blue/gray sclerae	Days
Type III	Autosomal recessive	Frequent fractures that heal with deformation; severe bone fragility; lower limb deformities; short stature	Normal or mildly blue/gray sclerae	Generally shortened
Type IV	Autosomal dominant	Increased susceptibility to fractures[a]	Normal sclerae; increased risk for aortic dilatation	Near normal

[a]Susceptibility to fractures progressively decreases during adolescence; pathologic fractures in adulthood are rare.

TABLE 19-2
PHYSICAL AND RADIOGRAPHIC CHARACTERISTICS OF ACHONDROPLASIA

Physical Examination
Disproportionate short stature
Disproportionate macrocephaly (head larger than expected for height and weight)
Frontal bossing
Midface hypoplasia
Widened, short, curved long bones (particularly proximal long bones)
Short, stubby digits
Kyphoscoliosis/lumbar lordosis

Skeletal Survey
Macrocranium with narrowing of the skull base
Flattened vertebral bodies
Proximal shortening of the long bones
Diminished interpediculate distance (lumbar spine)

an identifiable cause (teratogen exposure, abnormal positioning in utero, uterine constraint, genetic disease, central nervous system or neuromuscular disorder). Talipes equinovarus deformity and hip dislocations occur most frequently, but contractures of virtually any joint in the body may be present. Decreased fetal movement is also associated with other characteristic physical findings including intrauterine growth retardation, hypoplastic lungs, short umbilical cord, and facial anomalies (hypertelorism; micrognathia; low-set, deformed ears). Management consists of splinting, serial casting, physical therapy, and surgery when indicated. Prognosis depends on which and how many joints are involved, associated anomalies, and the presence of any underlying disorder.

Congenital Torticollis

Congenital torticollis involves shortening or contracture of one of the sternocleidomastoid muscles following abnormal in utero positioning or birth trauma with bleeding and subsequent fibrosis of the muscle. The condition is usually noted sometime after the first 2 weeks of life. Early in the course, a palpable mass is present in the "belly" of the muscle. Affected patients have limited range of motion at the neck, with the head tilted toward the shortened muscle and the chin rotated away from it. The rates of developmental hip dysplasia and metatarsus adductus are increased in infants with congenital torticollis. The majority of cases respond to repetitive passive stretching over several months. Persistent torticollis is associated with irreversible asymmetry of the face and skull; surgical release is indicated by 1 year of age if conservative therapy proves unsuccessful.

Congenital torticollis is by far the most common cause of head tilt in the infant and one of the most benign. Table 19-3 lists other conditions that should be considered in the differential diagnosis of head tilt; several may result in significant morbidity or death if treatment is delayed.

Klippel-Feil Syndrome

Klippel-Feil syndrome is a constellation of fusion of the cervical vertebrae, decreased cervical range of motion, short neck, and low hairline. The etiology is presently unknown. Individuals with minimal disease may remain asymptomatic and undiagnosed for life; more severe involvement presents with head tilt and facial asymmetry in infancy or early childhood. The limited range of motion at the neck predisposes patients to cervical spine injury; other serious conditions associated with Klippel-Feil syndrome include hearing loss, congenital heart defects, and renal anomalies. Radiographic findings in affected patients can include any of the following:

- Fusion of a variable number of cervical vertebrae
- Additional vertebral abnormalities (hemivertebrae; thoracic and/or lumbar involvement)
- Rib defects
- Elevation, medial deviation, and rotation of the scapulae
- Scoliosis

Developmental Hip Dysplasia

Developmental dysplasia of the hip (DDH) refers to an abnormal relationship between the head of the femur and the acetabulum that results in instability and/or dislocation at the hip joint. DDH is more common in females, first-born children, breech presentations, and patients with a positive family history. Severity ranges from *subluxatable* (partial dislocation induced on examination) to *dislocatable*

TABLE 19-3
DIFFERENTIAL DIAGNOSIS OF HEAD TILT

Neurologic—cranial nerve palsy (particularly cranial nerve IV); posterior fossa mass; cervical cord tumor; spasmus nutans; syringomyelia; hearing loss; seizure
Paroxysmal torticollis—dystonic disorder presenting in the first year of life with episodes of head tilt lasting several minutes at a time, accompanied by agitation, pallor, or vomiting. The condition is benign and self-limited, with spontaneous resolution by 3 years of age.
Muscular—cervical muscle trauma or inflammation
Vertebral[a]—atlantoaxial subluxation; hemivertebrae; Klippel-Feil syndrome

[a]In torticollis, due to vertebral abnormalities, the head and neck cannot be passively maneuvered into their correct anatomic positions.

(full dislocation induced on examination) to *dislocated* (abnormally positioned most of the time). Early diagnosis results in a better outcome; therefore, careful examination of the newborn is paramount. Signs suggestive of DDH include:

- asymmetry of the gluteal and/or thigh folds
- posterosuperior dislocation of the hip with adduction and posterior pressure (Barlow maneuver)
- abduction with a resulting "clunk" as the head relocates into the joint (Ortolani maneuver)
- foreshortening of the (affected) limb when the patient's ankles are held with the knees bent and the hips flexed (Galeazzi sign)
- limited hip abduction
- apparent shortening of the involved extremity

Ultrasonography is the diagnostic study of choice in the young infant; plain radiographs become positive at 4 to 6 months of age. Infants with suspected DDH should be referred for orthopedic consultation. Most subluxatable and dislocatable hips stabilize without intervention within the first 4 weeks of life. *Avascular necrosis of the femoral head,* the most serious complication, is more likely to occur when the child has been left untreated for longer than 6 months. Patients with DDH are at risk for degenerative hip arthritis later in life.

Subluxation of the Patella

Although acute partial or complete dislocation of the patella is rare before adolescence, the predisposition to sublux is thought to result from an underlying anatomic abnormality of the knee. The anomaly causes the patella to track laterally as the knee is flexed. Subluxation of the patella often resolves spontaneously in the field. Signs of a recently dislocated patella include swelling of the joint, tenderness along the medial side of the kneecap, and pain upon passive lateral movement of the patella, which can usually be displaced at least one third of the distance of its width. The most effective means of regaining function and preventing subsequent dislocation is strengthening of the quadriceps muscles with physical therapy. Patients with multiple dislocations may benefit from surgical intervention.

Talipes Equinovarus

Talipes equinovarus, or clubfoot, is a rare, multifactorial, debilitating deformity that consists of medial rotation of the tibia, fixed plantarflexion at the ankle, inversion of the foot, and forefoot adduction (metatarsus adductus). Without treatment, the foot becomes progressively more deformed, and ulcerations develop when the child is old enough to limp. Early intervention is essential for subsequent normal function and development. Initial treatment consists of splinting or serial casting; patients with unsatisfactory improvement require surgical repair, preferably at age 6 to 9 months. Approximately 15% of children with this condition have additional congenital malformations.

Metatarsus Adductus

Metatarsus adductus (in-toeing of the forefoot in the absence of hindfoot abnormalities) is a common, relatively benign condition caused by intrauterine positioning. Dorsiflexion and plantarflexion at the ankle joint are unrestricted. Cases in which the foot can be straightened with gentle pressure respond well to stretching exercises. More severe in-toeing is managed with serial bracing or casting. Surgery is rarely indicated.

Coxa Valga/Vara

Congenital coxa valga and coxa vara describe conditions in which the angle composed of the femoral head and femoral shaft is greater than or less than (respectively) the normal angle of 130 to 135 degrees. *Coxa valga* may be an isolated primary defect or may result from DDH or adductor spasticity. The condition, which is frequently asymptomatic, can be diagnosed by a careful hip examination demonstrating increased internal rotation and adduction. *Coxa vara* often becomes obvious in affected children between the ages of 2 and 6 years, when they begin to limp or "waddle" when walking. Abduction and internal rotation are restricted on examination; plain anteroposterior and frog leg lateral radiographs are diagnostic. Many cases correct spontaneously; surgical intervention is indicated for those that do not spontaneously correct.

Plano Valgus

Flat feet (plano valgus) that appear normally arched when the patient stands on his or her toes represent a benign, inherited condition that neither responds to nor requires treatment. Adolescent patients with associated knee or foot pain often benefit from longitudinal orthotic arch support inserts. Plano valgus that remains rigidly flat during plantarflexion requires surgical correction.

Femoral Anteversion

Medial femoral anteversion, the most common cause of in-toeing in children aged 3 to 8 years, is medial twisting of the distal femur relative to the proximal femur. As opposed to *tibial torsion,* in which the spiral occurs in the tibia, the patellae of patients with femoral anteversion are twisted in the medial direction when the patient walks. The resultant in-toeing increases in severity during the preschool years. Gradual resolution beginning at age 5 to

6 years is usually complete by 10 years of age. Femoral anteversion is a benign, self-limited condition; radiographs are not indicated.

Polydactyly

Postaxial polydactyly is the most common congenital digital anomaly of the hand. Rudimentary, pedunculated digits that contain no skeletal elements may be safely tied off. Others should be surgically removed. Polydactyly is usually an isolated defect but may occur as part of various genetic syndromes. A thorough history and careful physical examination are generally sufficient to rule out syndromic anomalies.

INFECTIONS OF THE BONE AND JOINT

Osteomyelitis

Bone infections require early recognition and aggressive treatment to result in a favorable outcome. Osteomyelitis usually results from *hematogenous seeding* of the metaphysis, an area of relative blood stasis and few phagocytes. Trauma seems to increase susceptibility. Other mechanisms of infection include *direct inoculation* (puncture wounds, animal bites) and *extension* from adjacent tissues. Two thirds of cases involve the femur or tibia. Incidence peaks in the neonatal period and again in older children (ages 9 to 11 years). The predominant organism in all age groups is *Staphylococcus aureus* (Table 19-4).

Infants present with a history of irritability, fever, and refusal to move the involved limb. Older patients complain of localized bony tenderness over the metaphysis and pain upon weight bearing or using the affected limb. Fever, malaise, and anorexia are often present as well. The physical examination may reveal soft tissue swelling, erythema, and warmth, although these signs appear late in the course. Sinus tracts may drain purulent fluid onto the skin surface. Range of motion generally remains intact in patients with osteomyelitis, as opposed to those with septic arthritis and epiphyseal disorders. The differential diagnosis includes traumatic injury, infarction (in patients with sickle cell disease), and malignant invasion of the bone.

Laboratory and radiographic studies assist in diagnosis and monitoring progress. The white blood count may or may not be elevated, but erythrocyte sedimentation rate (ESR) and C-reactive protein (CRP) concentrations are consistently high. CRP decreases within a week of initiating appropriate antimicrobial therapy; changes in the ESR are more closely correlated with disease resolution. The causative organism is recovered from blood cultures only approximately half of the time. When blood cultures are negative and the presentation is atypical, needle aspiration becomes imperative for recovery, identification, and sensitivity testing of the pathogen. Radiographs are initially normal but demonstrate periosteal elevation, radiolucent necrotic area, and/or new bone formation 2 to 3 weeks after infection. Radiographic improvement lags clinical resolution, so serial plain films are not useful. *Bone scans* become positive within 48 to 72 hours of infection. *Magnetic resonance imaging* (MRI) with contrast is incredibly sensitive for osteomyelitis. It is the diagnostic method of choice for differentiating infection from infarction in patients with sickle cell disease and for localizing involvement to the bone or soft tissue areas. MRI is also used to detect abscesses, particularly vertebral epidural and pelvic abscesses.

TABLE 19-4
OSTEOMYELITIS: CAUSATIVE ORGANISMS[a]

Neonate
Staphylococcus aureus
Group B *Streptococcus*
Escherichia coli

Empiric Therapy: nafcillin plus cefotaxime or tobramycin

Child and Adolescent: Hematogenous Osteomyelitis
S. aureus
Group A *Streptococcus*
Kingella kingae (patients younger than 3 years of age)
Haemophilus influenzae

Empiric Therapy: oxacillin or nafcillin
Alternate: clindamycin, first- or second-generation cephalosporins (cefotaxime if *H. influenzae* is suspected)

Patient with Sickle Cell Disease
S. aureus
Salmonella species

Empiric Therapy: oxacillin or nafcillin plus cefotaxime

Direct Inoculation
Pseudomonas aeruginosa (puncture wound through the shoe)
Empiric therapy: oxacillin or nafcillin plus ceftazidime
Anaerobic bacteria (animal bite)
Empiric therapy: clindamycin

Chronic Osteomyelitis
S. aureus

[a]Therapy based on specific organism and sensitivity testing.

Pelvic osteomyelitis, usually involving the ileum, occurs most commonly in boys during the middle childhood years. Nonspecific pain referred to the hip, thigh, or abdomen mimics the presentations of a myriad of other conditions. Delayed diagnosis and treatment is associated with increased morbidity. *S. aureus* is the usual pathogen. The diagnosis is suggested on bone scan and confirmed via MRI.

Treatment consists of intravenous antibiotics at doses that achieve bactericidal levels within the bone (Table 19-4). Therapy is narrowed when the organism and sensitivities are known. Four to 6 weeks of antimicrobial therapy is indicated for patients with hematogenous osteomyelitis. Oral antibiotics are appropriate once the patient is afebrile and significantly improved. Surgical therapy is reserved for unresponsive disease, chronic infection, abscesses, and cases requiring debridement.

The most common complication is recurrence of infection. If osteomyelitis involves the epiphyseal plate, growth deformities may occur. Septic arthritis may complicate the infection, particularly in infants (up to 50%). Abscess formation within the metaphyseal shaft is not uncommon; this risk is particularly high in patients with pelvic arthritis.

Pyogenic Arthritis

Septic arthritis, or purulent infection of the joint space, is more common and potentially more debilitating than osteomyelitis. In most cases, organisms enter the joint during episodes of bacteremia, although direct inoculation and spread from infected adjacent structures also occur. Causative organisms vary by age and mechanism of disease (Table 19-5). The incidence is highest in infants and young children; in these patients, the hip is the most commonly involved site. The knee is more frequently affected in older children. Risk factors include recent trauma, immunodeficiency, hemoglobinopathy, and diabetes mellitus.

TABLE 19-5
SEPTIC ARTHRITIS: CAUSATIVE ORGANISMS[a]

Neonate

Staphylococcus aureus
Group B *Streptococcus*
Escherichia coli

Empiric Therapy: nafcillin plus cefotaxime or tobramycin

Child and Adolescent: Hematogenous Arthritis

S. aureus
Group A *Streptococcus*
Streptococcus pneumoniae
Kingella kingae (patients younger than 3 years of age)
Haemophilus influenzae
Neisseria gonorrhoeae (sexually active adolescents)
Neisseria meningitidis

Empiric Therapy: oxacillin or nafcillin
Alternate: clindamycin, first- or second-generation cephalosporins (cefotaxime if *H. influenzae* is suspected)

Patient with Sickle Cell Disease

S. aureus
Salmonella species

Empiric Therapy: oxacillin or nafcillin plus cefotaxime

Direct Inoculation

Pseudomonas aeruginosa (puncture wound through the shoe)

Empiric therapy: oxacillin or nafcillin plus ceftazidime (or piperacillin plus gentamicin)

Anaerobic bacteria (animal bite)

Empiric therapy: clindamycin

Chronic Osteomyelitis

S. aureus

[a]Therapy based on specific organism and sensitivity testing.

Septic arthritis presents as a painful joint, often accompanied by fever, irritability, and refusal to bear weight. On examination, range of motion with passive movement is clearly limited and obviously painful. The joint may be visibly swollen, with overlying warmth and erythema; alternatively, external signs may be absent, particularly when the hip is involved. *Neisseria gonorrhoeae* should be considered in sexually active adolescents presenting with polyarthritis. Neonates may be incapable of mounting a febrile response; irritability, poor feeding, and obvious discomfort with diaper changes suggest the diagnosis.

The differential diagnosis of painful joint includes osteomyelitis, septic arthritis, reactive or postinfectious arthritis, viral arthritis (parvovirus, enterovirus, adenovirus, herpesvirus, rubella, and mumps), acute rheumatic fever, and toxic synovitis (among others). *Toxic synovitis* involves the acute onset of benign, self-limited sterile inflammation of the synovium, usually localized to the hip. Toxic synovitis is most common in children ages 3 to 9 years and often follows a viral upper respiratory illness. In contrast to septic arthritis, range of motion is minimally limited, the child is generally afebrile and will usually bear weight, the ESR is $<$40 mm per hour, and the peripheral white blood cell count is $<$12,000 per μL. Toxic synovitis is typically a diagnosis of exclusion; management consists of rest and anti-inflammatory medications for pain control.

A septic hip is an orthopedic surgical emergency. The standard of care for septic arthritis involves aspiration of the joint in an attempt to recover the causative organism. Gram stain may suggest the pathogen. Purulent or cloudy synovial fluid typically yields a white blood cell count in excess of $50{,}000 \times 10^3$ per μL. *N. gonorrhoeae* is notoriously difficult to recover; blood, cervical, rectal, and nasopharyngeal cultures may be additionally helpful. Overall, a third of synovial fluid samples grow no organisms; blood cultures are positive in less than half of confirmed cases. Imaging studies may be complimentary but are not considered diagnostic.

Delay in diagnosis and treatment results in permanent destructive changes and functional impairment, including avascular necrosis, deformity, and limb length discrepancies. Empiric intravenous antibiotic treatment is initiated following aspiration; conversion to oral therapy is appropriate when sensitivities are known and symptoms have substantially improved. Septic arthritis of the hip, knee, or shoulder requires specialized orthopedic management that may include drainage of the infected joint via aspiration, arthroscopy, or open surgical drainage (all hip, shoulder arthritis).

MUSCULOSKELETAL INJURY

Subluxation of the Radial Head

Subluxation of the radial head, or "nursemaid's elbow," is a common injury in young children. The history is often remarkable for a sudden strong jerking of the child's pronated hand, resulting in rapid forced extension at the elbow. The patient holds the arm close to the body and slightly flexed at the elbow, with pronation of the forearm. Motion at the elbow is limited. Point tenderness and swelling are notably absent. When history and physical findings are consistent with radial head subluxation, radiologic confirmation is unnecessary. Treatment consists of holding the patient's elbow at 90 degrees of flexion and firmly manipulating the forearm into supination. A successful reduction is usually accompanied by a "click" as the radial head pops back into place. Usually the child begins to move the arm normally within several minutes.

Fractures

Fractures in children require specialized evaluation and treatment because pediatric bones are fundamentally different from those of adults. Immature bones are *more porous* (limit fracture propagation); have *thicker periosteum* ("buckle" or greenstick fractures rather than displacement); are *relatively weaker* than ligaments and tendons (fractures more likely than sprains); and contain *growth plates* that, when disrupted, generate disordered growth patterns (deformity, limb length discrepancy). Epiphyseal fractures are categorized according to the Salter-Harris classification. Types I (transverse fracture limited to the physeal area of the growth plate) and V (crush injury) are not initially appreciated on plain films. Type I fractures should be suspected in children with point tenderness over an epiphyseal plate. Subsequent radiographs taken 7 to 10 days later will demonstrate periosteal reaction and new bone formation when a fracture is present. Most fractures can be adequately treated with external stabilization. Fractures that are unstable, misaligned, or through the growth plate often require operative reduction and fixation.

The "toddler's fracture" is a nondisplaced spiral fracture of the tibia resulting from a twisting injury, which is often unwitnessed. Spiral fractures used to be considered pathognomonic for abuse; however, subsequent research found that the toddler's fracture is actually one of the more common fractures in children age 3 years and younger. Spiral fractures are not always evident on plain films immediately following the injury, and localization of pain is often challenging in this age group. Occult fractures may come to light more than a week after the injury during more detailed evaluation of functional impairment.

Any condition that weakens the bone, such as OI, malignancy, long-term steroid use, infection, endocrine disorders, and certain inborn errors of metabolism, predisposes a patient to pathologic fractures.

Clavicular Fractures

Clavicular fractures are common in children, often resulting from a fall on the point of the shoulder or direct trauma to the clavicle. Most occur in the middle third of the bone. The majority of fractures are greenstick fractures with minimal or no displacement. Fractures of the medial third of the clavicle that are significantly displaced may be accompanied by injury to the subclavian vein or compression of the trachea, but this is rare and usually clinically evident. Fractures of the distal third of the clavicle also may be associated with significant complications. Orthopedic consultation is recommended for fractures occurring in the medial or distal third of the bone, fractures involving a growth plate, and fractures in which there is nonunion at the 2-week follow-up visit. All other clavicular fractures are adequately managed with pain control and immobilization of the arm in a sling (patients ≤12 years of age) or figure 8 strap during waking hours for 2 to 4 weeks.

Supracondylar Fracture of the Humerus

Supracondylar fracture of the humerus is most common in children under the age of 12 years. The mechanism of injury usually involves a fall on an outstretched arm with subsequent hyperextension at the elbow. The fragmented section of the humerus may be nondisplaced; if present, displacement may be anterior or (more commonly) posterior. Clinical signs of supracondylar fracture include swelling and pain in the region of the elbow, limited range of motion, and localized tenderness at the fracture site. Significant displacement is obvious on plain radiographs of the elbow. A nondisplaced fracture is suggested by misalignment of the anterior humeral line or the presence of a posterior fat pad. Computed tomography (CT) is recommended in questionable cases. Supracondylar fractures have a high complication rate, including neurovascular injury, damage to the brachial artery with necrosis of the musculature of the forearm, and compartment syndrome. Frequent monitoring of hand strength and peripheral pulses is indicated prior to and immediately following surgical reduction and/or fixation.

Acromioclavicular Separation

Acromioclavicular sprain (shoulder separation) is frequently accompanied by fracture of the distal clavicle in prepubertal patients but is more often an isolated injury in adolescents. The typical presentation involves a history of falling on the shoulder, pain with active and passive movement at the shoulder, and point tenderness over the acromioclavicular joint. Plain radiographs of the shoulders taken while the patient is grasping equal weights in each hand permit determination of differential separation between affected and unaffected joints. Management depends on the severity of the separation and whether there is associated ligamentous rupture and/or injury to the subclavian vessels or brachial plexus.

Shoulder Dislocation

Glenohumeral dislocation is an uncommon injury in preadolescent children; blunt trauma to the shoulder area is more likely to result in fracture in this age group. In adolescents, anterior shoulder dislocation presents with pain, obvious deformity (a "boxed-off" appearance of the shoulder), decreased range of motion, and swelling. Physical examination is significant for obvious displacement of the humeral head anterior to the glenoid fossa. Plain films of the shoulder should include posteroanterior, lateral, and axillary views; associated fractures of the humeral head are not uncommon. Films are repeated after closed reduction because the procedure itself may result in fractures. *Axillary nerve damage* complicates a minority of anterior dislocations; altered sensation over the lateral aspect of the shoulder (the "regimental badge" area) and absence of contraction of the deltoid on attempted abduction of the shoulder confirm axillary nerve involvement. The younger an individual is at initial dislocation, the higher the likelihood that dislocation will recur.

Ankle Sprain

The evaluation and management of pediatric ankle injuries are somewhat more specialized than those of adults. Eversion injuries in preadolescent patients often result in avulsion fractures at the growth plate, given that, as noted earlier, ligaments in this age group are stronger than growth plates. Isolated sprains are more common in postpubertal patients, particularly when the pain is isolated to the ligament and ankle films are negative. For adolescents, the degree of pain generally correlates with the severity of the ligamentous injury. The child with a significant ankle eversion injury and suspected Salter-Harris I fracture should avoid weight bearing (i.e., use crutches or a wheelchair) until follow-up films are available. Patients with isolated sprains are provided RICE instruction for the management of their injuries—rest, ice, compression, and elevation. Early physical therapy hastens resolution and improves outcome in these patients. Ankle injuries are reviewed in Chapter 25.

CONDITIONS OF THE BACK (CURVATURE, PAIN)

Scoliosis

Adolescent idiopathic scoliosis (lateral curvature and rotation of the spine) is diagnosed in otherwise healthy children with normal bones, muscles, and vertebral discs. Idiopathic scoliosis is not associated with back pain or fatigue; such symptoms warrant further investigation. All older children and adolescents should be screened with the *Adams forward-bending test* at each routine health maintenance visit. Progression of the curve is most rapid during the adolescent growth spurt. Management depends on the degree of curvature and the skeletal maturation and gender of the child. Severe scoliosis requiring intervention occurs more often in females; premenarchal females in particular should be treated aggressively. Curvatures less than 25 to 30 degrees need only be followed. More pronounced deformity (25 to 40 degrees) in a child who is still growing should be treated with external bracing until the growth spurt is completed. Bracing does not reduce the curve, but it does halt progression and is 85% effective if used correctly. Surgical intervention is recommended for curvatures >40 to 50 degrees following completion of the growth spurt. Curves of 50 degrees or greater are associated with decreased vital capacity and low functional pulmonary reserve. Occasionally, scoliosis may result from neuromuscular abnormalities or congenital deformities.

Kyphosis

Kyphosis is increased posterior convexity of the thoracic spine. Postural kyphosis can be corrected by the patient with hyperextension of the thoracic back while prone or standing. Fixed kyphosis (also called idiopathic kyphosis or *Scheuermann disease*) results from anterior wedging of adjacent vertebral bodies and is initially noted during puberty. Lumbar lordosis with protrusion of the abdomen is often present and may be accompanied by compensatory cervical lordosis as well. The clinical diagnosis is confirmed on lateral standing plain films of the thoracic spine.

For most affected patients, idiopathic kyphosis remains a benign, asymptomatic cosmetic deformity. Bracing may be recommended for patients who are still growing and have curvatures >45 to 60 degrees. Curvatures of 90 degrees or more are often associated with pain; physical therapy is indicated to improve strength and flexibility of the muscles in the thoracic area but does not alter the curvature. Patients with severe and/or painful curvature who have achieved skeletal maturity are candidates for surgical intervention. Neurologic and pulmonary complications are quite rare.

Back Pain

Back pain is an uncommon complaint in children in the absence of trauma. Musculoskeletal back pain is relatively rare, as opposed to adult complaints. A partial differential diagnosis of pediatric back pain is provided in Table 19-6. Laboratory and radiologic studies are guided by information gained through a careful history and thorough physical examination (Table 19-7).

Spondylolysis is a stress fracture of the pars interarticularis, the vertebral bony protrusion that joins the upper and

TABLE 19-6
DIFFERENTIAL DIAGNOSIS OF BACK PAIN IN CHILDREN

Musculoskeletal

- Musculoskeletal strain
- Spondylolysis
- Spondylolisthesis
- Disc herniation
- Nerve entrapment

Infection

- Vertebral osteomyelitis
- Discitis—most common in younger children; pain may be referred; presents with reluctance to rotate, flex, or extend the back
- Tuberculosis of the spine (Pott disease)

Bone/Spinal Neoplasms

- Changes in bowel/bladder control
- Muscle weakness
- Gait disturbances
- If malignant, constitutional symptoms (fever, night sweats, weight loss)

Rheumatologic Disorders

- Ankylosing spondylitis
- Arthritic syndromes

Multisystem Disease

Anomalies of the Spine and Spinal Cord

- Scheuermann disease

Referred Pain

- Urologic conditions (stones, obstruction)
- Gynecologic conditions
- Gastrointestinal conditions
- Slipped capital femoral epiphysis

Malingering/Psychogenic

lower joints. It is most commonly noted in vertebrae L4 and L5. Athletes who participate in competitive sports such as gymnastics, weight lifting, and football are susceptible to spondylolysis, which is often asymptomatic or mimics muscular strain. Bilateral fractures predispose an individual to *spondylolisthesis*, or anterior displacement of the involved vertebra. Spondylolisthesis presents with chronic, progressive pain over the lumbosacral area that worsens with active extension. Pain may radiate to the ipsilateral buttock or thigh; neurologic findings are absent unless the slippage is accompanied by disc herniation or nerve entrapment, whereupon hamstring contractures may be evident. The diagnosis is confirmed through detection of displacement on a standing lateral plain film of the lumbosacral spine. Affected patients benefit from bracing and physical therapy; anti-inflammatory medications are suggested for pain relief.

TABLE 19-7
BACK PAIN: SUGGESTED LABORATORY AND RADIOLOGIC EVALUATION

If systemic disease, rheumatologic conditions, referred pain, or neoplasms are suspected, consider:

- complete blood count with differential and smear
- erythrocyte sedimentation rate/C-reactive protein
- lactate dehydrogenase

Radiologic studies:

- Initial screening: plain radiographs of the back in the anteroposterior, lateral, and oblique views
- Bone scan
- CT with contrast
- Magnetic resonance imaging (if neurologic signs are present)

LEGG-CALVÉ-PERTHES DISEASE

Legg-Calvé-Perthes disease is defined as idiopathic avascular necrosis of the femoral head. Legg-Calvé-Perthes disease occurs more often in males (ages 4 to 8 years). The insidious development of a painless or mildly painful limp is the most common presenting complaint. When present, the pain may be referred to the knee or thigh, clouding the diagnostic picture. Abduction, flexion, and internal rotation are limited at the hip joint. Initial radiographic studies may appear normal; subsequent films demonstrate radiolucency of the epiphysis. Bone scans detect early impairment in the blood supply and fragmentation and flattening of the femoral head. Irregularities of the femoral head and marrow necrosis are evident on MRI. The goals of therapy consist of containment of the femoral head within the acetabulum, preservation of its spherical contour, and maintenance of normal range of motion and function. Younger children with minimal involvement and full range of motion may be observed. Orthotic bracing or surgery is necessary in older patients with significant changes in the femoral head. The amount and area of ischemic damage affect the prognosis. Collapse of the femoral head is the most serious acute complication; long-term disability is related to abnormal or asymmetric growth. Resolution occurs over approximately 2 years, as the ischemic bone is resorbed. Reossification is gradual and accompanied by continued (but not necessarily normal) growth.

SLIPPED CAPITAL FEMORAL EPIPHYSIS

Slipped capital femoral epiphysis (SCFE) is the gradual or acute separation of the proximal femoral growth plate, with the femur head slipping off the femoral neck and rotating into an inferior/posterior position. The cause is unknown but may be hormonal (the condition is most common during puberty) or due to excessive weight bearing (SCFE is more common in overweight individuals). It occurs slightly more often in males. Antecedent trauma is not a contributing factor. Although usually asymmetric at presentation, 25% of cases will eventually progress to bilateral involvement. The typical patient presents with a limp and pain, which may be located in the hip or groin region but often is referred to the knee. Limited internal rotation and limb shortening are present on examination. Epiphyseal displacement is evident on plain radiographs with the child's hips in the frog leg lateral position. Additional radiographic signs include physeal plate widening, decreased epiphyseal height, and a Klein line (drawn along the femoral neck) that does not intersect the lateral epiphysis. The primary goal of treatment is prevention of further misalignment. Pin fixation is effective in the acute setting. Chronic cases generally require osteotomy. Long-term complications include avascular necrosis and late degenerative changes similar to those seen with osteoarthritis.

OSGOOD-SCHLATTER DISEASE

Osgood-Schlatter disease involves inflammation, swelling, and tenderness over the tibial tuberosity. Repetitive mechanical forces result in tendonitis of the distal insertion of the infrapatellar tendon. Osgood-Schlatter disease typically occurs between the ages of 10 and 17 years, during the adolescent growth spurt, and may be uni- or bilateral. Stress from overuse and trauma are contributing factors. Pain is exacerbated with kneeling, running, jumping, or squatting; symptoms are relieved by rest. On physical examination, range of motion at the knee is intact, and there are no signs of joint effusion. Palpation of the tibial tuberosity produces tenderness, which may or may not be associated with localized swelling. Radiographs reveal irregularities of the tubercle ossification center and haziness of the adjacent tibial epiphysis. Most cases are mild and resolve with activity modification and stretching exercises. Severe cases may require casting for up to 6 weeks. Long-term morbidity is quite low; the disorder resolves when skeletal maturity is attained, although prominence of the tuberosity may persist.

GROWING PAINS

"Growing pains" are a form of functional muscular or joint pain most common in children between the ages of 8 and 12 years. Recurrent bilateral lower extremity pain is worse in the evenings and may awaken the child from sleep. The pain typically improves with local massage or application of a warming pad. Growing pains do not interfere with normal activity; children are asymptomatic during the day. Physical examination findings are normal by definition. Growing pains are benign and self-limited.

SOURCES

Bautista SR, Gholve P. Pediatric musculoskeletal infections: combating the major pathogens. *Pediatr Ann.* 2006;5:565–568.

Carson S, Woolridge DP, Colletti J, et al. Pediatric upper extremity injuries. *Pediatr Clin North Am.* 2006;53:41–67.

DeWolfe C. Back pain. *Pediatr Rev.* 2002;221.

Dinolfo EA. Fractures. *Pediatr Rev.* 2004;25:218–219.

Gutierrez K. Bone and joint infections in children. *Pediatr Clin North Am.* 2005;52:779–794.

Kronberg J, Small E. Tackling back pain in a young athlete. *Contemp Pediatr.* 2005;22:437–454.

Scherl SA. Common lower extremity problems in children. *Pediatr Rev.* 2004;25:52–61.

Sharif I. Current treatment of osteomyelitis. *Pediatr Rev.* 2005;26: 38–39.

QUESTIONS

1. A 6-year-old boy with a history of multiple (>40) fractures beginning in the neonatal period also has gray sclerae, discolored and decaying teeth, genu varum, and short stature. Which of the following conditions is the most likely complication this child will face in his adulthood?

A) Hearing loss
B) Autoimmune hepatitis
C) Severe scoliosis
D) Lower extremity paralysis and wheelchair dependence
E) Renal failure

2. Healthy, unaffected parents of an 18-month-old male with achondroplasia are considering another pregnancy. They question you regarding their risk of having another child with achondroplasia. In counseling them, you are correct in informing them that the risk is closest to which of the following?

A) 5%
B) <1%
C) 25%
D) 50%
E) 100%

3. An 8-month-old female with achondroplasia presents to the emergency department via ambulance with respiratory distress and recurrent apnea. Ankle clonus is present on physical examination. You learn from the mother that the patient seemed weaker than usual upon wakening and was difficult to rouse from her morning nap. Which of the following conditions is the most likely cause of her respiratory failure?

A) Pneumonia
B) Posterior fossa tumor

C) Compression of the brainstem
D) Hydrocephalus
E) Restrictive pulmonary disease

4. A mother brings her 1-month-old infant to your office because she is worried about his neck. The boy holds his head tilted to the right with his chin rotated to the left. A mass is palpated in the right sternocleidomastoid muscle. You are able to achieve normal anatomic positioning of the neck through passive stretching. Which of the following disorders is most often associated with this infant's condition?
A) Talipes equinovarus
B) Paroxysmal dystonia
C) Klippel-Feil syndrome
D) Developmental hip dysplasia
E) Polydactyly

5. The mother of a 6-week-old infant calls you apologetically to ask you if the infant's "leg wrinkles" are supposed to "match up." She brings her daughter to the office, where you confirm that the girl has asymmetric gluteal and thigh folds. You are not able to elicit a "clunk," but foreshortening of the right lower limb is evident when the patient is placed supine with her knees bent and hips flexed. Which of the following is the best procedure to confirm your suspicion of developmental hip dysplasia?
A) Examination by an experienced pediatric orthopaedist
B) Computed tomography
C) Plain radiograph of the hips with the legs extended
D) Plain radiograph of the hips in the frog leg position
E) Ultrasonography

6. You are called to the nursery to evaluate a newborn with a foot deformity. On physical examination of the infant, you note medial rotation of the tibia, fixed plantar flexion at the ankle, inversion of the foot, and forefoot adduction. No other obvious anomalies are found. The nurse asks you about treatment for the deformity. You are correct in telling her that initial treatment consists of which of the following?
A) Splinting and serial casting
B) Passive stretching 4 to 6 times per day
C) Corrective surgery before the age of anticipated ambulation
D) Pavlik harness therapy
E) The deformity is not correctable, but most affected children learn to ambulate with lower leg braces.

7. A new patient is in your office for her 5-year health maintenance visit. Her mother is concerned about the girl's in-toeing. Although the in-toeing does not appear to interfere with the child's ability to walk, run, or play, the mother is interested in having her daughter's legs "fixed" for cosmetic reasons. You observe that when the child walks, both patellae are medially rotated with respect to the normal anatomic position. Which of the following is the most appropriate next step in the management of this child?
A) Plain films of the hips in the frog leg position
B) Reassurance that the in-toeing will gradually resolve by the time the child reaches approximately 10 years of age
C) Plain films of the knees
D) Referral to a pediatric orthopedic surgeon
E) Referral to a physical therapist

8. A 3-year-old male in your office for his routine health maintenance visit has developed a waddling gait. He does not appear to be in any pain. Internal rotation is restricted in both hips. Which of the following is the most likely cause of this child's abnormal gait?
A) Developmental hip dysplasia
B) Slipped capital femoral epiphysis
C) Coxa vara
D) Coxa valgus
E) Legg-Calvé-Perthes disease

9. A 10-year-old boy presents to the emergency department with fever and refusal to bear weight on his right foot, which was punctured when he stepped on broken glass about 1 week ago. Radiographs of the foot are negative except for soft tissue swelling, and the patient is admitted to the hospital and started on intravenous nafcillin. His temperature continues to rise over the next 48 hours, and finally, he admits that he and a friend had gone to a construction site after hours despite being forbidden by his parents; while there, he stepped on a rusty nail, which punctured his foot through his tennis shoe. A MRI study is consistent with osteomyelitis. Following surgical debridement and biopsy to determine a causative organism, this patient should be placed on bactericidal dose(s) of which of the following antibiotics?
A) Levofloxacin
B) Oxacillin plus cefotaxime
C) Clindamycin
D) Nafcillin plus ceftazidime
E) Vancomycin

10. An 8-year-old patient with known sickle cell disease and frequent pain crises presents with a fever of 38.5°C and point tenderness over the proximal metaphyseal area of the tibia. Which of the following studies is most appropriate for differentiating local infarction from osteomyelitis?
A) Bone scan
B) Computed tomography without contrast
C) Computed tomography with contrast
D) MRI without contrast
E) MRI with contrast

11. You are lecturing at a noon conference for medical students and residents. Your topic is the management of osteomyelitis. You are correct in telling your audience each of the following EXCEPT:

A) Patients infected through hematogenous spread require 4 to 6 weeks of intravenous antibiotics.
B) Patients infected through hematogenous spread require 4 to 6 weeks of antibiotics at doses that produce bactericidal levels within the bone.
C) Patients infected through hematogenous spread who have negative blood cultures, no risk factors, and symptom resolution on empiric therapy do not require needle aspiration to identify the causative organism.
D) Empiric therapy against *Staphylococcus aureus* is indicated in all age groups, from neonate to adult.
E) Patients with pelvic osteomyelitis are at high risk for abscess formation.

12. A mother brings her 18-month-old previously healthy toddler to your office with a chief complaint of fever and refusal to walk. The child was well until yesterday, when he began limping. In the office, the patient is febrile to 39°C. He cries whenever you move his left leg and has decreased range of motion at the left hip. No erythema, warmth, or swelling is noted over the joint. The patient has a white blood count of 16×10^3 per μL, with an ESR of 42 mm per hour. Which of the following is the most appropriate next step in the management of this patient?

A) Needle aspiration of the metaphysis of the left femur
B) Needle aspiration of the left hip joint
C) Ultrasonography of the left hip
D) Computed tomography of the left hip
E) Plain radiograph of the hips in the frog leg position

13. A previously well, 7-year-old boy presents with a 2-day history of limp and right hip pain. There is no recent history of trauma or fever. He was diagnosed with a viral upper respiratory infection in the office the preceding week. Although the child walks with a limp, he is able to bear weight. Range of motion at the right hip is minimally restricted. The ESR is 15 mm per hour. Which of the following is the most likely cause of this patient's limp?

A) Acute rheumatic fever
B) Septic arthritis
C) Toxic synovitis
D) Reactive arthritis
E) Viral arthritis

14. A 13-year-old patient with a history of moderate blunt trauma to the upper body 9 days ago presents with the acute onset of severe left shoulder pain. His temperature in the emergency room is 38.5°C; the rest of his vital signs are stable. Examination of the left shoulder reveals warmth and swelling over the joint without overlying erythema and severe pain and restricted range of motion on passive movement of the joint. The joint is aspirated with recovery of cloudy fluid; results include a negative Gram stain and a white blood count in excess of $75 \text{ X } 10^3$/mcL. Which of the following is the most appropriate next step in the management of this patient?

A) Specific culture media to identify *Neisseria gonorrhoeae*
B) Bone scan
C) Empiric therapy with intravenous vancomycin until culture and sensitivity results are reported
D) Open surgical drainage of the joint
E) Empiric therapy with intravenous ceftazidime until culture and sensitivity results are reported

15. A previously well, 6-year-old boy presents with a 3-week history of progressively worsening limp. There is no history of fever, antecedent trauma, or upper respiratory infection. Examination of the right hip reveals limited range of motion upon abduction, flexion, and internal rotation. Plain radiographs are consistent with synovitis. Peripheral white blood count, ESR, and CRP are normal. Which of the following is the most likely cause of this child's limp?

A) Septic arthritis
B) Toxic synovitis
C) Slipped capital femoral epiphysis
D) Osgood-Schlatter disease
E) Legg-Calvé-Perthes disease

16. A 14-year-old hockey goalie presents to your office with a chief complaint of left knee pain. He denies any history of fever or trauma. He states that the pain is present when he kneels or squats to make a save. The physical examination is significant for swelling and point tenderness over the left tibial tuberosity. Range of motion at the knee is intact, and there is no evidence of joint effusion. Which of the following is the most likely cause of this patient's knee pain?

A) Osgood-Schlatter disease
B) Prepatellar bursitis
C) Patellofemoral syndrome
D) Septic arthritis
E) Patellar subluxation

17. A 10-year-old girl presents to your office for her routine health maintenance visit. A screening Adams forward-bending test is positive, with a rough estimate of 25 degrees of curvature by hand-held scoliometer. Plain films of the spine confirm a 30-degree lateral/

rotational curve. Which of the following is the most appropriate next step in the management of this patient?

A) Referral to an orthopaedic surgeon for possible surgery
B) Referral to an orthopaedic surgeon for possible bracing
C) Repeat spinal films in 6 months to evaluate for progression.
D) Referral to physical therapist for strengthening of thoracic extension muscles
E) Obtain pulmonary function testing to assess for restrictive pulmonary disease.

18. A 15-year-old competitive gymnast comes to your office complaining of progressive lower back pain of 2 months in duration. The pain is most severe when she is attempting back handsprings and backbends. She has no history of trauma to the area. Bowel and bladder habits are typical and have not changed. She denies lower extremity weakness and paresthesias. Her neurologic examination is normal. Range of motion is intact at the lower back, with tenderness noted on active extension. Which of the following is the most likely cause of this patient's back pain?

A) Disc herniation
B) Nerve entrapment
C) Spondylolisthesis
D) Spondylolysis
E) Muscle strain

19. A 12-year-old obese male presents to your office with the sudden onset of left hip pain and limp. He can recall no antecedent trauma or fever. The physical examination is significant for shortening of the left lower extremity and limited internal rotation at the left hip. Which of the following radiographic results is most likely to be present in this child?

A) Lytic lesions of the femoral neck
B) Effusion of the left hip joint
C) Fragmentation of the femoral head
D) Epiphyseal displacement of the femoral head
E) Avascular necrosis of the femoral head

20. A 9-year-old boy hopped off the third step of a stairway and landed on his friend's foot. He presents to your office with severe pain, swelling, and refusal to bear weight. Tenderness is diffuse over the swollen area but seems to be most severe over the epiphyseal plate of the distal tibia. Plain films of the ankle are negative. The most appropriate management of the child's injury at this time consists of which of the following?

A) Reassuring the family that no fracture is present
B) Rest, ice, compression with an elastic bandage, and elevation, with gradual return to normal activities as the pain subsides
C) Referral to a pediatric orthopaedic surgeon for further evaluation
D) Referral for physical therapy and strengthening of the muscles around the ankle
E) Deferral of weight bearing at least until follow-up films are obtained 7 to 10 days after the injury

21. A 16-year-old hockey player presents to the emergency department with severe shoulder pain after sliding shoulder-first into the boards. His right shoulder is swollen and appears to be "squared-off." He resists any attempt to check range of motion at the joint. Sensation over the lateral shoulder area is intact. Pre- and postreduction films are negative for fractures, and the patient is able to abduct his shoulder following reduction. This patient is at highest risk for which of the following complications of anterior shoulder dislocation?

A) Recurrence of dislocation
B) Axillary nerve damage
C) Radial nerve damage
D) Vascular injury
E) Occult fracture

22. An 8-year-old boy occasionally complains of bilateral lower extremity pain in the late evenings before bed. The pain does not interfere with ambulation, and it seems to improve with application of a warming pad. The patient is asymptomatic during the day and has continued with his normal activities. No abnormalities are noted on the physical examination. Which of the following is the most appropriate next step in the management of this patient?

A) Plain radiographs of the right and left lower leg bones
B) Reassurance and observation
C) Measurement of serum creatinine kinase concentration
D) Measurement of serum antinuclear antibody titers
E) Testing for human leukocyte antigen B27

23. A 3-year-old child was prevented from running into traffic when his father grabbed his left hand and jerked him sideways. The child began to cry immediately and refused to move his left arm, even after calming down. In your office, the boy holds his left arm close to his body, with the elbow slightly flexed and the forearm pronated. No swelling or point tenderness is noted on examination of the extremity, and distal pulses are normal. Which of the following is the most appropriate next step in the evaluation and management of this patient's injury?

A) Flexion of the elbow with lateral pressure on the humeral head
B) Plain radiograph of the clavicle
C) Supination of the forearm for reduction of the subluxation

D) Referral to an orthopaedic surgeon
E) Plain radiograph of the elbow

24. An 8-year-old boy sustains an injury to his right arm as a result of falling from a skateboard. He presents to the emergency department complaining of pain in his elbow, which he holds slightly flexed against his side. He resists any attempt to further flex or extend the joint, which is markedly swollen. The radial pulse in the right arm is attenuated. Plain radiographs of the elbow area are significant for posterior displacement of the fat pad with no obvious fracture. This patient has most likely sustained which of the following?
A) Subluxation of the radial head
B) Fracture of the distal ulna and/or radius
C) Anterior dislocation of the elbow
D) Nondisplaced supracondylar fracture of the humerus
E) Posterior dislocation of the elbow

25. A 12-year-old softball player collided with the fence in the outfield and is now complaining of pain over her shoulder region. Examination of the area reveals point tenderness and minimal swelling over the midclavicle. Range of motion is intact at the shoulder. The patient complains of severe pain upon active movement of the outstretched arm past the horizontal. Strength and sensation are intact in the upper extremity, and distal pulses are normal. Plain radiographs reveal a nondisplaced fracture of the medial third of the clavicle. Which of the following is the most appropriate next step in the management of this patient?
A) Discharge the patient without restriction of activity.
B) Obtain consultation for open fixation of the fracture.
C) Obtain consultation for closed reduction of the fracture.
D) Obtain computed tomography of the region to assess for interruption of the subclavian vein.
E) Discharge the patient in a figure 8 strap with adequate pain control.

ANSWERS

1. A
2. B
3. C
4. D
5. E
6. A
7. B
8. C
9. D
10. E
11. A
12. B
13. C
14. D
15. E
16. A
17. B
18. C
19. D
20. E
21. A
22. B
23. C
24. D
25. E

Dermatologic Disorders

20

CONGENITAL VASCULAR LESIONS

Port Wine Stains

Port wine stains are flat, nonpalpable, well-demarcated, dark-red skin lesions that are present at birth and found most commonly on the head or neck. They are the visible manifestation of congenital capillary malformations. *Sturge-Weber syndrome* (leptomeningeal angiomatosis) is a disorder of neurologic deterioration in which a port wine stain over the area innervated by the first division of the trigeminal nerve (CNV_1; forehead and periorbital region) is accompanied by vascular malformations of the underlying meninges and/or cerebral cortex. Affected children suffer progressive mental retardation, seizures, hemiparesis, and visual impairment; approximately one third develop glaucoma. *Tunable (pulsed) dye laser therapy* "fades" the port wine stain but does not address the underlying neurologic dysfunction. Lesions should be treated early in life to optimize cosmetic outcome. Control of seizures may limit subsequent developmental delay. Approximately 10% of children with a unilateral port wine stain over the dermatome innervated by CNV_1 will be affected with Sturge-Weber syndrome; this percentage is higher if the lesion is bilateral.

Strawberry Hemangiomas

Strawberry hemangiomas are benign, superficial tumors composed of small, closely packed proliferative vessels. They are not detectable at birth, instead becoming visible within the first month of life. The natural course of a strawberry hemangioma is rapid enlargement over 6 to 9 months, followed by gradual resolution throughout childhood. They may occur anywhere on the skin but are most common on the face, head, trunk, and back. Because they are benign and self-limited, treatment is unnecessary unless growth of the tumor interferes with development or functional ability. For example, a hemangioma that obstructs vision in a young infant requires aggressive therapy to prevent cortical blindness. A course of daily oral prednisone or prednisolone is effective in slowing or preventing further enlargement of the hemangioma and should be initiated during the first 6 months of life, when growth is most rapid. Corticosteroids may also be indicated for extensive facial hemangiomas with potential for subsequent disfigurement and lesions that frequently bleed or ulcerate. Vascular-specific pulsed dye laser therapy may be appropriate for use in small lesions. Surgical excision is reserved for cases in which the potential for scarring is outweighed by functional impairment or cosmetic deformity.

NEONATAL PUSTULAR LESIONS

Erythema toxicum neonatorum develops in the majority of full-term newborns; it is less common in premature infants. Small (2 to 3 mm) papules appear over the trunk, back, extremities, and occasionally the face, usually between 2 and 4 days of age. Within hours, the papules evolve into pustules surrounded by blotchy, irregular, erythematous macules. New lesions continue to appear and resolve over the next several days, with full resolution by 3 weeks of age. The lesions of erythema toxicum are filled with eosinophils, and peripheral eosinophilia may be noted on a differential white blood cell count obtained for another purpose during the outbreak. Erythema toxicum is a benign, self-limited condition that is easily recognized by experienced pediatricians; additional evaluation is unnecessary beyond assuring that the pustules are not due to a more serious neonatal disease.

Transient neonatal pustular melanosis is a chronic, benign, self-limited disorder consisting of recurrent outbreaks of papules and small hyperpigmented macules that may be surrounded by a rim of scale. The hands, feet, and face are typically involved, but lesions may be widespread. Episodes last weeks to months, with full resolution between outbreaks. This disorder rarely persists beyond approximately 3 years of age. In contrast to erythema toxicum, Wright stain of pustular fluid demonstrates predominately neutrophils.

A few significant neonatal diseases can present with erythematous pustular lesions. When uncertainty exists regarding the diagnosis, microscopic analysis of pustular contents permits differentiation of the above benign conditions from more serious illnesses (Table 20-1).

TABLE 20-1
MICROSCOPIC DIFFERENTIATION OF NEONATAL PUSTULAR DERMATITIS

Erythema toxicum neonatorum—predominance of eosinophils on Wright stain

Transient neonatal pustular melanosis—predominance of neutrophils on Wright stain

Staphylococcal folliculitis—Gram-positive cocci on Gram stain

Congenital candidiasis—pseudohyphae and budding yeast on potassium hydroxide preparation

Neonatal herpes simplex virus infection—multinucleated giant cells on Wright stain or Tzanck preparation

ATOPIC DERMATITIS

The pathogenesis, natural history, appearance, evaluation, and treatment of atopic dermatitis are presented in Chapter 9 and Figure 20-1.

SKIN INFECTIONS AND INFESTATIONS

Bacterial Infections

Bacterial infection of the skin is usually preceded by a break in the protective integument that permits entry of the pathogen. Given the normal colonization of human skin, *Staphylococcus aureus* and *Streptococcus* species are the most common infecting organisms, accounting for the majority of cellulitis, impetigo, and abscesses. *Cellulitis* is infectious inflammation of the dermis and subcutaneous tissue that presents clinically with tenderness, erythema, warmth, and edema. *Impetigo,* infection of the superficial skin layers, is classically categorized as *bullous* (Fig. 20-2) or *nonbullous* based on the method of inoculation and appearance of the lesions (Table 20-2); the distinction is less relevant clinically because *S. aureus* and *Streptococcus* species are routinely cultured from both types, with the result that they are treated identically. Impetigo is most common in preschool-aged children. *Abscesses* are deep soft tissue infections. Those that are associated with puncture wounds generally contain a combination of organisms, depending on the penetrating object. Objects that puncture the skin through a tennis shoe

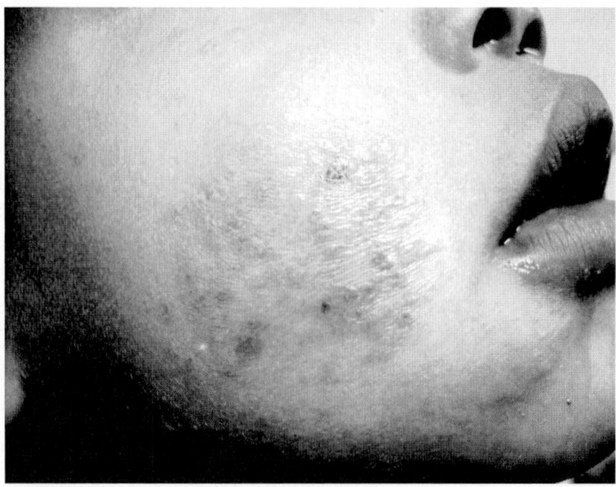

Figure 20-1 Atopic dermatitis in the infant: multiple grouped erythematous papules with associated scaling. (Courtesy of Paul S. Matz, MD, from Chung EK. *Visual Diagnosis in Pediatrics.* Philadelphia: Lippincott Williams & Wilkins; 2006:20.) (*See Color Insert.*)

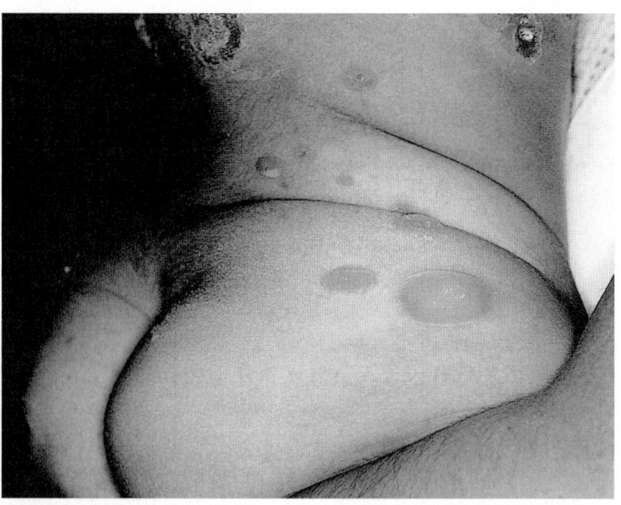

Figure 20-2 Bullous impetigo: large, clear bullae rupture, leaving remnants in a ring-shaped lesion around a central crusted sore. (From Fleisher GR. *Atlas of Pediatric Emergency Medicine.* Philadelphia: Lippincott Williams & Wilkins; 2003 with permission.) (*See Color Insert.*)

TABLE 20-2
BULLOUS AND NONBULLOUS IMPETIGO

	Bullous	Nonbullous
Causative organism(s)	*Staphylococcus aureus*	*S. aureus* or *Streptococcus* species
Source of infection	Pathogen spreads following colonization of the upper respiratory tract	Pathogen enters through a disruption in the skin
Appearance of lesions	Large, clear bullae rupture, leaving remnants in a ring-shaped lesion around a central crusted sore	Initial small pustules or vesicles rupture and becomes crusted with a honey-colored exudate
Pathophysiology	Exotoxin produced by *S. aureus* results in separation of the skin layers and formation of bullae	Direct infection of contiguous tissues; may spread to distal sites through scratching and autoinoculation

and sharp objects exposed to the elements are often contaminated with *Pseudomonas aeruginosa;* this organism should be suspected if the patient fails to measurably improve following several days of appropriate antibiotic therapy. Additional coverage should be considered if the wound results from a human or animal bite (Table 20-3). *Acute postinfectious glomerulonephritis* is a potential late sequela of inadequately treated group A streptococcal (GAS) skin infections (see Chapter 16). Other recognized complications of GAS disease include *necrotizing fasciitis* (a rapidly progressive infection of the deep fascia and subcutaneous tissue presenting with intense pain, induration, and possibly crepitus) and *toxic shock syndrome* (life-threatening invasive systemic disease progressing to shock and multisystem organ failure; carries a high mortality rate).

Staphylococcal scalded skin syndrome is a toxin-mediated illness that occurs most commonly in infants and toddlers. Although infection with the toxin-producing strain of *S. aureus* may not directly involve the skin, systemic dissemination of the toxin results in widespread epidermal erythema and blistering (Fig. 20-3). Application of

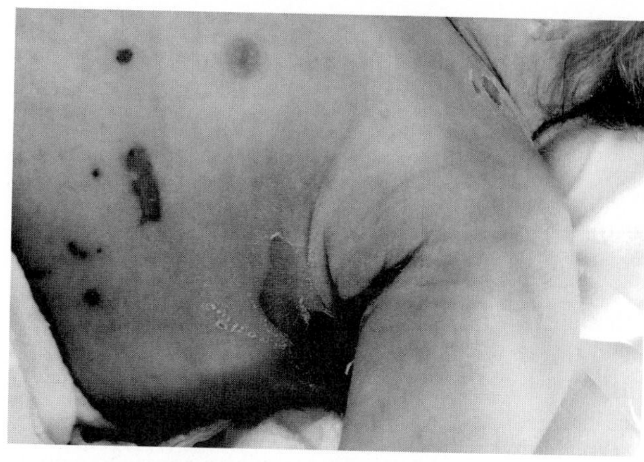

Figure 20-3 Staphylococcal scalded skin syndrome: a toxin-mediated reaction characterized by widespread epidermal erythema and blistering. (Courtesy of Gary Marshall, MD, from Chung EK. *Visual Diagnosis in Pediatrics.* Philadelphia: Lippincott Williams & Wilkins; 2006:480.) (*See Color Insert.*)

TABLE 20-3
BACTERIAL SKIN INFECTIONS: SUGGESTED ANTIBIOTIC THERAPY BASED ON SUSPECTED CAUSATIVE PATHOGENS

Infection Associated with:	Suspected Pathogens	Suggested Oral Treatment	Intravenous Alternative	+/− Prophylaxis
Superficial abrasion, laceration, or skin disruption	*Staphylococcus aureus*, *Streptococcus* species	Any one of the following: Cephalexin Dicloxacillin Erythromycin (in penicillin-allergic patients)	Any one of the following: Cefazolin Nafcillin	Prophylaxis not indicated
Puncture wound	*S. aureus*, *Streptococcus* species; if no response to treatment, consider *Pseudomonas aeruginosa*	Any one of the following: Cephalexin Dicloxacillin Erythromycin (in penicillin-allergic patients)	Same as above Ceftazidime if *P. aeruginosa* is suspected	Prophylaxis not indicated for wounds occurring <24 hours prior to presentation
Bite, human	*S. aureus*, *Streptococcus* species, anaerobic organisms	Amoxicillin-clavulanic acid OR Clindamycin plus trimethoprim-sulfamethoxazole (in penicillin-allergic patients)	Ampicillin-sulbactam	Prophylaxis indicated
Bite, dog	*S. aureus*, *Streptococcus* species, *Eikenella* species, *Pasteurella* species	Same as for human bites	Same as for human bites	Prophylaxis indicated
Bite, cat	*S. aureus*, *Streptococcus* species, *Pasteurella multocida*	Same as for human bites	Same as for human bites	Prophylaxis indicated

gentle tension pressure results in sloughing of the skin (Nikolsky sign). The underlying site of infection should be vigorously investigated (e.g., lungs, meninges, bone). Management involves intravenous antistaphylococcal antibiotics and supportive care; severely affected patients require intensive care similar to that provided for burn victims.

Viral Infections

Nongenital *warts* result from infection with different subtypes of human papillomavirus. The lesions are highly textured (hyperkeratotic), well-demarcated, flat or raised areas of clearly abnormal tissue. They may occur anywhere on the skin surface. Most warts in children spontaneously regress. If resolution or removal is desired for cosmetic reasons, multiple treatments are available (topical salicylic acid, liquid nitrogen, electrocautery, laser, or surgical removal).

Genital warts are discussed in Chapter 24.

Molluscum contagiosum is a benign superficial viral skin infection characterized by pearly white or waxy yellow dome-shaped lesions that range from 1 to 5 mm in diameter (Fig. 20-4). Most have a visible central umbilication. The DNA virus is spread through skin-to-skin contact and is highly contagious. Affected children may have a few or many lesions scattered over the face, trunk, extremities, buttocks, and genital region. Patients with atopic dermatitis can develop widespread cutaneous infection due to scratching and subsequent autoinoculation. In immunocompetent patients, molluscum contagiosum resolves within several months to a few years. Human immunodeficiency virus (HIV) infection should be considered in patients with extensive involvement. If the diagnosis is in doubt, removal of the central core permits detection of characteristic intracytoplasmic viral inclusion bodies. Treatment is unnecessary; however, lesions in sensitive areas and those that cause cosmetic distress can be removed via curettage. Topical agents that have proven benefit in the treatment of common warts have been tried with variable success.

Fungal Infections

Tinea corporis ("ringworm") is a fungal infection of the superficial stratum corneum. The pathogen may be acquired from a pet, from direct contact with an infected person, or through fomite transmission. One or more mildly pruritic annular lesions develop and enlarge, with erythematous, scaling, well-demarcated borders and central clearing (Fig. 20-5). In children, tinea corporis most commonly occurs on the face, trunk, or extremities. Most cases are diagnosed based on clinical presentation. Tinea corporis that does not respond to treatment with appropriate topical or systemic antifungal therapy may instead be misdiagnosed *granuloma annulare*. Granuloma annulare is a benign, self-limited dermatologic condition of unknown etiology that presents as an annular plaque of central clearing ringed with small, slightly erythematous papules.

Tinea pedis ("athlete's foot") is a fungal infection restricted to the outermost layer of the epidermis of the foot. It occurs almost exclusively in adolescents and adults. The disorder is characterized by fissuring and maceration of the interdigital (toe web) regions with associated scale. The involved area may be asymptomatic but is often pruritic. *Trichophyton rubrum* is the usual pathogen. A variant of this infection presents with chronic, diffuse scaling along the plantar surfaces of the feet. Examination of a potassium hydroxide preparation of skin scrapings reveals fungal elements; alternatively, fungal cultures may be obtained, but most cases are diagnosed clinically. Tinea pedis responds to broad-spectrum topical antifungal therapy (clotrimazole, ketoconazole). *Atopic dermatitis* involving the foot and/or toes may be mistaken for tinea pedis; however, patients with atopic changes are usually prepubertal, have a

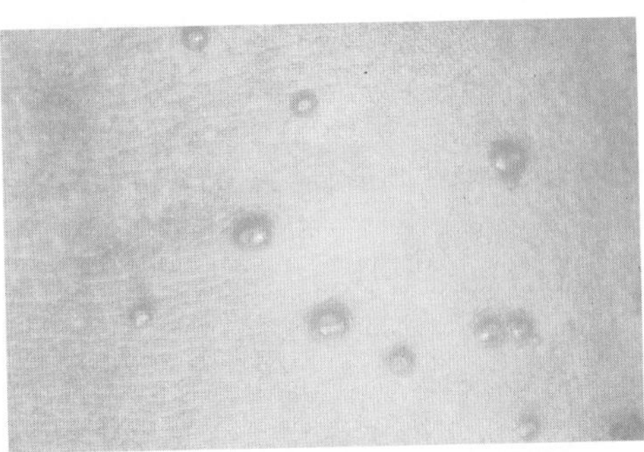

Figure 20-4 Molluscum contagiosum: pearly white dome-shaped lesions with central umbilication, ranging from 1 to 5 mm in diameter. (From Goodheart HP. *Goodheart's Photoguide of Common Skin Disorders: Diagnosis and Management.* 2nd ed. Philadelphia: Lippincott Williams & Wilkins; 2003:138 with permission.) (*See Color Insert.*)

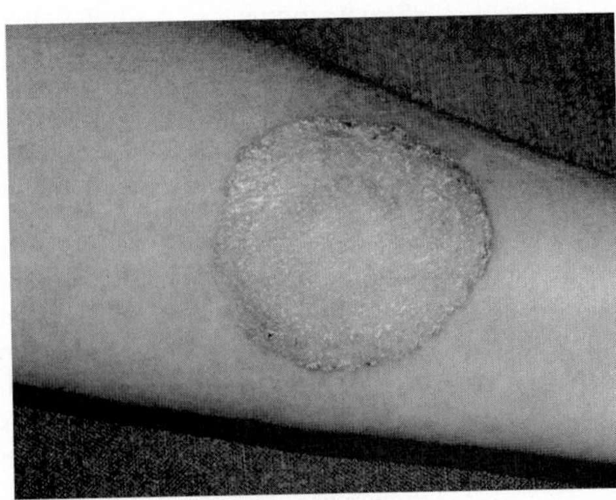

Figure 20-5 Tinea corporis: annular lesion with erythematous, scaling, well-demarcated borders and central clearing. (From Goodheart HP. *Goodheart's Photoguide of Common Skin Disorders: Diagnosis and Management.* 2nd ed. Philadelphia: Lippincott Williams & Wilkins; 2003:303 with permission.) (*See Color Insert.*)

positive history of atopy, and demonstrate sparring of the interdigital areas.

Tinea versicolor consists of hypo- or hyperpigmented scaly, oval macules 0.5 to several centimeters in diameter that may coalesce. The lesions result from infection of the superficial skin with *Pityrosporum ovale*. Tinea versicolor is uncommon before adolescence. This pathogen has a characteristic "spaghetti and meatballs" appearance when a potassium hydroxide preparation is examined under the microscope. Initial cosmetic treatment for this benign condition consists of topical selenium sulfide shampoo or cream, which is left on the skin for several minutes before being rinsed away. Topical ketoconazole is also effective. Oral antifungal agents may be necessary in patients with widespread involvement. Hypopigmented tinea versicolor is occasionally mistaken for *vitiligo*, a disorder of complete depigmentation of areas of the skin without associated superficial scaling.

INSECTS AND INFESTATIONS

Papular Urticaria

Papular urticaria results from hypersensitivity to insect bites or stings (usually dog or cat fleas; occasionally mosquitoes). The reaction presents as recurrent episodes of pruritic, erythematous papules, many with a small, central depression, that are clustered together. The lesions last approximately 7 to 10 days. Papular urticaria is most common in preschool-aged children; older household members are rarely affected. Itching can be addressed with a mild topical corticosteroid or oral antihistamine if severe. The most effective treatment is elimination of the flea infestation or prevention of bites and stings.

Scabies

Scabies is an infestation of the skin with the mite *Sarcoptes scabiei*. The organism spreads through skin-to-skin contact or contact with infected bedding. The mite burrows under the skin, producing a small vesicle or papule. As the female mite advances, she lays her eggs and deposits fecal pellets in the skin along a visible *linear burrow*; these burrows are pathognomonic for the infestation (Fig. 20-6). They are typically concentrated on the finger webs, palms, wrists, belt line, and, in infants, the feet and toes. The lesions are intensely pruritic and may cause unexplained fussiness in infants. Usually, multiple family members are symptomatic at the same time. The mites can be recovered by placing a drop of mineral oil over a vesicle or burrow and scraping with a #15 blade; when the scrapings are placed on a slide beneath a cover slip, the mite, eggs, and/or feces are clearly visible at ten times the magnification.

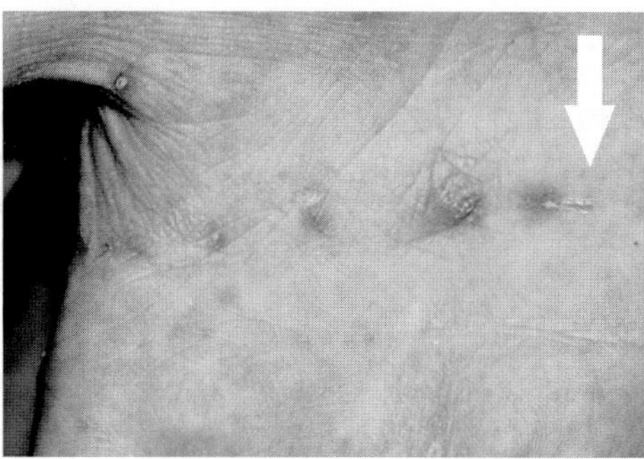

Figure 20-6 Scabies: papular lesions in a linear distribution across the palm with a visible linear burrow. (From Goodheart HP. *Goodheart's Photoguide of Common Skin Disorders: Diagnosis and Management*. 2nd ed. Philadelphia: Lippincott Williams & Wilkins; 2003:305 with permission.) (*See Color Insert.*)

Permethrin 5% cream is the most effective scabicide available; it should be applied to all household and other close contacts from the neck down and left on overnight, regardless of whether they are symptomatic. A scabicide cream should be applied to the head and scalp as well in infants. Lindane is a less desirable alternative due to reports of mite resistance and neurotoxicity in infants. The lesions may remain pruritic for up to 2 weeks after treatment; retreatment is unnecessary.

Topical permethrin, which is also used to treat pediculosis and is the main ingredient in many insect repellents, is rarely systemically toxic in humans when used appropriately. Permethrin 5% formulations are not approved for use in children younger than 2 years of age or in pregnant or nursing women.

Pediculosis

Pediculosis is infestation with lice. Pubic lice are discussed in Chapter 24. "Head lice" are extremely contagious. The lice spread through direct head-to-head contact or through sharing combs or caps. Infestation with head lice causes significant pruritus; scratching may lead to excoriation, secondary skin infection (impetigo), and cervical and/or occipital lymphadenopathy. The adult louse is mobile, feeds on blood from the scalp every 4 to 6 hours, and cannot survive without feeding for more than 24 to 48 hours. Adult lice lay eggs at the base of the hair shaft. Nymphs (immature lice) emerge 7 to 10 days later, leaving empty white "nits" behind. Nymphs mature and can begin to reproduce and lay eggs within 1 to 2 weeks. The diagnosis of head lice requires detection of both adult lice and attached eggs. Permethrin 1% cream rinse should be applied to clean, dry hair, left in place for 10 minutes, and then thoroughly rinsed away. This kills adult and nymph-stage lice, but eggs remain viable, necessitating a second course of treatment 7 to 10 days later. Resistance to permethrin is increasing.

Alternative therapies include malathion lotion 0.5% (massaged into dry hair and scalp and removed 8 to 12 hours later), which kills both live lice and those inside eggs, and permethrin 5% cream (applied to hair and scalp and removed after 8 to 12 hours, with a second application 7 to 10 days later). Neither nits nor eggs, which are tightly attached to the hair shaft, are contagious; however, most school systems still require the child to be "nit-free" before returning to the classroom. Special combs are available for removal of the nits.

HAIR LOSS

Tinea Capitis

Tinea capitis is a superficial fungal infection of the scalp that is usually due to *Trichophyton tonsurans.* Tinea capitis is characterized by a single or multiple areas of patchy hair loss; the involved skin is covered with fine scale and contains visible broken ("black dot") hairs within follicles. Associated posterior and/or occipital lymphadenopathy is commonly noted. A *kerion* is a tender, boggy, erythematous mass that may be mistaken for a secondary bacterial infection but is actually a local inflammatory reaction to the fungal pathogen.

Tinea capitis must be treated with an oral antifungal agent; topical treatment does not eradicate fungal elements within the hair shaft. *Griseofulvin* is preferred as a first-line therapy given its safety profile; adverse effects, including severe neutropenia and aplastic anemia, are serious but rare.

Tinea capitis can be differentiated from *trichotillomania,* the loss of hair due to habitual or pathologic hair pulling or twisting, by the presence of irregular borders and hair shafts broken off at different lengths within the same area in the latter disorder.

Alopecia Areata

Alopecia areata is characterized by the sudden and total loss of hair within an affected region. The underlying skin is devoid of any hair remnants but appears otherwise normal; overlying scale, "black dot" hairs, and associated lymphadenopathy are notably absent. Alopecia areata runs in families and is thought to be autoimmune in origin. The hair often regrows after a time, although episodic hair loss remains chronic.

NEUROCUTANEOUS SYNDROMES

Phakomatoses are neurocutaneous disorders characterized by lesions in the nervous system, skin, and eyes. The two most common of these autosomal dominant conditions are neurofibromatosis and tuberous sclerosis.

Neurofibromatosis

Of the several variants of neurofibromatosis, types 1 (*von Recklinghausen disease;* Table 20-4) and 2 (*bilateral acoustic neurofibromatosis*) are the most common in children. Neurofibromatosis type 1 is a clinical diagnosis based in part of the presence of six or more café-au-lait spots of a certain size (Fig. 20-7). *Lisch nodules* (hamartomas of the iris) typically predate *neurofibromas,* which are not usually detected until late childhood or adolescence. Patients with von Recklinghausen disease may require treatment for associated seizures, learning disorders, renovascular hypertension, and scoliosis. Tibial dysplasia (thinning of the cortex and medullary sclerosis) results in noticeable lower extremity anteromedial bowing within the first year of life and predisposes the patient to pathologic fractures. Neurofibromas that cause functional impairment are surgically removed; however, most will recur.

Bilateral acoustic neuromas are the hallmark of type 2 neurofibromatosis. Complications include hearing loss

TABLE 20-4
DIAGNOSIS OF NEUROFIBROMATOSIS TYPE 1

Two or more of the following must be present:

1. Six or more café-au-lait spots, >0.5 cm in size in children (>1.5 cm in adolescents or adults)
2. Axillary or inguinal freckling
3. Two or more Lisch nodules (hamartomas) in the irises
4. Two or more neurofibromas or one plexiform neurofibroma
5. A distinctive osseous lesion, such as sphenoid dysplasia
6. Optic gliomas
7. Affected first-degree relative diagnosed with neurofibromatosis type 1 based on the above criteria

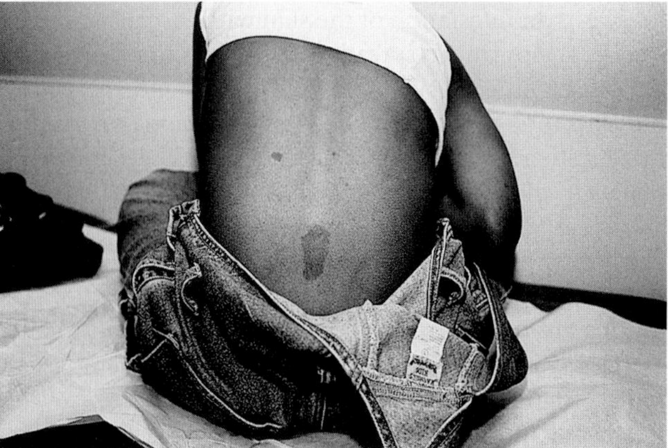

Figure 20-7 Café-au-lait spots: flat, nonpalpable hyperpigmented macules. (From Chung EK. *Visual Diagnosis in Pediatrics.* Philadelphia: Lippincott Williams & Wilkins; 2006:473 with permission.) (*See Color Insert.*)

and vestibular disorientation. Brain magnetic resonance imaging demonstrates bilateral eighth cranial nerve masses. Neurofibromas, meningiomas, schwannomas, and astrocytomas are also associated with type 2 neurofibromatosis. Cataracts and retinal hamartomas are not uncommon. Surgical debulking is appropriate when hearing impairment becomes pronounced. Cochlear implants have restored hearing in some patients.

Tuberous Sclerosis

Tuberous sclerosis complex is a progressive neurocutaneous disorder with extremely variable expressivity. The genetic defect interferes with normal production of tuberin, a protein involved in the suppression of tumors, resulting in widespread growth of hamartomas in skin, organs, and bone. Sporadic cases are more common than inherited ones. *Ash-leaf spots* (flat, hypopigmented macules) are the earliest visible sign of tuberous sclerosis; 90% of affected newborns are born with at least one ash-leaf spot, which is best visualized through Wood lamp examination. These macules may be found in unaffected infants as well. Other characteristic findings that develop later in childhood include shagreen patches (areas of leathery skin thickening representing connective tissue nevi), cutaneous angiofibromas (raised red papules; Fig. 20-8), periungal and gingival fibromas, and microcephaly. Angiofibromas may occasionally be mistaken for acne lesions; however, acne is rare in prepubertal children. Neuroimaging demonstrates the distinctive periventricular knoblike areas of localized swelling, or "tubers." Subependymal nodules, giant cell astrocytomas, and tumors of the kidney, heart, and retina may also be present. Mental retardation and seizures, particularly *infantile spasms*, are common in severely affected individuals; others may have only mild learning disorders. Treatment consists of antiepileptic therapy and surgical removal of related tumors when indicated.

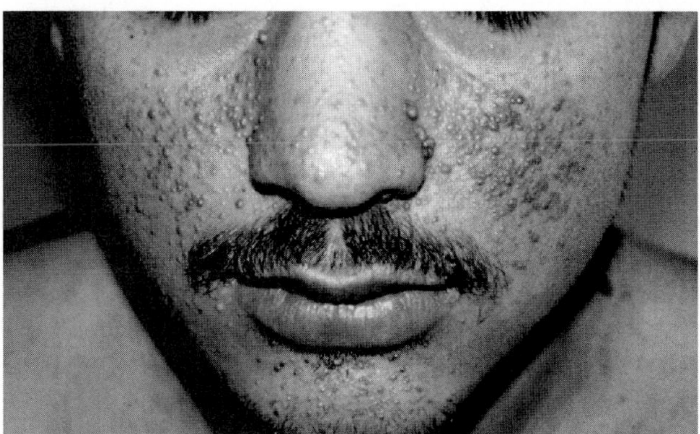

Figure 20-8 Angiofibromas: raised red papules in a patient with tuberous sclerosis. (From Goodheart HP. *Goodheart's Photoguide of Common Skin Disorders: Diagnosis and Management*. 2nd ed. Philadelphia: Lippincott Williams & Wilkins; 2003 with permission.) (*See Color Insert.*)

PIGMENTED LESIONS

Urticaria Pigmentosa

Urticaria pigmentosa is a rare disease that usually presents within the first year of life with pigmented papules (abnormal collections of mast cells in the skin) that wheal and flare when stroked. At least half of affected children also display *dermatographism*, the formation of erythema and edema following rubbing of apparently uninvolved areas of skin. The lesions continue to appear throughout infancy but eventually lose the ability to urticate and become asymptomatic. No treatment is necessary beyond periodic control of symptoms with an antihistamine such as hydroxyzine.

Malignant Melanoma

Malignant melanoma remains rare in the pediatric population but is being diagnosed with increasing frequency in adolescents. The main long-term consequences of sun exposure, the effects of which are cumulative, are premature aging of the skin and malignancy (basal or squamous cell carcinomas, malignant melanomas). Characteristics of pigmented cutaneous lesions that should prompt suspicion of melanoma include these "ABCDs:"

- Asymmetry
- Border that is uneven or notched
- Color variation within the lesion (brown, red, blue, white, black)
- Diameter >6 mm

Lesions meeting any of these criteria should be evaluated and managed by an experienced dermatologist, who is often better able to clinically differentiate between melanoma and benign skin lesions such as dysplastic nevi, halo nevus, blue nevus, and melanocytic nevi.

ACNE VULGARIS

Comedones result from obstruction and progressive enlargement of the follicle. Open comedones are commonly called "blackheads," and closed comedones are referred to as "whiteheads." Papules and pustules are *inflammatory lesions*. *Nodulocystic* acne consists of inflammatory lesions that are >0.5 cm in diameter; these sores may involve multiple follicles. Acne is classified clinically as mild, moderate, or severe:

- *Mild acne* consists of mostly open and closed comedones and a few small inflammatory lesions, with involvement of less than one fourth of the face.

- Many inflammatory papules and pustules are present in *moderate acne,* and approximately half of the face is involved.
- *Severe acne* includes nodulocystic lesions, which are associated with a high incidence of scarring, and involves >75% of the face.

Common topical agents, their formulations and usage, and their adverse effects are listed in Table 20-5. Mild comedonal acne is initially treated with benzoyl peroxide; if inflammatory lesions are present, a combination topical agent (e.g., benzoyl peroxide and clindamycin) may be a reasonable first choice. If the response is unsatisfactory, addition of a topical retinoid should be considered. Moderate acne is best treated with combination medication and a topical retinoid product, although these should not be put on at the same time due to inactivation of the retinoid by benzoyl peroxide. Oral antibiotics are indicated for severe acne with extensive inflammatory lesions, in combination with a topical retinoid. Oral antibiotics should also be considered in patients with moderate acne who have an unsatisfactory response to topical agents alone and patients with extensive acne involving the face, shoulders, and back. Oral isotretinoin is reserved for patients with nodulocystic acne and scarring. Regardless of the therapy used, patients should be counseled not to expect significant improvement in their acne for 6 to 8 weeks.

CONTACT DERMATITIS

Exposure to poison ivy, oak, or sumac is one of the most common causes of contact dermatitis in children and adolescents. These plants contain urushiol; following initial sensitization, contact with this substance results in the development of extremely pruritic linear vesicles and papules. The fluid within the vesicles does not contain urushiol, and direct contact with this fluid does not produce the characteristic rash. Washing the contaminated skin with soap and water within 15 minutes of exposure prevents or limits the delayed cutaneous reaction. Oral prednisone is indicated for *Rhus* dermatitis that is extensive, severe, or involves a sensitive area (the face or periorbital region). Corticosteroid treatment should be continued

TABLE 20-5
TOPICAL THERAPY FOR ACNE VULGARIS

Product	Indication	Formulation	Adverse Effects
Benzoyl peroxide	Mild-to-moderate, comedonal and/or inflammatory acne	Over-the-counter or prescription creams, lotions, ointments, washes, and gels	Superficial irritation of the skin
Topical antibiotics (erythromycin, clindamycin)	Mild-to-moderate inflammatory acne	Prescription; single-agent medications available, but most often the antibiotic is combined with benzoyl peroxide for an additive effect	Increased antibiotic resistance when used in isolation (this is negated when the antibiotic is formulated in combination with benzoyl peroxide)
Topical retinoids (tretinoin)	Most effective in treating comedonal acne or as an adjunct therapy to the above	Prescription creams, liquids, or gels	Superficial skin irritation, dryness
Oral antibiotics (tetracycline, erythromycin, doxycycline, minocycline)	Moderate-to-severe inflammatory acne or widespread lesions	Prescription oral agents	Gastric upset, photosensitivity, vaginal candidiasis
Oral combination (estrogen/progestin) birth control pills	Used mostly as adjunct therapy; may have more of a role in patients who cannot tolerate other forms of oral therapy	Prescription	Possibility of decreased efficacy for preventing pregnancy when combined with long-term oral antibiotic therapy; sexually active patients should continue to use barrier contraception in addition to oral contraception pills
Isotretinoin	Severe nodulocystic acne with scarring; recalcitrant acne	Prescription from approved providers only	Highly teratogenic; hair loss, dry skin; questionable potential for exacerbating depression

for 12 to 21 days; shorter courses may result in recurrence of symptoms.

ICHTHYOSIS VULGARIS

Ichthyosis vulgaris is an autosomal dominant chronic dermatitis that is particularly common in patients with atopic dermatitis. Inability of the stratum corneum to retain moisture results in the development of fine, mosaic-like scales over the lower extremities and buttocks that usually become evident between 6 months and 5 years of age. Hyperlinearity of the palms and soles and keratosis pilaris over the extensor surfaces of the extremities are associated features. These cutaneous manifestations often persist despite optimal treatment of the eczema. Frequent application of an emollient may improve retention of moisture. Second-line therapy consists of a topical alpha-hydroxy acid to both hydrate the skin and promote detachment of the scales. Other topical agents that may prove beneficial include urea-containing emollients, propylene glycol, and salicylic acid.

PSORIASIS

Psoriasis is an autosomal dominant chronic dermatitis with variable penetrance. Disease manifestations typically become evident in late childhood, adolescence, or early adulthood. The rash is characterized by well-demarcated, round or oval plaques with overlying thick, white, adherent scales (Fig. 20-9). Removal of the scale results in pinpoint bleeding (Auspitz sign). The lesions are often moderately pruritic. Commonly involved areas of skin include the scalp, eyebrows, ears, elbows, and knees. Local trauma may precipitate the development of the plaques. A minority of patients exhibit changes in the nails (thickening, pitting, or yellowish discoloration). Management consists of medication to decrease the size and thickness of the plaques and symptomatic treatment of the associated pruritus.

PITYRIASIS ROSEA

Pityriasis rosea is a benign, self-limited dermatitis that occurs most commonly in older children and adolescents. The rash is characterized by a multitude of 1- to 2-cm oval, scaly, salmon-colored patches covering the trunk, back, and thighs in a "Christmas tree" pattern (alignment of the ovals with their long axes oriented along dermatomal lines). The rash may be preceded by mild, nonspecific constitutional symptoms and/or a "herald patch," a scaly, oval macule 3 to 5 cm in diameter with central clearing that is often mistaken for tinea corporis. The rash intensifies over 10 to 14 days, with gradual fading and resolution within 8 to 10 weeks. Secondary syphilis may be clinically indistinguishable from pityriasis rosea; sexually active patients should be screened for this disease with nontreponemal testing for *Treponema pallidum*.

ERYTHEMA MULTIFORME

Erythema multiforme (EM) is a clinically distinct cutaneous hypersensitivity reaction that follows exposure to certain medications and childhood infections (e.g., herpes labialis). The initial cutaneous sign is the symmetric eruption of "target lesions" over the dorsum of the hands and feet as well as the extensor surfaces of the arms and legs. *Target lesions* begin as erythematous papules that evolve into dusky-colored bullae 5 to 10 mm in diameter, each surrounded by an erythematous ring (Fig. 20-10). New

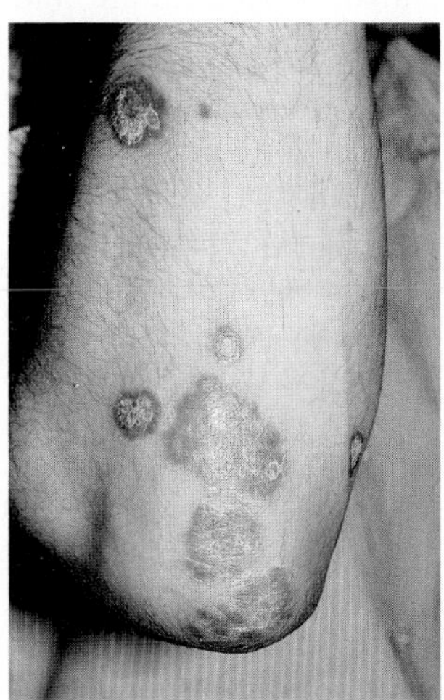

Figure 20-9 Psoriasis: well-demarcated, round or oval plaques with overlying thick, white, adherent scales. (From Goodheart HP. *Goodheart's Photoguide of Common Skin Disorders: Diagnosis and Management*. 2nd ed. Philadelphia: Lippincott Williams & Wilkins; 2003:54 with permission.) (*See Color Insert.*)

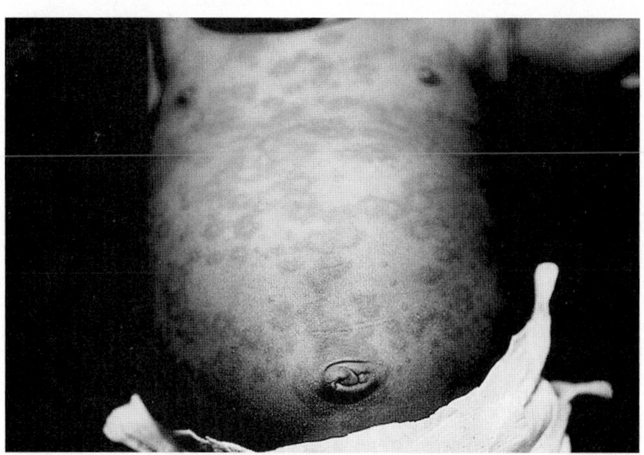

Figure 20-10 Erythema multiforme: "target lesions" (dusky-colored bullae 5 to 10 mm in diameter, each surrounded by an erythematous ring). (From Chung EK. *Visual Diagnosis in Pediatrics*. Philadelphia: Lippincott Williams & Wilkins; 2006:434 with permission.) (*See Color Insert.*)

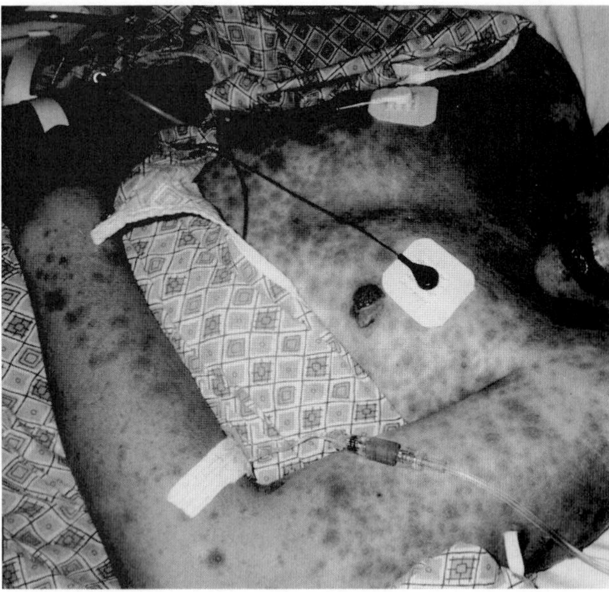

Figure 20-11 Stevens-Johnson syndrome: widespread epidermal erythema and purpuric lesions; note the hemorrhagic crusting of the oral mucosa. (From Chung EK. *Visual Diagnosis in Pediatrics*. Philadelphia: Lippincott Williams & Wilkins; 2006:481 with permission.) (*See Color Insert.*)

crops of lesions continue to appear for up to 3 weeks and may be accompanied by low-grade fever, malaise, and myalgia. Mucous membranes are only minimally involved. Therapy is supportive and symptomatic; the condition is self-limited and rarely progressive unless the inciting medication is not discontinued.

Stevens-Johnson syndrome (also called erythema multiforme major) is a severe form of progressive EM characterized by widespread epidermal erythema and shedding and hemorrhagic crusting and necrosis involving the oral, conjunctival, and urethral mucous membranes (Fig. 20-11). Affected children appear very ill, with high fevers, vomiting and diarrhea, and arthralgia. Extensive disruption of the integument results in fluid and electrolyte imbalances and impaired local immunity. Management goals consist of preventing secondary infection, maintaining hydration, preserving metabolic homeostasis, and controlling pain. *Mycoplasma* pneumonia is the most common infectious cause of Stevens-Johnson syndrome in older children and adolescents.

SOURCES

Bloomfield D, Adam HM. Head lice. *Pediatr Rev*. 2002;23:34–35.

Chung EK. *Visual Diagnosis in Pediatrics*. Philadelphia: Lippincott Williams & Wilkins; 2005.

Conlon JD, Drolet BA. Skins lesions in the neonate. *Pediatr Clin North Am*. 2004;51:863–888.

Goodheart HP. *Goodheart's Photoguide of Common Skin Disorders*. 2nd ed. Philadelphia: Lippincott Williams & Wilkins; 2003.

Krowchuk DP. Managing adolescent acne: a guide for pediatricians. *Pediatr Rev*. 2005;26:244–255.

Sagerman PJ. Wounds. *Pediatr Rev*. 2005;26:43–49.

QUESTIONS

1. The physical examination of a newborn infant who will be joining your practice reveals a unilateral port wine stain over the dermatome innervated by the first division of the right trigeminal nerve. In counseling the parents, you are correct in telling them all of the following EXCEPT:

A) Pulsed laser therapy will address both the visible capillary malformations and similar lesions affecting the meninges.
B) Their child may have Sturge-Weber syndrome.
C) Their child's chance of having Sturge-Weber syndrome would be greater if the birthmark was bilateral.
D) The birthmark will not enlarge in relation to the child's growth.
E) The lesion may darken during adolescence or adulthood.

2. A 12-day-old former full-term infant is brought to the clinic for evaluation of his poor feeding and rash. He was well until 2 days ago, when his parents noticed increased fussiness and decreased appetite. Vital signs are stable in the clinic; the infant is fussy but consolable. The physical examination is significant for a well-nourished infant with signs of mild dehydration and several vesiculopustular lesions scattered over his scalp, trunk, and perioral region. The Wright stain demonstrates multinucleated giant cells. Fluid from a lesion is obtained for viral culture, and polymerase chain reaction testing of the cerebrospinal fluid is negative for herpes simplex virus DNA. Which of the following represents the most appropriate treatment for this patient?

A) Intravenous acyclovir for 7 days
B) Intravenous acyclovir for 14 days
C) Intravenous acyclovir for 21 days
D) Oral acyclovir for 14 days
E) Oral acyclovir for 21 days

3. Which of the following neonatal pustular disorders is correctly matched with its anticipated microscopic analysis result?

A) Neonatal herpes simplex virus infection—Gram-positive cocci on Gram stain
B) Staphylococcal folliculitis—multinucleated giant cells on Wright stain or Tzanck preparation
C) Congenital candidiasis—pseudohyphae and budding yeast on potassium hydroxide preparation

D) Erythema toxicum neonatorum—predominance of neutrophils on Wright stain
E) Transient neonatal pustular melanosis—predominance of eosinophils on Wright stain

4. A 3-day-old full-term newborn girl presents to your clinic for evaluation of her rash. The mother is concerned about the blisters on her trunk but remarks that she is feeding well, does not seem to be fussy, and has not felt feverish. Examination of the skin reveals blotchy erythematous macules with central pustules scattered over the trunk and extremities. No other abnormalities are noted on the physical examination. In discussing these lesions with the mother, you would be correct in telling her which of the following?
A) Microscopic analysis is necessary to confirm the diagnosis.
B) Skin biopsy is necessary to confirm the diagnosis.
C) The lesions are likely to resolve and recur in outbreaks over the next 3 years.
D) No specific therapy is required.
E) She should call you immediately if the lesions spread to the face.

5. A 2-month-old African-American infant is in your office for his regular health maintenance visit and immunizations. He is feeding well by report and has appropriate growth. The physical examination is within normal limits except for scattered hyperpigmented macules with minimal scaling over his face and extremities. His mother, a nurse, states that she noticed similar "freckles" when he was born and was surprised when they went away; in fact, this is the third time she has noticed this rash, which usually begins as pustules. In discussing the lesions with the child's mother, you are correct in telling her all of the following EXCEPT:
A) Fluid from the pustules would most likely be filled with neutrophils.
B) The child has a benign condition.
C) The child does not need to be isolated from other children when the rash is present.
D) The child has a self-limited condition.
E) Specific therapy is recommended for cosmetic purposes only.

6. An 18-month-old boy presents to your office for evaluation of his rash. He has numerous 2-mm papules and vesicles scattered over his palms, wrists, and waist as well as in the webs of his fingers. Many of the sores are associated with linear burrows and excoriations. Neither his parents nor his older sister are complaining of pruritic lesions. His parents are convinced that he does not have scabies because "we keep a clean, hygienic house." The best method of recovering evidence of an active infestation with *Sarcoptes scabiei* is which of the following?
A) Place a drop of mineral oil on one of the lesions and obtain scrapings for low-magnification (10×) microscopic analysis.
B) Place a drop of mineral oil on one of the lesions and obtain scrapings for high-magnification (25×) microscopic analysis.
C) Apply scotch tape to the lesion overnight and view the tape the following morning under low-power magnification.
D) Apply scotch tape to the lesion overnight and view the tape the following morning under high-power magnification.
E) Obtain blood for immunoglobulin M–specific antibodies against *Sarcoptes scabiei.*

7. You have just diagnosed a 4-year-old girl with scabies. She lives with her mother, her maternal aunt, and her 8-year-old sister, none of whom report pruritic lesions. Which of the following provides the most effective treatment of this child's infestation with the least chance of recurrence?
A) 1% permethrin cream applied from head to toe overnight for the patient, with treatment of additional household members and close contacts if they develop symptoms
B) 5% permethrin cream applied from head to toe overnight for the patient, with treatment of additional household members and close contacts if they develop symptoms
C) 5% permethrin cream applied from head to toe overnight for the entire household and close contacts
D) Lindane lotion applied from head to toe overnight for the patient, with treatment of additional household members and close contacts if they develop symptoms
E) Lindane lotion applied from head to toe overnight for the entire household and close contacts

8. A 24-month-old boy has developed recurrent episodes of 2- to 3-mm pruritic erythematous papules and pustules. The sores are located in clusters on his ankles and lower legs. Many lesions contain a small central punctate depression. Resolution takes place over 7 to 10 days. This patient's recurring rash is most consistent with which of the following?
A) Punctate psoriasis
B) Papular urticaria
C) Scabies
D) Verruca vulgaris
E) Punctate keratitis

9. An 8-year-old boy has been sent home from school with head lice. The frantic mother calls you to ask how she should proceed in ridding the child of his

infestation. The most appropriate first-line treatment consists of which of the following?
A) Prescription malathion 0.5% lotion
B) Prescription permethrin 5% cream
C) Over-the-counter permethrin 1% cream rinse
D) Prescription lindane shampoo
E) Over-the-counter lindane shampoo

10. A 3-year-old girl who was sent home from day care with head lice has been properly treated with over-the-counter permethrin 1% cream rinse. Her care center refuses to allow her to return until she has completed a second treatment in 7 days and been certified as nit free by her pediatrician. Her mother is afraid to expose the girl to her siblings and the neighborhood children. You are correct in telling the mother which of the following?
A) The girl remains contagious until she has been retreated 7 to 10 days later.
B) The girl remains contagious until the empty nits are removed.
C) The girl remains contagious until she has been retreated 7 to 10 days later AND the empty nits have all been removed.
D) If no mobile lice are visible, the child is no longer contagious and will not become contagious unless she becomes reinfested.
E) If no mobile lice are visible, the child is not presently contagious and will not become contagious for another 7 to 10 days.

11. A mother brings her 7-year-old son to your office for you to evaluate "some bumps he got while he was at overnight camp." The child has eight lesions scattered over his chest and extremities. All are 2- to 4-mm, firm, pearly white, dome-shaped lesions, each with a central umbilication. You are correct in telling the boy and his mother all of the following EXCEPT:
A) The lesions are unlikely to resolve without treatment.
B) The lesions are caused by a virus.
C) The pathogen responsible for the lesions is spread through direct skin-to-skin contact.
D) New lesions may continue to appear.
E) The lesions contain a central white core.

12. A 6-year-old girl has several areas of thickened skin over the dorsal region of the first through third toes on both feet. The areas occasionally itch. The involved skin is mildly erythematous; the skin of the interdigital webs appears normal. Her mother states that the rash has been present for about 3 months. They have topical medicine at home for the child's atopic dermatitis and mupirocin left over from her brother's bout of impetigo, but they have not applied any medicine or emollients to date. This child's rash is most likely to respond to which of the following agents?
A) Topical mupirocin
B) Topical triamcinolone
C) Topical ketoconazole
D) Topical clotrimazole
E) Oral terbinafine hydrochloride

13. A 3-year-old boy is brought to the clinic by his mother for a follow-up visit. He was clinically diagnosed with tinea corporis 3 weeks ago and prescribed a topical antifungal agent. When compared with the description from the previous visit, the 2.5-cm diameter annular lesion on his left thigh consisting of an area of central clearing ringed with small, distinct papules appears to be unchanged in size and appearance. This patient's condition is most consistent with which of the following?
A) Resistant tinea corporis
B) Partially treated tinea corporis
C) Granuloma annulare
D) Atopic dermatitis
E) Psoriasis

14. A 15-year-old boy who is an outdoor lifeguard is in your office for evaluation of a skin condition. He has noticed light-colored oval lesions on his back and shoulders for the past 6 weeks. The involved areas are covered with a fine scale and coalesce across his upper back. A potassium hydroxide preparation is made with scrapings from the scale of one of the ovals. Which of the following are you most likely to see upon microscopic examination of the specimen?
A) Normal stratum corneum
B) Ruptured cells with inclusion bodies
C) Branching fungal hyphae; no spores
D) Short fungal hyphae and spores resembling "spaghetti and meatballs"
E) Multinucleated giant cells

15. A 4-year-old boy presents to the clinic with a chief complaint of hair loss. The examination reveals an 8-cm diameter scaly area of hair loss located in the left parieto-occipital region. The affected skin contains hair shafts broken off at the scalp. Lymph nodes are palpable in the left occipital and posterior cervical regions. Which of the following is the most appropriate treatment for this child's hair loss?
A) 2.5% selenium sulfide shampoo applied daily for 10 minutes and then rinsed away, for 2 weeks
B) 1% selenium sulfide shampoo applied daily for 10 minutes and then rinsed away, for 2 weeks
C) Topical ketoconazole twice a day until the rash has resolved, then daily for 1 additional week
D) Oral griseofulvin daily for 2 weeks
E) Oral griseofulvin daily for 6 weeks

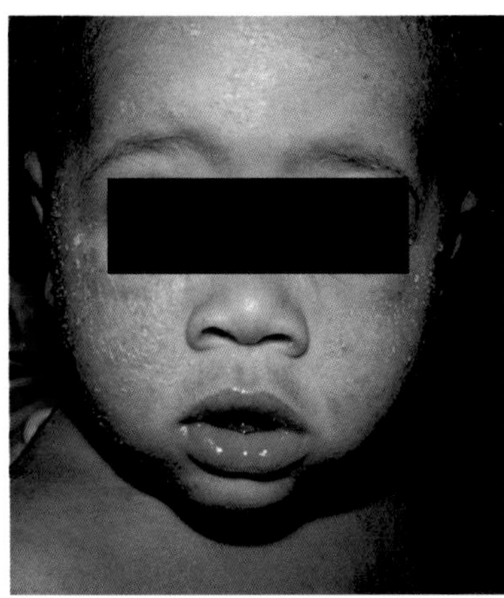

Figure 9-1 Atopic dermatitis in an infant. (From Goodheart HP. *Goodheart's Photoguide of Common Skin Disorders: Diagnosis and Management*. 2nd ed. Philadelphia: Lippincott Williams & Wilkins; 2003 with permission.) (This figure appears in black and white on page 116.)

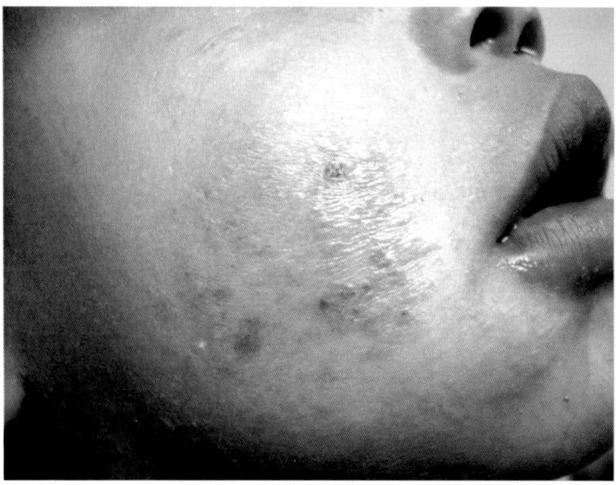

Figure 20-1 Atopic dermatitis in the infant: multiple grouped erythematous papules with associated scaling. (Courtesy of Paul S. Matz, MD, from Chung EK. *Visual Diagnosis in Pediatrics*. Philadelphia: Lippincott Williams & Wilkins; 2006:20.) (This figure appears in black and white on page 366.)

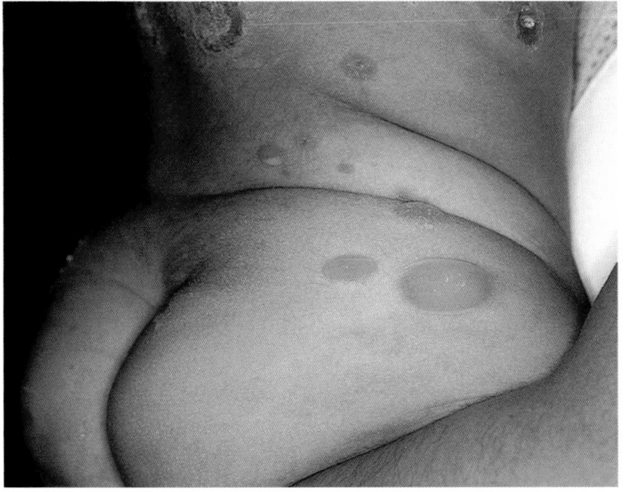

Figure 20-2 Bullous impetigo: large, clear bullae rupture, leaving remnants in a ring-shaped lesion around a central crusted sore. (From Fleisher GR. *Atlas of Pediatric Emergency Medicine*. Philadelphia: Lippincott Williams & Wilkins; 2003 with permission.) (This figure appears in black and white on page 366.)

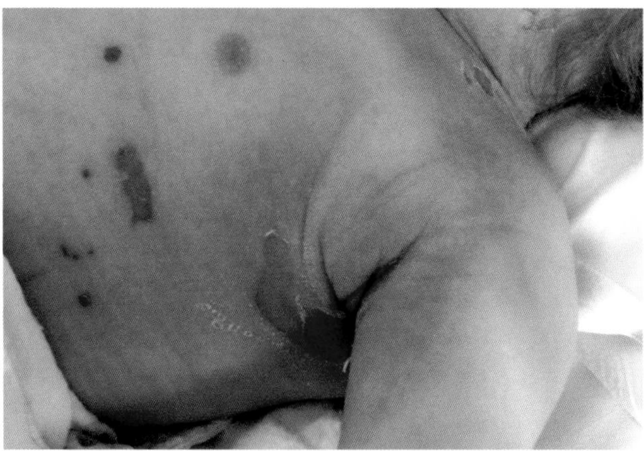

Figure 20-3 Staphylococcal scalded skin syndrome: a toxin-mediated reaction characterized by widespread epidermal erythema and blistering. (Courtesy of Gary Marshall, MD, from Chung EK. *Visual Diagnosis in Pediatrics*. Philadelphia: Lippincott Williams & Wilkins; 2006:480.) (This figure appears in black and white on page 367.)

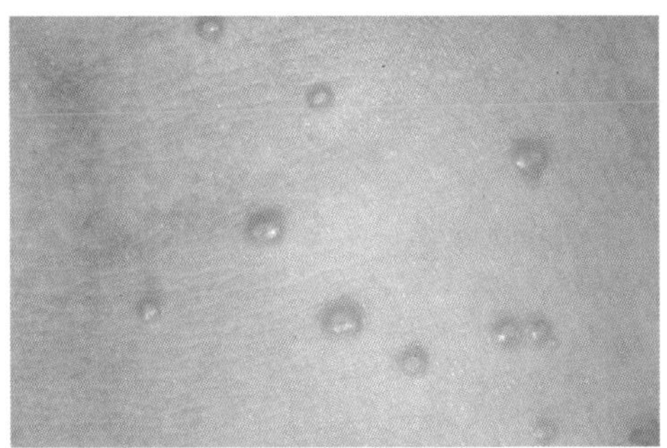

Figure 20-4 Molluscum contagiosum: pearly white dome-shaped lesions with central umbilication, ranging from 1 to 5 mm in diameter. (From Goodheart HP. *Goodheart's Photoguide of Common Skin Disorders: Diagnosis and Management*. 2nd ed. Philadelphia: Lippincott Williams & Wilkins; 2003:138 with permission.) (This figure appears in black and white on page 368.)

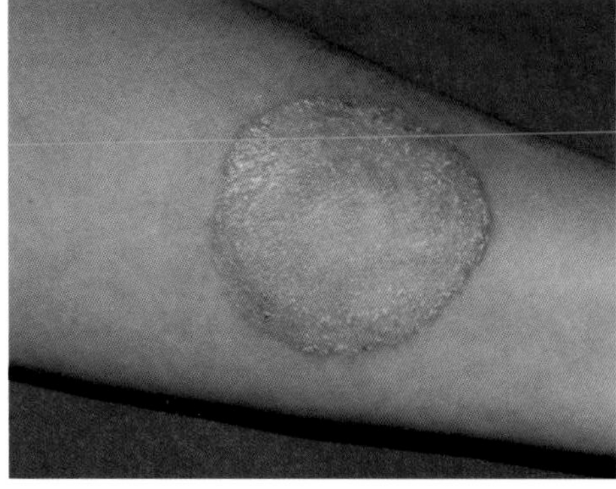

Figure 20-5 Tinea corporis: annular lesion with erythematous, scaling, well-demarcated borders and central clearing. (From Goodheart HP. *Goodheart's Photoguide of Common Skin Disorders: Diagnosis and Management*. 2nd ed. Philadelphia: Lippincott Williams & Wilkins; 2003:303 with permission.) (This figure appears in black and white on page 368.)

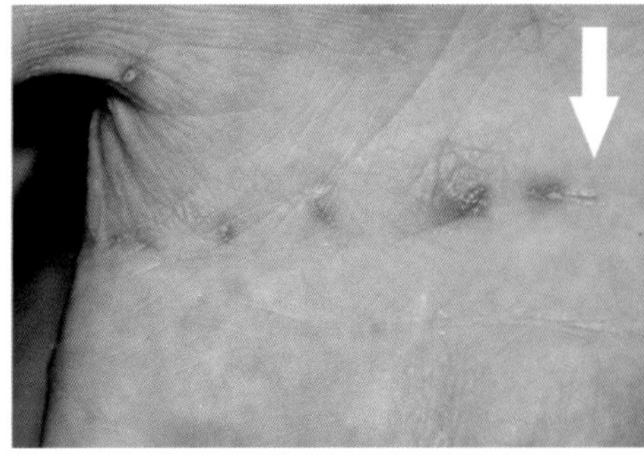

Figure 20-6 Scabies: papular lesions in a linear distribution across the palm with a visible linear burrow. (From Goodheart HP. *Goodheart's Photoguide of Common Skin Disorders: Diagnosis and Management*. 2nd ed. Philadelphia: Lippincott Williams & Wilkins; 2003:305 with permission.) (This figure appears in black and white on page 369.)

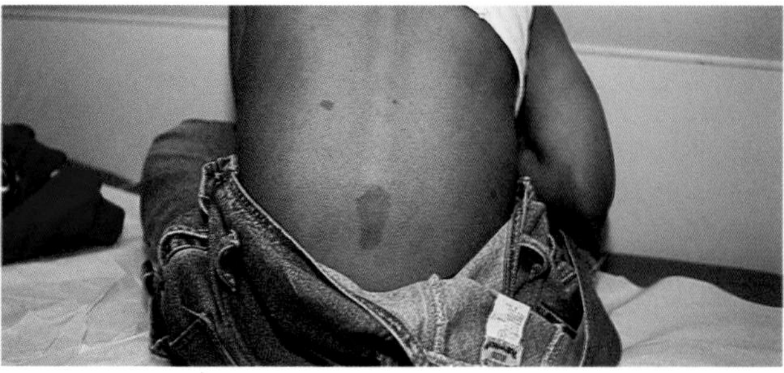

Figure 20-7 Café-au-lait spots: flat, nonpalpable hyperpigmented macules. (From Chung EK. *Visual Diagnosis in Pediatrics*. Philadelphia: Lippincott Williams & Wilkins; 2006:473 with permission.) (This figure appears in black and white on page 370.)

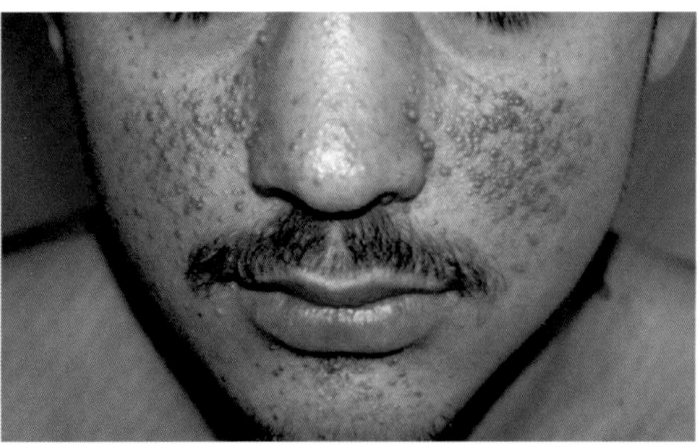

Figure 20-8 Angiofibromas: raised red papules in a patient with tuberous sclerosis. (From Goodheart HP. *Goodheart's Photoguide of Common Skin Disorders: Diagnosis and Management*. 2nd ed. Philadelphia: Lippincott Williams & Wilkins; 2003 with permission.) (This figure appears in black and white on page 371.)

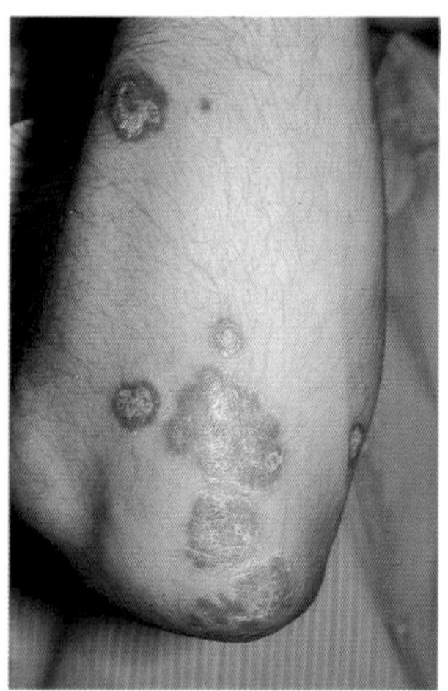

Figure 20-9 Psoriasis: well-demarcated, round or oval plaques with overlying thick, white, adherent scales. (From Goodheart HP. *Goodheart's Photoguide of Common Skin Disorders: Diagnosis and Management*. 2nd ed. Philadelphia: Lippincott Williams & Wilkins; 2003:54 with permission.) (This figure appears in black and white on page 373.)

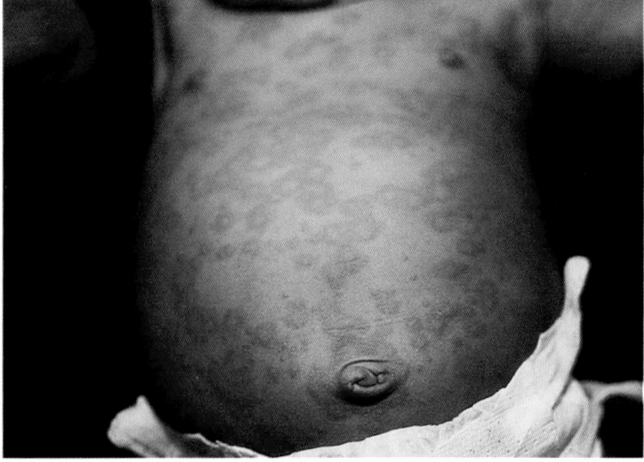

Figure 20-10 Erythema multiforme: "target lesions" (dusky-colored bullae 5 to 10 mm in diameter, each surrounded by an erythematous ring). (From Chung EK. *Visual Diagnosis in Pediatrics*. Philadelphia: Lippincott Williams & Wilkins; 2006:434 with permission.) (This figure appears in black and white on page 373.)

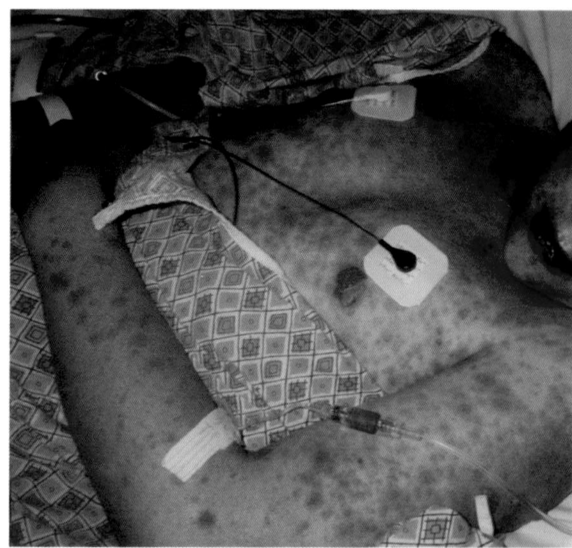

Figure 20-11 Stevens-Johnson syndrome: widespread epidermal erythema and purpuric lesions; note the hemorrhagic crusting of the oral mucosa. (From Chung EK. *Visual Diagnosis in Pediatrics*. Philadelphia: Lippincott Williams & Wilkins; 2006:481 with permission.) (This figure appears in black and white on page 374.)

16. A 3-year-old girl presents with an area of hair loss located behind her right ear. The involved skin contains hair of varying lengths and has indistinct borders; scale and lymphadenopathy are absent. The child refuses to allow her hair to be tied back in a ponytail when she goes to school or bed, although she will wear a barrette in the front of her hair. This child's hair loss is most likely due to which of the following?
A) Trichotillomania
B) Tinea capitis
C) Kerion of the scalp
D) Alopecia areata
E) Telogen effluvium

17. A 2-week-old infant with mastitis presents with widespread erythema and blistering of the epidermis. A Nikolsky sign is present. Blood is obtained for laboratory studies and culture. Fluid from a lumbar puncture is clear, with three white blood cells and no organisms on Gram stain. Which of the following is the most appropriate empiric antibiotic choice for this infant?
A) Oral cephalexin
B) Intravenous cefazolin
C) Oral clindamycin
D) Intravenous ceftazidime
E) Intravenous imipenem

18. An 8-year-old boy presents to the emergency department for management of a dog bite to the face. The wound is appropriately cleansed and repaired. Tetanus immune status is addressed, and the dog is located by Animal Control authorities. The patient has no known drug allergies. Which of the following is indicated for prophylaxis against wound infection in this child?
A) Oral clindamycin
B) Oral trimethoprim-sulfamethoxazole
C) Oral amoxicillin-clavulanic acid
D) Oral cephalexin
E) Prophylaxis is not indicated in this patient.

19. An 8-year-old girl presents to the emergency department for management of a cat bite on her left hand. The wound is appropriately cleansed and treated. Tetanus immune status is addressed, and the cat is located by Animal Control authorities. The girl is allergic to penicillin. Which of the following is indicated for prophylaxis against wound infection in this child?
A) Oral amoxicillin-clavulanic acid
B) Oral trimethoprim-sulfamethoxazole
C) Oral clindamycin
D) Oral clindamycin and oral trimethoprim-sulfamethoxazole
E) Intravenous clindamycin and oral trimethoprim-sulfamethoxazole

20. A 6-year-old boy visiting his grandfather's farm sustains a puncture wound to his left thigh from a rusty nail on a fencepost. The boy's mother cleansed and irrigated the wound as best she could and treated it with topical over-the-counter antibiotic cream. Five days later, the mother brings the child to the emergency department, where he is diagnosed with cellulitis and admitted to the hospital for intravenous nafcillin. Forty-eight hours later, the infection appears clinically unchanged, and the patient becomes febrile to 39.0°C. This patient's infection is most likely due to which of the following organisms?
A) *Streptococcus viridans*
B) Group A beta-hemolytic *Streptococcus*
C) *Pasteurella multocida*
D) *Eikenella* species
E) *Pseudomonas aeruginosa*

21. Which of the following conditions is not a recognized complication of infection with group A beta-hemolytic *Streptococcus*?
A) Scalded skin syndrome
B) Toxic shock syndrome
C) Necrotizing fasciitis
D) Postinfectious glomerulonephritis
E) All of the above are recognized complications of infection with group A beta-hemolytic *Streptococcus*.

22. A mother brings her 3-year-old son to the clinic for evaluation of his spreading rash. He was well until 3 days ago, when she noticed a few small fluid-filled bumps on his left arm. Later in the afternoon, the bumps were replaced by thick, honey-colored scabs. The scab-covered lesions are now spreading along his left arm; several new sores have also appeared on his right thigh. The child is afebrile and is acting well. Your examination of the child is consistent with the mother's description, with a total involved area of about 36 cm^2. Which of the following is the most appropriate initial therapy for the child's lesions?
A) Over-the-counter antibiotic ointment twice a day for 10 to 14 days
B) Prescription mupirocin ointment two to three times a day for 7 to 10 days
C) Over-the-counter clotrimazole ointment twice a day for 10 to 14 days
D) Prescription ketoconazole ointment twice a day for 10 to 14 days
E) Over-the-counter hydrocortisone ointment twice a day for 10 to 14 days

23. A 7-year-old boy is in your office for his routine health maintenance visit. His examination is significant for seven hyperpigmented macules scattered over his trunk, back, and extremities. All are >0.5 cm in diameter. Axillary freckling is noted bilaterally. This patient's

skin findings are most consistent with which of the following conditions?
A) Neurofibromatosis type 2
B) Peutz-Jeghers syndrome
C) von Recklinghausen disease
D) Crohn disease
E) Tuberous sclerosis

24. A 3-year-old boy born to a father with neurofibromatosis type 1 now has six café-au-lait spots, each of which is >0.5 cm in diameter. Which of the following is not a recognized feature of this child's disorder?
A) An increased incidence of tibial dysplasia within the first year of life
B) An increased risk of scoliosis
C) The appearance of Lisch nodules prior to the development of neurofibromas
D) The appearance of multiple neurofibromas prior to the age of 4 years
E) An increased risk of optic gliomas

25. You are called to the newborn nursery to examine a newborn who will be joining your practice. The mother tells you that there is a family history of tuberous sclerosis and asks you if there is a way to tell whether the baby is affected. You are correct in telling the mother which of the following?
A) The diagnosis of tuberous sclerosis cannot be made until central nervous system tumors develop later in childhood.
B) The diagnosis of tuberous sclerosis cannot be made until Lisch nodules are noted on the iris after the first year of life.
C) The diagnosis of tuberous sclerosis can be reliably excluded if the patient does not have a shagreen patch at birth.
D) The diagnosis of tuberous sclerosis can be reliably excluded if the patient has a normal head circumference at birth.
E) Ninety percent of newborns affected with tuberous sclerosis have at least one ash-leaf spot at birth.

26. A 5-month-old patient has just been diagnosed with infantile spasms based on the clinical appearance of his seizures and characteristic hypsarrhythmia on electroencephalogram. Which of the following is the most appropriate next study in the evaluation of this patient?
A) Examination of the infant's skin under a Wood lamp
B) Echocardiography
C) Electrocardiogram
D) Renal sonogram
E) Computed tomography of the head with intravenous contrast

27. A 9-month-old boy is brought to your office by his parents for evaluation of his "bug bites." The parents tell you that the boy has numerous bites on his trunk, back, legs, and arms, which initially look like blisters but eventually turn brown and "freckle." The child's examination is significant for a well-nourished, well-developed male with multiple small, blotchy, pigmented macules scattered about his trunk and back. The lesions wheal and flare when stroked by the examiner. Dermatographism is present as well. This child's skin findings are most indicative of which of the following?
A) Skin allergies
B) Urticaria pigmentosa
C) Food allergies
D) Lichen planus
E) Lichen striatus

28. Documented early warning signs of malignant melanoma in a pigmented cutaneous lesion include all of the following EXCEPT:
A) Asymmetry of the lesion
B) Diameter of the lesion >6 mm
C) Bleeding from the lesion
D) Border of the lesion that is irregular and/or notched
E) Presence of multiple colors of pigment within the lesion

29. A father and mother bring their 6-week-old daughter to your office for evaluation of a red mass on her arm that is rapidly enlarging. The area of skin appeared normal at birth; the parents first noted the enlarging bright-red bump when the girl was 2 weeks old. The physical examination is significant for a well-nourished, well-developed, content infant with a palpable, 2.5 cm in diameter, bright-red, compressible mass on her left upper arm that does not interfere with range of motion. Which of the following is the most appropriate initial management of this patient's mass?
A) Biopsy under local anesthesia
B) Biopsy under general anesthesia
C) Intravenous solumedrol
D) Observation
E) Oral prednisone

30. A 2-month-old boy has a strawberry hemangioma involving his right upper eyelid that is enlarging and threatening his field of vision. Which of the following is the most appropriate initial management of this patient's tumor?
A) Observation
B) Vascular-specific pulsed dye laser therapy
C) Surgical excision
D) Serial intralesional steroid injections
E) A course of oral steroids

31. A 7-year-old boy who is well-known to your practice (microcephaly, poor academic achievement, and refractory seizures) presents for evaluation of his "pimples." The skin examination is significant for multiple small erythematous papules scattered across his cheeks and also located in the nasolabial folds. No comedones are present. This child's skin lesions are most likely to consist of which of the following?
A) Sebaceous adenoma
B) Acne vulgaris
C) Gram-negative folliculitis
D) Keratosis pilaris
E) Rosacea

32. Oral antibiotic therapy is indicated for which of the following patients?
A) A 15-year-old girl with moderate inflammatory acne involving the face
B) A 15-year-old girl with inflammatory acne involving the face, shoulders, and back
C) A 15-year-old girl with moderate comedonal acne involving the face
D) A and B
E) A, B, and C

33. A previously well 6-year-old boy with a recent episode of "fever blisters" presents with a rash of 4 days in duration. His mother denies any history of fever, nausea, vomiting, changes in appetite, cough, or headache. Vital signs are stable in the office. The physical examination is significant for a well-nourished, well-developed, cooperative child in no acute distress. He has two small erosive lesions on his left buccal mucosa and one on his right; when questioned, he admits that "they hurt a little bit." Multiple erythematous macules 5 to 10 mm in diameter are concentrated on his hands and feet, with inclusion of the palms and soles; most of the lesions are dusky in color and surrounded by an erythematous ring. This patient's rash is most consistent with which of the following?
A) Bullous impetigo
B) Eczema herpeticum
C) Erythema multiforme
D) Stevens-Johnson syndrome
E) Toxic epidermal necrolysis

34. A 15-year-old girl diagnosed last week with "walking pneumonia" presents today with fever, mouth pain, and difficulty eating. She finished her azithromycin 4 days ago, about the same time that she developed her mouth sores and diarrhea. Her temperature in the office is 39.0°C; vitals are otherwise stable. Her examination is significant for an uncomfortable-appearing adolescent female with obvious conjunctival injection; extensive erosive lesions of the oral and labial mucosa; and many dusky macules 5 to 10 mm in diameter scattered over her face, hands, feet, and the extensor surfaces of her arms and legs. Many are surrounded by an erythematous ring, and a few have necrotic centers. This patient's illness is most consistent with which of the following?
A) Inadequately-treated *Mycoplasma pneumoniae* infection
B) Stevens-Johnson syndrome
C) Disseminated *Mycoplasma pneumoniae* infection
D) *Neisseria meningitidis* sepsis
E) Rocky Mountain spotted fever

35. You are "on call" for your practice over the July 4th weekend when a mother calls you because she found her son playing in a natural area that contained a plant she thinks is poison ivy. You would advise her of all of the following EXCEPT:
A) Contact with poison ivy following initial sensitization produces a characteristic contact dermatitis consisting of intensely pruritic linear vesicles and papules.
B) Washing the child's skin with soap and water may prevent or lessen the severity of the rash.
C) The child's clothes should be washed in order to remove any residual urushiol.
D) Oral prednisone is reserved for patients with extensive or severe contact dermatitis and those with involvement of sensitive areas.
E) The child should be isolated from other children as the vesicles rupture because the fluid within the vesicles can sensitize others to poison ivy.

36. A mother brings her 3-year-old son to your office for evaluation of his chronic dry skin. The child was diagnosed with atopic dermatitis in infancy that is currently controlled with daily application of emollients; moderate-potency topical steroids are added during exacerbations. However, even when his eczema is well controlled, the skin of his legs and buttocks is covered with a mosaic of fine, dry scales. This patient's condition is most consistent with which of the following?
A) Ichthyosis vulgaris
B) Misdiagnosis of eczema
C) Vitamin E deficiency
D) Acrodermatitis enteropathica
E) Psoriasis

37. A 5-year-old patient with atopic dermatitis who uses emollients daily is in your office for evaluation of his chronic rash. You diagnose him with ichthyosis vulgaris. Which of the following topical agents is most appropriate for initial therapy of this patient's ichthyosis vulgaris?
A) Moderate-potency topical steroids
B) Lactic acid or another alpha-hydroxy acid–containing agent
C) Mupirocin
D) Tacrolimus
E) Tretinoin

38. A 12-year-old boy is brought to your office by his parents for evaluation of his rash. His mother states that he has had "dry knees and elbows" for the past year. Over the past 2 months, he has developed thick white "scabs" on his knees and elbows that do not respond to topical emollients. The examination is significant for a well-appearing, cooperative child with plaques over the extensor surfaces of his knees and elbows ranging from 3 to 5 cm in diameter. Removal of the thick, white, adherent scale results in pinpoint hemorrhaging. Similar lesions are noted behind both ears. This patient's rash is most consistent with which of the following?

A) Ichthyosis vulgaris
B) Atopic dermatitis
C) Psoriasis
D) Nummular eczema
E) Tinea corporis

39. A 16-year-old patient presents with hundreds of slightly scaly, 1- to 2-cm, salmon-colored oval macules covering his chest, back, abdomen, and thighs. The longitudinal axes of the ovals seem run parallel to dermatomal skin lines. Which of the following is the most appropriate initial laboratory test in the evaluation of this patient's condition?

A) No further evaluation is necessary for this patient's benign, self-limited dermatitis.
B) Monospot and Epstein-Barr virus titers
C) Human immunodeficiency virus (HIV) enzyme-linked immunosorbent assay (ELISA)
D) Nontreponemal tests for *Treponema pallidum*
E) Serum antibody titers to *Borrelia burgdorferi*

ANSWERS

1. A	14. D	27. B
2. B	15. E	28. C
3. C	16. A	29. D
4. D	17. B	30. E
5. E	18. C	31. A
6. A	19. D	32. D
7. C	20. E	33. C
8. B	21. A	34. B
9. C	22. B	35. E
10. E	23. C	36. A
11. A	24. D	37. B
12. B	25. E	38. C
13. C	26. A	39. D

21 Collagen, Vascular, and Other Multisystem Diseases

SYSTEMIC LUPUS ERYTHEMATOSUS

Systemic lupus erythematosus (SLE) is a multisystem autoimmune disorder characterized by widespread connective tissue inflammation and arteriolar vasculitis. SLE develops when autoantibodies are elaborated against various nuclear proteins, cytoplasmic contents, and connective tissue. Antigen-antibody immune complexes become deposited in the walls of small arteries, resulting in inflammation and necrosis. This *immune complex vasculitis* is the basic pathologic lesion responsible for the extensive and variable multiorgan clinical manifestations of SLE.

SLE is uncommon in children, usually presenting after the second decade of life. The peak incidence of SLE in the pediatric population occurs during early adolescence. The disorder is far more common in females. Black and Hispanic patients tend to have more severe disease.

The diagnosis of SLE is based on clinical criteria (Table 21-1). Disease onset may be insidious or acute and rapidly progressive. Fever, malaise, and weight loss are frequent constitutional complaints. Skin findings are present in 80% of affected adolescents, the most frequent being the characteristic erythematous maculopapular eruption over the cheeks and nose in a *malar* or "butterfly" distribution, with sparing of the nasolabial folds. *Discoid* lesions are initially erythematous but eventually atrophy and scar. They can be widespread but are often localized to the face and scalp, where they result in hair loss. Patients with lupus frequently develop papulosquamous lesions on the dorsa of the hands that arise *between* the knuckles. Arthritis of the hands, wrists, elbows, shoulders, knees, and ankles produces pain out of proportion to physical findings; in fact, the arthritis of SLE is neither erosive nor deforming. Central nervous system involvement may present at any time over the course of the disease.

TABLE 21-1
DIAGNOSTIC CRITERIA FOR SYSTEMIC LUPUS ERYTHEMATOSUS (SLE)*

Four of 11 criteria must be met for the diagnosis of SLE:

- Malar (butterfly) rash
- Discoid lupus rash
- Photosensitivity
- Oral ulcerations
- Arthritis
- Renal disorder (hematuria, proteinuria)
- Neurologic disorder
- Serositis
- Hematologic disorder (anemia, leukopenia, thrombocytopenia)
- Immunologic disorder (anti-dsDNA, anti-Smith, antiphospholipid antibodies)
- Antinuclear antibody test

*American College of Rheumatology 1982; revised 1997.

Lupus nephritis is usually present at diagnosis. Renal involvement is classsified as normal (type I, 6%, renal failure extremely rare), mesangial (type II, 20%, renal failure rare), focal proliferative (type III, 23%, renal failure uncommon), diffuse proliferative (type IV, 40%, progressive renal failure common, high mortality), and membranous disease (type V, renal failure uncommon).

SLE should be considered in any patient with unexplained fevers and multiple organ system involvement, arthritis, or nephritis. It is also part of the differential for all cases of new-onset heart block, especially those occurring among females who have a family history of SLE. Lupus may resemble acute rheumatic fever if specific criteria are present [arthritis, carditis, prolonged PR interval, fever, elevated erythrocyte sedimentation rate (ESR)]; however, evidence of an antecedent group A streptococcal infection is lacking. Cutaneous findings in juvenile dermatomyositis are very similar to those in SLE, but in the former, characteristic inflammatory changes (*Grotton papules*) overlie the knuckles on the dorsa of the hands.

When a rheumatologic disorder such as SLE is suspected based on clinical presentation, a serum antinuclear antibody (ANA) titer should be obtained. Many healthy individuals are low-level ANA positive, particularly females and family members of those with positive titers. Thus, ANA should not be used as a screening tool to identify connective tissue or autoimmune disease in healthy individuals. In the absence of characteristic findings (fever, rash, photosensitivity, alopecia, mucous membrane lesions, serositis, arthritis), ANA testing has no role in detecting an asymptomatic condition. Furthermore, the presence of a measurable ANA titer does not confer additional risk for the development of subsequent connective tissue disease. The ANA is often positive in other rheumatologic and nonrheumatologic disorders such as sclerosis, dermatomyositis, psoriasis, viral infections, tuberculosis, idiopathic thrombocytopenic purpura, and autoimmune hepatitis.

Disease severity is quantified through clinical data and serologic markers, particularly complement levels. Anemia, leukopenia, and thrombocytopenia are characteristic. Complement levels, including C3 and C4 are generally depressed or decreasing, especially during active disease. Anti-Smith antibody is very specific for lupus but is only present in approximately one third of affected patients. Elevation in the level of double-stranded DNA antibody correlates with renal involvement. Antiphospholipid antibodies include anticardiolipin antibodies and lupus anticoagulants, which are associated with an increased risk of thrombosis despite prolonging the in vitro partial thromboplastin time. Circulating anti-Ro/SS-A and anti-La/SS-B antibodies in an SLE-affected mother may cause neonatal lupus syndrome and complete congenital heart block in her fetus.

Treatment is long term, multifactorial, and dependent on the specific organs affected and severity of disease. Careful attention must be paid to nutritional status and fluid balance. Limiting sun exposure and using appropriate sun block improve skin conditions. Aggressive characterization and treatment of kidney disease, including biopsy and frequent imaging, are invaluable in minimizing renal morbidity. Hypertension is a relatively common complication that is usually well controlled with conventional therapy.

Anti-inflammatory therapy remains the mainstay of pharmacologic treatment. Oral prednisone is prescribed as needed for maintenance therapy; high-dose oral or intravenous pulse therapy (methylprednisolone) is preferable during acute exacerbations. Methotrexate or cyclophosphamide may be beneficial as steroid-sparing maintenance therapy in many patients. Patients with SLE who require chronic systemic or high-dose pulse corticosteroid therapy are at risk for the development of avascular necrosis, which usually involves the femoral head. Other major complications of corticosteroid therapy are detailed in Chapter 30.

Overall, prognosis and quality of life are improving; currently, the majority of patients with SLE have good long-term survival and normal or near-normal function. Renal disease is the most significant sequela; renal failure is the leading cause of death after infection. Libman-Sacks endocarditis is a serious cardiac complication. Central nervous system disease, when present, is associated with slow but progressive deterioration in mental capacity.

VASCULITIC SYNDROMES

Henoch-Schönlein Purpura

Henoch-Schönlein purpura (HSP) is an immunoglobulin A (IgA)-mediated vasculitis involving the skin, gastrointestinal tract, joints, and kidneys. It is most common in children 3 to 10 years of age, peaks in the winter months, and is often preceded by a viral or group A streptococcal upper respiratory infection. The characteristic nonthrombocytopenic palpable purpuric rash is the most classic and consistent sign of HSP. The lesions begin as macules and papules, develop primarily in dependent areas (the buttocks and legs), and may be accompanied by edema. Gastrointestinal involvement is usually significant, including diffuse colicky abdominal pain (out of proportion to physical signs), vomiting, diarrhea, and occult or obvious lower tract bleeding. Vague abdominal complaints may precede the rash by several weeks. Intussusception is the most common serious gastrointestinal complication of HSP. Arthritis or arthralgia, particularly of the knees and ankles, occurs in the majority of patients and may also precede the rash. Approximately half of patients develop self-limited glomerulonephritis, which may present as many as 3 months after the onset of the rash. Patients with isolated hematuria typically regain normal renal function. The presence of proteinuria portends a worse prognosis; a larger proportion of these patients develop irreversible changes in renal function that may progress to chronic renal failure. Renal biopsy reveals deposition of IgA complexes in the mesangial cells of the kidney. The diagnosis of HSP is based on clinical course and findings. An abnormal platelet count suggests other diagnoses (e.g., idiopathic thrombocytopenic purpura). Treatment is symptomatic and supportive; corticosteroids may be helpful if gastrointestinal symptoms and renal involvement are severe, but there is no conclusive evidence that their use lessens the duration or severity of the disease. The prognosis for full recovery within 4 to 12 weeks is excellent. Long-term complications parallel the severity of renal involvement. HSP may recur over the following months or years, with subsequent episodes being significantly milder.

Kawasaki Syndrome

Kawasaki disease is a systemic vasculitis of medium-sized blood vessels characterized by high fever, lymphadenopathy, and mucocutaneous lesions. It occurs almost exclusively in infants and young children and is more common in males. An infectious etiology (*Coronavirus*) has been suggested but not confirmed. Current criteria for diagnosis are noted in Table 21-2. Children with Kawasaki syndrome are typically very irritable (more so than would be expected given their symptoms), with temperatures as high as 40°C. The rash is composed of many polymorphous 1- to 2-cm lesions that cover the trunk and proximal extremities; the entire skin surface below the neck may be involved. The rash desquamates within days. Fever, rash, lymphadenopathy, and lesions of the lips and mouth arise during the first week (*acute febrile phase*); coronary aneurysms may develop over the next few weeks (*subacute phase*), and the disease resolves over 2 to 3 months (*convalescent phase*).

Kawasaki disease is a clinical diagnosis. Other conditions that may present in a similar manner include several

TABLE 21-2
CRITERIA FOR DIAGNOSIS OF KAWASAKI DISEASE

Unexplained fever for 5 days or more, together with four of the following five signs on physical examination (or by history):

1. Bilateral, nonexudative conjunctival injection
2. Changes of lips and oral cavity (dry, red, fissured lips; injected pharynx; or strawberry tongue)
3. Changes of peripheral extremities (erythema or indurative edema of hands and feet; periungal desquamation)
4. Polymorphous rash (primarily on trunk)
5. Acute nonsuppurative enlargement of at least one cervical lymph node to ≥1.5 cm in diameter

infectious diseases (measles, scarlet fever, toxic shock syndrome, and Rocky Mountain spotted fever), Stevens-Johnson syndrome, and juvenile idiopathic arthritis. The broad differential and marked irritability of the patient often lead to extensive laboratory assessment. Leukocytosis, thrombocytosis, elevation of the ESR, and sterile pyuria are consistent with Kawasaki disease. Cerebrospinal fluid, if obtained, may be normal but more often demonstrates isolated mononuclear pleocytosis.

Acquired cardiovascular pathology is the most serious long-term consequence of Kawasaki disease. Twenty-five percent of untreated patients are affected, as well as up to 5% of those who receive early and appropriate care. Overall prognosis is tied to severity of cardiac involvement. Myocardial instability may be associated with arrhythmias, infarction, or congestive heart failure within days of presentation. Aneurysms and coronary artery disease persist and may result in sudden cardiac death months to years later. Echocardiography performed at diagnosis permits detailed evaluation of the myocardium, valves, and arteries, serving as a baseline for comparison with future studies. Restriction of athletic activities is recommended based on residual coronary artery involvement (Table 21-3).

The two primary goals of management are reducing inflammation and preventing formation of coronary artery aneurysms. Intravenous immunoglobulin (IVIG) therapy results in rapid and profound improvement and significantly reduces the risk of coronary artery aneurysms. High-dose oral aspirin is administered until several days after the resolution of fever; low-dose aspirin is continued thereafter until the end of the convalescent phase. It can safely be discontinued after this time provided coronary artery architecture remains normal. Patients with persistent aneurysms should continue aspirin therapy indefinitely.

TABLE 21-3
RESTRICTION OF ATHLETIC ACTIVITY IN PATIENTS WITH A HISTORY OF KAWASAKI DISEASE

No coronary involvement—no restriction

Minor residual abnormalities—low static, moderate dynamic sports only

Persistent coronary aneurysm or stenosis—low-intensity competitive sports only

Intermittent exercise-induced myocardial ischemia—competitive sports prohibited

JUVENILE IDIOPATHIC ARTHRITIS

Juvenile idiopathic arthritis [JIA; formerly termed juvenile rheumatoid arthritis (JRA)] consists of a group of loosely related immunologic disorders characterized by *chronic synovitis*. As is true of most rheumatologic conditions, JIA occurs more commonly in girls. Individuals with a positive family history of autoimmune disorders are at increased risk for JIA. Certain human leukocyte antigen (HLA) types are more closely associated with specific forms of disease (e.g., HLA-DR4 with severe, erosive arthritis). Tests for rheumatoid factor are usually negative in patients with JIA.

The International League Against Rheumatism has established the following criteria for the diagnosis of JIA:

- Age younger than 16 years at onset of disease
- Objective signs of arthritis (limited range of motion, tenderness or pain with motion, increased warmth) in at least one joint for >6 consecutive weeks
- Exclusion of other causes of arthritis (infection, reactive arthritis, mechanical abnormality, inherited diseases, malignancy, and other rheumatic or connective tissue disorders)

Noteworthy clinical manifestations are listed in Table 21-4.

TABLE 21-4
SIGNS AND SYMPTOMS SUGGESTIVE OF JUVENILE IDIOPATHIC ARTHRITIS

Joint-Related Symptoms	Systemic Manifestations
Morning stiffness	Asymptomatic uveitis (in oligoarticular and polyarticular JIA)
Gelling (stiffness after inactivity)	Fatigue
Guarding	Anorexia
Deformity	Failure to thrive
	Rash
	Irritability
	Lymphadenopathy
	Hepatosplenomegaly
	Pericarditis

Systemic JIA constitutes approximately 10% of all cases, occurs equally in both genders, and peaks in onset between 1 and 6 years of age. It presents with daily or twice-daily brief, high, spiking fevers accompanied by a faint, blanching, evanescent pink or salmon-colored rash. These children appear quite ill during the febrile episodes but are otherwise asymptomatic. Lymphadenopathy and hepatosplenomegaly are often present at diagnosis; 30% will have pericarditis. These systemic symptoms may precede the onset of arthritis by weeks to months. Elevated white blood cell and platelet counts, anemia, and a high sedimentation rate are characteristic. Tests for ANA and rheumatoid factor are generally negative; serum ferritin levels are high. Systemic JIA is *not* associated with chronic uveitis. Approximately half of affected individuals experience complete resolution of disease within a year of diagnosis; a significant minority of the others develops severe destructive arthritis despite abatement of systemic symptoms.

Oligoarticular JRA accounts for approximately 5% of cases of childhood idiopathic arthritis. Girls outnumber boys in a ratio of 4:1. The arthritis most commonly affects large joints such as the knees and ankles, causing the child to ambulate with a limp that is most pronounced upon rising in the morning. Approximately 70% patients with oligoarticular JRA will go into remission after several years of active arthritis. Oligoarticular JRA is currently subdivided into two distinct categories:

- In *persistent oligoarthritis*, four or fewer joints are involved over the course of illness. This form is most common in girls between 1 and 5 years of age. Patients are usually ANA positive and have a high risk of developing chronic uveitis.
- *Extended oligoarthritis* is less common than the persistent form. Symptoms develop in more than four joints during the first 6 months of disease. These patients are typically rheumatoid factor–positive adolescents. Erosive joint changes similar to those seen with adult disease may occur. Radiographs show soft tissue swelling early; later, narrowing of the joint spaces occurs; and finally, bony erosions appear.

Lyme disease in particular may mimic oligoarthritic JIA; other conditions to consider include Legg-Calvé-Perthes disease, toxic synovitis, and septic arthritis. Joint aspiration is helpful in differentiating JIA from septic arthritis; in the latter, the white blood cell count of the aspirated fluid is typically >50,000 per μL, with a marked predominance of neutrophils. In JIA, synovial fluid analysis reveals a much lower white blood cell count (5,000 to 30,000/μL).

Polyarteritis (formerly called polyarticular JRA) involves five or more joints within the first 6 months of disease. Girls predominate, with a ratio of 3:1. Joint involvement may include small and large joints as well as the temporomandibular joint and cervical vertebrae. Rheumatoid factor may be present, usually in adolescents, who go on to develop disease similar to adult rheumatoid arthritis. Those without rheumatoid factor have a better prognosis; half will eventually go into remission. Fewer patients are ANA positive, but those who are positive are at risk for uveitis.

Uveitis, also called iritis or iridocyclitis, is inflammation of any of the structures of the anterior chamber of the eye. *Synechia* is defined as adhesion between the iris and either the cornea or lens due to chronic inflammation; it manifests as an irregular pupil. Other possible complications of chronic uveitis include cataracts and glaucoma. Uveitis is entirely asymptomatic and can lead to vision loss but, if discovered early by slit lamp examination, is usually well controlled by corticosteroid eye drops and mydriatics. Occasionally oral prednisone or methotrexate is required. Ophthalmologic surveillance is recommended every 3 to 6 months for several years in all patients with JIA, even those who are ANA-negative.

JIA is a chronic disease; a multidisciplinary approach provides the best opportunity for limiting morbidity and preserving function. Most patients with JIA experience little permanent disability and remain in remission for long periods. Treatment consists of pharmacologic intervention to curb inflammation and physical therapy to maintain strength and range of motion. Nonsteroidal anti-inflammatory drugs (NSAIDs) may be sufficient treatment for patients with mild disease affecting only a few joints. These medications provide symptomatic relief of joint pain but do not affect the course of disease and may take up to 3 months to achieve maximal effect. Adverse effects of chronic NSAID use are detailed in Chapter 30. Most patients with JIA are best managed when NSAIDs are used in conjunction with an agent that retards progressive destruction of the joints. Glucocorticoids, methotrexate, and etanercept (a tumor necrosis factor receptor antagonist) have all been shown to slow radiographic progression of arthritis in children. Short courses of high-dose corticosteroids are reserved for serious systemic manifestations of JIA such as pleuritis or pericarditis. Low-dose steroids can be used to provide rapid functional and symptomatic relief from severe polyarthritis. Intra-articular steroids are occasionally offered to patients with involvement of a single joint. Methotrexate is generally well tolerated in children and may be administered via oral or subcutaneous route. Anorexia, oral ulcers, and abdominal pain are the most frequently reported adverse effects in this setting. JIA with severe joint involvement may lead to cartilage destruction, joint deformity, and leg length discrepancy. Surgery is rarely indicated; if at all possible, it is delayed until growth is complete. Autologous stem cell transplantation has been performed in a small number of patients.

The *enthesis* is the tissue attaching tendon to bone. In *enthesitis-related JIA*, the arthritis is accompanied by inflammation of the enthesis as well. This distinction is important because children with enthesitis are frequently HLA-B27 positive, which places them at increased risk for evolution of their disease into one of the recognized *spondyloarthropathies* (e.g., ankylosing spondylitis, reactive arthritis, and arthritis associated with inflammatory bowel disease). Spondyloarthropathies are more common in boys. Rheumatoid factor and ANA tests are usually negative.

Ankylosing spondylitis is most common in adolescent boys. It initially presents with lower extremity oligoarthritis and enthesitis limited to knees and/or ankles. Localized tenderness is noted at involved sites of tendinous attachment. *Sacroiliitis* is a key diagnostic feature of ankylosing spondylitis that may be noted at presentation but usually occurs much later. Spinal involvement should be suspected when range of motion during forward flexion is limited. Plain radiographs may be positive, but magnetic resonance imaging is the most sensitive study for sacroiliitis. The white blood count and ESR are mildly elevated. Ninety percent of affected individuals are HLA-B27 positive.

Reactive arthritis is joint inflammation that occurs during or immediately after gastrointestinal or genitourinary infection. The arthritis is acute in onset, asymmetric, and usually limited to large joints. Reactive arthritis is thought to represent an autoimmune reaction that results when sensitized T cells react with antigens present in the joints. The condition is self-limited; joint pain typically responds to NSAIDs. *Reiter syndrome* is a form of reactive arthritis characterized by a triad of features: *urethritis* (which is generally asymptomatic and associated with *Chlamydia trachomatis* infection), nonexudative *conjunctivitis*, and *arthritis*. Reiter syndrome is more common in males but is known to occur in females with *Chlamydia* urethritis or cervicitis.

Postinfectious arthritis may be misdiagnosed as reactive arthritis. Postinfectious arthritis usually follows a nonspecific viral infection and is thought to be due to deposition of viral antigen-containing immune complexes in the joint. Clinical evidence of arthritis is minimal, with the main complaint being pain. Organisms commonly implicated in the development of postinfectious arthritis include parvovirus, *Mycoplasma pneumoniae*, *Streptococcus* species, Epstein-Barr virus, and varicella.

Arthritis associated with *inflammatory bowel disease* is more common in patients with Crohn disease. Both large and small joints are affected, but the spine is generally spared. Approximately 70% of patients with enteropathic-related arthritis are positive for HLA-B27. In some patients, the joint complaints predate gastrointestinal symptoms, and the child is initially diagnosed with enthesitis-related JIA.

DERMATOMYOSITIS

Juvenile dermatomyositis (JDM) is an inflammatory disease involving the skin, striated muscle, and occasionally the gastrointestinal tract. Deposition of immune complexes within the walls of the vessels leads to inflammation, ulceration, bleeding, and eventual fibrinous repair. Onset is typically between 2 and 10 years of age and may be acute, subacute, or insidious. The condition is more common in females and has a strong heritable component.

Patients report a history of malaise, fatigue, weight loss, and intermittent fevers. The diagnosis is virtually assured when progressive proximal muscle weakness is accompanied by the characteristic violaceous dermatitis of the eyelids (*heliotrope*) and cheeks in a malar distribution. Symmetric, scaly, flat-topped erythematous papules and plaques (*Grotton papules*) overlie the extensor surfaces of the interphalangeal joints of the fingers, the elbows, and the knees. Skin changes may occur before, in conjunction with, or after the onset of muscle weakness. Chronic involvement of the skin leads to calcium deposition, cutaneous striation, and scarring. Proximal muscles are often tender as the weakness sets in. In severe disease, weakness affects muscle groups responsible for swallowing, phonation, and respiration. Oropharyngeal, chest wall, and respiratory muscle weakness predisposes patients to aspiration. Chronic, unabated myositis results in significant muscle atrophy. Serum concentrations of muscle-derived enzymes (e.g., creatinine kinase, aldolase, aspartate aminotransferase, lactate dehydrogenase) are uniformly elevated. Approximately one half of affected individuals have positive ANA titers.

Treatment consists of appropriate physical therapy and pharmacologic immunosuppression. As long as muscle-derived enzyme concentrations remain high, activity is limited, and the primary aim of therapy is prevention of contractures with positioning and splints. High-dose prednisone is prescribed in an attempt to control the inflammatory response. Once evidence of muscle destruction begins to abate, steroid doses are tapered, and strengthening exercises are gradually added. Patients with resistant disease may benefit from short courses of intravenous corticosteroids or steroid-sparing drugs such as methotrexate or cyclophosphamide. Dermatomyositis patients undergoing chronic systemic corticosteroid therapy may develop *steroid myopathy*, characterized by the insidious onset of proximal muscle weakness. Steroid myopathy may be mistaken for exacerbation of the patient's underlying myositis; however, the former is painless and is not associated with elevations in serum muscle enzyme concentrations.

The majority of children diagnosed with dermatomyositis recover with no permanent disability within a few years. Approximately 25% develop a chronic relapsing course with readily responsive exacerbations. Resistant disease progresses to severe calcinosis of the skin and muscle necessitating eventual wheelchair dependence. Spontaneous perforation of the gastrointestinal tract, although rare, is the leading cause of death.

SCLERODERMA

Scleroderma is a rare autoimmune connective tissue disorder characterized by induration and thickening of the skin due to excessive production of collagen. Skin biopsy confirms the diagnosis. Scleroderma is categorized as localized or systemic. *Systemic scleroderma* involves multiple organ systems and is rare in the pediatric population. The lesions of *localized scleroderma* initially present as 2- to 6-cm sharply demarcated areas of violaceous-hued skin. As excess collagen is laid down, the lesion loses its color, becoming thick, waxy, and hypopigmented. The areas evolve for a few years but eventually "burn out," leaving atrophic scars. Localized scleroderma is much more common in children and has a better outcome; it is self-limited, lasting an average of 3 to 5 years. Localized scleroderma occurs in three distinct forms:

- *Linear scleroderma*—thick, bandlike lesions with a predilection for the scalp and extremities. When abnormal tissue spans a joint, functional impairment and deformity result. Scalp lesions are often located in the frontoparietal region, involve the face, and are associated with hair loss (*coup de sabre*). Linear scleroderma may involve underlying muscle or bone.
- *Morphea*—one or two discrete lesions only, often found on the trunk, face, or scalp. The abnormal tissue is limited to the skin.
- *Generalized*—widespread or coalescent lesions

Various topical, intralesional, systemic, and ultraviolet therapies have proven benefit; treatment is specialized and best undertaken by a dermatologist.

MARFAN SYNDROME

Marfan syndrome (MS) is an inherited multisystem connective tissue disorder resulting from mutation of the fibrillin gene on chromosome 15. Inheritance is autosomal dominant with full penetrance but extremely variable expressivity. Thirty percent of cases arise from new mutations. Because the fibrillin gene is very large and the mutation can occur in multiple sites, genetic testing is variably reliable, and the diagnosis remains primarily a clinical one (Table 21-5).

TABLE 21-5
CLINICAL DIAGNOSIS OF MARFAN SYNDROME: THE REVISED GHENT CRITERIA[a]

In patients without a family history of Marfan syndrome, two major criteria are required for diagnosis, with involvement of a third organ system (minor criterion).

In patients with a known family history of Marfan syndrome, only one major criterion is required for diagnosis, with involvement of a second organ system (minor criterion).

Major Criteria (features that are specific to Marfan syndrome and rarely occur in the general population)

Aortic root enlargement/aneurysm
Aortic dissection
Ocular lens dislocation
Lumbosacral dural ectasia
Presence of at least four major skeletal features:
- Pectus carinatum
- Significant pectus excavatum
- Arm span-to-height ratio >1.05
- Scoliosis or spondylolisthesis
- Decreased extension at the elbows
- Pes planus
- (And others)

Minor Criteria (features that are present with increased frequency in patients with Marfan syndrome but also occur in the general population)

Organ System	Examples
Skeletal system	Joint hypermobility High, arched palate with crowded teeth
Ocular system	Abnormally flat cornea Increased axial length of globe
Cardiovascular system	Mitral valve prolapse Pulmonary artery dilatation
Pulmonary system	Spontaneous pneumothorax
Dermatologic signs	Unprovoked stretch marks Incisional hernias
Nondiagnostic features: arachnodactyly	

[a]Revised from De Paepe A, Devereux RB, Dietz H, et al. Revised diagnostic criteria for the Marfan syndrome. *Am J Med Genet.* 1996;62:417–426.

The majority of patients with MS have cardiac anomalies, the most serious of which is *aortic root dilatation*, which is associated with sudden cardiac death. Mitral valve prolapse is a minor diagnostic feature for MS; significant mitral regurgitation may require pharmacologic intervention. Patients with no aortic root dilatation or mitral regurgitation may participate in low- and moderate-intensity static sports and low-intensity dynamic sports. All but low-intensity competitive sports are prohibited in patients with aortic root dilatation; strenuous exercise should be avoided in an effort to prevent progressive dilation and eventual rupture.

Patients with suspected or confirmed MS should be referred for cardiology and ophthalmologic consultation for specialized assessment and management of cardiovascular and ocular issues.

HYPERMOBILITY SYNDROMES

Hypermobility syndrome is characterized by musculoskeletal complaints related to generalized joint laxity in individuals with no underlying genetic or acquired connective tissue pathology. Hypermobility syndrome is a diagnosis of exclusion. Patients present with joint pain, the location and severity of which are determined by the repetitive activity that provokes the discomfort. The pain is self-limited but recurs with similar activities. Myalgia and joint stiffness/swelling are notably absent. The diagnosis of hypermobility syndrome rests on assignment of a Beighton score of 4 or more:

- Apposition of the thumb to the forearm (1 point for each side)
- Extension of the fifth finger beyond 90 degrees (1 point for each side)
- Extension of the elbow beyond 10 degrees (1 point for each side)
- Extension of the knee beyond 10 degrees (1 point for each side)
- Forward flexion of the trunk, palms placed flat on the floor with knees straight (1 point)

Patients with hypermobility syndrome should be reassured that their condition is benign. Joint pain related to repetitive activity responds to NSAIDs; alternatively, the patient may choose forms of exercise that do not exacerbate symptoms.

Ehlers-Danlos syndrome is actually a collection of connective tissue disorders characterized by hyperextensibility of the joints, hyperextensibility of the skin, and poor wound healing. The skin is described as soft and stretchy. Patients exhibit easy bruising, abnormal scar formation (thin, "cigarette paper" scars), and recurrent spontaneous joint dislocations. Ehlers-Danlos syndrome is associated with an increased risk for dilation and rupture of the ascending aorta.

SARCOIDOSIS

Sarcoidosis is a multisystem inflammatory disease that affects the skin, bones, joints, and organs, primarily the lungs. The presentation in older children and adolescents is identical to that in adult patients. Pulmonary manifestations predominate, including granulomatous infiltration of the lungs and hilar lymphadenopathy. A distinct form of sarcoidosis involving children younger than 4 years of age entails a triad of findings: a *rash* consisting of flat, reddish plaques; *uveitis*; and *arthritis*. Biopsy of the lesions confirms the diagnosis through demonstration of the characteristic noncaseating granulomas. Immunosuppressant therapy is the mainstay of management.

SOURCES

Goldmuntz EA, White PH. Juvenile idiopathic arthritis: a review for the pediatrician. *Pediatr Rev*. 2006;27:e24–e32.

Klein-Gitelman MS, Miller ML. Systemic lupus erythematosus. In: Behrman RE, Kliegman RM, Jenson HB, eds. *Nelson textbook of pediatrics*. 17th ed. Philadelphia: WB Saunders; 2004:809–813.

Lodish MB. Weeks of weakness, then reddish bumps on prominences. *Contemp Pediatr*. 2006;23:24–25.

Milana C, Chandran L. What's new in Kawasaki disease? *Contemp Pediatr*. 2006;23:40–47.

Miller ML, Pachman LM. Vasculitis syndrome: Henoch-Schönlein purpura. In: Behrman RE, Kliegman RM, Jenson HB, eds. *Nelson textbook of pediatrics*. 17th ed. Philadelphia: WB Saunders; 2004:826–828.

Morel KD, Hogeling M, Eichenfield LF. More than skin deep: cutaneous signs of systemic disease. *Contemp Pediatr*. 2005;22:26–37.

Rosenberg AM. Juvenile onset spondyloarthropathies. *Curr Opin Rheumatol*. 2000;12:425–429.

Siegel DM. Antinuclear antibody testing. *Pediatr Rev*. 2003;24:320–321.

Waseem M, Pinkert H. A febrile child who has "red eyes" and a rash. *Pediatr Rev*. 2003;24:245–248.

QUESTIONS

1. A 14-year-old African-American girl presents to your office for evaluation of her facial rash. Her physical examination is significant for an erythematous maculopapular eruption over the cheeks and nose, with sparing of the nasolabial folds. Asymmetric papulosquamous lesions are noted on the dorsa of the hands between the knuckles. Urinalysis reveals hematuria. Which of the following is the most likely diagnosis in this patient?

A) Systemic lupus erythematosus
B) Juvenile dermatomyositis
C) Acute rheumatic fever
D) Localized scleroderma
E) Pauciarticular juvenile idiopathic arthritis

2. You are providing a lecture to first-year pediatric interns concerning systemic lupus erythematosus. You would be correct in informing the young medical doctors of all of the following EXCEPT:

A) Systemic lupus erythematosus is a clinical diagnosis.
B) The arthritis of systemic lupus erythematosus is progressive, erosive, and deforming.
C) Antinuclear antibody titers are sensitive but not specific for systemic lupus erythematosus.
D) Systemic lupus erythematosus may present initially with isolated heart block.
E) Circulating anti-Ro/SS-A and anti-La/SS-B antibodies in an SLE-affected mother may cause neonatal lupus syndrome and/or complete congenital heart block in her fetus.

3. Antinuclear antibody titers would be least useful as a screening test in which of the following patients?

A) A 7-year-old girl with a symmetric, photosensitive facial rash and diffuse tenderness of both thighs
B) A 7-year-old girl with twice-daily fevers and swelling and decreased range of motion involving the left knee
C) A 14-year-old girl whose mother has systemic lupus erythematosus
D) A 12-year-old girl with first-degree heart block
E) A 6-year-old girl with arthritis of the left wrist and right knee and urine that is positive for blood and protein

4. A 12-year-old girl presents with a fever of 38.5°C, shortness of breath, and swelling of the right knee and elbow. Her physical examination reveals a new heart murmur. The girl's erythrocyte sedimentation rate and platelet counts are elevated. Which of the following studies represents the best option for differentiating acute rheumatic fever from systemic lupus erythematosus in this patient?

A) Measurement of the PR interval on electrocardiogram
B) Serum C-reactive protein concentration
C) Antinuclear antibody titer
D) Streptococcal antibody titers
E) Aspiration of a swollen joint

5. A father brings his 4-year-old son to your office for evaluation of his multiple bruises. The child has recently recovered from a nonspecific viral respiratory illness but was otherwise well until 3 days ago, when he began complaining of episodic abdominal pain. Vital signs are within normal limits in the office. The examination is significant for a well-nourished, cooperative child who appears comfortable. Palpable purpuric lesions are present over the buttocks and lower extremities. No abnormalities or pain are noted on examination of the abdomen. A stool sample obtained during digital rectal examination is positive for occult blood. A complete blood count is obtained in the office and demonstrates mild elevation of the white blood count and normal hemoglobin and platelet levels. Which of the following is the most likely diagnosis in this patient?

A) Physical abuse
B) Intussusception
C) Retrocecal appendicitis
D) Hemolytic-uremic syndrome
E) Henoch-Schönlein purpura

6. A 3-year-old boy is brought to your office by his mother, who is concerned because she saw frank blood in his stool. The boy has recently completed a course of antibiotics for group A streptococcal pharyngitis. He was otherwise well until 2 days ago, when he began complaining of bilateral knee pain. Vital signs are stable in the office. The physical examination reveals moderate diffuse abdominal tenderness, decreased range of motion and pain with movement in both knees, and a purpuric rash over the buttocks and legs. When you leave the room to order a few laboratory tests, the medical student who is shadowing you asks what you think the diagnosis is. In an effort to jog her memory, you would be correct in telling her all of the following about the patient's condition EXCEPT:

A) Elevation of the serum immunoglobulin A (IgA) concentration is required for the diagnosis.
B) It is an IgA-mediated disease involving the skin, gastrointestinal tract, and joints.
C) Intussusception is the most common serious gastrointestinal complication of this patient's disease.
D) The patient's platelet count will be normal despite the presence of the purpuric lesions.
E) The patient's prognosis for full recovery in 4 to 12 weeks is excellent.

7. A mother brings her 18-month-old febrile daughter to the clinic for her second visit in the past 5 days. The girl has a temperature of 38.8°C today; her temperature 5 days ago was 39°C. She is extremely irritable. The physical examination is significant for nonexudative conjunctivitis, fissured lips, and a polymorphous rash over her trunk and extremities. Cervical lymphadenopathy is present, with one of the nodes measuring >1.5 cm in diameter. Which of the following studies is most important in the initial assessment of this patient?

A) Urinalysis
B) Echocardiography
C) Electrocardiography
D) Lumbar puncture
E) Measles antibody titers

8. An emergency department physician calls you over the weekend to let you know that he has diagnosed one of your patients with Kawasaki disease. The patient is scheduled for intravenous immunoglobulin therapy during the night. Which of the following statements regarding recommendations for pharmacologic management of this patient's condition is TRUE?

A) Aspirin should be avoided in this patient due to an increased risk for the development of Reye syndrome.
B) Daily low-dose aspirin therapy should be started in this patient today and continued until hospital discharge.
C) Daily high-dose aspirin therapy should be started in this patient today and continued until the patient has been afebrile for several days; then the patient should be switched to daily low-dose aspirin therapy at least until the end of the convalescent period.
D) Daily high-dose aspirin therapy should be started in this patient today and continued at least until the end of the convalescent period.
E) Daily high-dose aspirin therapy should be started in this patient today and continued until hospital discharge.

9. A 2-year-old boy has twice-daily brief episodes of high fever accompanied by a faint, blanching, evanescent pink or salmon-colored rash. He appears completely well when he is not febrile. He is now complaining of left knee pain; the joint is swollen and warm, and range of motion is limited. The liver edge is palpable two fingerbreadths below the costal margin, and the spleen tip is palpable. You suspect systemic juvenile idiopathic arthritis. Which of the following statements regarding this condition is FALSE?

A) Juvenile idiopathic arthritis cannot be definitively diagnosed until joint findings have been present for 6 weeks.
B) Aspiration of the joint would be beneficial for differentiating juvenile idiopathic arthritis from septic arthritis.
C) This patient should be evaluated for evidence of pericarditis.
D) You would expect to find elevated antinuclear antibody titers and positive rheumatoid factor in this patient if he has systemic juvenile idiopathic arthritis.
E) You would expect this patient to have elevations in the serum white blood count, platelet count, and erythrocyte sedimentation rate if he has systemic juvenile idiopathic arthritis.

10. Which of the following laboratory results is most closely tied to the development of uveitis in patients with juvenile idiopathic arthritis?

A) Elevated serum ferritin concentration
B) Human leukocyte antigen B27
C) Serum white blood count >20,000 per μL
D) Presence of rheumatoid factor
E) Positive antinuclear antibody titers

11. A 5-year-old girl with clinical evidence of arthritis involving her left knee joint that has persisted for >6 weeks is diagnosed with pauciarticular juvenile rheumatoid arthritis. Six months later, plain radiographs of the joint demonstrate narrowing of the intra-articular space and erosive cartilage changes. The progression of this patient's disease places her at risk for which of the following sequelae?

A) Limb length discrepancy
B) Loss of ambulation
C) Frozen joint
D) Joint malignancy
E) Toxic synovitis

12. Patients with enthesitis-related juvenile idiopathic arthritis who are positive for human leukocyte antigen B27 are at increased risk for subsequent development of all of the following conditions EXCEPT:

A) Ankylosing spondylitis
B) Spondylolisthesis
C) Inflammatory bowel disease–related arthritis
D) Psoriatic arthritis
E) Osteoarthritis

13. A 17-year-old adolescent presents with a swollen left ankle of 3 days in duration. He denies any history of trauma or constitutional symptoms. The physical examination is significant for a cooperative, well-appearing male with swelling, warmth, and tenderness with movement of the left ankle. No other joint abnormalities are present. The patient is also noted to have bilateral nonexudative conjunctivitis. Which of the following studies is the most appropriate next step in the evaluation of this patient?

A) Human leukocyte antigen B27
B) Urine culture
C) Leukocyte esterase testing of first-void urine
D) Rheumatoid factor
E) Analysis and culture of synovial fluid from the left knee

14. The mother of an 8-year-old boy newly diagnosed with inflammatory bowel disease (IBD) has read on the Internet that patients with this disease may develop arthritis. All of the following statements concerning IBD-related arthritis are correct EXCEPT:

A) IBD-related arthritis is more common in patients with Crohn disease.
B) IBD-related arthritis involves both large and small joints.
C) IBD-related arthritis is more common in patients who are positive for human leukocyte antigen B27.
D) IBD-related arthritis typically involves the sacral region of the vertebral column.
E) IBD-related arthritis is more common in patients with enthesitis-related juvenile idiopathic arthritis.

15. A 15-year-old girl who is playing on an organized volleyball team for the first time presents with recurrent joint pain in her right shoulder, which she uses to serve and spike the ball. She denies stiffness or myalgia. The pain improves with rest and ibuprofen. The physical examination is significant for increased range of motion at the shoulder joint. The patient has a Beighton scale score of 6; she can appose both thumbs to the forearms and hyperextend both elbows and knees beyond 10 degrees. Scars from previous injuries appear normal, and the skin is not hyperextensible. This patient's joint pain is most consistent with which of the following diagnoses?

A) Ankylosing spondylitis
B) Marfan syndrome
C) Ehlers-Danlos syndrome, hypermobility type
D) Classic Ehlers-Danlos syndrome
E) Hypermobility syndrome

16. A 2-year-old girl complains of recurrent pain in her legs. Her mother thinks the pain is localized to her knees. She says that her child seems to bruise easily. The physical examination is significant for a Beighton score of 9 and abnormally thin scars with the appearance of "cigarette paper." This child's pain is most likely due to which of the following?

A) Ehlers-Danlos syndrome
B) Hypermobility syndrome
C) Juvenile idiopathic arthritis
D) Oligoarthritic juvenile rheumatoid arthritis
E) Growing pains

17. A 9-year-old girl is in your office for evaluation of her leg pain. Her mother states that her daughter was well until about 3 weeks ago, when she began complaining of pain in her anterior thighs. Now the child has begun avoiding her regular activities (such as dance class and physical education at school) because her legs hurt and she feels weak. The physical examination is significant for normal muscle tone in the lower extremities and normal findings at the hip, knee, and ankle joints. Violaceous dermatitis of the eyelids (heliotrope) and cheeks is noted in a malar distribution. Which of the following studies is most likely to be abnormal in this patient?

A) Antinuclear antibody titers
B) Serum muscle enzyme concentrations
C) Rheumatoid factor
D) Human leukocyte antibody B27
E) Anti-Smith antibodies

18. You are providing a lecture about pediatric inflammatory muscle conditions to a group of medical students. In discussing juvenile dermatomyositis, you would be correct in telling them all of the following EXCEPT:

A) Proximal muscle weakness is a key feature of the diagnosis.
B) Skin changes may occur before, in conjunction with, or after the onset of muscle weakness.
C) Grotton papules are symmetric, scaly, flat-topped erythematous papules and plaques located between the interphalangeal joints of the fingers.
D) Serum concentrations of muscle-derived enzymes (e.g., creatinine kinase, aldolase, aspartate aminotransferase, lactate dehydrogenase) are uniformly elevated.
E) Spontaneous perforation of the gastrointestinal tract, although rare, is the leading cause of death.

19. A 9-year-old girl presents with a solitary, 3-cm, flat oval lesion on her trunk. The lesion is erythematous and slightly violaceous in color. Borders are sharply demarcated. There is no history of trauma, insect bite, or fever. You suspect localized morphea. Which of the following offers the best description of the natural history of the lesion?

A) Recurrent ulceration and bleeding with eventual scarring
B) Malignant transformation requiring local excision
C) Gradual resolution over 3 to 6 months with no scaring
D) Evolution to an ivory-colored, firm, waxy lesion with eventual atrophy
E) Central necrosis and eventual calcium deposition within the lesion

20. A 12-year-old girl presents to your office for evaluation of her recurrent chest pain. Her mother says that the girl experiences chest pain with vigorous exercise that resolves with rest. The physical examination is significant for a well-nourished, well-developed, well-appearing cooperative child. The palate is highly arched, with crowded dentition. Fingers are long and spidery. A systolic click is present that varies in timing with positional changes. Which of the following features completes the diagnostic criteria for Marfan syndrome in this patient?

A) Pectus excavatum
B) Scoliosis
C) Generalized joint hypermobility
D) History of recurrent incisional hernias
E) Family history of Marfan syndrome

ANSWERS

1. A	8. C	15. E
2. B	9. D	16. A
3. C	10. E	17. B
4. D	11. A	18. C
5. E	12. B	19. D
6. A	13. C	20. E
7. B	14. D	

22

Disorders of the Eye

EVALUATION OF THE EYE

A detailed *history, visual acuity testing,* and thorough *examination* will suggest a diagnosis and direct the clinician toward further studies, management, and/or referral for specialized treatment (Table 22-1). The examination of the eye may include any of the following, depending on the age of the child:

- *Visual acuity testing,* for each eye separately and together (ages 3 years and above)
- Inspection of the structures surrounding the eye (skin and lids)
- Inspection of the conjunctiva (bulbar and/or tarsal), sclera, cornea, iris, and pupil
- Pupil size, symmetry, constriction to light, accommodation
- Corneal light reflex test
- Cover test
- Detection of the red reflex (neonates and infants)
- Fundoscopic examination

Visual acuity is assessed in patients 3 years of age and older with Snellen eye charts consisting of Allen figures (pictures of objects and animals) in young preschoolers, tumbling E symbols in 4- and 5-year-old patients, and HOTV or assorted letters in older children. Visual acuity of 20/40 or better is considered normal in children aged 3 to 5 years; referral is indicated for patients with poor acuity or those with a difference in visual acuity between the eyes of greater than one line.

VISION, AMBLYOPIA, AND STRABISMUS

Development of optimal vision requires that two *normally aligned* eyes receive *equal stimulation* with *clear retinal images. Amblyopia* refers to decreased vision that develops due to abnormal stimulation of the visual centers in the brain. Amblyopia may occur throughout childhood, but abnormalities that arise during the period of critical *visual development (birth to 4 months of age)* carry a high risk of permanent loss of vision. The earlier this condition is diagnosed and treated, the better the outcome. Development of the visual axis is largely complete by 8 years of age, so intervention thereafter is unlikely to produce significant improvement of the amblyopia.

Strabismus, or ocular misalignment, is the most common cause of amblyopia. When the eyes are not properly aligned, visual centers in the brain suppress the images from one eye and do not develop normally, resulting in decreased vision in that eye. Children with strabismus require patching of their "good" eye to force visual stimulation and appropriate brain development. Surgical correction of the alignment is indicated for some forms of strabismus. Young infants may

TABLE 22-1
PEDIATRIC VISION SCREENING RECOMMENDATIONS OF THE AMERICAN ACADEMY OF OPHTHALMOLOGY

Age	Examination	Referral
Newborn	Corneal light reflex test Red reflexes	Abnormal red reflexes Any other ocular abnormality
By age 6 months	Fixation to light or small toys Monocular occlusion Corneal light reflex test Cover/uncover test Red reflexes	Aversion to occlusion Strabismus Nystagmus Abnormal red reflexes Any other ocular abnormality
Age 3 to 4 years	Visual acuity Corneal light reflex test Fundus examination	Visual acuity of at least 20/40 in each eye and no more than one line difference between the two eyes on vision testing Strabismus Any other ocular abnormality
Age 5 or older	Visual acuity Corneal light reflex test Cover/uncover test Fundus examination	Visual acuity of 20/40 or less in one or both eyes Strabismus Any other ocular abnormality

Source: Communication of the American Academy of Ophthalmology, San Francisco, CA; 2001.

appear to have crossed or "wandering" eyes, especially when fatigued. Strabismus that persists beyond 2 months of age (or aversion to monocular occlusion beyond 6 months of age) is more likely to be pathologic and warrants referral to an ophthalmologist.

Pseudostrabismus is the false appearance of strabismus in a child who has normal alignment. Flat, wide nasal bridges or skin folds in the medial corners of the eyes may give the mistaken impression that the eyes are crossed (esotropia). The corneal light reflex test and the cover test can be used to differentiate pseudostrabismus from true strabismus.

Amblyopia may also result from:

- *anisometropia,* a significant difference (two Snellen lines or greater) in the refractive errors of the two eyes, such that the image from the eye with the larger error becomes suppressed
- *visual deprivation* due to interference with the formation of clear retinal images (ptosis, cataracts)

Treatment of amblyopia involves removal of any obstacles obstructing formation of a clear image on the retina, correcting refractive errors, and patching the dominant eye to force development of the contralateral visual axis. Children with amblyopia, anisometropia, or bilateral visual acuity lower than expected for their age should be referred. Visual impairment in school-age patients can lead to problems in reading or other academic tasks when the child is unable to visually decipher information presented on the page or board.

Significant vision loss negatively impacts early childhood development. Conditions such as congenital cataracts, cortical blindness, severe myopia, retinopathy of prematurity, and ocular malformations can all affect infant vision. Both gross and fine motor development are typically delayed by several months; for example, the blind infant may not walk independently until 24 to 36 months of age. These children have no visual motivation to reach for or move toward objects. The inability to see does not permit interpretation of body language and other social cues, which affects both social and emotional development. Speech and language development is typically spared.

NYSTAGMUS

Nystagmus is the presence of rapid, involuntary, rhythmic eye movements. The oscillations may be horizontal, vertical, or rotational. Nystagmus is best evaluated and managed by an ophthalmologic specialist. Four forms of nystagmus encountered in pediatric practice include:

- *congenital motor nystagmus* (inherited; occurs within the first month of life; associated with normal or near-normal vision)
- *congenital sensory nystagmus* (later onset; occurs secondary to early, severe vision loss; has a "roving" or "searching" quality)
- *acquired nystagmus* (strong association with central nervous system abnormality)
- *spasmus nutans* (acquired between 3 and 18 months; associated with rhythmic head nodding; disappears by age 4 years; generally benign but occasionally associated with a chiasmal or suprachiasmal mass)

DISORDERS OF THE LIDS

Hordeolum/Chalazion/Blepharitis

A stye (external hordeolum) occurs when a bacterial abscess, usually caused by *Staphylococcus aureus,* forms within either a sebaceous (Zeis) or sweat (Moll) gland associated with the lash follicles on the eyelids. A small area of erythema and swelling comes to a point at a pustule or papule on the lid margin. Styes usually resolve spontaneously within a week. Warm compresses several times a day may hasten resolution; occasionally topical antibiotics are prescribed if there is significant involvement of the lid margin.

An *internal hordeolum* is a bacterial abscess, usually due to *S. aureus,* located in a meibomian gland within the tarsal plate. These sebaceous glands open onto the lid margin and secrete a lipid substance that prevents evaporation of the tear film covering the eye. An internal hordeolum has more diffuse swelling, may be erythematous, and presents with a pustule either at the lid margin or along the inner tarsal conjunctiva. Treatment is similar to that for a stye.

A *chalazion* is a sterile inflammatory reaction to an accumulation of lipid materials in the meibomian gland. The well-circumscribed area of swelling may be located in either an upper or lower lid and typically is neither painful nor erythematous. Chalazions that do not resolve within 1 month of therapy (warm compresses, baby shampoo eyelid washes) warrant referral to an ophthalmologist for incision and drainage.

Blepharitis is inflammation of the eyelid. It may be infectious or secondary to meibomian gland dysfunction and is usually accompanied by conjunctival injection. Infectious (staphylococcal) blepharitis presents with itching, erythema, and crusting of the lid margin at the bases of the lashes. Topical antibiotics are prescribed; the lids and lashes should be washed twice a day with baby shampoo. Meibomian gland dysfunction has a similar presentation and is treated with lash hygiene and gland massage.

Ptosis

Ptosis ("drooping" of the upper lid) may be uni- or bilateral and congenital or acquired. *Congenital ptosis* that interferes with vision results in amblyopia and should be surgically repaired. If the abnormality is purely cosmetic, surgery can be delayed until the patient is older. *Acquired ptosis* may be secondary to third nerve palsy, myasthenia gravis, or muscular dystrophy and warrants an urgent evaluation to rule out serious pathology. Patients with ptosis should be referred to an ophthalmologist for management of the eye abnormality.

DISORDERS OF THE LACRIMAL DUCT SYSTEM

Nasolacrimal Duct Obstruction

Normal opening of the Hasner valve (at the junction of the distal lacrimal duct with the posterior nose) occurs during the first few weeks of life, about the time that the lacrimal gland begins secreting tears. *Nasolacrimal duct obstruction* results when this valve fails to open. Infants with nasolacrimal duct obstruction present with chronic tearing, matted lashes, and mucus accumulation at the medial canthus. Nasolacrimal duct obstruction may be uni- or bilateral. Approximately 50% of cases resolve spontaneously by 6 months of age. Those that do not resolve by age 12 months should be probed. In the meantime, management consists of duct massage in both superior and inferior directions. A topical antibiotic is added if there are signs of infection such as conjunctival injection and purulent discharge.

Dacryocystitis

Dacryocystitis (infection of the lacrimal sac) presents with redness, swelling, and tenderness below the nasal canthal area. It occurs primarily in infants but also may afflict older patients. Mild infections are treated with massage and an oral first-generation cephalosporin; more serious cases require hospitalization for intravenous antibiotics.

CONJUNCTIVITIS

Neonatal Conjunctivitis

Neonatal conjunctivitis is defined as inflammation of the conjunctiva that occurs within the first month of life. The time of onset and clinical manifestations may suggest a specific infectious organism, which should be confirmed through laboratory testing (Table 22-2). Empiric treatment with topical erythromycin and intravenous cefotaxime should begin immediately after laboratory samples are obtained. Patients with suspected herpes simplex virus (HSV) type 2 infections require additional therapy as listed in Table 22-2. Any infant who presents with neonatal conjunctivitis and an abnormal red reflex warrants urgent examination by an ophthalmologic specialist to assess for corneal or intraocular pathology. Other indications for referral include inflammation limited to one eye, lid swelling that interferes with vision, and minimal improvement within 48 hours of initiating treatment. All newborns receive prophylaxis shortly after birth with ophthalmic silver nitrate, erythromycin, or povidone-iodine. Proper hand washing by caretakers limits the incidence of contact inoculation within the nursery.

Pediatric Conjunctivitis

Conjunctivitis, often called "pink eye," is a nonspecific term that denotes inflammation of the conjunctiva. Many conditions may be associated with conjunctivitis (corneal abrasion, chemical exposure, systemic disease, uveitis). However, most cases of pediatric conjunctivitis are viral, bacterial, or allergic. Frequent hand washing and limiting exposure to others help prevent the spread of infectious conjunctivitis.

Treatment decisions are based on clinical presentation (Table 22-3). Referral to an ophthalmologist is indicated for pediatric conjunctivitis that:

- is severe
- does not improve within a week of initiating empiric therapy
- is associated with contact lens use (increased risk of bacterial corneal ulceration)
- is associated with decreased vision
- is associated with an abnormal red reflex
- is associated with corneal involvement (keratitis)
- is associated with uveitis
- is unilateral and HSV infection or foreign body is suspected

In contrast, *uveitis* is inflammation of any of the structures of the intraocular uveal tract (iris, ciliary body, and choroid). The conjunctival injection associated with uveitis is often concentrated around the iris. Symptoms include eye pain, photophobia, and possibly decreased vision. Uveitis may be associated with systemic disease (juvenile idiopathic arthritis, inflammatory bowel disease) or infection (toxoplasmosis).

PERIORBITAL AND ORBITAL CELLULITIS

The connective tissue that forms the periosteum of the bones surrounding the orbit reflects into the eyelids, effectively forming a *septum* that divides each lid into an anterior part and a posterior part. This septum acts as a barrier to prevent microbes from gaining access to the orbital space. Infections anterior to this septum are termed "preseptal" or *periorbital*. Infections posterior to the septum are *orbital*.

Infection of any of the paranasal sinuses (frontal, maxillary, ethmoid) can spread to the orbit or periorbital area, but this is particularly true for *ethmoid* sinus infections. The lamina papyracea is a thin bony area separating the orbit from the ethmoid sinus. Infections of the ethmoid sinus mucosa can spread to the bone (subperiosteal abscess), pass through naturally occurring dehiscences in the lamina papyracea, or track along the path of the ethmoidal arteries.

TABLE 22-2
MICROBIOLOGY, DIAGNOSIS, AND TREATMENT OF NEONATAL CONJUNCTIVITIS

Etiology	Time of Onset	Typical Presentation	Laboratory Results[a]	Treatment	Key Points
Chemical conjunctivitis (usually secondary to silver nitrate prophylaxis)	Within 6 to 24 hours of instillation	Bilateral conjunctival injection with clear, watery discharge	No organisms on scraping; negative cultures	None (spontaneous resolution within days)	
Neisseria gonorrhoeae	Days of life 2 to 4	Bilateral copious, purulent discharge; notable lid edema; marked conjunctival injection	Gram-negative intracellular diplococci on scraping; positive culture	Uncomplicated conjunctivitis: single-dose cefotaxime or ceftriaxone Systemic disease: 7 to 14 days of the above	■ Complications: corneal ulceration/perforation ■ Screen for invasive disease ■ Treat even if asymptomatic ■ Parent(s) should be evaluated and treated
Chlamydia trachomatis	Days of life 5 to 14	Bilateral mild-to-moderate injection and eye discharge ± lid swelling; conjunctival friability and pseudomembrane formation in severe cases	Cytoplasmic inclusion bodies/positive immunofluorescent assay on scraping; positive culture	Oral erythromycin for 14 days	■ Pseudomembrane may be present under lid ■ Screen for pneumonia ■ Oral erythromycin to prevent/treat pneumonia ■ Parent(s) should be evaluated and treated
Group B streptococci (also other streptococci, staphylococci, *Escherichia coli*)	Days of life 4 to 7	Usually bilateral conjunctival injection with purulent discharge ± lid swelling	Positive Gram stain; positive culture	Topical erythromycin or polymyxin B-trimethoprim	
Haemophilus influenzae	Days of life 4 to 10	Usually bilateral, marked (possibly hemorrhagic) conjunctival injection with clear or serosanguinous drainage	Gram-negative coccobacillus on scraping; positive culture	Topical polymyxin B-trimethoprim and intravenous cefotaxime	■ May present with violaceous hue over lids
Herpes simplex virus (HSV) type 2	Days of life 6 to 14	Typically unilateral moderate conjunctival injection with serous drainage	Multinucleated giant cells, intranuclear inclusion bodies on scraping; positive culture (may take up to 10 days)	Topical trifluorothymidine and intravenous acyclovir	■ Often infects the cornea as well (keratitis) ■ May cause secondary bacterial ulcers ■ May be associated with systemic HSV infection and/or encephalitis

[a]Laboratory samples include conjunctival scraping (to examine for cellular elements) and swabbing the conjunctiva for culture.

TABLE 22-3
INFECTIOUS AND ALLERGIC CONJUNCTIVITIS: PRESENTATION AND TREATMENT

	Viral[a]	Acute Bacterial	Allergic
Onset	May be bilateral or start in one eye and spread to the other	Typically starts in one eye and spreads to the other	Bilateral; more common in the spring; often associated with allergic rhinitis
Injection	Diffuse; mild to severe; may be hemorrhagic if adenovirus	Diffuse; variable severity; may be hemorrhagic if *Haemophilus influenzae*	Diffuse; variable severity but usually minor
Discharge	Clear; often copious	Mucopurulent; eyes may stick together in the morning	Clear; often copious
Lid involvement	Variable	Variable; may be violaceous hue with *H. influenzae*	Often minimal
Pain	Mild	Mild to moderate	None
Itching	Usually absent	Absent	Present
Causes	Adenovirus (less commonly others)	*H. influenzae, Streptococcus pneumoniae, Moraxella catarrhalis, Staphylococcus* species	Type 1 hypersensitivity reaction
Treatment	None (spontaneous resolution)	Topical polymyxin B-trimethoprim or bacitracin-polymyxin B or fluoroquinolone	Topical antihistamines; oral antihistamines; mast cell stabilizers (alone or in combination)

[a]Does not include herpes simplex virus and varicella infections, which require specialized ophthalmologic management.

Periorbital Cellulitis

Periorbital (preseptal) cellulitis may result from:

- infection of any of the structures anterior to the septum, including both the skin around the eye (bacterial cellulitis introduced via trauma or impetigo) and structures in the lids (e.g., hordeolum, chalazion, dacryocystitis)
- hematogenous spread secondary to bacteremia (most common in children ≤18 months of age)

The child with periorbital cellulitis due to hematogenous seeding may have a history of upper respiratory symptoms followed by high fever and the rapid development of swelling and marked erythema. The lids often swell shut, and the tissue around the eye may be quite tender. However, there is no true eye pain, and extraocular movements and visual acuity remain intact. Cellulitis due to the traumatic introduction of skin flora is more insidious in onset and generally less severe.

A lumbar puncture is indicated for patients who are young and appear toxic or who have meningeal signs. Computed tomography is necessary if orbital infection cannot be excluded based on the physical examination. Blood cultures may reveal the causative organism.

S. aureus and group A streptococci should be considered if direct inoculation has occurred. Therapy consists of intravenous nafcillin or a first-generation cephalosporin, or clindamycin for penicillin-allergic patients. Periorbital cellulitis from hematogenous seeding is most likely due to *Streptococcus pneumoniae*. *Haemophilus influenzae* should be considered in nonimmunized children. Intravenous cefuroxime or cefotaxime, with added vancomycin if there is evidence of meningitis, is the empiric treatment of choice. Oral amoxicillin-clavulanic acid is appropriate for mild cases when good follow-up is assured. All patients with isolated periorbital cellulitis should complete a 10-day course of antibiotics.

Orbital Cellulitis

Orbital cellulitis may result from:

- complications of acute sinusitis, such as subperiosteal or orbital abscesses
- hematogenous spread
- direct inoculation via trauma

Clinical manifestations of orbital cellulitis include eye pain, proptosis, restriction of extraocular eye movements (particularly upward gaze paralysis), and decreased visual acuity. Edema and erythema involving the region around the eye may progress rapidly. Systemic signs (fever, toxicity) range from minimal to severe.

Patients with suspected orbital infections require orbital computed tomography to ascertain the extent of involvement and locate potential abscesses that may benefit from surgical drainage. Any material obtained from an abscess or infected paranasal sinuses is analyzed with Gram staining and culture. *S. pneumoniae, H. influenzae,* and *Moraxella catarrhalis* are the most common pathogens implicated in acute sinusitis and may all cause orbital infections. Other bacteria to consider include *S. aureus, Streptococcus pyogenes,* and anaerobes normally found in the upper respiratory tract. An appropriate choice for empiric therapy is a second- or third-generation intravenous cephalosporin plus clindamycin if anaerobic organisms are suspected. Patients may be switched to an oral agent to complete a 14- to 21-day course when sensitivities are known and the eye examination returns to normal.

A serious complication of orbital cellulitis is *cavernous sinus thrombosis*, thrombophlebitis of the orbital veins that extend into this vascular watershed area. Affected patients experience the rapid onset of severe headache, eye pain, loss of vision, and meningismus. They appear profoundly ill with high, spiking fevers. The physical examination may be significant for proptosis or loss of voluntary eye movements. Fortunately, this complication is rare.

INTRAOCULAR DISORDERS

Cataracts

Cataracts are lens opacifications. Congenital cataracts may be idiopathic or associated with intrauterine infections, particularly rubella. Congenital cataracts blur the retinal image during the critical period of visual development. Timely diagnosis and treatment (usually surgery) are necessary to prevent profound, irreversible amblyopia. The clinical hallmark of congenital cataract is *leukocoria*.

Leukocoria is defined as a white pupil. Abnormalities in the cornea may cause a blurring of the red reflex, but a true white pupil results from a disorder at or behind the pupil. Two pediatric conditions that can cause leukocoria are cataracts and *retinoblastoma*. Leukocoria merits referral to an ophthalmologist for immediate evaluation. Documenting normal bilateral red reflexes is an essential part of the eye examination during infancy.

Glaucoma

Glaucoma occurs when increased intraocular pressure causes optic nerve damage and atrophy. Congenital glaucoma usually presents before 6 months of age with some combination of tearing, photophobia, and blepharospasm (spasmodic involuntary eyelid closure or blinking). It is frequently bilateral. The elastic nature of the infant eye permits marked corneal enlargement that may be visually evident. Corneal edema results in tearing and cornea clouding, indicated by a dull red reflex and possibly blurring of the demarcation lines of the pupil and iris. Any resultant optic nerve damage and vision loss are irreversible. Surgery is usually required to improve outflow and reduce the pressure.

Glaucoma that develops after the age of 3 years does not produce eye enlargement and may remain asymptomatic. Chronic steroid therapy is associated with glaucoma; regular monitoring of intraocular pressure is indicated in these cases. Approximately a third of children with Sturge-Weber syndrome develop glaucoma, which is more likely if the port wine stain involves the upper lid.

Papilledema/Papillitis

Papilledema is the term used to describe edema of the optic disc that is secondary to increased intracranial pressure. *Papillitis (optic neuritis)* is inflammation of the optic nerve, which is often accompanied by disc edema. Most cases in children involve a postviral autoimmune response and resolve spontaneously within a few weeks. In older patients, optic neuritis may be a manifestation of multiple sclerosis. *Pseudopapilledema* is blurring of the optic disc margins *not* associated with disc edema; it is usually incidental and benign. The distinguishing clinical manifestations of these conditions are outlined in Table 22-4.

NEOPLASMS THAT AFFECT VISION

Vision loss may result from primary intraocular (retinoblastoma), metastatic (neuroblastoma, lymphoid tumor), or extraorbital tumors (glioma of the optic nerve/chiasm, craniopharyngioma). The decline in vision is usually insidious. Intracranial masses, neurodegenerative diseases, and phakomatoses may also produce chronic vision loss. Sudden loss of vision is more likely to result from infection of the brain or inner eye structures, trauma (retinal detachment), or intracranial bleeding.

Retinoblastoma is a malignant tumor of the retina. Leukocoria is a common presenting sign of retinoblastoma. Other findings may include strabismus, glaucoma, pain, conjunctivitis, hyphema (blood in the anterior chamber), periorbital inflammation, and vision loss (retinal detachment or vitreous hemorrhage). Retinoblastoma may be inherited or sporadic. In the heritable form, a mutation at chromosome location 13q14 is inherited, and a subsequent mutation occurs at the other allele to result in disease. Patients with this form present early in life (approximately 12 months of age) with bilateral disease. The sporadic form is usually unilateral and presents at approximately age 24 months; sporadic mutations occur in both normal inherited alleles. Genetic screening should be performed on both parents, and siblings of patients with hereditary retinoblastoma should be closely followed. Patients with hereditary retinoblastoma

TABLE 22-4
DISTINGUISHING CLINICAL FEATURES OF PAPILLEDEMA, PAPILLITIS, AND PSEUDOPAPILLEDEMA

	Papilledema	Papillitis	Pseudopapilledema
Symptoms	Headache, vomiting, behavior changes, lethargy	Vision loss, pain with eye movement	None
Visual acuity	Normal (unless long-standing with resulting optic nerve atrophy)	Significantly reduced	Normal
Appearance of disc	Blurred disc margins; no spontaneous venous pulsations[a]	Blurred disc margins; spontaneous venous pulsations may be present	Blurred disc margins; spontaneous venous pulsations may be present

[a]Spontaneous pulsations (associated with collapse and refilling of the veins of the optic disc) indicate that intracranial pressure is not significantly elevated. Their absence is less specific because some people do not have them even at normal central nervous system pressures.

are at an increased risk of developing secondary tumors later in life.

RETINOPATHY OF PREMATURITY

Retinopathy of prematurity (ROP) describes the abnormal vascularization of the retina in preterm infants who receive oxygen therapy. These abnormal vessels may hemorrhage, resulting in fibrotic areas that predispose to retinal detachment and blindness. Hyperoxia and low birth weight (<1,500 g) are the two highest risk factors for the development of ROP. Other contributing conditions include early gestational age, respiratory distress syndrome, and intracranial hemorrhage.

Current guidelines (joint statement issued by the American Academy of Pediatrics, American Association for Pediatric Ophthalmology and Strabismus, and American Academy of Ophthalmology) recommend an initial screening for high-risk infants at age 4 to 6 weeks (or 31 to 33 weeks postconceptual age) by an experienced ophthalmologist. High-risk infants include preterm infants weighing <1,500 g, infants born at a gestation age of ≤28 weeks, and infants with an unstable course requiring hyperoxia. Thereafter, management depends on the stage of ROP at diagnosis and ranges from serial examinations to obliteration of the abnormal vessels with laser or cryotherapy. Patients with a history of ROP are at increased risk for strabismus and amblyopia later in life.

EYE TRAUMA

Corneal Abrasions

Corneal abrasions involve the traumatic removal of the epithelial layer covering the cornea. Symptoms include the sudden onset of marked pain, excessive tearing, and refusal to open the eye. Older patients often complain of a "foreign body" sensation. Preverbal children may present with extreme irritability and refusal to open the eye. Instillation of topical anesthetic drops significantly decreases pain and permits the patient to open the eye for evaluation. Following an initial inspection to rule out foreign body or corneal injury, examination of the eye under blue light or Wood lamp following instillation of fluorescein should reveal the abrasion. Treatment involves patching (12 to 48 hours) to promote healing and comfort and topical antibiotic drops (for 2 to 4 days) to prevent infection. Corneal abrasions associated with contact lens use require consultation with an ophthalmologist to rule out bacterial corneal ulcer.

Significant Eye Trauma

The patient with a history of trauma to the eye warrants a thorough evaluation to determine the nature and extent of the injury. Trauma to the eye may be blunt or penetrating. A *perforating* injury that results in rupture of the globe usually presents with global deformity, an irregular pupil/iris, intraocular bleeding, and distorted vision, although occasionally a conjunctival laceration is the only finding. Immediate evaluation and repair by a knowledgeable specialist is crucial to limiting morbidity and retaining residual vision, if possible.

Patients with *traumatic hyphema* due to blunt trauma present with eye pain and possibly blurred vision, depending on the amount of bleeding. Bright red blood is evident in the inferior aspect of the anterior chamber of the affected eye, beneath the cornea. Large hyphemas may partially obscure the iris and pupil. The child with significant hyphema due to trauma should be admitted to the hospital for ophthalmologic management and bed rest, with the head of the bed elevated 45 degrees. Ocular medications are administered in

TABLE 22-5
POTENTIAL INJURIES RESULTING FROM BLUNT TRAUMA TO THE EYE

Traumatic Iritis
- Symptoms: photophobia, pain, blurry vision, tearing
- Signs: injected sclera; possibly constricted pupil

Lens Subluxation
- Symptoms: pain, blurred vision, diplopia
- Signs: a visible edge of the lens

Vitreous Hemorrhage
- Symptoms: sudden appearance of spots, floaters, or loss of vision
- Signs: absent red reflex (due to intraocular bleeding)

Detached Retina
- Symptoms: a "curtain effect," flashes of light, and/or floaters
- Signs: defects in the visual field

Blowout Fracture (fracture of the orbital floor)
- Symptoms: diplopia, pain
- Signs: any of the following: ptosis, a "sunken" eyeball, limited ocular mobility, cheek numbness

an attempt to provide comfort and limit inflammation. The most significant sequela of traumatic hyphema is glaucoma, which develops when outflow from the anterior chamber is disrupted.

Clinical manifestations of other injuries resulting from *blunt trauma* to the eye are provided in Table 22-5. All are indications for immediate ophthalmology consultation.

SOURCES

American Academy of Pediatrics Committee on Practice and Ambulatory Medicine, Section on Ophthalmology, American Association of Certified Orthoptists, American Association for Pediatric Ophthalmology and Strabismus, and American Academy of Ophthalmology. Eye examination in infants, children, and young adults by pediatricians. *Pediatrics*. 2003;111:902–907.

Levine LM. Pediatric ocular trauma and shaken infant syndrome. *Pediatr Clin North Am*. 2003;50:137–148.

Miller KM, Apt C. The eyes. In: Rudolph CD, Rudolph AM, Hostetter MK, et al., eds. *Rudolph's pediatrics*. 21st ed. New York: McGraw-Hill; 2003:2351–2418.

Neuman MI, Eriksson E. Facial trauma. In: Fleisher GR, Ludwig S, Henretig FM, eds. *Textbook of pediatric emergency medicine*. 5th ed. Philadelphia: Lippincott Williams & Wilkins; 2006: 1475–1484.

Olitsky SE, Nelson LB. Disorders of eye movement and alignment. In: Behrman RE, Kliegman RM, Jenson HB, eds. *Nelson textbook of pediatrics*. 17th ed. Philadelphia: WB Saunders; 2004: 2092–2096.

Section on Ophthalmology, American Academy of Pediatrics, American Academy of Ophthalmology, American Association for Pediatric Ophthalmology and Strabismus. Screening examination of premature infants for retinopathy of prematurity. *Pediatrics*. 2006; 117:572–576.

Tingley DH. Vision screening essentials: screening today for eye disorders in the pediatric patient. *Pediatr Rev*. 2007;28:54–62.

Wilson WG. Retinoblastoma. *Pediatr Rev*. 2007;28:37–38.

QUESTIONS

1. An infant born at 26 weeks of gestation has a hospital course complicated by necrotizing enterocolitis and intraventricular hemorrhaging. What are the current recommendations regarding screening for retinopathy of prematurity in this patient?
A) This infant does not require screening for retinopathy of prematurity.
B) This infant should be screened at 2 weeks of life and every week thereafter.
C) This infant should receive an initial screening at 4 to 6 weeks of age.
D) This patient should be screened when all intercurrent illnesses have been stabilized.
E) This patient should be screened within 1 week of weaning to room air.

2. An 18-month-old boy is brought to the emergency department with a chief complaint of "swollen eye." The patient's history is significant for 3 days of runny nose and cough. In the past 12 hours, the upper and lower lids of the patient's right eye have swollen shut and become markedly inflamed. The patient has a temperature of 103.9°F and appears quite ill. An orbital computed tomography reveals right-sided periorbital soft tissue swelling with inflammatory changes. All orbital and subperiosteal tissues are normal. A lumbar puncture is negative for pleocytosis, and no organisms are noted on Gram stain. Blood cultures are obtained. The most appropriate empiric antibiotic regimen for this patient is:
A) oral amoxicillin-clavulanic acid and oral clindamycin
B) intravenous cephalexin and intravenous clindamycin
C) intravenous cefotaxime
D) intravenous cefotaxime and intravenous vancomycin
E) intravenous cephalexin and intravenous clindamycin

3. An infant is born with a port wine stain covering the left forehead and cheek and involving the left upper lid. The most likely ophthalmologic complication associated with this patient's condition is:
A) congenital cataract
B) anisometropia
C) nystagmus
D) glaucoma
E) ptosis

4. Which of the following is a true statement regarding nasolacrimal duct obstruction?
A) Infants with nasolacrimal duct obstruction present with chronic conjunctivitis.
B) Infants with nasolacrimal duct obstruction require antibiotic prophylaxis until resolution of their blockage.
C) Infants with nasolacrimal duct obstruction are at increased risk for the development of dacryocystitis.
D) Infants with nasolacrimal duct obstruction that has not resolved spontaneously by 6 months of age should be probed.
E) Infants with nasolacrimal duct obstruction are more likely than their peers to develop significant amblyopia.

5. A full-term infant discharged at 48 hours presents to your office for a 1-week routine health maintenance appointment. You notice bilateral upper and lower lid swelling with thin, watery discharge. Moderate conjunctivitis and a pseudomembrane are noted on inversion of the upper lids. The rest of the examination is normal. The mother notes that the child's eye became swollen and began "tearing" yesterday. Which of the following is the most likely etiologic agent of this child's conjunctivitis?
A) *Neisseria gonorrhea*
B) *Chlamydia trachomatis*
C) Group B streptococcus
D) *Haemophilus influenzae*
E) Herpes simplex virus type 2

6. During the initial newborn examination of a full-term infant, inspection of the patient's eyes with the ophthalmoscope reveals bilateral white pupils. Which of the following intrauterine conditions is most closely associated with this bilateral leukocoria in the neonate?
A) Congenital rubella
B) Congenital retinoblastoma
C) Congenital glaucoma
D) Ophthalmia neonatorum
E) Congenital human immunodeficiency virus

7. A 13-year-old girl presents to your office with complaints of blurry vision in her left eye for 5 days and eye pain behind the left eye for 2 days. The eye discomfort decreases when the patient holds her eyes still. The patient has 20/30 vision in her right eye and 20/200 vision in her left eye. Funduscopic examination reveals blurred optic disc margins; spontaneous venous pulsations are present and appear normal. This patient's visual loss is most likely due to which of the following?
A) Papilledema
B) Optic neuritis
C) Pseudopapilledema
D) Retinal detachment
E) Optic glioma

8. A 14-year-old adolescent presents to the emergency department following a baseball game during which he was hit in the right eye with a bat. The patient is complaining of eye pain and double vision. He is unable to look up with his right eye. The eyeball appears slightly sunken in the orbit. This patient has most likely sustained which of the following?
A) Lens subluxation
B) Vitreous hemorrhage
C) Detached retina
D) Blowout fracture
E) Traumatic hyphema

9. A 4-month-old infant presents for well child care and immunizations. His mother notes that the child has had increasing tearing from both eyes in the past 3 weeks and seems uncomfortable in the bright sunlight. He has also developed episodes of "blinking" in which he closes the eyes for a few seconds several times in a row. This occurs two to three times a day. This child's symptoms merit urgent referral to an ophthalmologist to evaluate for which of the following?
A) Congenital glaucoma
B) Congenital cataracts
C) Congenital retinoblastoma
D) Congenital third nerve palsy
E) Congenital strabismus

10. A 7-year-old girl presents to your office with conjunctivitis that has not cleared during 5 days of topical polymyxin B-trimethoprim eye drops. Her mother notes that she is becoming very sensitive to light and complains of eye pain. Her visual acuity tests at 20/50; 2 years ago at her kindergarten assessment, she tested 20/30 in both eyes. On examination, you note that the conjunctival injection is diffuse but slightly more concentrated around the iris. What systemic disease is most likely to be associated with this patient's ocular condition?
A) Systemic lupus erythematosus
B) Wegener granulomatosis
C) Tuberous sclerosis
D) Riley-Day syndrome
E) Juvenile idiopathic arthritis

11. Which of the following patients does not meet the criteria for referral to an ophthalmologist for evaluation and management?
A) A 4-year-old girl with 20/20 vision in her left eye and 20/30 vision in her right eye
B) A 16-year-old male adolescent who wears contacts and develops eye pain and conjunctivitis

C) A 3-month-old infant with intermittent strabismus on examination
D) A 10-day-old infant with unilateral conjunctival injection, serous eye drainage, and keratitis
E) A 6-month-old infant with rhythmic eye oscillations in one eye when the other eye is occluded

12. A 3-month-old patient has isolated ocular malformations resulting in near-total blindness. Which of the following developmental tracts is likely to be most affected by his visual impairment between now and age 3 years?
A) Social development
B) Emotional development
C) Language development
D) Motor development
E) Attachment to a primary caregiver

13. A 13-year-old boy who was hit in the eye with a baseball during practice is brought to the emergency department by his parents. There is no history of altered consciousness, vomiting, or additional head trauma. The left periorbital soft tissues are markedly edematous. The patient is able to open the eye with difficulty (due to the swelling), and extraocular movements are intact. Pupillary responses are normal. Bright red blood is noted in the inferior aspect of the anterior chamber, partially obstructing the iris. The ophthalmologist on call is currently evaluating another patient in a hospital across town; he is expected within the hour. Which of the following represents the best management of this patient in the interim?
A) Administer intravenous ceftriaxone
B) Patch the eye under moderate pressure
C) Admit the patient to the intensive care unit for sedation
D) Discharge the patient with strict instructions to follow-up with an ophthalmologist within 24 hours
E) Elevate the head of the bed 45 degrees and limit patient activity to bed rest

ANSWERS

1. C	6. A	11. A
2. C	7. B	12. D
3. D	8. D	13. E
4. C	9. A	
5. B	10. E	

Disorders of the Ear, Nose, and Throat

23

EVALUATION OF HEARING

Universal newborn hearing screening is discussed in Chapter 5. Before the institution of universal newborn screening, congenital hearing loss was diagnosed at an average age of 15 months. Most infants with congenital hearing impairment acquire prelinguistic language skills at the expected times; that is, they smile, coo, babble, and understand gesture games at the same ages as their normal-hearing peers. The period between 6 and 24 months of age is critical in the development of the auditory system and the foundation for normal speech. Formal audiologic assessment is indicated for children with one or more defined risk factors for hearing loss (Table 23-1), infants who fail newborn hearing screening tests, patients with early language and/or global developmental delay, and children whose parents are concerned about their child's ability to hear. A review of audiologic testing procedures used in children is contained in Table 23-2. Although specific tests are more or less appropriate depending on the age of the patient, evaluation for hearing loss is possible in patients of all ages and developmental levels. It is thought that early identification and intervention are beneficial for optimizing speech and language abilities in infants and children with hearing loss. The onset of hearing impairment beyond the age of 5 years has much less of an impact on language development than earlier hearing loss.

Tympanometry does not measure hearing ability; rather, it is a method of evaluating the function of the middle ear. Tympanometry measures *compliance* of the tympanic membrane and ear canal *volume*. Tympanometry is useful for documenting poor membrane mobility suggestive of middle ear effusion, detecting membrane perforation, or assessing the patency of tympanostomy tubes. It can be performed in patients of all ages but is technically difficult in the very young. The absence of a pressure peak in the setting of normal canal volume is consistent with fluid in the middle ear.

TABLE 23-1
RISK FACTORS FOR CHILDHOOD HEARING LOSS

Risk Factors for Congenital Hearing Loss

Neonatal intensive care unit admission lasting longer than 48 hours
Prolonged mechanical ventilation or extracorporeal membrane oxygenation
Intrauterine growth retardation
Perinatal asphyxia
Syndromic anomalies or craniofacial anomalies
Family history of hearing loss in childhood
Clinical evidence of congenital infection

Risk Factors for Acquired Hearing Loss

Parental concern regarding hearing or language development
Bacterial meningitis
Neonatal factors—hyperbilirubinemia requiring exchange transfusion; persistent pulmonary hypertension of the newborn requiring mechanical ventilation; extracorporeal membrane oxygenation
Syndromes associated with progressive hearing loss (e.g., neurofibromatosis)
Neurodegenerative disorders
Head trauma
Recurrent or persistent otitis media with effusion for at least 3 months

HEARING LOSS

Hearing loss in children may be peripheral or central. In *central hearing loss,* the deficit results from disordered function of central nervous system auditory processing centers; generation and transport of the auditory impulse remain intact. Central hearing loss is rare in children. *Peripheral hearing loss,* which is more common, is due to abnormalities of the ear (outer, middle, or inner) and/or the auditory nerve. Peripheral hearing loss is further classified as conductive, sensorineural, or mixed (Table 23-3).

In isolated *conductive hearing loss* (CHL), generation and transmission of sound through the external ear canal, tympanic membrane, middle ear, and/or ossicles are impaired. Cochlea and auditory nerve function remain intact. Signs of mild CHL ("ignoring" behavior and increasing television or radio volume) are subtle and may initially be missed, delaying diagnosis. Many forms of CHL improve or resolve with medical or surgical intervention. In children, *otitis media with effusion is the most common cause of CHL.*

TABLE 23-2
TECHNIQUES FOR EVALUATION OF HEARING IN INFANTS AND CHILDREN

Behavioral Testing Procedures require the patient to perform a behavior in response to an auditory stimulus. Behavioral procedures are considered the "gold standard" for detection of hearing loss in patients older than 6 months of age; however, they are less reliable in younger infants and children with neurologic abnormalities. Certain physical disabilities such as cerebral palsy may interfere with a child's ability to produce a behavioral response despite normal hearing.

Behavioral Observation Audiometry (BOA)
- Chronologic or developmental age: birth to 6 months
- Speakers located on both right and left sides of the patient provide auditory stimulus
- Technician observes for changes in behavior following standardized auditory stimuli
- Detects moderate-to-severe hearing loss
- Normal result does not exclude subtle or unilateral hearing loss
- Does not allow differentiation of conductive hearing loss from sensorineural hearing loss

Visual Reinforcement Audiometry (VRA)
- Chronologic or developmental age: 6 to 36 months
- Speakers located on both right and left sides of the patient provide auditory stimulus
- Patient is rewarded with an interesting visual reward (e.g., puppet) when he or she looks toward the sound, which conditions the patient to localize the sound
- Different decibel levels of sound can be tested to detect a "threshold" and give a rough estimate of the severity of hearing loss
- Does not exclude subtle or unilateral hearing loss
- Does not allow differentiation of conductive hearing loss from sensorineural hearing loss

Conditioned Play Audiometry
- Chronologic or developmental age: 3 to 5 years
- Involves placement of headphones, so unilateral hearing loss can be detected
- Capable of detecting subtle hearing loss
- Ability to measure bone conduction thresholds permits differentiation of conductive hearing loss from sensorineural hearing loss

Conventional Audiometry
- Chronologic or developmental age: ≥5 years
- Standardized auditory stimulus is delivered via headphones, with child raising a hand or pressing a button when he or she hears the sound
- Capable of detecting subtle and unilateral hearing loss
- Ability to measure bone conduction thresholds permits differentiation of conductive hearing loss from sensorineural hearing loss

Electrophysiologic Testing Procedures do not require a voluntary action on the part of the patient for assessment. Auditory brainstem response (ABR) is considered the "proxy gold standard" for evaluation of hearing in the child younger than 6 months of age. Both ABR and otoacoustic emissions (OAE) are more reliable for newborn screening when they are performed after the first 48 hours of life. These tests are noninvasive, easy to perform, quick, and relatively inexpensive.

OAE
- Can be performed in patients of any age
- Tests outer hair cell function of the cochlea
- Allows detection of unilateral hearing loss
- Abnormal results are obtained in the presence of middle ear effusion
- Does not provide information regarding the severity of hearing loss
- Results will be normal in a patient with hearing loss due to abnormalities of the auditory nerve or central nervous system auditory processing centers

ABR
- Accepted as a proxy gold standard for assessment of hearing in infants <6 months of age (including newborns)
- Can be performed in patients of any age; however, patients >6 months may require sedation
- Measures surface brainwave patterns generated in response to a standardized auditory stimulus
- Does not measure hearing directly, but does provide a indirect approximation of ear-specific hearing thresholds, including subtle impairment
- Permits assessment of neurologic auditory function through the level of the lower brainstem
- Permits differentiation of conductive hearing loss and sensorineural hearing loss
- Results may be unreliable or difficult to interpret in patients with underlying neurologic abnormalities

In contrast, *sensorineural hearing loss* (SNHL) involves malfunction of the inner ear (cochlea) or auditory nerve (rare). Tympanometry results are normal, and the outer and middle ear structures appear normal. Electrophysiologic tests are used to localize impairment to the cochlea or auditory nerve. The presence of middle ear fluid leads to abnormal results on otoacoustic testing; when tympanometry is normal in patients who fail otoacoustic tests, SNHL is

TABLE 23-3
CAUSES OF HEARING LOSS IN CHILDREN

Conductive/Congenital
Aural stenosis/atresia
Malformation of the ossicles

Conductive/Acquired
Cerumen impaction
Otitis media (with or without effusion)
Tympanic membrane perforation
Cholesteatoma
Otitis externa
Tympanosclerosis
Traumatic ossicular disruption[a]
Bacterial meningitis

Sensorineural/Congenital
Genetic hearing loss (50%)
- Nonsyndromic genetic hearing loss
  - Various abnormalities in the connexin-26 gene
- Syndromic genetic hearing loss (less common than nonsyndromic hearing loss)
  - Alport syndrome
  - Waardenburg syndrome
  - Treacher-Collins syndrome
  - Usher syndrome
  - Pendred syndrome
  - Jervell and Lange-Nielsen syndrome

Congenital infection (50%)
- Cytomegalovirus
- Less commonly rubella, toxoplasmosis, syphilis

Sensorineural/Acquired or Progressive
Bacterial meningitis
Mumps
Trauma to the temporal bone with associated cochlear or auditory nerve injury
Acoustic trauma (sudden or cumulative; irreversible)
Ototoxicity secondary to medication
- Aminoglycosides
- Furosemide
- Cisplatin
- Salicylic acid (high-dose)

Hypoxic injury
Hyperbilirubinemia
Radiation exposure

[a]Presents with the sudden onset of moderate-to-severe hearing loss following trauma; the tympanic membrane remains intact and appears normal.

highly probable. Congenital SNHL is more common than acquired SNHL.

Full audiologic assessment includes a combination of age-appropriate tests to assess the functioning of each component of the auditory system and ascertain the type and degree of impairment. Children with confirmed hearing loss merit referral to a pediatric otolaryngologist experienced in the evaluation and treatment of hearing loss. Consultation with a clinical geneticist is appropriate for patients who may have syndromic or nonsyndromic genetic disorders. A screening urinalysis should be obtained in children, particularly boys, with newly diagnosed hearing loss; the presence of protein or urine is suspicious for Alport syndrome.

Hearing loss severity is classified according to hearing thresholds:

- 0 to 15 dB: normal hearing
- 16 to 25 dB: borderline hearing loss
- 26 to 40 dB: mild hearing loss
- 41 to 55 dB: moderate hearing loss
- 56 to 70 dB: moderate-to-severe hearing loss
- 71 to 90 dB: severe hearing loss
- $>$90 dB: profound hearing loss

Hearing impairment not only impacts speech and language skills, but it also adversely affects cognitive, social, and emotional development. The child with borderline hearing loss may misunderstand questions in class and respond inappropriately to teachers and peers. Children with mild-to-moderate hearing loss may be misidentified as poor listeners or as having behavior problems in class; they have trouble communicating effectively with others and may develop poor self-esteem. More severe hearing loss is usually identified sooner; early intervention preserves the patient's ability to communicate with others, assists with development of normal speech, and prevents social isolation.

Patients with borderline-to-mild hearing loss benefit from sound amplification (e.g., hearing aids, FM system assistive listening devices) and preferred seating in the classroom. Amplification is essential for patients with moderate and severe hearing loss, who also require special educational intervention. The educational needs of children with severe-to-profound hearing loss are best met within special classrooms with the use of sign language and other programs designed specifically for the deaf student. Cochlear implants are reserved for the patient $\geq$12 months of age whose hearing cannot be improved with amplification. These implants are appropriate regardless of whether the hearing impairment is congenital or acquired.

EAR PAIN

Otogenic causes of ear pain (otitis media, otitis externa, foreign body, or trauma) are generally obvious upon examination of the outer ear, external canal, and tympanic membrane. Tumor is a rare cause of ear pain in children. A nonotogenous source must be considered when the ear canal and tympanic membrane appear normal. Ear pain may be referred from the teeth, temporomandibular joint (TMJ), salivary glands, and cervical lymph nodes. Dental conditions, such as abscesses, impacted molars, and teething, are the most common source of referred pain to the ear. Dental radiographs may identify an underlying abnormality. Malocclusion or mechanical disturbance at the TMJ presents with severe pain radiating to the ear, temporalis, cheek, and neck areas. Examination reveals tenderness of the joint and associated muscles; abnormal lateral movement or an audible or palpable "click" may be noted upon opening or closing the joint. Finally, referred ear pain may be a feature of acute tonsillitis, postoperative adenotonsillectomy, and parotitis.

OTORRHEA

In children, otorrhea most commonly results from otitis externa or otitis media with perforation of the tympanic membrane. Table 23-4 lists other potential causes of otorrhea. Traumatic *fracture of the temporal bone* should be suspected in the patient with a consistent history and any of the following: persistent clear drainage through a perforation in the tympanic membrane, moderate-to-severe SNHL, and vertigo.

DISORDERS OF THE EXTERNAL EAR

Congenital Malformations

Preauricular tags and preauricular pits are relatively common anomalies in newborns. Although most occur in isolation, a significant minority present as part of a syndromic complex [e.g., CHARGE association (coloboma of the eye, heart defect, retardation of growth, genital anomalies, and ear abnormalities)]. Neonates with congenital malformations of the external ear should be examined carefully for other dysmorphic features. If additional anomalies are found or if the patient has a family history of hearing loss or malformation of the ear or kidney, consultation with a clinical geneticist is indicated for further evaluation, counseling, and management. Renal ultrasonography and chromosomal analysis are usually obtained in this setting. Newborns with benign family histories and otherwise normal physical examinations do not require additional evaluation.

TABLE 23-4
POTENTIAL CAUSES OF OTORRHEA IN CHILDREN

Nonbloody Otorrhea

Perilymph fistula

Trauma to the temporal bone (temporal bone fracture with leakage of cerebrospinal fluid)

First branchial cleft sinus formation

Bloody Otorrhea

Local trauma

Formation of friable granulation tissue around new or occluded tympanostomy tubes

Nonbloody or Bloody Otorrhea

Acute suppurative otitis media with perforation of the tympanic membrane

Otitis externa

Cholesteatoma

Foreign body in the ear canal

Tumor (rare)

Auricular Hematoma

Blunt or shearing trauma to the external ear can result in auricular hematoma. The collection of blood may be located between the skin and perichondrium (the thick fibrous layer of connective tissue surrounding the cartilage). Alternatively, the blood may be trapped between the perichondrium and cartilage. Trauma to the external ear results in pain, swelling, ecchymosis, and localized fluctuance. The potential for irreversible disfigurement is high in cases of auricular hematoma. Evacuation of the collected blood with fine-needle aspiration prevents subsequent tissue necrosis and cosmetic deformity.

Otitis Externa

Otitis externa ("swimmer's ear") is inflammation of the external auditory canal that is generally infectious in nature. Otitis externa is usually unilateral but may involve both ears simultaneously. The affected patient presents with severe ear pain that is exacerbated by gentle tugging on the tragus or pinna. Discharge is purulent and often tinged with blood. The entire canal is markedly erythematous and edematous; swelling and cellular debris may obscure the tympanic membrane. Suctioning often removes enough material to permit visualization of the tympanic membrane, which remains translucent and mobile, allowing differentiation of otitis externa and suppurative otitis media with perforation. *Furunculosis* may occasionally be mistaken for otitis externa; in the former, signs of cellulitic infection are localized to a specific region of the canal.

Pathogens most commonly implicated in otitis externa are *Pseudomonas aeruginosa*, *Staphylococcus* species, and Gram-negative rods (*Klebsiella*, *Proteus* species). Fungal infections are less common but do occur. Placement of an ear wick, followed by instillation of topical antibiotic drops with or without hydrocortisone, typically results in marked improvement by the time the wick is removed 48 to 72 hours later. Appropriate antibiotic choices include neomycin/polymyxin B, ciprofloxacin, ofloxacin, gentamicin, and tobramycin.

Foreign Body

Foreign bodies become lodged in the ear canal due to self-insertion during play or trauma; insects may rarely crawl into the external canal as well. Patients present with persistent ear pain, otorrhea (which is often foul smelling and does not clear with topical antibiotic use), and less commonly hearing loss and cervical lymphadenopathy. Foreign bodies are often clearly visible but may be obscured by cerumen or purulent discharge. If foreign body is suspected based on the history and examination, computed tomography (CT) and/or otic microscopy under sedation may be required if the excess material cannot be cleared by suctioning. Disc batteries and vegetable matter should be removed immediately. Most small objects can be grasped with forceps or dislodged with irrigation. Irrigation is contraindicated in cases of vegetable matter in the canal, which readily swells when hydrated.

DISORDERS OF THE MIDDLE EAR

Acute Otitis Media

Acute otitis media (AOM) is infection of the middle ear chamber involving a bacterial or viral pathogen. AOM is the most commonly diagnosed disease of childhood and accounts for more outpatient prescriptions than any other pediatric condition. Incidence peaks in children 6 to 18 months of age, with gradual tapering thereafter. It is diagnosed more frequently during the winter months. AOM is associated with underlying *eustachian tube dysfunction*, so recurrence is common. Recurrent and chronic otitis media are associated with temporary CHL; children who suffer from these conditions during the critical period for language development (ages 6 to 24 months) are at risk for language disorders and social delay. Risk factors for AOM and strategies for prevention are listed in Table 23-5.

TABLE 23-5
ACUTE OTITIS MEDIA: RISK FACTORS AND PREVENTION

Predisposing Factors
Male gender
Family history of recurrent otitis media
Atopic disease
Immunodeficiency
Craniofacial anomalies (particularly cleft palate)
Child care attendance
Older siblings
Environmental smoke exposure
Pacifier use
Bottle feeding
Specific genetic disorders (trisomy 21; Crouzon syndrome)
Onset of first ear infection prior to 6 months of age
Low socioeconomic status

Strategies for Prevention
Breastfeeding
Limitation of days of child care attendance
Limitation of the number of children to which the patient is exposed at child care
Remaining up to date on immunizations (particularly heptavalent pneumococcal, influenza vaccines)
Limiting environmental smoke exposure
Discouraging pacifier use
Early weaning to a cup in bottle-fed infants

The middle ear chamber is normally aerated. Most cases of AOM are preceded by a few days of upper respiratory symptoms. Associated inflammation and edema narrow and partially occlude the lumen of the eustachian tube. The air in the middle ear space is resorbed, resulting in a relative vacuum; bacteria-filled fluid from the nasopharynx is drawn into the middle ear, where the organisms multiply and stimulate an inflammatory response. Infants and young children present with fever, fussiness, interrupted sleep, and/or poor feeding. Patients who are old enough to verbalize complain of significant ear pain that often interferes with sleep. Fever and irritability are often present as well.

The clinical criteria required for a diagnosis of AOM include a bulging, nonmobile tympanic membrane *and* evidence of local or systemic inflammation. Thus, both *visualization of the tympanic membrane* and *assessment of mobility* (via insufflation or tympanogram) are necessary elements of the evaluation. The tympanic membrane is normally gray and translucent, with a visible light reflex and identifiable ossicular landmarks. The membrane moves easily when positive and negative pressures are applied, and the tympanogram forms a peaked wave. Patients with AOM present with variable combinations of the following: erythema of the tympanic membrane; a bulging membrane, evidenced by loss of the light reflex and bony landmarks; opaque middle ear fluid; and decreased mobility. The tympanogram demonstrates decreased wave amplitude and may be flat. AOM is occasionally confused with *viral myringitis* (ear pain and erythema of the tympanic membrane associated with viral upper respiratory illness; normal membrane mobility). Pain control is adequate treatment for this benign, self-limited condition. In *bullous myringitis,* which may complicate cases of isolated AOM, a large bulla forms on the tympanic membrane. Patients with bullous myringitis have particularly severe otalgia. Myringotomy with incision of the bulla is not required for treatment but does result in rapid relief of the pain. Decisions regarding antimicrobial therapy are identical to those for uncomplicated bacterial AOM.

The vast majority of bacterial AOM is due to infection with *Streptococcus pneumoniae,* nontypeable *Haemophilus influenzae,* and *Moraxella catarrhalis* (Table 23-6). Because more antibiotics are prescribed for AOM than any other pediatric condition and because antibiotic resistance is a growing concern, the Centers for Disease Control and Prevention recently issued consensus recommendations regarding the treatment of AOM. Patients younger than 24 months of age, patients thought to be at risk for poor follow-up, ill-appearing patients, and patients with chronic

TABLE 23-6
COMMON PATHOGENS IN ACUTE OTITIS MEDIA

Streptococcus Pneumoniae
- Currently causes 25% to 40% of bacterial AOM (decreased percentage due to universal immunization with heptavalent pneumococcal vaccine)
- Spontaneous resolution in 20% of cases
- Increasingly resistant to penicillin through alteration of penicillin-binding proteins; increasing the dose of the medication overcomes resistance in many cases

Haemophilus Influenzae
- Currently causes 35% to 50% of bacterial AOM
- Spontaneous resolution in 50% of cases
- Fifty percent of isolates produce beta-lactamases (increasing the dose does not overcome resistance)

Moraxella Catarrhalis
- Currently causes 10% to 15% of bacterial AOM
- Spontaneous resolution in 80% of cases
- Nearly 100% of isolates produce beta-lactamases

Other Bacterial Pathogens
- Group A *Streptococcus*
- *Staphylococcus aureus*
- *Mycoplasma pneumoniae*

Viral Pathogens
- Currently cause approximately 25% to 30% of AOM
- Common pathogens include adenovirus, respiratory syncytial virus, rhinovirus, influenza, parainfluenza

illnesses (including immunodeficiencies) or recurrent, severe, or perforated AOM should be prescribed antibiotics. High-dose amoxicillin (70 to 90 mg/kg/day) is the recommended first-line treatment. Patients who have been treated with antibiotics within the last month and those who have not improved within 48 hours are eligible for second-line therapy with amoxicillin/clavulanic acid, an oral second- or third-generation cephalosporin, or intramuscular ceftriaxone. A second-line agent is also appropriate for initial therapy in the child with clinical manifestations suggesting a resistant organism (e.g., AOM associated with conjunctivitis). Children who are older than 24 months with less severe disease may be offered the choice of immediate antibiotic therapy versus pain control and watchful waiting. Those children in whom antibiotics are initially withheld are provided a prescription to fill 48 hours later if there has been no improvement. Ten days of therapy are recommended for affected children younger than 2 years of age; shorter courses (5 to 7 days) are equally effective in older individuals. Patients with disease that does not respond to multiple (three consecutive) daily doses of parenteral ceftriaxone should be referred for diagnostic and therapeutic tympanocentesis. Decongestants and antihistamines are of no benefit in the management of AOM. Of note, 80% of cases of untreated AOM resolve within 2 weeks, compared with 95% of cases managed with antimicrobial therapy.

Otitis media with effusion (OME) follows virtually all cases of AOM. OME is defined as fluid within the middle ear space in the absence of systemic or local signs of infection. The presence of fluid translates to poor mobility of the tympanic membrane, which is often retracted. The fluid may be straw or amber colored, and bubbles or an air-fluid level may be visible on examination. OME persists for a variable length of time (Table 23-7) but is considered *chronic* when the fluid is present for longer than 3 months. Chronic OME is unlikely to resolve spontaneously. Patients with AOM should undergo follow-up examination of the affected ear 6 weeks later, with another visit 6 weeks thereafter if the fluid has not cleared. Patients with chronic OME are assessed for hearing loss and referred for possible *tympanostomy tube* placement. Tympanostomy tubes are generally indicated for bilateral OME that persists for >3 to 4 months and unilateral OME persisting for >6 months. If hearing loss is present, speech and language assessment should be pursued.

Tympanostomy tube should also be considered in patients with *recurrent AOM* (three episodes within 6 months or more than four episodes within 12 months). Children with persistent effusions are particularly susceptible to recurrent episodes of AOM. Recurrent AOM may also be associated with underlying predisposing conditions, including allergic rhinitis, cleft palate, immunodeficiency, sinus disease, and primary ciliary dyskinesia. First-line therapy (high-dose amoxicillin) is appropriate for subsequent episodes of AOM as long as at least 1 to 2 months have passed since the last infection. Placement of tympanostomy tubes significantly reduces the incidences of both recurrent AOM and persistent OME. It is the most commonly performed pediatric surgical procedure in the United States. The average life of a tympanostomy tube is approximately 14 months. Short- and long-term complications of tympanostomy tube placement are listed in Table 23-8.

Perforation of the tympanic membrane occurs in 5% of AOM and is the most common complication. Most spontaneous perforations resolve within 24 to 72 hours; this should be verified and documented on a follow-up examination. Oral antimicrobial therapy is generally adequate for treatment; topical drops are occasionally added. Prolonged perforation or persistent drainage that is unresponsive to appropriate

TABLE 23-7
PERSISTENCE OF MIDDLE EAR FLUID AFTER ACUTE OTITIS MEDIA

30% with complete resolution 2 weeks after initial infection
50% to 60% with complete resolution 4 weeks after initial infection
70% to 80% with complete resolution 8 weeks after initial infection
90% with complete resolution 12 weeks after initial infection

TABLE 23-8
COMPLICATIONS OF TYMPANOSTOMY TUBES

Indwelling Tympanostomy Tubes

Obstruction

Otorrhea during subsequent episodes of acute otitis media

Premature extrusion

Long-Term Sequelae (after tube extrusion)

Myringosclerosis[a]

Persistent perforation of the tympanic membrane

Tympanic membrane atrophy

Chronic retraction of the tympanic membrane and cholesteatoma formation

[a]Myringosclerosis consists of localized sclerosis of the tympanic membrane. It is the most common long-term complication of tympanostomy tubes. Myringosclerosis is not associated with hearing loss.

TABLE 23-9
POTENTIAL COMPLICATIONS OF OTITIS MEDIA

Intratemporal Complications

Otitis media with effusion

Perforation of the tympanic membrane

Chronic suppurative otitis media

Cholesteatoma

Facial nerve palsy

Mastoiditis

Subperiosteal abscess

Tympanosclerosis

Hearing loss

Intracranial Complications (exceedingly rare)

Meningitis (most common of the rare)

Epidural empyema or abscess

Subdural empyema or abscess

Lateral sinus thrombosis

Otitic hydrocephalus

antibiotic therapy warrants referral to an otolaryngologist. Tuberculosis should be considered in the patient with otorrhea through multiple perforations.

Chronic suppurative otitis media (CSOM) presents as persistent or recurrent foul-smelling, purulent otorrhea through a perforation in the tympanic membrane accompanied by localized signs of infection (e.g., erythema of the tympanic membrane). CSOM most frequently follows AOM but may also be associated with persistent perforation (from prior tympanostomy tubes) and cholesteatoma. The majority of cases are caused by *P. aeruginosa; Staphylococcus* is another common isolate. Ofloxacin or ciprofloxacin drops produce resolution in the majority of patients. Approximately 10% require surgical intervention, usually tympanomastoidectomy (removal of mastoid air cells and reconstruction of the tympanic membrane).

Cholesteatoma is a complication of persistent OME. Retraction of the tympanic membrane leads to the formation of a "retraction pocket" lined with epidermal tissue and filled with keratin debris, which remains chronically infected. Granulation tissue may be noted around the edges of the keratin mass. Affected children present with persistent otorrhea that is unresponsive to antimicrobial therapy. At least half of patients have associated CHL. Other possible complications include ossicular disruption, facial nerve paralysis, and mastoiditis with subperiosteal abscess formation. Antipseudomonal drops are prescribed to prevent infection; however, surgical excision is necessary to prevent continued enlargement and destruction of adjacent tissue.

The air cells within the mastoid bone are a direct extension of the aerated middle ear, so it is not surprising that mastoiditis may complicate AOM. *Acute mastoiditis* is usually due to *S. pneumoniae* or *H. influenzae; M. catarrhalis* is rarely implicated. The classic presentation involves a patient with signs and symptoms of AOM (e.g., fever, ear pain), edema/erythema/tenderness over the mastoid region, and lateral protrusion of the pinna. Mastoid radiographs are sensitive for opacification of the mastoid air cells and loss of septae; however, CT of the temporal bone is the procedure of choice due to detailed views of the air cells and bony septae and the ability to detect subperiosteal abscesses. Such abscesses may be detected clinically when bogginess is noted over the mastoid bone and the pinna is laterally displaced. Management of uncomplicated mastoiditis consists of myringotomy (for drainage of the middle ear and pathogen identification) and broad-spectrum empiric intravenous antimicrobial therapy (ceftriaxone, ampicillin-sulbactam). Abscesses, if present, should be drained. Mastoiditis that develops in the setting of CSOM is more likely to result from pseudomonal or staphylococcal organisms.

Tympanosclerosis is generalized scarring of the tympanic membrane due to recurrent AOM. It is usually not associated with perceptible hearing loss or changes in sound perception. Table 23-9 provides a summary of intratemporal and intracranial complications of otitis media.

DISORDERS OF THE NOSE

Congenital Malformations

Choanal atresia is the abnormal postnatal persistence of a bony or membranous septum that restricts the flow of air between the nasal passages and the oropharynx. Choanal atresia is usually unilateral; affected infants present with intermittent cyanosis that is relieved by crying. The discovery of choanal atresia (through failure to pass a nasogastric tube or nasal suction catheter) should prompt a search for other congenital anomalies, particularly those that occur in association with CHARGE sequence. Because neonates are obligate nose breathers, infants with bilateral choanal atresia develop severe respiratory distress shortly after birth. Endotracheal intubation bypasses the lesion in the acute setting; definitive repair requires surgical intervention. *Piriform aperture stenosis* is a less common structural cause of congenital nasal obstruction that also presents with severe respiratory distress in the immediate newborn period.

Choanal atresia should be differentiated from other structural (tumors) and nonstructural (gastroesophageal reflux disease) causes of nasal obstruction or congestion in the neonate. The most common cause is *nonspecific rhinitis*, a self-limited condition of unknown etiology best managed with saline drops and a bulb syringe. CT permits detailed views of the nasal structures and is beneficial for ruling out anatomic abnormalities as the source of obstruction.

Epistaxis

Most bleeding from the nose in children results from nasal trauma (including nose picking), excessive dryness, or local chemical or inflammatory irritation. Less common causes of epistaxis are listed in Table 23-10. Bleeding that originates from the Kiesselbach plexus in the anterior nose is easily identifiable on examination of the nose; external nasal compression is generally adequate to stop the bleeding, but cautery with silver nitrate may be necessary in some instances. Application of topical antimicrobial ointment provides moisture and prevents low-grade infectious inflammation. Epistaxis that does not respond to conservative measures is treated with placement of an anterior nasal pack. Nasal endoscopy is required to pinpoint the source of posterior nasal bleeding; a posterior nasal pack should be placed while the patient is awaiting consultation with an otolaryngologist.

TABLE 23-10
DIFFERENTIAL DIAGNOSIS OF RECURRENT EPISTAXIS

Recurrent nasal trauma
Excessive dryness
Upper respiratory infection
Allergic rhinitis
Sinusitis
Chemical irritation
Foreign body
Bleeding diathesis
Leukemia
Tumors
Polyps
Hemangioma
Cocaine use

Isolated *posttraumatic epistaxis* typically resolves spontaneously within several minutes of the injury. If the injured individual is not in distress, is breathing without difficulty, and does not have any obvious nasal deformity, a follow-up visit should be scheduled within a day or two to assess for a *septal hematoma*. Bleeding into the nasal septum results in significant pain, nasal obstruction, septal deviation, and a soft, bulging, erythematous submucosal mass occluding one or both sides of the nose. Visualization of the mass often requires examination with an otoscope and speculum. Patients with septal hematoma are at risk for tissue necrosis and permanent "saddle nose" cosmetic deformity. Prompt intervention (incision and drainage and prophylactic oral antibiotics) restores blood flow to cartilaginous tissue and prevents abscess formation.

Juvenile nasopharyngeal angiofibroma is a benign, markedly vascular tumor of the posterior nose; it is found almost exclusively in adolescent males. Patients present with the gradual onset of nasal obstruction; profuse, persistent epistaxis; and occasionally cranial neuropathies and a palpable mass in the cheek, soft palate, or temporalis region. Plain radiographs (basal sinus view) demonstrate anterior bowing of the posterior wall of the maxillary sinus on the same side as the lesion. CT and magnetic resonance imaging provide detailed views of the tumor and adjacent tissues. Biopsy is contraindicated. The tumor is surgically removed following embolization.

Adolescents who regularly snort *cocaine* and other illicit substances develop local vasoconstriction and reactive congestion and hyperemia. Prolonged use is associated with avascular necrosis and eventual perforation of the nasal septum.

Rhinitis

Allergic rhinitis is discussed in greater detail in Chapter 9. Table 23-11 provides an overview of some of the more frequent causes of rhinitis in children. Upper respiratory infection (URI) is the most common cause of rhinitis in all age groups. Infants and young children average between three and ten acute viral URIs a year. Many viruses and serotypes of those viruses are associated with cold symptoms; most are spread through direct or indirect (fomite) contact with infected *nasal* secretions. Saliva (coughing) is much less infectious. Cold viruses can live on inanimate objects for up to a few days. Although colds occur more commonly during the winter months, neither cold weather nor sudden change in weather increases susceptibility to viral URIs.

There is no scientific evidence that cough and cold preparations lessen the severity of symptoms or the duration of the illness. However, they are widely administered by parents. *Topical decongestants* decrease nasal congestion through local vasoconstriction and reduction of

TABLE 23-11
DIFFERENTIAL DIAGNOSIS OF RHINITIS IN CHILDREN

Acute

Seasonal allergic rhinitis

Symptoms: clear, thin rhinorrhea; nasal congestion; postnasal drip with cough; sneezing; watery eyes; pruritus (nose, eyes, palate, throat); symptoms recur at roughly the same time every year

Signs: pale, bluish nasal mucosa; enlarged, boggy turbinates; bilateral clear rhinorrhea; pharyngeal cobblestoning; "allergic shiners"; transverse nasal crease due to frequent "allergic salute"

Evaluation: increased eosinophils on nasal smear; serum eosinophilia, specific immunoglobulin E (IgE) antibodies; positive skin prick allergy tests

Acute viral rhinitis

Symptoms: rhinorrhea, congestion, fever

Signs: consistent with acute upper respiratory infection

Foreign body

Symptoms: acute or chronic, persistent purulent nasal discharge with or without epistaxis; unilateral nasal obstruction

Signs: foul-smelling, purulent, possibly bloody discharge; bromhidrosis (generalized body odor); possibly visualization of the foreign body in the nose

Chronic

Perennial allergic rhinitis

Symptoms: clear, thin rhinorrhea; nasal congestion; postnasal drip with cough; sneezing; watery eyes; pruritus (nose, eyes, palate, throat); symptoms present year round

Signs: pale, bluish nasal mucosa; enlarged, boggy turbinates; bilateral clear rhinorrhea; pharyngeal cobblestoning; "allergic shiners"; transverse nasal crease due to frequent "allergic salute"

Evaluation: increased eosinophils on nasal smear; serum eosinophilia, specific IgE antibodies; positive skin prick allergy tests

Chronic infectious rhinosinusitis

Symptoms: chronic mucopurulent nasal discharge; nasal congestion; postnasal drip with cough; headache; facial pain

Signs: tenderness over the involved sinuses

Vasomotor rhinitis

Symptoms: nasal obstruction; profuse rhinorrhea; intermittent sneezing; symptoms exacerbated with sudden temperature changes

Signs: profuse watery rhinorrhea; edema and hypertrophy of the nasal mucosa

Rhinitis medicamentosa

Symptoms: nasal congestion

Signs: hypertrophy of nasal mucosa

Cause: rebound effect from overuse of topical decongestants

Nasal Foreign Body

Nasal polyps

Symptoms: nasal obstruction

Signs: clear rhinorrhea; otoscopic visualization of a soft, semitransparent mass partially or fully obstructing the nose

Associated conditions: Nasal polyps are found in approximately 40% of children with cystic fibrosis; other conditions associated with nasal polyps include asthma, chronic allergic rhinitis, and chronic rhinosinusitis.

tissue edema. Topical decongestants should not be administered for >72 hours because of the potential for rebound congestion. This is a particularly dangerous development in infants younger than 3 to 6 months of age, who are still dependent on nasal airflow for breathing. *Oral decongestants* are not associated with rebound congestion. Adverse effects of systemic decongestants include anorexia, agitation, tachycardia, poor sleep, palpitations, and rarely dystonic reactions.

Although histamine release is not a feature of the common cold, first-generation *antihistamines* may be beneficial in drying the nasal mucosa through anticholinergic mechanisms. However, the effect is minimal at best. They may provide comfort through mild sedation of the patient, although some children develop paradoxic excitability. Other potential adverse effects include respiratory depression, ataxia, arrhythmias, dry mouth, blurred vision, and urinary retention, although these are less common than central nervous system sedation. First-generation antihistamines (e.g., diphenhydramine, hydroxyzine, chlorpheniramine) should not be administered to children with asthma unless there is clinical evidence of allergy. Second-generation antihistamines do not possess significant anticholinergic properties.

Nasal Polyps

Polyps are soft, semitransparent mass lesions that develop in the nose in response to chronic inflammation. Nasal polyps are an unusual finding in an otherwise healthy child; they are usually associated with underlying pathophysiology (e.g., chronic allergic rhinitis, chronic infectious rhinosinusitis). Between 40% and 50% of patients with cystic fibrosis eventually develop nasal polyps; in some cases, polyps are the presenting feature of the disease. Clinical manifestations of polyps include chronic rhinorrhea and progressive nasal obstruction. Surgical removal resolves the obstruction, but the masses tend to recur if underlying inflammation is left unchecked.

SINUS DISORDERS

Acute Sinusitis

The maxillary and ethmoid sinuses are present at birth; sphenoid sinuses develop later in childhood, and frontal sinuses are not present until adolescence. The spectrum of pathogens responsible for sinusitis is virtually identical to that for AOM. Sinusitis is often difficult to diagnose in the young child because the classic symptoms of headache, facial pain, and sinus tenderness may be absent or difficult to articulate. In older patients, the primary complaint may be toothache, sore throat, or persistent cough. *Acute bacterial sinusitis* has two common clinical presentations: (a) persistent respiratory symptoms (>10 to 14 days) without improvement, including either nasal discharge (clear or purulent) or a daytime cough; and (b) initially severe symptoms of high fever and purulent nasal discharge for at least 3 days. Older patients usually complain of headache or facial pain; periorbital edema, altered sense of smell, and fetid breath are common. Sinus tenderness is typically present on physical examination. In contrast, acute viral rhinosinusitis produces a few days of low-grade fever and variable degrees of clear, mucoid, or purulent rhinorrhea that resolves by the tenth day of illness.

Sinusitis is primarily a clinical diagnosis. Plain films of the sinuses may be useful in older children when there is a poor response to therapy and the diagnosis is in doubt; findings of sinus opacification, mucosal thickening, or air-fluid levels are consistent with sinusitis. CT is unnecessary in acute disease. However, limited CT of the sinuses is the preferred diagnostic procedure for evaluation of chronic sinusitis, also permitting assessment of contiguous structures for predisposing anatomic abnormalities. Nasal swab and throat cultures are noncontributory; sinus aspiration is the only way to identify the causative organism. The procedure is poorly tolerated in children and is reserved for recurrent or resistant disease, sinusitis in the patient who is allergic to multiple antibiotics, and immunocompromised patients, in whom there is a need to identify the organism for treatment. Antibiotic coverage is similar to that for AOM, although treatment should continue for 10 to 21 days. The addition of topical or systemic decongestants, mucolytic agents, and nasal saline irrigation may provide symptomatic relief in older patients. Intranasal corticosteroids have been used with variable success. Patients who are prone to sinusitis should consistently practice good nasal hygiene.

Complications from acute sinusitis are uncommon but include bony erosion, optic neuritis, orbital cellulitis, and intracranial extension. Intraorbital and intracranial extension (brain abscess) is occasionally associated with frontal sinusitis in adolescents and adults.

Chronic Sinusitis

Chronic sinusitis is defined as signs and symptoms of disease that persist beyond 90 days. Chronic sinusitis should be suspected in the individual with a persistent cough that does not respond to maximal asthma therapy but transiently improves with antibiotics. Responsible pathogens include those implicated in acute bacterial sinusitis (*S. pneumoniae*, nontypeable *H. influenzae*, and *M. catarrhalis*) as well as *Staphylococcus aureus*, other streptococcal species, anaerobic bacteria, and fungi. High-dose amoxicillin, amoxicillin/clavulanic acid, broad-spectrum cephalosporins, and clindamycin are all appropriate empiric antimicrobial choices. As opposed to acute disease, adjunct therapies (e.g., decongestants, mucolytics) provide no benefit in the management of chronic sinusitis.

Sinus Trauma

Fractures of the nasal bones and mandible are more common than sinus fractures in pediatric trauma patients. CT of the head and facial bones is the preferred study for evaluation of traumatic injuries to the bones and soft tissues of the face. Frontal sinus fractures of the anterior table may or may not be accompanied by posterior table fractures. Isolated, nondisplaced anterior plate fractures heal without intervention. Displaced fractures require surgical reduction and fixation to prevent cosmetic deformity. Fractures through the posterior table place the individual at risk for leakage of cerebrospinal fluid through the fracture and subsequent central nervous system infection. Open reduction with sinus obliteration is indicated in the majority of these cases to limit the potential for central nervous system complications.

DISORDERS OF THE THROAT

Pharyngitis

Most cases of acute pharyngitis in the pediatric population are viral in origin (Table 23-12). Viral pharyngitis may occasionally be accompanied by mild, self-limited pneumonia; affected individuals do not appear toxic and rarely require respiratory support. Adenovirus is responsible for 15% to 20% of isolated pharyngitis in children. *Pharyngoconjunctival fever*, characterized by 4 to 5 days of fever, pharyngitis, conjunctivitis, preauricular and cervical lymphadenopathy, and rhinitis, is a clinically distinct presentation of adenoviral infection.

Group A beta-hemolytic *Streptococcus* (GAS) is the leading cause of bacterial pharyngitis in school-age children; it is uncommon in younger age groups. The diagnosisis suggested by a constellation of the following: fever, palatal petechiae, tonsillar enlargement and exudates, tender cervical lymphadenitis, and scarlet fever rash. Rhinorrhea is notably absent. The abdominal pain that accompanies GAS pharyngitis may occasionally be severe and focal enough to be mistaken for appendicitis. GASis discussed in detail in Chapter 10. *Neisseria gonorrhoeae* should be considered in the sexually active patient with pharyngitis and obvious patches of erythema if the rapid strep screen is negative. Symptoms develop approximately 5 to 7 days after participation in oral sex. Although the pharyngitis is self-limited, resolving in 10 to 12 weeks, infected patients are at risk for disseminated disease, and sexual contacts should be identified and treated. Management is identical to that for genital disease. Unless GAS or *N. gonorrhoeae* is suspected, routine throat culture is of no benefit; the results provide no information concerning the etiology of intercurrent sinusitis, pneumonia, meningitis, or peritonsillar or retropharyngeal abscess.

TABLE 23-12
PARTIAL LIST OF VIRUSES KNOWN TO CAUSE ACUTE PHARYNGITIS IN INFANTS AND CHILDREN

Rhinovirus
Respiratory syncytial virus
Adenovirus
Enterovirus
Parainfluenza
Influenza viruses
Epstein-Barr virus
Cytomegalovirus
(among others)

Peritonsillar and Retropharyngeal Abscesses

Peritonsillar abscess is a polymicrobial infection of the peritonsillar tissues with resultant abscess formation. Although it may occur at any age, peritonsillar abscess is most common in adolescents and young adults. The microbiology, clinical manifestations, and treatment of peritonsillar abscess are provided in Table 23-13.

Retropharyngeal abscess is most common in preschool-age children; immunocompromise should be suspected when this illness is diagnosed in older children and adolescents. Most cases are preceded by an upper respiratory illness such as pharyngitis or tonsillitis.

ABNORMALITIES OF THE ORAL MUCOSA AND GLANDS

Cold panniculitis ("popsicle panniculitis") is the formation of erythematous plaques and subcutaneous nodules on the buccal mucosa following prolonged exposure to cold (frozen) objects. The overlying skin is normal. Cold panniculitis on the skin surface results from extended contact with an external cold source such as snow or an ice pack. Ill-defined erythematous plaques and bluish nodules develop over several hours to a few days. Cold panniculitis is similar in appearance to *buccal cellulitis;* however, the latter is usually unilateral and accompanied by tenderness, warmth, and fever.

A *ranula* is a mucin-filled pseudocyst found under the tongue in the region of the sublingual gland. The mass is usually soft and bluish in color. Ranulas develop when the sublingual gland duct becomes obstructed or disrupted. They are neither infectious nor inflammatory. Excision of the cyst and accompanying sublingual gland is required for definitive treatment; the recurrence rate following needle aspiration alone is unacceptably high.

Parotitis (inflammation of the parotid gland) in children is usually viral, but bacterial pathogens and noninfectious conditions can also cause parotitis (Table 23-14). Given the position of the parotid gland, other conditions that cause preauricular swelling should be considered in the differential diagnosis. Preauricular lymphadenopathy may result from parotitis; infection of the skin over the cheek, lateral lid, or temporal region; chronic conjunctivitis (due to infection with *Chlamydia trachomatis* or adenovirus); *Parinaud oculoglandular syndrome* (cat scratch disease); atypical *Mycobacteria* infection; and tumor. The most common cause of preauricular swelling in children is reactive lymphadenopathy secondary to adenoviral conjunctivitis.

CLEFT LIP AND PALATE

Cleft palate may occur in isolation but is often associated with other congenital anomalies (cleft lip), genetic disorders (Pierre-Robin syndrome), or anomaly sequences

TABLE 23-13

COMPARISON OF THE MICROBIOLOGY, CLINICAL MANIFESTATIONS, AND MANAGEMENT OF PERITONSILLAR ABSCESS AND RETROPHARYNGEAL ABSCESS

Features	Peritonsillar Abscess	Retropharyngeal Abscess
Age of typical patient	Older child/adolescent	3 to 5 years of age
Microbiology	Polymicrobial infections with aerobic and anaerobic organisms: Group A *Streptococcus* *Streptococcus viridans* Group C *Streptococcu* *Staphylococcus aureus* *Anaerobic streptococci* *Prevotella* species *Bacteroides* species *Fusobacterium* species *Peptostreptococcus* species	
Symptoms	Fever Malaise Severe sore throat Pain with eating and drinking Dysphagia Difficulty swallowing Drooling Trismus (difficulty opening the mouth) Muffled voice Neck pain on the involved side Neck swelling on the involved side	Fever Sore throat Pain with eating Neck pain on the involved side Neck swelling on the involved side
Signs	Pharyngeal and tonsillar erythema Tonsillar exudate Enlargement at the superior pole of the involved tonsil Deviation of the uvula away from the involved tonsil	Resistance to moving the neck, particularly associated with hyperextension Torticollis Respiratory distress, stridor, and toxic appearance are rare Neck stiffness Cervical lymphadenopathy Retropharyngeal bulge Posterior pharyngeal erythema
Diagnostic studies	Radiographic studies are usually unnecessary *Soft tissue films* of the neck reveal generalized distortion of tissues but do not localize the abscess *Computed tomography* can be used to rule out retropharyngeal abscess, localize the abscess, and evaluate for local extension if this is suspected	*Soft tissue films* of the neck demonstrate prevertebral swelling *Computed tomography* (with intravenous contrast) is the radiographic study of choice for confirming the diagnosis (localizing the abscess), differentiating an abscess from cellulitis, and evaluating contiguous structures
Medical management	Clindamycin (oral, intravenous) OR ampicillin-sulbactam (intravenous) OR amoxicillin/clavulanic acid (oral)	Clindamycin (intravenous) OR third-generation cephalosporin (intravenous) OR ampicillin-sulbactam (intravenous)
Surgical management	Needle aspiration or incision and drainage are reserved for the rare patient with severe disease and/or impending respiratory compromise	Transoral surgical drainage is indicated if the patient does not improve following 24 to 48 hours of appropriate antimicrobial therapy

TABLE 23-14
CAUSES OF PAROTITIS IN THE PEDIATRIC POPULATION

Acute viral parotitis

- Most common in children ≤10 years of age
- Presents with visible swelling of the parotid gland (which may obscure the angle of the jaw) and edema/erythema surrounding the opening of the parotid duct; the swelling is most pronounced on the second or third day, with gradual resolution over the following week
- The skin overlying the swollen gland appears normal; erythema is not present.
- Accompanying symptoms include pain with chewing, fever, malaise, anorexia.
- Parainfluenza and influenza viruses, coxsackievirus, Epstein-Barr virus, and echovirus can each infect the parotid gland
- Mumps should be considered in unimmunized patients.

Acute bacterial parotitis

- Much less common than acute viral parotitis
- Affects mostly neonates and children older than 10 years of age
- The parotid gland is swollen and tender to palpation, and the overlying skin is warm and erythematous.
- The patient may appear toxic; significant temperature elevation is common.
- Massage of the gland produces purulent material through the parotid duct orifice
- *Staphylococcus aureus* is the most commonly isolated pathogen.
- Treatment consists of adequate hydration, sialogogues to promote salivary flow, regular massage of the gland to clear purulent material, and antimicrobial therapy with coverage for *S. aureus.*

Chronic infectious parotitis

- Pathogens include human immunodeficiency virus, tuberculosis, atypical *Mycobacterium*, *Toxoplasma gondii*, and *Bartonella henselae.*

Noninfectious parotitis

Recurrent idiopathic parotitis of childhood (peak age and presentation similar to that for acute viral parotitis, with attacks recurring every 3 to 4 months)

Obstruction of the salivary duct by a stone

Rheumatic disease (e.g., systemic lupus erythematosus)

Drug and toxin exposures

(22q11 deletion syndrome). The cleft may be complete, affecting both bony and soft palate, or isolated to the latter. Immediate management issues focus on feeding, compensating for swallowing dysfunction, and preventing CHL; virtually all patients with cleft palate develop persistent OME necessitating tympanostomy tube placement. Cleft repair is undertaken in the latter half of the first year of life. *Velopharyngeal insufficiency* (VPI), the most significant long-term sequela of cleft palate, results from abnormal insertion or dysfunction of the palatine muscles. Surgical repair of the cleft does not appear to prevent the development of VPI. Children with VPI may not be identified until later in childhood, when they are found to have hypernasal speech and nasal emissions (escape of air through the nose during speech); attempts to compensate often result in associated articulation disorders.

Patients found to have a bifid uvula should be evaluated for *submucous cleft palate,* a mild variant of cleft palate in which the mucous membrane is almost fully intact. Like cleft palate, submucous cleft palate may be isolated or syndromic. Notching at the midline of the posterior palate is palpable and often visible. Approximately one half of affected patients develop persistent OME. The prevalence of VPI is lower in patients with submucous cleft. Both cleft palate and submucous cleft are associated with an increased incidence of postadenoidectomy VPI.

Cleft lip (with or without cleft palate) and isolated cleft palate are compared in Table 23-15. Infants with isolated cleft lip can typically breastfeed or be fed with a traditional bottle. Bottle feeding may also be possible in the infant with a cleft that is limited to the soft palate. However, infants with complete cleft palate must be fed with a compressible bottle.

DISORDERS OF THE TEETH

The typical age at eruption of the first tooth is approximately 6 months, with a range of 3 to 16 months. Eruption of the eight anterior teeth is usually complete by 12 months of age. Dental eruption may be delayed beyond

TABLE 23-15
COMPARISON OF CLEFT LIP (WITH OR WITHOUT CLEFT PALATE) AND ISOLATED CLEFT PALATE

Cleft Lip (with or without cleft palate)	Isolated Cleft Palate
More common	Less common
More common in boys	More common in girls
Multifactorial inheritance	At least half of cases due to underlying chromosomal abnormality
Typically an isolated defect	Often associated with other malformations (craniofacial, ophthalmologic, skeletal)

this period in healthy children; as long as the teeth that erupt are normal in appearance, delayed dental eruption has no pathologic significance. Referral to a pediatric dentist for radiographic confirmation of the presence of normal teeth is appropriate if there is lingering concern. Conditions such as calcium deficiency, hypothyroidism, and hypothalamic failure with associated growth hormone insufficiency are rare causes of delayed dental eruption. Most children have their complete set of primary teeth by the age of 3 years.

The eruption of abnormal-appearing teeth is usually indicative of underlying pathology. *Hypohidrotic ectodermal dysplasia* is an X-linked recessive disorder characterized by the following: *abnormal dentition* (widely spaced, peg-shaped teeth; rarely absence of teeth); *hypohidrosis* (diminished perspiration resulting in heat intolerance and unexplained high fevers); and *hypotrichosis* (decreased amount of hair).

The addition of *fluoride* to community water sources has had a major impact on the incidence of dental caries in the United States. Bacteria in the mouth produce an acid that dissolves the matrix of tooth enamel, eventually forming a cavity. Fluoride protects teeth by enhancing tooth mineralization, reversing tooth demineralization, and inhibiting acid-producing bacteria responsible for caries. Because the protective effects of fluoride are limited to erupted teeth, the Centers for Disease Control and Prevention have stated that fluoride supplementation is unnecessary in children younger than 6 years of age. Similarly, fluoride supplements are not recommended for pregnant women. Fluoride-containing toothpaste should be reserved for children who are old enough to spit the majority of the paste out following brushing. Parents are counseled to clean the teeth of younger children with a soft cloth or brush following meals. In children older than 6 years who are at high risk for dental caries, topical fluoride is probably more effective than oral fluoride supplements.

Infants and toddlers who are put to bed with bottles or allowed to breastfeed for prolonged periods at night are at risk for the development of "nursing bottle" caries. The maxillary incisors are affected sooner than the lower teeth. Protective factors include cleaning or brushing the teeth before bedtime, eliminating nighttime feedings, and weaning to a cup soon after the age of 12 months.

When most of the tooth has been destroyed through cavity formation, infection of the exposed pulp may extend into the periapical tissues of the periodontal ligament, forming a *dental abscess*. The presentation of dental abscess consists of fever, facial swelling, and tenderness to palpation of the tooth. The location of facial swelling depends on the tooth involved (swelling below the jaw with mandibular abscess; periorbital edema with maxillary dental abscess). Dental abscesses are polymicrobial, with a predominance of anaerobic organisms. Most dentists prefer to treat the underlying abscess prior to repairing or removing the tooth. Penicillin provides appropriate coverage for dental abscess; erythromycin or clindamycin is recommended in penicillin-sensitive individuals.

DISORDERS OF THE NECK

Hoarseness

Hoarseness can be defined as any abnormal change in vocal quality. The differential diagnosis of hoarseness is provided in Table 23-16. Acute alterations are more likely to result from trauma or infectious conditions; structural lesions typically cause insidious changes in voice quality. The timing of the onset of hoarseness may suggest congenital versus acquired abnormalities. Hoarseness following extubation in children is usually due to subglottic stenosis.

If the diagnosis remains in doubt following a careful history and physical examination, direct visualization of the larynx with flexible laryngoscopy is indicated. Radiographic imaging studies are less helpful in children than adults because most hoarseness in the pediatric population is mucosal or functional in origin rather than secondary to a structural lesion. Chest radiographs, CT, and magnetic resonance imaging permit assessment for mass lesions. Barium swallow is indicated if the hoarseness is associated with dysphagia or symptoms of reflux. Definitive treatment depends on the diagnosis.

Cervical Lymphadenopathy

Acute reactive lymphadenopathy is extremely common in the pediatric population. Lymph nodes are considered normal in size in children when the diameter is 1 cm or

TABLE 23-16
CONDITIONS KNOWN TO CAUSE CHANGES IN VOICE QUALITY

Acute Hoarseness

- Infections
  - Acute laryngitis (viral)
  - Acute laryngotracheobronchitis (viral croup)
  - Bacterial laryngotracheitis
  - Epiglottitis
- Trauma
  - Traumatic hematomas and nodule formation
  - Trauma to the recurrent laryngeal nerve during thoracic surgery
  - Traumatic breech delivery
- Postintubation
  - Subglottic stenosis
  - Dysfunction of the arytenoid muscle following traumatic intubation
- Vocal strain
  - Responds to rest and vocal retraining
- Miscellaneous
  - Left atrial enlargement
  - Caustic ingestion
  - Smoke inhalation

Chronic Hoarseness

- Structural lesions
  - Laryngeal clefts
    - Affected infants present with hoarseness, wheezing, or stridor; increased secretions; feeding difficulties; and failure to thrive. Small clefts may be managed with antireflux therapy; large clefts require surgical repair.
  - Laryngeal webs
    - Congenital webs present with an atypical cry in infancy and hoarseness later in life. They occur more often in patients with chromosome 22q11 deletion syndrome. Intubation, trauma, and surgery may be associated with the development of acquired laryngeal webs.
- Tumors
  - Laryngopapillomas
    - Benign tumors most often discovered in children 1 to 4 years of age
  - Malignant tumors
    - A rare cause of hoarseness in the pediatric population
- Gastroesophageal reflux
- Allergic rhinitis
- Chronic sinusitis
- Neurologic disease
  - Peripheral
    - Disorders of the recurrent laryngeal nerve
  - Central
    - Arnold-Chiari malformation, posterior fossa tumor, cerebral agenesis
- Metabolic disease
  - Hypothyroidism
  - Hypocalcemia
- Genetic syndromes
  - De Lange syndrome
  - Williams syndrome
  - Farber disease
- Miscellaneous
  - Aberrant great vessels
  - Recreational abuse of inhalants

less. Lymph node enlargement that is rapid, persistent, or symptomatic requires medical evaluation. The diagnosis of *acute cervical lymphadenitis* (infection of the lymph node) is largely clinical. Acute adenitis presents with rapid enlargement of the node over 1 to 2 days, fever, and tenderness to palpation; the involved node remains mobile. The overlying skin may become erythematous. Children ages 1 to 5 years are disproportionately affected. Oral antibiotics (semisynthetic penicillins or second- or third-generation cephalosporins) are sufficient for empiric therapy unless the patient appears toxic. Nodes that are fluctuant or resistant to therapy should be incised and drained, with samples provided for Gram stain and culture. If there is a question of abscess formation, ultrasonography or CT may be indicated.

Lymph nodes enlargement that slowly progresses or persists for over 1 to 2 months is more consistent with a chronic inflammatory condition or malignancy. Factors that should accelerate assessment for a malignant process are listed in Table 23-17. A suggested evaluation of lymph node enlargement that persists for ≥12 weeks without improvement in well-appearing patients without constitutional symptoms is presented in Table 23-18.

TABLE 23-17
DIFFERENTIAL DIAGNOSIS OF CHRONIC LYMPHADENOPATHY

Infection
Atypical mycobacteria
Tuberculosis
Cat scratch disease
Human immunodeficiency virus
Epstein-Barr virus
Cytomegalovirus
Toxoplasma gondii
Brucellosis
Tularemia
Fungal pathogens (e.g., histoplasmosis)
Chronic infection of the head or neck (or other areas drained by the cervical lymph nodes)

Malignancy
Features suspicious for malignancy include:
- Slowly progressive or persistent enlargement over a few months
- Constitutional symptoms (fever, malaise, weight loss, night sweats)
- Firm or fixed node(s) (rather than mobile nodes)
- Enlargement of nodes in the posterior cervical triangle or supraclavicular region
- Matted nodes that traverse the sternocleidomastoid muscle

Immune Deficiency
Chronic granulomatous disease

Infiltrative Disorders
Sarcoidosis

TABLE 23-18
EVALUATION OF CHRONIC LYMPHADENOPATHY IN THE WELL-APPEARING PATIENT

Place a Mantoux skin test. If positive, proceed as per Chapter 10 (***Mycobacterium tuberculosis***).
If negative, obtain serology studies for *Bartonella henselae* infection. If positive, proceed as per Chapter 10 (***Bartonella henselae***).
If negative, or if the patient becomes symptomatic during evaluation, consider further testing to elucidate the cause [complete blood count; serology studies for Epstein-Barr virus, cytomegalovirus, toxoplasmosis, human immunodeficiency virus; throat culture, antistreptolysin O titers; chest radiographs; computed tomography of the node(s)].
If etiology remains undiagnosed, excisional biopsy is indicated.

Neck Masses

Neck masses may be congenital, reactive/inflammatory, or neoplastic in children (Table 23-19); reactive cervical lymphadenopathy is by far the most frequent cause, although this finding is rare in young infants. Neck mass in the neonate or infant is most likely to be congenital; however, infectious lymphadenitis, tumor (teratoma), and congenital goiter should also be considered in this age group.

TONSILLECTOMY AND ADENOIDECTOMY

A summary of the recommended indications for tonsillectomy, adenoidectomy, and adenotonsillectomy is provided in Table 23-20. Hypertrophy of the tonsils and/or adenoids can have significant consequences, including obstructive sleep apnea (and its sequelae), hyponasal speech, obstruction of the nasal passages, exclusive mouth breathing, adenoidal facies, and problems with dentition.

Most children with no surgical complications can now be discharged the day of the procedure; however, patients younger than 3 years of age and those with a history of severe obstructive sleep apnea syndrome, chronic systemic illness, craniofacial abnormalities, and

TABLE 23-19
DIFFERENTIAL DIAGNOSIS OF NECK MASS IN CHILDREN

Congenital

Thyroglossal duct cyst

- The most common congenital neck mass
- A small, round neck mass located in the midline anywhere between the base of the tongue and the inferior edge of the thyroid gland
- Asymptomatic initially; detection typically delayed until the child is older than 2 years of age
- May present with sudden painful enlargement, warmth, and erythema when the cyst becomes infected
- May present with chronic drainage through a sinus tract in the midline of the neck
- Large cysts can rarely cause dysphagia
- Dermoid and cervical thymic cysts are less common causes of midline congenital neck masses

Branchial cysts

- Second most common cause of congenital neck mass
- Usually detected in infancy when fistula or sinus drainage occurs along the anterior border of the inferior portion of the sternocleidomastoid muscle
- Branchial cysts not associated with external drainage enlarge slowly and are usually not diagnosed until adulthood
- Infection of a branchial cyst results in rapid enlargement, warmth, erythema, and tenderness

Congenital vascular lesions

- Collectively represent the third most common cause of congenital neck mass
- Cystic hygroma—mobile, nontender cystic mass discovered in the posterior cervical triangle on newborn examination
- Hemangiomas—soft, nontender, mobile lesions with a reddish or bluish hue that are not present at birth but develop in the first 2 to 3 weeks of life

Sternocleidomastoid pseudotumor of infancy

- Firm, discrete mass within the belly of the sternocleidomastoid muscle typically detected in the first few weeks of life
- Often associated with congenital torticollis; patients with torticollis require physical therapy to prevent head tilt

Inflammatory

Acute suppurative cervical lymphadenitis

- Usually secondary to lymphatic seeding of the draining node from the upper respiratory tract, teeth, gums, or facial skin
- In neonates, may result from otitis media, bacteremia, or cellulitis; common causative organisms include *Staphylococcus aureus* and group B *Streptococcus*
- Pathologic organisms in children more likely to be *S. aureus* or group A *Streptococcus*; anaerobic organisms should be considered if the primary infection is a dental abscess

Neoplastic

Malignancies known to present with neck mass (due to primary tumor or involvement of lymph nodes) include Hodgkin disease, non-Hodgkin lymphoma, thyroid tumors, rhabdomyosarcoma, and neuroblastoma.

neuromuscular disease affecting pulmonary function require inpatient observation following surgery. Immediate complications include respiratory distress following extubation and hemorrhage, which usually occurs in the first 24 hours but may be delayed by as much as a few weeks. The development of VPI following surgical removal of the adenoids is related to removal of tissue from the posterior pharynx. In this setting, VPI may be self-limited, resolving within a few weeks. Persistent VPI requires surgical repair. Patients with cleft palate or submucosal cleft palate and patients with craniofacial abnormalities and Down syndrome are at increased risk for the development of VPI following adenotonsillectomy.

TABLE 23-20
INDICATIONS FOR TONSILLECTOMY, ADENOIDECTOMY, AND ADENOTONSILLECTOMY

Tonsillectomy

Recurrent *severe* pharyngitis

Recurrent peritonsillar abscess

Tonsillar asymmetry accompanied by constitutional symptoms (suspected malignancy)

Recurrent tonsillar hemorrhage

Adenoidectomy

Repeat tympanostomy tube placement for persistent otitis media with effusion or recurrent acute otitis media

Chronic inflammation or recurrent infection of the adenoids

Chronic sinusitis

Adenotonsillectomy

Obstructive sleep apnea syndrome (first-line therapy in the majority of children)

SOURCES

American Academy of Pediatrics. Policy statement: oral health risk assessment timing and establishment of the dental home. *Pediatrics*. 2003;111:1113–1116.

American Academy of Pediatrics Subcommittee on Management of Acute Otitis Media, American Academy of Family Physicians. Clinical practice guideline: diagnosis and management of acute otitis media. *Pediatrics*. 2004;113:1451–1465.

Bernius M, Perlin D. Pediatric ear, nose, and throat emergencies. *Pediatr Clin North Am*. 2005;52:195–214.

Centers for Disease Control and Prevention. Recommendations for using fluoride to prevent and control dental caries in the United States. *MMWR Morbid Mortal Wkly Rep*. 2001;50:1–42.

Cotton RT. The ear, nose, pharynx, and larynx. In: Rudolph CD, Rudolph AM, Hostetter MK, et al., eds. *Rudolph's pediatrics*. 21st ed. New York: McGraw-Hill; 2003:1239–1282.

Dudas R. Retropharyngeal abscess. *Pediatr Rev*. 2006;27:e45–e46.

Gerber MA. Diagnosis and treatment of pharyngitis in children. *Pediatr Clin North Am*. 2005;52:729–747.

Ghanem T, Rasamny JK, Park SS. Rethinking auricular trauma. *Laryngoscope*. 2005;115:1251–1255.

Gigante J. Tonsillectomy and adenoidectomy. *Pediatr Rev*. 2005;26: 199–203.

Gregg RB, Wiorek LS, Arvedson JC. Pediatric audiology: a review. *Pediatr Rev*. 2004;25:224–234.

Hendley JO. Clinical practice: otitis media. *N Engl J Med*. 2002;347: 1169–1174.

Joint Committee on Infant Hearing. Year 2000 Position Statement. Principles and guidelines of early hearing detection and intervention programs. Available at http://www.aap.org/policy/jcihyr2000.pdf.

Kamat DM. "Popsicle" panniculitis. *Consultant for Pediatricians*. 2006; 5:729.

Kelly LF. Pediatric cough and cold preparations. *Pediatr Rev*. 2004; 25:115–123.

King JF. When a child is born deaf. *Contemp Pediatr*. 2006;23:73–60.

Krol DM, Keels MA. Oral conditions. *Pediatr Rev*. 2007;28:15–22.

Lewis CW, Milgrom P. Fluoride. *Pediatr Rev*. 2003;24:327–336.

Paradise JL, Bluestone CD. Tympanostomy tubes: a contemporary guide to their judicious use. *Pediatr Rev*. 2005;26:60–66.

Pelton SI. Otitis media: re-evaluation of diagnosis and treatment in the era of antimicrobial resistance, pneumococcal conjugate vaccine, and evolving morbidity. *Pediatr Clin North Am*. 2005;52: 711–728.

Pfeiffer WF. A multicultural approach to the patient who has a common cold. *Pediatr Rev*. 2005;26:170–175.

Siegel RM, Bien JP. Acute otitis media in children: a continuing story. *Pediatr Rev*. 2004;25:187–193.

Sokol J, Hyde M. Hearing screening. *Pediatr Rev*. 2002;23:155–162.

Stone KE. Otitis externa. *Pediatr Rev*. 2007;28:77–78.

Twist CJ, Link MP. Assessment of lymphadenopathy in children. *Pediatr Clin North Am*. 2002;49:1109–1025.

QUESTIONS

1. A 16-year-old adolescent who was an unsecured front-seat passenger in a head-on motor vehicle collision is brought to the emergency department with multiple facial lacerations. Computed tomography of the head and facial bones demonstrates a displaced fracture of the anterior table of the left frontal sinus accompanied by a nondisplaced posterior table fracture. Surgical reduction and obliteration of the involved sinus is indicated to prevent which of the following complications?

A) Leakage of cerebrospinal fluid
B) Paralysis of the facial nerve
C) Bell palsy
D) Cavernous sinus thrombosis
E) Superior vena cava syndrome

2. A 14-year-old adolescent presents with the sudden onset of high fevers and focal seizures. He was well until about a week ago, when he was diagnosed with sinusitis and placed on a 5-day course of azithromycin. Computed tomography of the head demonstrates bilateral frontal, ethmoid, and maxillary sinusitis. There is no history of trauma or rash. This patient's neurologic signs are most likely due to which of the following?

A) Herpes simplex virus
B) Intracranial extension of frontal sinusitis
C) Bacterial meningitis
D) Aseptic meningitis
E) Arboviral encephalitis

3. A mother brings her previously well 3-year-old son to your office for evaluation of his fever. Three days ago, the child developed a fever to 39.6°C. He has also been complaining of a sore throat. The physical examination is significant for bilateral nonpurulent conjunctivitis of the palpebral and bulbar conjunctivae, pharyngitis with tonsillar exudates, clear rhinorrhea, and anterior cervical lymphadenopathy. This child's illness is most likely due to infection with which of the following pathogens?

A) Measles
B) Epstein-Barr virus
C) Adenovirus

D) Group A streptococcal pharyngitis
E) Cytomegalovirus

4. Which of the following hearing tests does not permit detection of unilateral hearing loss?
A) Distortion product otoacoustic emissions
B) Transient evoked otoacoustic emissions
C) Conventional audiometry
D) Visual reinforcement audiometry
E) Conditioned play audiometry

5. An 8-year-old boy is at risk for sensorineural hearing loss. Which of the following is the most appropriate initial diagnostic study for the differentiation of conductive hearing loss from sensorineural hearing loss in this patient?
A) Distortion product otoacoustic emissions
B) Transient evoked otoacoustic emissions
C) Tympanometry
D) Visual reinforcement audiometry
E) Conventional audiometry

6. A mother brings her 16-year-old son to your office for evaluation of his hearing. Lately she has begun accusing the boy of ignoring her; she has also noticed that he often increases the volume of the television so that he can hear it. The family history is significant for an uncle who developed hearing loss is his early thirties. Which of the following is the most appropriate initial test in this patient?
A) Urinalysis
B) Tympanometry
C) Renal ultrasonography
D) Otoacoustic emissions testing
E) Magnetic resonance imaging of the brain

7. A 12-year-old girl is in your office for evaluation of her ear pain. Her mother tells you that she was well until several weeks ago, when she developed intermittent ear pain and "ringing" in her left ear. Her symptoms have steadily progressed, and she now rates her ear pain as "severe." No abnormalities are noted upon examination of the external ear and tympanic membrane. There is tenderness to palpation of the temporalis and masseter regions on the left. A palpable "click" is present in the preauricular area upon opening of the mouth. This patient's ear pain is most likely due to which of the following conditions?
A) Tumor involving the temporal bone
B) Temporomandibular joint malocclusion
C) Trauma to the temporal bone
D) Acute tonsillitis
E) Idiopathic arthritis

8. A 10-year-old girl was the rear passenger in a car involved in a motor vehicle collision in which it was hit from the passenger side. The girl sustained a brief loss of consciousness and required repair of a large laceration above her right ear. At a follow-up visit 7 days later, the mother tells you that she has noticed clear fluid draining from the right ear. A perforation is noted in the right tympanic membrane. Conventional audiometry demonstrates moderate hearing loss in the right ear. This child's otorrhea is most likely due to which of the following conditions?
A) Traumatic perforation of the tympanic membrane
B) Perilymph fistula
C) Temporal bone fracture
D) Acute labyrinthitis
E) Acute suppurative otitis media

9. A full-term infant is the product of an uncomplicated pregnancy and delivery. A preauricular pit is identified on the right. The remainder of the physical examination is unremarkable; no dysmorphic features are noted. The parents deny any family history of childhood hearing loss, renal anomalies, or malformations of the ear. When they question you about the significance of the preauricular pit, you are correct in counseling them that the most appropriate next course of action is which of the following?
A) Full-scale audiologic assessment
B) Renal sonogram
C) Computed tomography of the ear and temporal bone
D) No further diagnostic study is indicated.
E) Head sonogram

10. A 9-year-old girl who is a year-round competitive swimmer presents to your office complaining of severe left-sided ear pain. Examination of the external canal reveals widespread erythema and edema. Visualization of the tympanic membrane is obstructed by copious amounts of purulent and bloody debris. Gentle suctioning permits visualization of about one fourth of the tympanic membrane, which appears grey and translucent. Which of the following is most appropriate for the immediate management of this patient?
A) Topical gentamicin drops
B) Oral cefixime
C) Oral ciprofloxacin
D) Thorough irrigation of the canal to remove all visible debris
E) Placement of a wick and instillation of neomycin/polymyxin B/hydrocortisone drops

11. An 18-month-old girl presents with right-sided purulent and occasionally bloody drainage that has persisted for 2 weeks despite a course of topical gentamicin drops. You remain unable to visualize the tympanic membrane due to retained debris, despite suctioning. Which of the following is the most appropriate next course of action in this patient?

A) Referral for otic microscopy
B) Irrigation of the external canal
C) Re-treat with topical ciprofloxacin
D) Re-treat with topical neomycin/polymyxin B
E) Prescribe a course of oral amoxicillin/clavulanic acid

12. Which of the following interventions does not reduce the overall risk of developing otitis media in infants and young children?
A) Breastfeeding rather than bottle feeding
B) Encouraging pacifier use
C) Limiting environmental smoke exposure
D) Caring for the child at home rather than at a day care center
E) Early weaning to a cup

13. A parent brings his 14-month-old daughter to your weekend clinic because she woke up crying this morning and is very fussy. He thinks she might have an ear infection, although she has never been diagnosed with this condition before. In your office, the child is afebrile and appears generally well but fussy. She has scant clear rhinorrhea. Examination of the ear reveals erythema of the tympanic membrane, well-visualized ossicular landmarks, and normal mobility. Which of the following is the most appropriate management of this patient?
A) Oral amoxicillin
B) Oral amoxicillin/clavulanic acid
C) Topical or oral medication for pain control
D) Topical neomycin/polymyxin B drops
E) Topical ciprofloxacin drops

14. Which of the following tympanometry results is most consistent with middle ear effusion?
A) High-amplitude pressure peak
B) Early pressure peak
C) Delayed pressure peak
D) Absence of pressure peak
E) "Mountain peak" at 0 dekapascals of pressure

15. You are providing a lecture to a group of medical students regarding acute otitis media (AOM) in children. You would be correct in informing the students of all of the following EXCEPT:
A) Approximately half of cases of AOM due to *Haemophilus influenzae* will resolve spontaneously.
B) Approximately 80% of cases of AOM due to *Moraxella catarrhalis* will resolve spontaneously.
C) Approximately 20% of cases of AOM due to *Streptococcus pneumoniae* will resolve spontaneously.
D) Although 80% of cases of untreated AOM resolve within 2 weeks, 95% of cases managed with antimicrobial therapy resolve within 2 weeks.
E) Perforation of the tympanic membrane occurs in approximately 15% of AOM.

16. A 16-month-old boy is brought to the office by his mother because she believes the child has an ear infection. He has had two previous episodes of acute otitis media, the last being 4 months prior. He was well until 2 days ago, when he developed clear rhinorrhea and a nonproductive cough. This morning, his temperature was elevated to 38.3°C. Examination of the ear reveals a bulging, erythematous membrane with decreased mobility. Which of the following is the most appropriate choice for treatment of this child's ear infection?
A) Amoxicillin 70 to 90 mg per kg a day divided twice a day for a total of 10 days
B) Amoxicillin 70 to 90 mg per kg a day divided twice a day for a total of 5 to 7 days
C) Amoxicillin 25 to 50 mg per kg a day divided three times a day for a total of 10 days
D) Amoxicillin 25 to 50 mg per kg a day divided three times a day for a total of 5 to 7 days
E) Myringotomy and oral medications for pain control

17. Approximately what percentage of children with acute otitis media will be free of middle ear fluid 4 weeks after initial treatment?
A) 25%
B) 50%
C) 75%
D) 90%
E) 100%

18. An 18-month-old child is diagnosed with his third episode of otitis media within the past 3 months. His mother asks you about referral for tympanostomy tube placement. You would be correct in telling her all of the following EXCEPT:
A) Placement of tympanostomy tubes significantly reduces the incidence of recurrent acute otitis media in children.
B) Placement of tympanostomy tubes significantly reduces the incidence of persistent otitis media with effusion in children.
C) Her son does not meet the recommended criteria for referral to an otolaryngologist.
D) Tympanostomy tube placement is the most commonly performed pediatric surgical procedure in the United States.
E) Tympanostomy tubes remain in place for an average of about 14 months.

19. A 3-year-old girl has had 3 weeks of persistent purulent drainage from her right ear that is sometimes tinged with blood. Examinations prior to development of the drainage showed persistent otitis media with effusion. The drainage resolved during a course of ciprofloxacin drops but recurred almost immediately. Physical examination of the child is significant for a cooperative, well-appearing, afebrile girl with a retraction pocket of the right tympanic membrane. Granulation tissue is noted around the edges of the retracted area. Which of the following is required for definitive treatment of this child's otorrhea?

A) Intravenous ceftazidime
B) Topical hydrocortisone drops
C) Antifungal otic drops
D) Surgical excision
E) Tympanomastoidectomy

20. A 2-year-old boy presents to the emergency department for evaluation of his fever and ear pain. The child was well until 3 days ago, when he developed a cough and rhinorrhea. His ear began hurting yesterday morning; he was seen by his doctor, who provided him with a prescription for azithromycin. When the boy awoke this morning, he was complaining of severe ear pain. His temperature is currently elevated to 38.7°C. The left tympanic membrane is erythematous and bulging; the child has tenderness to palpation of the area behind the involved ear, with fluctuance noted, and lateral displacement of the pinna. Which of the following studies is indicated for further evaluation of this patient?

A) Ultrasonography of the mastoid area
B) Needle aspiration of the mastoid area
C) Magnetic resonance imaging of the mastoid area
D) Plain radiographs of the mastoid area
E) Computed tomography of the mastoid area

21. Which of the following conditions is associated with an increased incidence of acute otitis media?

A) Allergic rhinitis
B) Sinus disease
C) Immotile cilia syndrome
D) Immunodeficiency
E) All of the above

22. A 1-day-old infant has recurrent intermittent episodes of cyanosis that are relieved by crying. You are unable to pass a suction catheter through the left naris. The examination is significant for a vigorous male infant with appropriate weight for gestation age; the left ear is short and wide and does not appear to have a lobe. This infant should also be evaluated for which of the following conditions?

A) Aniridia
B) Congenital heart defect
C) Intracranial calcifications
D) Agenesis of the corpus callosum
E) Situs inversus

23. A 3-year-old boy who was diagnosed with acute otitis media in your office 48 hours ago returns because he is still febrile and complaining of ear pain. The physical examination is significant for erythema and bulging of the tympanic membrane, which has decreased mobility. Neither the physical findings nor the patient's symptoms have improved after 2 days of high-dose amoxicillin. Which of the following is the most appropriate next course of action in this patient?

A) Continue high-dose amoxicillin and prescribe codeine for improved pain control
B) Refer the patient for diagnostic and therapeutic myringotomy
C) Change the patient from amoxicillin to amoxicillin/clavulanic acid
D) Change the patient from amoxicillin to azithromycin
E) Continue high-dose amoxicillin and prescribe topical numbing drops for improved pain control

24. A 13-year-old boy presents to the emergency department with profuse epistaxis that is not responsive to external nasal pressure. The patient has noticed increasing nasal obstruction on the right over the past several months and has developed right-sided facial paresthesias. He denies fever, pain, rhinorrhea, and weight loss. Examination of the anterior aspect of the nose does not result in localization of the bleeding. This patient's epistaxis is most likely due to which of the following?

A) Excessive dryness
B) Local trauma
C) Rhabdomyosarcoma
D) Juvenile nasopharyngeal angiofibroma
E) Hemangioma

25. A 2-year-old previously well child with persistent bilateral otitis media with effusion is referred for a full audiologic assessment prior to consultation with a pediatric otolaryngologist. You would expect his results to be most consistent with which of the following?

A) Conductive hearing loss
B) Sensorineural hearing loss
C) Mixed hearing loss
D) No hearing loss
E) Central hearing loss

26. A 17-year-old male is in the clinic for evaluation of nasal obstruction. He has been diagnosed with allergies in the past, but treatment with oral antihistamines has not resulted in improvement of his symptoms. Examination of the nose reveals hyperemic nasal mucosa, mucoid rhinorrhea, and perforation of the anterior nasal septum. This patient's nasal symptoms most likely result from which of the following?

A) Juvenile nasopharyngeal angiofibroma
B) Frequent cocaine use
C) Hereditary hemorrhagic telangiectasia
D) Inadequately treated perennial allergies
E) Human immunodeficiency virus

27. A mother brings her 3-year-old son to your office for evaluation of persistent rhinorrhea. She states that the child was well until about a week ago, when he awoke one morning with greenish, blood-tinged nasal discharge from the right nostril. The drainage has persisted. She also complains that the child smells terrible even though she bathes him daily. The boy has no recent history of fever, cough, or ear pain. Which of the following is the most likely cause of this patient's rhinorrhea?
A) Acute infectious rhinitis
B) Nasal foreign body
C) Vasomotor rhinitis
D) Perennial allergic rhinitis
E) Rhinitis medicamentosa

28. A 9-year-old girl is brought to the emergency department following a motor vehicle accident. She was a front-seat unrestricted passenger in a low-impact head-on collision. Her examination is normal, other than some dried blood in the left naris. Early the following morning, the child returns to the emergency department with severe nose pain and is not able to breathe through her nose. The otoscopic examination reveals a deviated septum and a bulging, erythematous mass obscuring the right and most of the left side of the nose. Which of the following courses of action is most appropriate in the management of this patient?
A) External compression with ice pack
B) Bilateral anterior nasal packs
C) Incision and drainage; oral antibiotics
D) Reassurance and follow-up 48 to 72 hours later
E) Outpatient referral to an otolaryngologist

29. A 5-year-old child is brought to your office by her mother for evaluation of chronic nasal drainage. The child has had bilateral clear rhinorrhea for 8 weeks, associated with sneezing, nasal congestion, and itching of the eyes. She received a clinical diagnosis of allergic rhinitis 1 month ago and was started on loratadine, which has produced no change in her symptoms. Which of the following is the best initial test for differentiating allergic rhinitis from other forms of rhinitis?
A) Serum immunoglobulin E–specific antibodies
B) Conjunctival smear for eosinophils
C) Nasal swab for culture
D) Nasal smear for eosinophils
E) Nasal smear for neutrophils

30. Which of the following is not an adverse effect of systemic decongestant use in infants and young children?
A) Irritability
B) Palpitations
C) Disordered sleep
D) Tachycardia
E) Sedation

31. A working mother whose 14-month-old son has just been diagnosed with an acute viral upper respiratory infection expresses frustration that he has been out of day care with illness so much. She thinks he may have "some sort of immune defect." Review of his chart confirms five separate acute viral upper respiratory infections since the age of 6 months. The child has never been placed on antibiotics and recovers fully between episodes of illness. Which of the following is the most appropriate next step in the management of this patient?
A) Reassurance
B) Quantitative serum immunoglobulin studies
C) Qualitative serum immunoglobulin studies
D) Waters view of the sinuses
E) Analysis of nasal smear for eosinophils

32. A 30-month-old girl is a mouth breather due to chronic nasal congestion. She was born at the 50th percentile for weight but has steadily dropped to well below the third percentile. Bilateral nasal polyps are noted on otoscopic examination of the nose. Which of the following is the most appropriate next diagnostic study in the evaluation of this patient?
A) Serum zinc concentration
B) Sweat chloride test
C) Computed tomography of the head
D) Serum ferritin level
E) Renal ultrasonography

33. A 6-year-old boy presents with a fever of 39°C and purulent nasal discharge. Mild periorbital edema, fetid breath, and tenderness to palpation of the area overlying the maxillary sinuses are noted on physical examination. The child has no significant past medical history and has not been treated with antibiotics within the past 3 years. Which of the following is the most appropriate initial treatment of this patient?
A) Topical decongestants
B) Systemic decongestants
C) A 14-day course of oral amoxicillin
D) A 14-day course of oral amoxicillin/clavulanic acid
E) A 14-day course of oral clindamycin

34. You diagnosed a previously well 6-year-old girl with acute bacterial sinusitis 2 weeks ago. You provided a prescription for 14 days of high-dose amoxicillin. Her symptoms initially improved, but she is now having increased purulent nasal discharge. You examination remains consistent with the diagnosis of acute bacterial sinusitis. Which of the following is the most appropriate next course of action in this patient?
A) Obtain a Waters view radiograph of the sinuses.
B) Obtain sinus aspirates for Gram stain and culture.
C) Prescribe a 21-day course of amoxicillin.

D) Prescribe a 14- to 21-day course of amoxicillin/clavulanic acid.
E) Prescribe a 14- to 21-day course of azithromycin.

35. A 16-year-old girl presents to the emergency department with a 3-day history of a temperature to 39°C, a severe sore throat, right-sided neck pain, difficulty swallowing, and a muffled voice. Examination of the oropharynx is significant for deviation of the uvula to the left and enlargement of the superior pole of the right tonsil. This patient's clinical presentation is most consistent with which of the following?
A) *Neisseria gonorrhoeae* pharyngitis
B) Infectious mononucleosis
C) Acute group A beta-hemolytic streptococcal pharyngitis
D) Retropharyngeal abscess
E) Peritonsillar abscess

36. A 4-year-old girl with no significant past medical history presents with fever and sore throat. The fever began 3 days ago. Her sore throat has become progressively worse; she now refuses to eat. Her neck appears swollen on the right side; she is holding her neck in slight flexion and rotation to the right. The physical examination is significant for a toxic-appearing child who refuses to open her mouth; cervical lymphadenopathy; and tenderness to palpation of the right side of the neck. Soft tissue films demonstrate prevertebral swelling. Which of the following is the most appropriate next step in the management of this patient?
A) Intravenous cefotaxime
B) Intravenous cephalexin
C) Intravenous vancomycin
D) Oral amoxicillin/clavulanic acid
E) Intravenous imipenem

37. A 3-year-old girl presents with ill-defined erythematous plaques and subcutaneous nodules over the buccal mucosa bilaterally. The child has not been febrile, and the lesions do not keep her from eating and drinking. The overlying skin appears normal, and there is no associated warmth. Upon further questioning, the mother is most likely to confirm a history of which of the following?
A) Bug bites to the face
B) Eating popsicles
C) Thick, scaly plaques over the knees and elbows
D) Desquamation of the hands and feet
E) Intermittent joint pain

38. You are examining a newborn infant born with cleft palate; the upper lip is intact. The student who is shadowing you asks how isolated cleft lip compares with cleft lip and palate. You would be correct in telling him which of the following?
A) Cleft lip (with or without cleft palate) is more common in females.
B) Cleft palate is less likely than cleft lip (with or without cleft palate) to be associated with an underlying chromosomal or genetic abnormality.
C) Cleft lip (with or without cleft palate) is typically an isolated defect (i.e., not associated with other congenital malformations).
D) Cleft lip (with or without cleft palate) occurs more frequently in patients with chromosome 22q11.2 deletion syndrome.
E) Isolated cleft lip is more likely to be associated with velopharyngeal insufficiency than isolated cleft palate.

39. A woman who has delivered a full-term infant with a cleft affecting both the hard and soft regions of the palate is planning on breastfeeding her infant. Which of the following represents the most appropriate method of providing breast milk for this infant?
A) Place the infant at the breast for feeding.
B) Obtain breast milk via a pump and feed it to the infant through a nasogastric tube.
C) Obtain breast milk via a pump and feed it to the infant in a traditional bottle.
D) Obtain breast milk via a pump and feed it to the infant in a compressible bottle.
E) This infant should be fed exclusively with formula.

40. A 5-year-old boy is referred to your office for a preoperative physical examination. He is scheduled to undergo removal of his tonsils and adenoids the following day. You note a bifid uvula and palpable notching at the midline of the posterior pharynx. Your findings increase the risk of which of the following surgical complications?
A) Adult-onset respiratory distress syndrome
B) Aspiration pneumonia
C) Difficulty with extubation
D) Retropharyngeal abscess
E) Velopharyngeal insufficiency

41. The mother of a 9-month-old girl asks how she should be caring for her daughter's teeth and whether the child should take fluoride supplements. You would be correct in informing her of all of the following EXCEPT:
A) Oral fluoride supplements are probably more effective at preventing cavities than topical fluoride applications.
B) The addition of fluoride to community water sources has had a major impact on the incidence of dental caries in the United States.
C) Since the protective effects of fluoride are limited to erupted teeth, fluoride supplementation is unnecessary in children younger than 6 years of age.
D) Fluoride-containing toothpaste should be reserved for children who are old enough to spit the majority of the paste out following brushing.

E) Parents are counseled to clean the teeth of children younger than 24 months with a soft cloth or brush following meals.

42. A 19-month-old boy presents with extensive dental caries of his maxillary incisors and molars. He has been put to bed with a milk-filled bottle since the age of 9 months. Which of the following interventions will be most effective in preventing further deterioration of the child's teeth?
A) Substitute water for the milk in the bottle.
B) Discontinue bottle feeding at night.
C) Substitute juice for the milk in the bottle.
D) Application of a fluoride sealant to the teeth
E) Brushing with a fluoride-containing toothpaste prior to bedtime

43. A 16-year-old adolescent presents to the urgent care center with tooth pain. He had been well until his tooth began to bother him about 2 weeks ago; the pain has become progressively worse. In the clinic, the patient is febrile to 38.5°C. Nonerythematous swelling is noted beneath the jaw on the right. The first mandibular molar on the right is cavitated and exquisitely tender to touch. The patient has no known drug allergies. Which of the following is the most appropriate management of this patient?
A) Admission for intravenous penicillin
B) Administration of oral penicillin and emergent referral to an oral surgeon
C) Administration of oral penicillin and referral to a dentist within the next few days
D) Admission for intravenous clindamycin
E) Immediate removal of the tooth in the urgent care center

44. A 5-year-old previously healthy boy presents with a 12-week history of an enlarged lymph node in the right anterior cervical triangle. The node measures 2 cm × 2.5 cm and is mobile and nontender. There is no history of fever, malaise, or night sweats. Despite a 10-day course of amoxicillin, the node has neither increased nor decreased in size. Which of the following is the most appropriate next step in the management of this patient?
A) Excisional biopsy
B) Fine-needle aspiration biopsy
C) Obtain serology for *Bartonella henselae*
D) Placement of a Mantoux skin test
E) Serum antistreptolysin O titers

45. A 15-year-old adolescent who has spent the summer on his grandfather's dairy farm now has an 8-week history of cervical lymphadenopathy. He is complaining of undulating fevers, myalgias, and anorexia. Physical examination reveals enlargement of both the liver and spleen. This patient's history of illness and clinical presentation are most consistent with which of the following?
A) Rat bite fever
B) Tularemia
C) Infectious mononucleosis
D) Lymphadenitis due to atypical *Mycobacteria*
E) Brucellosis

46. A 3-year-old boy with acute otitis media who has been on high-dose amoxicillin for 48 hours develops rapid enlargement of a lymph node located in the anterior cervical triangle on the same side as the ear infection. The child remains febrile but nontoxic appearing, and the appearance of the tympanic membrane is unchanged from the initial visit. The lymph node is firm, mobile, and tender to palpation; it measures 2.5 cm in diameter. Which of the following is the most important next step in the management of this patient?
A) Change the antibiotic to amoxicillin/clavulanic acid
B) Change the antibiotic to clindamycin
C) Obtain an sonogram of the anterior neck
D) Refer the patient for needle aspiration biopsy of the lymph node
E) Refer the patient for tympanocentesis

47. Which of the following patients should be kept overnight for observation following removal of his or her tonsils and adenoids?
A) A 20-month-old girl
B) An 8-year-old girl with severe obstructive sleep apnea
C) A 5-year-old with Becker-type muscular dystrophy
D) B and C
E) A, B, and C

48. An 18-month-old girl who has transferred from another practice is in your office for her routine health maintenance visit. The girl is not yet saying any words; her parents report that she rarely verbalizes anymore, and her babbling contains few consonants. A review of the child's chart shows that she failed the newborn screening test in the hospital; a follow-up test was scheduled but never completed. The child smiled, cooed, and babbled at the expected times and played gesture games with interest. Gross and fine motor skills are intact. Which of the following statements regarding further management of this patient is TRUE?
A) A urine sample should be obtained to screen for hematuria.
B) The child should be referred for speech therapy, but audiology testing is not indicated because early language milestones have been achieved.
C) This child's hearing loss is probably congenital.
D) The child should be referred for global developmental testing.
E) The child should be referred for behavioral therapy.

49. You are providing a lecture to medical interns about hearing loss in the pediatric patient. You would be correct in telling them each of the following about the effects of hearing loss on development EXCEPT:

A) Hearing impairment in the infant and toddler years negatively impacts speech and language development.
B) Hearing impairment that is acquired after the age of 5 years has less of an effect on speech and language development.
C) Isolated hearing impairment in children negatively impacts cognitive development.
D) Isolated hearing impairment in children negatively impacts gross motor development.
E) Isolated hearing impairment in children negatively impacts emotional development.

50. The parents of a 1-month-old girl with congenital hearing loss are interested in referral for possible placement of a cochlear implant. Which of the following statements regarding cochlear implants is correct?

A) Cochlear implants are a less desirable alternative to sign language.
B) Cochlear implants should be placed in patients with congenital hearing loss prior to the age of 3 months.
C) Cochlear implants are only beneficial in patients with congenital hearing loss.
D) Cochlear implants are only beneficial in patients with acquired hearing loss.
E) Cochlear implants are reserved for the patient who cannot benefit from sound amplification.

ANSWERS

1. A	18. C	35. E
2. B	19. D	36. A
3. C	20. E	37. B
4. D	21. E	38. C
5. E	22. B	39. D
6. A	23. C	40. E
7. B	24. D	41. A
8. C	25. A	42. B
9. D	26. A	43. C
10. E	27. B	44. D
11. A	28. C	45. E
12. B	29. D	46. A
13. C	30. E	47. E
14. D	31. A	48. C
15. E	32. B	49. D
16. A	33. C	50. E
17. B	34. D	

Adolescent Medicine

24

Adolescence begins with the onset of puberty. For practical purposes, adolescence encompasses the ages of 11 to 20 years, including early (11 to 13 years), middle (14 to 17 years), and late (17 to 20 years) adolescence. It is a period of marked physical, emotional, and cognitive growth. These tracks of development do not progress strictly in parallel; that is, an adolescent who appears to be an adult physically may still have significant psychosocial or cognitive milestones to achieve.

ADOLESCENT HEALTH MAINTENANCE VISIT

Currently, the American Academy of Pediatrics (AAP) advises annual health maintenance visits during the adolescent years. Important elements of the office visit include the interview/history, anticipatory guidance, physical examination, laboratory assessment, preventive health services, and formulation of a treatment plan (if needed).

Interview and Anticipatory Guidance

Ideally, the parent and child should be interviewed together to evaluate family dynamics, explore past medical and family history, and gather nonsensitive health-related information. During this time, the physician may discuss his or her approach to the adolescent visit. Additional time should be set aside to interview and evaluate the adolescent alone. This allows the physician to discuss confidentiality issues with the patient and encourages the frank discussion of more sensitive issues. Laws regarding *confidentiality* and *consent* vary from state to state. Generally, issues that represent a serious threat to the adolescent's health must be disclosed. The physician may also seek the patient's permission to disclose information to the parents when he or she deems it in the best interest of the child. For instance, patients may be willing to discuss issues related to their sexual behavior, drinking, or drug use with their parents in the presence of a supportive physician that they would never bring up at home. Depending on the state, adolescents under the age of 18 years can provide consent for their own health care regarding: (a) contraception, prenatal care, and sexually transmitted diseases (STDs); and (b) issues related to mental health and/or substance abuse evaluation and treatment. In addition, various states grant "mature" or "emancipated" minors (those who have children, are married, or are living apart from their parents) the right to consent to or decline health care.

The interview also permits the physician to evaluate the functional status of the adolescent regarding self-image and identity, peer relationships, family relationships, school and/or work, and sexuality. The HEADSS interview is a useful tool for this purpose (Table 24-1). Adolescents who are "stressed" or "under pressure" in any of these areas may present with nonspecific somatic complaints. The physician should strive to be nonjudgmental and avoid lecturing. Interview techniques that may prove helpful in eliciting more complete and honest information include open-ended questions and statements of reflection, restatement, and clarification. Questions about peer behavior regarding sex or substance use are beneficial for initiating discussion of the patient's own behavior. The physician should be supportive of the patient's positive health choices and the patient him- or herself, while also identifying and discussing unhealthy behaviors.

Anticipatory guidance is an integral part of every routine adolescent health maintenance visit. Topics include anticipated physical and emotional changes, nutrition and exercise, sexual behavior (e.g., abstinence, STD and pregnancy prevention), substance use/abuse (e.g., tobacco,

TABLE 24-1
THE ADOLESCENT PSYCHOSOCIAL HISTORY: HEADSS[a]

Home (family members, relationships, and living arrangements)
Education (academic performance/educational goals)
Activities (peer relationships, work and recreational activities)
Drugs (substance use/abuse, including tobacco, alcohol, steroids, inhalants, and illicit drugs)
Sexuality (dating, sexual activity, contraception, sexual orientation)
Suicide (depression, anxiety, other mental health concerns)

[a]Some experts suggest that a second "E" should be added to remind physicians to screen for behaviors associated with **E**ating disorders and that a third "S" should be included to prompt questions concerning **S**afety [the potential for abuse or violent behavior (e.g., domestic violence, gang membership, owning a firearm)].

alcohol, illicit drugs, inhalants, steroids), and injury prevention (e.g., seat belts, bicycle helmets, drinking and driving, firearm safety).

Physical Examination

The younger/middle adolescent should be asked whether he or she prefers to be examined alone or in the presence of the parent. Younger adolescents may feel more comfortable during the examination with a parent in the room. Any areas of concern on the review of systems should be addressed by a comprehensive physical examination. Growth parameters (e.g., height, weight, body mass index), sexual maturity rating (SMR), and blood pressure should be recorded. Blood pressure measurements gradually rise to adult levels during adolescence, and hypertension may become apparent. Since height percentage affects blood pressure, tables exist that give normal blood pressure ranges for different genders, ages, and heights. Blood pressure that is greater than two standard deviations above normal on three separate occasions warrants further investigation. Vision screening should be performed every 2 to 3 years, and hearing should be tested at least once during adolescence.

Laboratory Assessment

Hemoglobin or hematocrit should be measured at the initial adolescent visit and/or at the end of puberty. Normal levels for females remain steady (hematocrit 36% to 44%), but male levels gradually increase to male adult levels (40% to 50%). A urinalysis is also performed at this time. Cholesterol screening is recommended at least once during adolescence. Cholesterol measurements rise gradually throughout adolescence to adult levels. Tuberculin testing should be considered for at-risk individuals.

Other laboratory parameters that change throughout adolescence include creatinine and alkaline phosphatase. Creatinine rises to adult levels by the end of adolescence. A transient elevation in the alkaline phosphatase level may occur during peak growth velocity; this is a physiologic response to the growth spurt and does not signify disease.

Screening tests recommended for sexually active adolescents are listed in Table 24-2.

TABLE 24-2
SCREENING TESTS FOR SEXUALLY ACTIVE ADOLESCENTS

Female: annual Pap smear, cervical specimens for *Neisseria gonorrhoeae/Chlamydia trachomatis*, vaginal wet mount

Male: leukocyte esterase urine screen

Consider for both: syphilis serology, human immunodeficiency virus (HIV) screening

Preventive Health

Recommended adolescent immunizations are listed in Table 24-3.

Formulation of Treatment Plan/Adherence

The adolescent should be an active participant in the formulation of any treatment plan. Adolescents generally dislike being told what to do and are more likely to be compliant if they are a part of the discussion. Parents should be included whenever possible because parental involvement is associated with increased compliance. Other factors that may improve compliance include use of a treatment calendar and dosing that is synchronized with the patient's other activities. Factors that often limit compliance include patient issues (e.g., embarrassment, denial, rejection of authority), disease characteristics (e.g., lack of symptoms, absence of short-term consequences), and treatment specifics (e.g., time commitment, multiple treatments or doses, convenience, cost, side effects, availability, pain).

TABLE 24-3
ADOLESCENT IMMUNIZATION GUIDELINES (ADVISORY COMMITTEE ON IMMUNIZATION PRACTICES)

Immunization	Indications
Hepatitis A	Adolescents at risk for hepatitis A (traveling to or working or living in area or population with high rate of hepatitis A) Adolescents at risk for severe complications (patients with chronic liver disease or those who receive clotting factors; patients who use some illicit drugs; males who engage in sex with other males)
Hepatitis B	Adolescents age 11 to 12 years or older who have not been previously vaccinated
Influenza	Adolescents at risk for severe complications
Measles, mumps, rubella	Adolescents who did not receive two doses of the vaccine at age ≥12 months
Pneumococcal polysaccharide	Adolescents at increased risk for the disease or its complications
Tetanus/diphtheria	Adolescents age 11 to 12 years or older who have not received a booster within the past 5 years
Varicella	Adolescents with no history of vaccination or disease
Meningococcal (conjugate)	Adolescents entering middle school, high school, or college
Human papillomavirus	Effective in females ≥9 years old

Noncompliance should be considered in any adolescent patient with highly variable or subtherapeutic drug levels. Advice regarding alteration of life habits (e.g., diet, exercise, smoking) generally has the lowest compliance. Ideally, at least one medical representative should accept long-term care of the patient in order to provide stability of services and continuity of care.

PHYSIOLOGIC GROWTH AND PUBERTAL DEVELOPMENT

The onset and progression of puberty are dependent on changes in gonadotropin secretion (Fig. 24-1).

The five (Tanner) stages of sexual maturity are described in Table 24-4. Figures 24-2 and 24-3 summarize the course of pubertal development in males and females, respectively.

In males, the onset of puberty typically ranges from ages 9.5 to 13.5 years but may be occurring earlier, especially in the black population. *Testicular enlargement* (>2.5 mm prepubertal length) is the earliest sign of puberty, followed sequentially by *pubarche* (the start of pubic hair growth), *penile growth*, and *peak height velocity*. Gynecomastia, the temporary development of breast tissue in some males, occurs most frequently during genital SMR stage 3 to 4, may be asymmetric, is not abnormal, and resolves spontaneously.

In females, the onset of puberty ranges from ages 8 to 13 years but may be occurring earlier, especially in the black population. *Breast budding* is the earliest sign of puberty, followed sequentially by *pubarche*, *peak height velocity*, and *menarche*. The average age of menarche in the United States is 12 years and 4 months but ranges from 10 to 15 years of age. Menarche is strongly associated with Tanner stage 4 breast development; vaginal bleeding that occurs in the setting of stage 2 or earlier breast development is likely to be pathologic. When present, *physiologic leukorrhea* is

TABLE 24-4
SECONDARY SEX CHARACTERISTICS: TANNER SEXUAL MATURITY RATING (SMR) SCALE

Stage	Description
Breast Development (Females)	
Stage I	Preadolescent; elevation of papilla only
Stage II	Breast bud beneath the areola; enlargement of areolar diameter
Stage III	Further enlargement and elevation of breast and areola
Stage IV	Projection of areola to form secondary projection above contour of breast
Stage V	Mature stage; smooth breast contour
Note: Stages IV and V may not be distinct in some patients	
Genital Development (Male)	
Stage I	Preadolescent
Stage II	Enlargement of scrotum and testes; skin of scrotum reddens and changes in texture
Stage III	Enlargement of penis, particularly length; further growth of testes and scrotum
Stage IV	Increased size of penis with growth in thickness and development of glans; further enlargement of testes and scrotum and increased darkening of scrotal skin
Stage V	Adult genitalia
Pubic Hair (Male and Female)	
Stage I	Preadolescent (no pubic hair)
Stage II	Sparse growth of longer, slightly pigmented hair, chiefly at base of penis or along labia
Stage III	Increasingly darker, coarser, and more curled hair spreads over junction of pubis
Stage IV	Adult-type pubic hair with no spread to medial surface of thighs
Stage V	Adult in quantity and type with spread to thighs

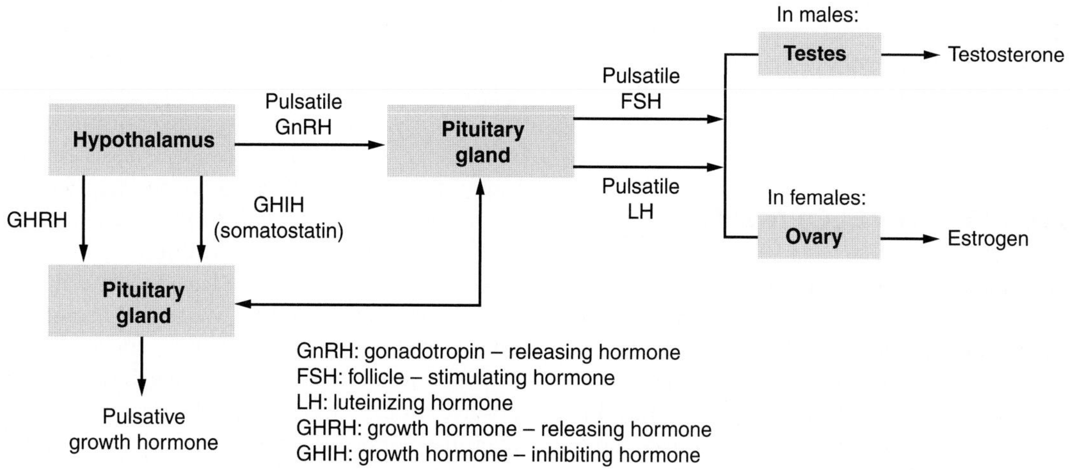

Figure 24-1 Simplified schematic representation of pubertal hormone secretion.

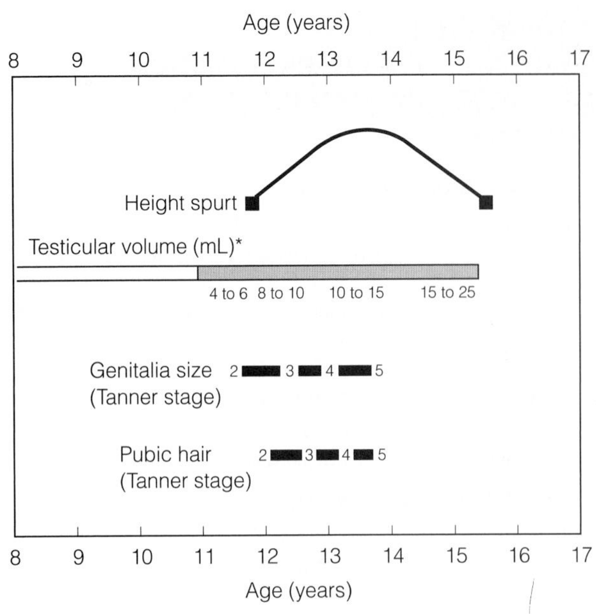

Figure 24-2 Sequence of pubertal events in the average (American) male. (From Marino BS, Fine KS. *Blueprints Pediatrics.* 4th ed. Philadelphia: Lippincott Williams & Wilkins; 2006 with permission.)

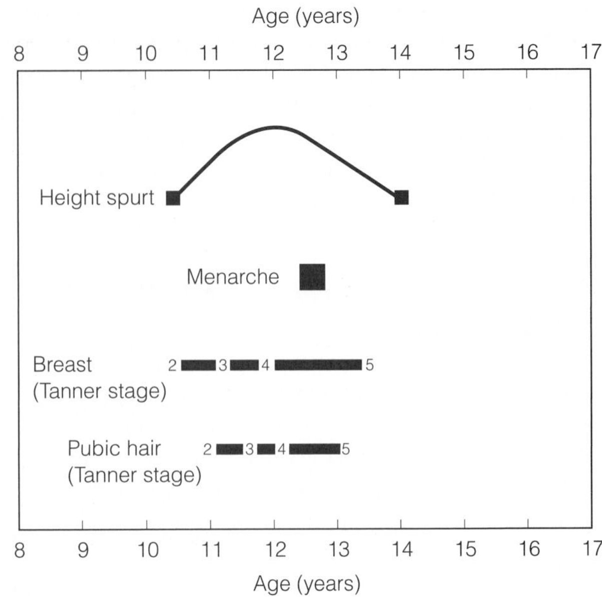

Figure 24-3 Sequence of pubertal events in the average (American) female. (From Marino BS, Fine KS. *Blueprints Pediatrics.* 4th ed. Philadelphia: Lippincott Williams & Wilkins; 2006 with permission.)

typically followed by menarche within 6 months. During the first 2 years of menstruation, infrequent and/or irregular menstrual periods (due to anovulatory cycles) are not uncommon. Asymmetric breast development is neither uncommon nor abnormal.

The average growth rate of prepubertal children is approximately 6 cm (2.4 inches) a year. This increases to a peak growth velocity of 8 cm (3.1 inches) a year in girls and 9 cm (3.5 inches) a year in boys. Peak height velocity occurs during genital SMR stage 4 in boys (vs. breast SMR stage 3 in girls). The pubertal growth spurt typically lasts approximately 2 to 4 years. Children who enter puberty relatively early tend to be, on average, shorter as adults than their later-maturing peers. Of note, skeletal age is more closely concordant with pubertal development than chronologic age. Therefore, during adolescence, bone age may be up to 2 years more or less than actual age without being abnormal.

Short stature, tall stature, precocious puberty, and delayed puberty are discussed in Chapter 11.

PSYCHOSOCIAL DEVELOPMENT

Important psychosocial tasks of adolescence include the achievement of independence, development of appropriate peer relationships, and development of a strong self-identity. An adolescent's psychological development takes place within the framework of *family* and *peer* relationships. Important family dynamics to consider include the make-up of the family (e.g., intact two-parent, single-parent, extended), cultural background and socioeconomic status, parenting style, and sources of stress. Whenever possible, it is beneficial to identify the family's primary method of dealing with conflict, including stress related to the redefinition of family roles and the increasing relative importance of peer relationships. Parents who can adjust to, responsibly guide, encourage, and accept their child's attempts to gain independence (including taking risks and testing limits) greatly facilitate the maturation process and lay the groundwork for the child to re-engage with the family after this stage is complete. It is also important for parents to model the behaviors they wish to instill in their child. Children with parents who engage in smoking, excessive drinking, violence, or other high-risk behaviors are more likely to try these activities themselves.

Peer groups play a very important role during adolescent psychosocial development. Adolescents tend to seek out and bond with peers who dress and behave like them and have similar likes and dislikes. Peer groups may strongly influence the adolescent's opinions and behaviors relating to smoking/alcohol/drug use, sex, education, and violence. Acceptance and inclusion by peers assist in the development of a positive self-image; conversely, adolescents who are socially isolated ("loners") are at risk for depression and other psychological difficulties.

Formation of a *positive self-image* is an important task of adolescence that cannot be overstated. Parents can assist in this regard by accepting their child, spending time enjoying activities with the child, and praising the child's strengths and positive choices. Adolescents who develop a poor self-image often have difficulty with family and peer relationships, are at increased risk for school underachievement and depression, and are more likely to engage in high-risk behaviors.

COGNITIVE DEVELOPMENT

Physicians who treat adolescents must have a thorough understanding of cognitive development. Medical explanations and recommendations that are not offered in a manner consistent with the adolescent's level of cognitive achievement are unlikely to be effective. Early adolescents are typically "concrete" thinkers; they tend to see the world in absolutes and have a limited ability to understand abstractions, complicated relationships, cause and effect, long-term consequences, and their own vulnerability/mortality. This results in increased risk-taking behavior and propensity to engage in behaviors such as smoking and poor diet, which may eventually have significant health consequences. In late adolescence, most patients develop the capacity for "formal operational" thought, which involves understanding multiple viewpoints, thinking and planning ahead, and delaying gratification.

ADOLESCENT SEXUAL BEHAVIOR

Development of a sexual identity is an important part of adolescence. Masturbation often begins during early adolescence as the body starts to mature. Interest in the opposite sex progresses from increased nonphysical contact early in adolescence to more exploratory physical behavior, including both coital and noncoital sexual acts (i.e., oral sex). Homosexual experimentation may also occur during this period of development. The emotional ability and desire to sustain a monogamous intimate sexual relationship is typically a late-adolescent development.

A surveillance study by the Centers for Disease Control and Prevention (Youth Risk Behavioral Survey, 1999) reveals that approximately two thirds of high school seniors of each gender reported that they had engaged in sexual intercourse. Many adolescents are receptive to discussions with their personal physician about safe sex practices and contraception. The health maintenance visit in early adolescence provides an invaluable opportunity to discuss contraception and encourage abstinence as the most effective method of preventing STDs and unwanted pregnancies, because most young people in this age group are not yet sexually active.

Specific physician and parental aspects of promoting adolescent sexual health are discussed in detail in Chapter 28.

GYNECOLOGY

The female genital and pelvic examinations, including appropriate specimen collection, play an important role in the health maintenance of sexually active adolescents, the diagnosis of STDs, and the evaluation of unexplained abdominal and/or pelvic pain (Table 24-5). *Genital tract outflow obstruction* occurs when there is a congenital/anatomic abnormality that prevents the passage of endometrial bleeding. Abdominal pain may be accompanied by constipation, urinary retention, and an abdominal mass. *Endometriosis* is a condition in which uterine tissue is located outside the uterine cavity, usually in the pelvis or abdomen. Patients experience chronic or cyclic pelvic pain, abnormal uterine bleeding, and/or painful defecation. A bimanual examination just prior to the start of menses may be significant for posterior uterine or cul-de-sac tenderness. Often, the family history is positive for endometriosis.

TABLE 24-5
GYNECOLOGIC CAUSES OF ABDOMINAL AND/OR PELVIC PAIN

Acute
Ectopic pregnancy
Spontaneous abortion
Pelvic inflammatory disease (PID)
Ruptured ovarian cyst
Ovarian/adnexal torsion
Endometritis
Chronic
Endometriosis
Chronic pelvic pain (due to previous PID)
Congenital outflow tract obstruction (e.g., imperforate hymen)
Cyclic Pain
Dysmenorrhea
Endometriosis
Mittelschmerz

The examination begins with inspection of the external genital hair and skin for Tanner SMR, irritation, warts, or other lesions. The hymen is examined for evidence of trauma and for patency. Vaginal fluid samples for pH and wet mount are collected if there is a complaint of vaginal discharge. The speculum examination allows visualization of the vaginal walls, cervix, cervical os, and any cervical discharge. A Pap smear should be collected yearly in the sexually active patient or at the age of 18 years in the abstinent patient. Endocervical swabs are collected for STD testing if indicated. The bimanual examination includes palpation of the cervix, uterus, posterior fornix, and ovaries for tenderness and/or masses.

Dysmenorrhea

Dysmenorrhea refers to cramping lower midline abdominal pain associated with menstrual periods. The pain may also be experienced in the lower back and anterior thigh areas. Prostaglandins released following ovulation stimulate uterine contractions, vasoconstriction, ischemia, and pain. Dysmenorrhea is an important cause of episodic school absence in the adolescent female population.

- *Primary dysmenorrhea* begins with or just before the start of menstrual flow, is worse during the first day or two, and resolves before cessation of flow. It is by far the most common form of dysmenorrhea in adolescents, typically beginning 6 to 20 months after menarche. It may be accompanied by other "premenstrual" symptoms such as nausea, bloating, fatigue, headache, diarrhea, and labile mood. The differential diagnosis of primary dysmenorrhea includes pelvic inflammatory disease (PID), inflammatory bowel disease, irritable bowel syndrome, and cystitis.
- *Secondary dysmenorrhea* begins earlier in the cycle, from days to weeks before the onset of blood flow, and lasts for the duration of bleeding. It is more likely to be present from the beginning of menarche. Secondary dysmenorrhea may be associated with endometriosis, uterine fibroid tumors, pelvic adhesions, genital outflow tract obstruction, or presence of an intrauterine device.

Examination of the external genitalia is indicated in all patients with dysmenorrhea in order to rule out distal genital outflow tract obstruction (i.e., imperforate hymen). A trial of an over-the-counter nonsteroidal anti-inflammatory drugs (NSAIDs) (e.g., ibuprofen, naproxen, ketoprofen) is appropriate in patients who have symptoms consistent with primary dysmenorrhea, have normal external genitalia, and are not sexually active. Patients should chart their periods, begin the medicine at the start of symptoms or menstrual flow, and continue for 1 to 3 days. Oral contraceptive pills (OCPs) are a reasonable second-line therapy for patients who do not experience a significant reduction in their pain. NSAIDs inhibit prostaglandin production; OCPs prevent ovulation (and thereby the stimulus for prostaglandin release). Acetaminophen is not thought to be beneficial in reducing the symptoms of dysmenorrhea because it does not affect prostaglandin levels.

A pelvic examination with STD testing is recommended for sexually active patients with dysmenorrhea. Pelvic or transvaginal ultrasonography is helpful in ruling out anatomic abnormalities and fibroids. Patients with severe pain, pain that does not respond to the medical management outlined earlier, pain that results in significant impairment, or symptoms consistent with endometriosis should be referred for laparoscopy.

Dysfunctional Uterine Bleeding

Normal menstrual cycles are 28 (±7) days in length, with 5 (±3) days of bleeding and up to 80 mL of blood loss. Dysfunctional uterine bleeding (DUB) is defined as irregular or prolonged endometrial bleeding in the absence of any pelvic abnormality. The most common cause of DUB in the adolescent population is *anovulation*; thus, DUB occurs more frequently in the first few years after the onset of menstruation, when anovulatory cycles are common. DUB secondary to anovulation is typically irregular and painless. Any uterine bleeding that lasts longer than 10 days is considered pathologic. Descriptive patterns of DUB are as follows:

- *Metrorrhagia* is bleeding that occurs at irregular intervals.
- *Menorrhagia* is prolonged bleeding that occurs at regular intervals.
- *Menometrorrhagia* is prolonged, heavy bleeding that occurs at regular intervals.

Conditions that increase the likelihood of anovulation (and therefore DUB) include anorexia nervosa, chronic disease, hypothyroidism (or less commonly hyperthyroidism), pituitary tumor, late-onset adrenal hyperplasia, stress, excessive exercise, and *polycystic ovarian syndrome* (PCOS). In PCOS, anovulation is associated with clinical evidence of androgen excess such as acne, facial hair, and occasionally clitoral enlargement. Obesity and insulin resistance are common, as is *acanthosis nigricans*, a velvety brown thickening of skin in the neck, axilla, and groin regions. On ultrasonography, the ovaries may appear normal or exhibit multiple small cysts. Patients with PCOS are treated with OCPs, spironolactone, and medroxyprogesterone acetate every few months to induce withdrawal bleeding.

DUB may also be caused by conditions not associated with anovulation. Coagulation disorders are a less common but significant cause of DUB (see Chapter 15). Disorders that affect platelet number (thrombocytopenia) or function (von Willebrand disease) result in menses that are regularly cyclical but prolonged and/or very heavy. Infection with *Neisseria gonorrhoeae* has been associated with menometrorrhagia.

The differential diagnosis of DUB includes ectopic pregnancy, threatened abortion, trauma, PID, and congenital outflow tract anomalies.

The history should include questions about personal menstrual history, sexual history, family history, and review of symptoms to narrow the differential. If the patient is sexually active, the history is atypical for anovulatory DUB, or a structural abnormality is suspected, a bimanual pelvic examination is indicated. A screening hematocrit is required in all patients with DUB. Other tests to consider include a complete blood count, thyroid function tests, pregnancy test, and coagulation studies.

An algorithm for the management of DUB is provided in Figure 24-4.

Amenorrhea

Amenorrhea is the absence of menses. It may be primary or secondary.

- *Primary amenorrhea* is defined as the absence of spontaneous uterine bleeding by age 16 years OR in any girl who has been breast SMR stage 5 for at least 1 year. Possible

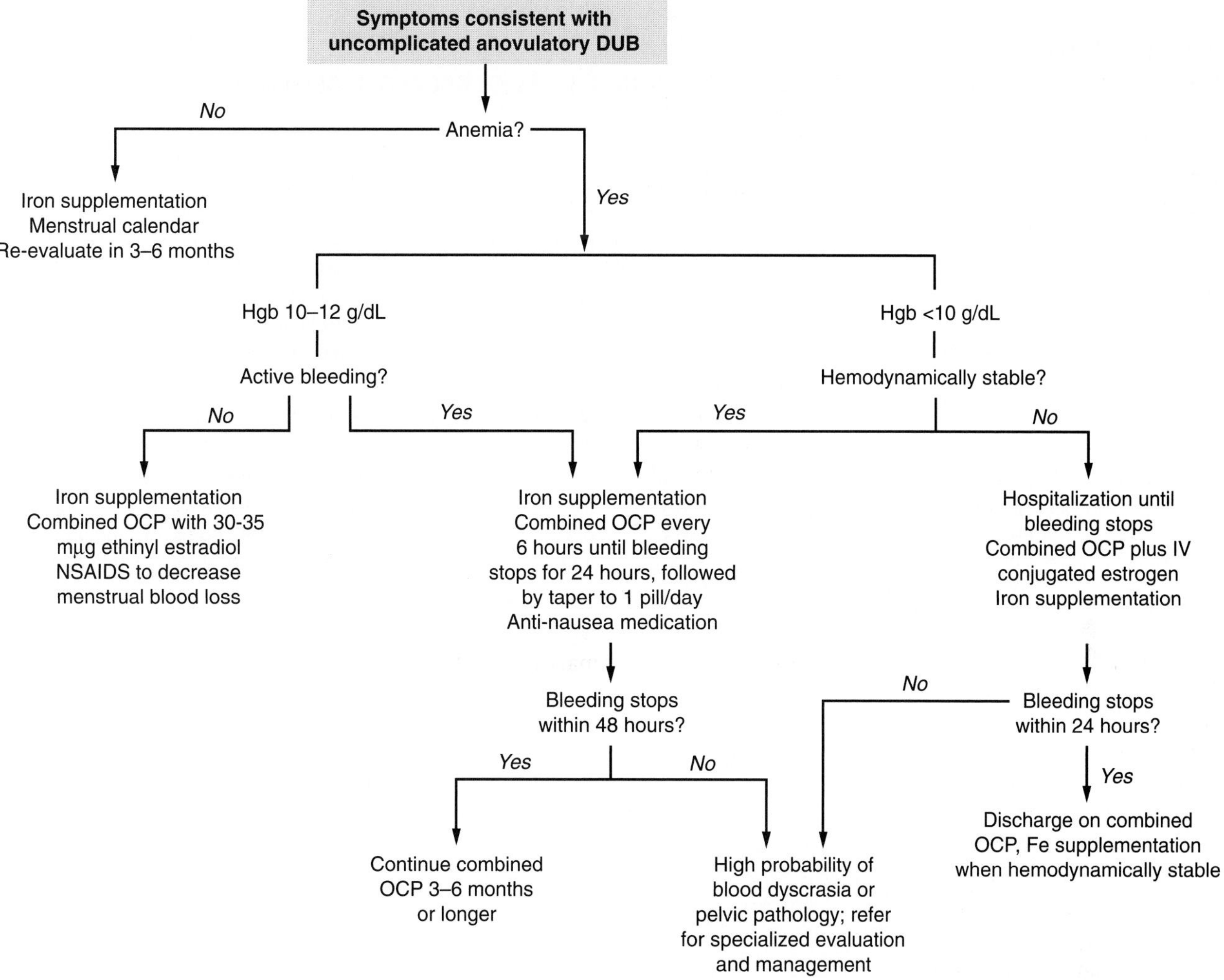

Figure 24-4 Treatment algorithm for anovulatory dysfunctional uterine bleeding (DUB). Hgb, hemoglobin; OCP, oral contraceptive pill; NSAIDs, nonsteroidal anti-inflammatory drugs; IV, intravenous.

causes include disorders of the hypothalamic-pituitary tract, ovarian dysfunction, adrenal disease, anatomic abnormalities of the genital tract, pregnancy, and Turner syndrome or other genetic disorders.

- *Secondary amenorrhea* is the cessation of previously normal menstrual uterine bleeding for a period of time equal to three previous cycles. Secondary amenorrhea typically results from disruption of a previously functioning hypothalamic-pituitary-ovarian axis. Possible causes include tumors (craniopharyngioma, pituitary tumor), reduced energy intake or excessive output (anorexia nervosa, female athlete triad), and psychological stress. PCOS, pregnancy, endocrine disorders (thyroid dysfunction, diabetes), and chronic illness have also been associated with amenorrhea.

Primary amenorrhea due to hypothalamic, pituitary, or ovarian failure is treated with conjugated estrogen and cycles of progestin to induce withdrawal bleeding. The management of secondary amenorrhea associated with the female athlete triad is provided in Chapter 25.

SEXUALLY TRANSMITTED DISEASES

Most infections with STDs are asymptomatic, so adolescents should be questioned regarding their sexual activity at each health maintenance visit and offered STD screening and treatment as needed. Screening is indicated at least once a year, within 3 months of acquiring a new partner, and in the setting of suggestive symptoms. Nucleic acid amplification tests, which have good sensitivity/specificity and can be used with urine as well as urethral/cervical specimens, offer a noninvasive alternative for detecting sexually transmitted pathogens. The most prevalent causative organisms of STDs in adolescents are listed in Table 24-6. *Patients who test positive for one or more STDs should be encouraged to be tested for others as well, including human immunodeficiency virus (HIV) and syphilis* (see Chapter 10). In most cases, sexual partners should also be evaluated and treated. Adolescents who are or are considering becoming sexually active should be counseled to use latex or polyurethane condoms with each act of anal and vaginal intercourse to reduce the risk of contracting an STD.

TABLE 24-6
COMMON SEXUALLY TRANSMITTED DISEASES IN THE ADOLESCENT POPULATION

Causative Organism (Disease)	Conditions	Diagnosis	Effective Treatment
Neisseria gonorrhoeae (gonorrhea)	*Males* Epididymitis Prostatitis *Females* Menometrorrhagia Endocervicitis Salpingitis PID *Both Genders* Urethritis Proctitis Pharyngitis Conjunctivitis Gonococcal arthritis Disseminated gonococcal infection Perihepatitis	Gram stain for Gram-negative intracellular diplococci Culture on Thayer-Martin (Martin-Lewis) medium or chocolate agar DNA probe NAATs All *N. gonorrhoeae* isolates should be tested for beta-lactamase production.	Sexual contacts of persons infected with *N. gonorrhoeae* should also be screened and treated. Ciprofloxacin (oral) Ofloxacin (oral) Levofloxacin (oral) Ceftriaxone (parenteral) Cefoxitin plus probenecid (parenteral) Spectinomycin (parenteral) Patients with disseminated disease (arthritis, endocarditis, meningitis, bacteremia/sepsis) are treated with ceftriaxone.
Chlamydia trachomatis (chlamydia)	*Males* Epididymitis *Females* Cervicitis PID *Both Genders* Urethritis Proctitis Pharyngitis Perihepatitis Reiter syndrome[a]	Culture DFA/EIA DNA probe NAATs	Sexual contacts of persons infected with *C. trachomatis* should also be screened and treated. Azithromycin (oral, single dose) Doxycycline (oral)
Trichomonas vaginalis (trichomoniasis)	*Males* Nongonococcal urethritis *Females* Vaginitis *Both Genders* Asymptomatic	Microscopy Culture Immunochromatography Nucleic acid probe	Sexual contacts of persons infected with *T. vaginalis* should also be screened and treated. Metronidazole (oral, single dose)
Herpes simplex virus (herpes)	*Males* Urethritis *Females* Cervicitis *Both* Herpetic lesions Dysuria	Tzanck smear (giant multinucleated cells) Viral culture EIA Immunofluorescence DNA probe PCR	Genital herpes is not curable. Sexual contacts of persons infected with genital herpes should also be screened. Genital herpes may be prevented by the use of condoms.
Human papillomavirus (genital warts)	*Females* Cervical dysplasia Cervical cancer *Both Genders* Asymptomatic Anogenital warts	Clinical diagnosis (anogenital warts) Pap smear (screening for cervical dysplasia) Molecular probes (detect organism in cervical cells)	Human papillomavirus is not curable.

[a]Reiter syndrome consists of conjunctivitis, dermatitis, urethritis, and reactive arthritis (see Chapter 21).
PID, pelvic inflammatory disease; NAATs, nucleic acid amplification tests (NAATs have good sensitivity/specificity, can be used on urine as well as urethral/cervical specimens, and generally test for both *N. gonorrhoeae* and *C. trachomatis*); DFA, direct fluorescent antibody; EIA, enzyme immunoassay; PCR, polymerase chain reaction.

Male Urethritis

Urethritis, or inflammation of the urethra, is often asymptomatic in males. As noted in Table 24-7, urethritis is generally classified as "gonococcal" or "nongonococcal" (NGU) for treatment purposes. All male patients with urethritis should be tested for *N. gonorrhoeae* and *Chlamydia trachomatis*. If a causative organism is isolated in nongonococcal urethritis, it is typically *Chlamydia*. Other organisms (i.e., *Ureaplasma urealyticum, Trichomonas vaginalis*) are not routinely tested for but should be considered in cases of treatment failure. Both are sensitive to metronidazole. Herpes simplex virus (HSV) type 2 may also cause urethritis.

Vaginitis

Vaginitis is inflammation of the vaginal lining. Vaginitis may be due to bacteria (anaerobes such as *Peptostreptococcus, Bacteroides, Gardnerella vaginalis, Mycoplasma hominis*), *T. vaginalis*, or fungi (typically species of *Candida*). Presentation, diagnosis, treatment, and complications are outlined in Table 24-8. Bacterial vaginosis and *T. vaginalis* are more common in sexually active adolescents. Abstinent adolescents with vaginal inflammation are most likely suffering from vulvovaginal candidiasis; predisposing conditions include diabetes, pregnancy, and broad-spectrum antibiotic therapy.

In contrast, leukorrhea is a clear-to-white, thin, mucoid vaginal discharge that may begin up to 6 months before menarche and continue for a few years. It is a normal physiologic occurrence. If the patient is not sexually active and the history is consistent with leukorrhea, no further workup is needed. A thin panty shield may help if the discharge is bothersome; daily tampon use should be avoided.

Cervicitis

Cervicitis, or inflammation of the cervix, may be caused by any of the organisms listed in Table 24-6. Although often asymptomatic, cervicitis can produce mucopurulent discharge and be mistakenly diagnosed as vaginitis. In addition to the discharge, patients may complain of pain with sexual intercourse (*dyspareunia*) and bloody spotting afterwards. The

TABLE 24-7
PRESENTATION, DIAGNOSIS, TREATMENT, AND COMPLICATIONS OF SEXUALLY TRANSMITTED URETHRITIS IN MALES

Characteristic	Gonococcal Urethritis	Nongonococcal Urethritis
Typical presentation	Asymptomatic, OR Purulent urethral discharge, dysuria, urinary frequency, meatal edema/erythema	Asymptomatic, OR Milder urethral discharge (mucoid or purulent), dysuria, urinary frequency
Diagnosis (A) or (B) at right, plus at least one of the following: ■ Mucoid or purulent urethral discharge ■ Positive leukocyte esterase test on first void urine ■ $\geq$10 WBCs per high-power field on first void urine	(A) Gram-negative intracellular diplococci on smear of urethral discharge Same on culture Positive NAAT	(B) $\geq$5 WBCs per field on intraurethral smear and no Gram-negative intracellular diplococci Positive leukocyte esterase test on first void urine and negative gonorrhea test (NAAT or other tests for *Chlamydia* may be positive or negative)
Treatment	Recommended: Single dose of any of the following: Cefixime 400 mg PO Ceftriaxone 125 mg IM Ciprofloxacin 500 mg PO Ofloxacin 400 mg PO Levofloxacin 250 mg PO Alternatives: spectinomycin, other fluoroquinolones	Recommended: azithromycin 1 gm PO (single dose) OR doxycycline 100 mg PO bid for 7 days Alternatives: erythromycin, ofloxacin, levofloxacin
Complications	Epididymitis	Epididymitis, Reiter syndrome

WBC, white blood cells; NAAT, nucleic acid amplification test; PO, oral; IM, intramuscular; bid, twice a day.

TABLE 24-8
VAGINAL DISCHARGE: PRESENTATION, DIAGNOSIS, TREATMENT, AND COMPLICATIONS

Characteristic	Bacterial Vaginosis	*Trichomonas Vaginalis*	Vulvovaginal Candidiasis	Leukorrhea
Typical presentation	Asymptomatic, OR foul smell; increasing discharge following sexual intercourse	Asymptomatic, OR itching, vaginal discharge, dysuria	Intense vulvovaginal itching, burning; tissue erythema	No symptoms other than discharge
Discharge characteristics	Slight to moderate, thin, gray-white, foul-smelling (fishy) discharge	Profuse, bubbly or frothy, greenish discharge	Thick, curdlike, white; adherent	Thin, white, mucoid, odorless discharge
Diagnosis (vaginal pH, wet prep examination of discharge, "whiff" test[a])	pH >4.5 >20% clue cells[b] Whiff test positive	pH >4.5 White blood cells (WBCs), trichomonads Whiff test usually negative	pH 4–4.5 WBCs, budding yeast, pseudohyphae Whiff test negative	pH <4.5 Vaginal epithelial cells; no inflammation Rod-shaped lactobacilli on Gram stain
Treatment	Recommended:[c] metronidazole PO (500 mg bid for 7 days) or intravaginally (qd for 5 days) OR Clindamycin cream qhs for 7 days Sexual partners not routinely treated	Recommended: metronidazole OR Tinidazole 2 g PO (single dose) Alternative: metronidazole 500 mg PO bid for 7 days Sexual partners should be treated	Recommended: intravaginal butoconazole, clotrimazole, or miconazole OR Fluconazole 150 mg PO (single dose) Replacement of diaphragms, if used All underwear washed in hot water	None
Complications	In pregnant women, increased incidence of preterm labor and other adverse outcomes	None significant	None significant, but may be recurrent	None

[a]Fishy odor is released when specimen of vaginal secretions is mixed with drop of 10% potassium hydroxide.
[b]Clue cells: squamous epithelial cells for the vaginal lining that become coated with bacteria and develop blurred borders.
[c]Pregnant women with bacterial vaginosis should receive *oral* metronidazole or clindamycin rather than intravaginal therapy.
PO, oral; qd, once daily; qhs, daily at bedtime; bid, twice a day.

collection of endocervical swabs for culture, DNA probe, or nucleic acid amplification test (NAAT) often produces bleeding as well. Of note, *C. trachomatis* and *N. gonorrhoeae* cause cervicitis rather than vaginitis and, if left untreated, result in PID.

Pelvic Inflammatory Disease

PID is defined as infectious inflammation of the ascending genital tract proximal to the cervix. Specific diagnoses include endometritis, salpingitis, oophoritis, tubo-ovarian abscesses, peritonitis, and perihepatitis (*Fitz-Hugh-Curtis syndrome*). PID is a polymicrobial infection; *N. gonorrhoeae, C. trachomatis,* and bacteria also associated with bacterial vaginosis (e.g., *Bacteroides*) have all been implicated in the development of PID. Endocervical specimens should be collected for *N. gonorrhoeae* and *C. trachomatis* testing as previously described. Adolescents who develop PID have a significantly elevated risk of fertility problems, ectopic pregnancy, and/or chronic pelvic pain.

PID is a clinical diagnosis. Adolescents should be presumed to have PID if:

- They are sexually active, AND
- They are experiencing pelvic or lower abdominal pain due to no other known cause, AND
- They exhibit one or more of the following signs on examination: cervical motion tenderness, uterine tenderness, and adnexal tenderness.

Additional findings that support the diagnosis of PID include the following:

- Mucopurulent cervical or vaginal discharge*
- Large number of white blood cells in vaginal secretions*
- Laboratory evidence of infection with *C. trachomatis* or *N. gonorrhoeae*

TABLE 24-9
RECOMMENDED TREATMENTS FOR PELVIC INFLAMMATORY DISEASE

Treatments	Inpatient	Outpatient
Recommended	Cefotetan IV OR Cefoxitin IV PLUS Doxycycline PO or IV	Levofloxacin 500 mg PO qd for 14 days OR Ofloxacin 400 mg PO qd for 14 days WITH OR WITHOUT Metronidazole 500 mg PO bid for 14 days
Alternative	Clindamycin IV PLUS Gentamicin IV or IM	Single dose of either ceftriaxone 250 mg IM or cefoxitin 2 g IM and probenecid 1 g PO PLUS Doxycycline 100 mg PO bid for 14 days WITH OR WITHOUT Metronidazole 500 mg PO bid for 14 days

IV, intravenous; PO, oral; qd, once daily; bid, twice a day; IM, intramuscular.

- Elevated C-reactive protein and/or erythrocyte sedimentation rate
- Oral temperature ≥101°F

* Either or both virtually always present.

Recommended inpatient and outpatient treatment regimens are detailed in Table 24-9. Partners should be evaluated and treated. Patients who require admission for intravenous antibiotic therapy may be discharged on oral therapy to complete a 14-day course when they no longer meet the criteria for inpatient therapy.

The Centers for Disease Control and Prevention recommends hospitalization if any of the following are present:

- A surgical emergency cannot be ruled out.
- Pregnancy
- Illness does not respond to or patient cannot tolerate oral therapy.
- Patient is severely ill.
- Documented tubo-ovarian abscess

Fitz-Hugh-Curtis syndrome is a variant of PID manifested by right upper quadrant pain, which may be the sole presenting symptom. It is most closely associated with *C. trachomatis* infection. The pain may be referred to the shoulder and/or accompanied by nausea. Fitz-Hugh-Curtis syndrome should be suspected in the adolescent female patient with right upper quadrant pain, signs of PID, and no radiologic or laboratory evidence of hepatitis, gallbladder disease, or pancreatitis. If necessary, diagnostic laparoscopy confirms the diagnosis. No additional treatment is indicated beyond that recommended for PID.

Herpes Simplex Virus

Genital herpes is an incurable STD that becomes latent and recurs over time. Although HSV2 causes the majority of cases, HSV1 is implicated as well. Patients first notice a burning sensation in the affected area, followed by the appearance of the characteristic 1- to 2-mm vesicles on erythematous bases that then ulcerate over several days. Fever and malaise are common during the primary infection. Genital herpes is generally a clinical diagnosis; laboratory confirmation is unnecessary in typical cases. Oral antiviral medication (acyclovir) will shorten the duration of the disease and viral shedding if administered early, while new lesions are still forming. Treatment of the primary episode does not affect the rate of recurrence. Antivirals also shorten the duration of recurrent episodes if taken at the first sign of symptoms. Daily use of suppressive therapy should be considered in patients who have more than six recurrences per year, patients who have severe recurrences, patients who are in relationships with HSV-negative partners, and patients who are immunocompromised. Transmission can occur during primary infections, recurrences, and periods of asymptomatic shedding. Most patients who become infected are exposed to the virus through contact with an asymptomatic partner. Condom use substantially decreases the likelihood of genital HSV transmission.

Human Papillomavirus

Human papillomavirus (HPV) is the most prevalent STD in the United States. Although HPV may cause anogenital warts and cervical dysplasia, *most HPV infections are asymptomatic*. The warts can be treated topically, with laser, or surgically, but the infection can never be eradicated. Certain HPV genotypes (16 and 18) are associated with an increased risk of cervical cancer. The Food and Drug Administration recently approved the first HPV vaccine, which is now recommended for routine administration in girls 9 years of age and older.

Pediculosis Pubis

Although pediculosis pubis is not technically a sexually transmitted infection, this parasitic infestation is usually acquired via sexual contact. Sustained contact with bedding contaminated with *Phthirus pubis* is an alternate means of spread. Unlike other parasitic skin infestations, *P. pubis* affects all racial and ethnic groups equally. Viable eggs that attach to the hair shaft may hatch up to 10 days after deposition. The lice can survive up to 36 hours without a blood meal. Symptoms include intense itching at the site of the bites, which are usually found in the pubic and perianal regions but may also involve the hairy areas above the waist. The "crabs" are easily visible on physical examination of the pruritic areas. Treatment consists of topical permethrin 1% to 5%.

TABLE 24-10
COMPARISON OF THE AVAILABLE FORMS OF CONTRACEPTION

Contraception	Failure Rate: Ideal/Typical	Advantages	Disadvantages
Male condom	3%/12%	Cost Availability Decreases risk of STDs Reversible form of birth control	Must be used with each act of sexual intercourse Relatively higher rate of contraception failure Possible latex allergy
Female barrier contraceptives	5%/23%	Useful when male partners refuse to wear condoms Reversible form of birth control	More expensive than male condoms Difficult to use correctly Questionable reduction in STD risk
Estrogen/progestin (combined) contraceptive pill	0.1%/4%	Safe and effective Predictable, controlled menstrual cycles Reduction in acne Reduced risk of ovarian, endometrial cancer Reduced risk of PID Reduced incidence of benign breast changes Rapidly reversible	Requires daily administration Side effects may include weight gain Use with caution in smokers Contraindicated in certain populations of patients[a] Extremely rare but serious side effects including thromboembolism, cardiovascular disease, and cholelithiasis
Progestin-only pill	0.5%/7%	May be useful if estrogen is contraindicated or not tolerated	Decreased efficacy/higher failure rate
Depo-medroxyprogesterone acetate (DMPA)	0.3%/0.3%	Convenient (requires only four injections per year) Safe and effective Safe for smokers Decreased risk of endometrial cancer May be used during breast feeding and immediately after delivery	Not immediately reversible Side effects include amenorrhea, breakthrough bleeding, and weight gain Contraindications include thromboembolic disorders, abnormal vaginal bleeding, pregnancy, liver disease, intracranial hypertension
Combination hormonal injections	0.2%/<1%	Safe and effective Convenient Predictable, controlled menstrual cycles Rapidly reversible Theoretically same health benefits as combined OCPs	Must return for reinjection during specified time Theoretically has same contraindications and complications as combined OCPs
Transdermal patch	Ideal failure rate comparable to OCPs/higher compliance	Better compliance than OCPs Otherwise advantages similar to combined OCPs	Theoretically similar to combined OCPs

[a]Contraindicated in woman with history of thromboembolism and those with cerebral vascular or coronary artery disease; hypercoagulability; hepatic, breast, or endometrial carcinomas; abnormal vaginal bleeding; and pregnancy, breastfeeding, or immediately postpartum. Relative contraindications include breast nodules, brittle diabetes, elevated triglycerides/cholesterol, heart or kidney disease, migraines, and depression.
STD, sexually transmitted disease; PID, pelvic inflammatory disease; OCP, oral contraceptive pills.

CONTRACEPTION AND PREGNANCY

Despite a recent, highly publicized drop in the teenage pregnancy rate, the United States still leads the industrialized world in pregnancy, abortion, and birth rates in those younger than 20 years of age. At least 80% of teenage pregnancies are unintentional. Factors associated with increased rates of teenage pregnancy include poverty, frequent sexual activity, abuse, and acceptance of teenage pregnancy within the culture. Teenage mothers are significantly more likely to drop out of school, live in poverty, require public assistance, and become pregnant again during adolescence. Pregnant adolescents who receive good prenatal care and counseling are not at any increased risk for adverse health events during pregnancy.

About a third of patients who ask their physician to prescribe birth control are already sexually active. Table 24-10 lists the forms of contraception available, compares their effectiveness, and discusses advantages and disadvantages of each. Of note, the risk of morbidity and mortality due to pregnancy and delivery is greater than that associated with any of the contraceptive methods listed below.

Contraceptive methods that require minimal effort rather than repeated action each day or with each episode of intercourse generally have lower rates of failure because they are less user dependent. Condoms and daily oral birth control pills have the highest rates of noncompliance. There are multiple reasons why adolescents may be reluctant to use birth control, including misconceptions about the safety and efficacy of birth control options; fear that their parents will find out that they are sexually active; the mistaken belief that a pelvic examination is required prior to initiating birth control; belief that pregnancy/STDs will not happen to them; barriers to access/availability; and pressure from peers or their partner.

HIGH-RISK BEHAVIORS

Delinquency

Juvenile delinquency is defined as the performance of illegal acts by a minor. Males make up the majority of juvenile arrests for crimes such as theft/burglary/robbery and assault. Females are more often arrested for prostitution or running away, but there has been a marked increase in the number of girls arrested for violent crime over the past 10 years. Factors believed to be associated with an increased risk for delinquent behavior in the adolescent are listed in Table 24-11. Delinquent patients are likely to suffer from health conditions associated with inadequate care (e.g., dental decay) or suboptimal management (e.g., asthma, poor eyesight), injuries, substance abuse, smoking, STDs, pregnancy, and depression.

A status offender is a minor who commits behaviors that would not be defined as illegal in an adult, such as truancy, running away, acting beyond the parental control, and curfew violation.

TABLE 24-11
FACTORS ASSOCIATED WITH AN INCREASED RISK OF DELINQUENCY IN THE ADOLESCENT

Medical
Significant head trauma
Attention deficit disorder
Learning disability
Prenatal alcohol/illicit drug exposure

Familial
Parental psychiatric illness
Family history of alcoholism
Family history of criminal behavior
Family conflict
Child abuse

Social
Association with delinquent peers[a]
Gang involvement
Low socioeconomic status

School
Early academic failure
Lack of commitment to education

Individual
Low self-esteem
Serious delinquent behaviors (violence toward animals, setting fires) at an early age

Protective Factors
High intelligence
Resilient temperament
Supportive social relationships with adults
Commitment to education

[a]The strongest predictor of delinquent behavior.

Injury

Accidental injury is the leading cause of adolescent morbidity and mortality in the United States. Motor vehicle collisions cause the majority of injury deaths. Risky behavior that contributes to vehicular death includes driving under the influence of alcohol or drugs, speeding, riding or driving without a seat belt, and the performance of illegal traffic maneuvers. Drowning is the second leading cause of unintentional injury and death in adolescents, followed by accidental firearm deaths.

Although accidental injuries as a group result in the greatest morbidity and mortality during adolescence, intentional violence against others (homicide) and oneself (suicide) are the second and third leading causes of death in the adolescent population. Violent teens are more likely than their peers to have been a victim of physical abuse, to have witnessed domestic violence within the home, to be described as impulsive, and to have poor social skills. The most successful violence prevention programs are those that identify at-risk individuals and their families at an early age and intervene to limit family violence (e.g., abuse, corporal punishment) and exposure to violent media while teaching and supporting nonviolent resolution skills (e.g., negotiation, mediation).

The Female Rape Victim

Rape is sexual intercourse that occurs against a person's will, either through the use or threat of force or because the person is unable to resist or consent (e.g., intoxication, severe mental retardation). Although rape is considered a medical emergency, the psychological consequences are tremendous, life altering, and long lasting. *Rape trauma syndrome* describes three stages of adjustment that occur in victims of rape:

- The *acute reaction phase* begins during the assault and lasts days to weeks; may involve a flat affect or visible distress and anxiety; victim is disoriented and experiences feelings of shame, anger, guilt, and humiliation; may experience difficulty sleeping/eating
- The *outward adjustment/avoidance stage* lasts days to weeks; uses denial and suppression to cope; experiences depression and may withdraw from family and friends; experiences nightmares and flashbacks
- The *integration/resolution stage* victim begins to process the experience and emotions rather than suppressing them; integration of the experience helps the individual progress from self-image of victim to one of a survivor

The history and physical examination of a rape victim ideally should be undertaken by a physician knowledgeable in the evaluation of rape victims, gathering of evidence, and reporting; in a private, quiet area; in the presence of a supportive companion (if desired); and in an unhurried manner that allows the patient to discuss emotions, ask questions, receive answers and referrals, and benefit from anticipatory counseling.

Any patient who has been raped should be offered STD prophylaxis and counseled regarding the risk/benefit of HIV postexposure prophylaxis. If the patient is not currently using a form of birth control, she should be offered an option for the prevention of pregnancy. The most commonly used form of postcoital contraception (*Plan B*) consists of two 0.75-mg levonorgestrel pills taken 12 hours apart within 3 days after unprotected intercourse; this reduces the risk of pregnancy by approximately 90%. Plan B was approved by the FDA in 2006 for over-the-counter use by women 18 years of age or older. An alternative called the *Yuzpe* method uses two doses of levonorgestrel 0.5 mg together with at least 100 μg of ethinyl estradiol, also administered 12 hours apart within 72 hours of unprotected intercourse.

EATING DISORDERS

Anorexia and bulimia are eating disorders that can develop in adolescents. Obsession with thinness, binge eating, and purging behaviors may be found in the obese as well as

TABLE 24-12
SUGGESTED LABORATORY TESTS FOR ADOLESCENTS WITH EATING DISORDERS

	Study	Suspected Result
All patients	Complete blood count	Neutropenia; also anemia and thrombocytopenia
	Serum electrolytes	Hypokalemia/alkalosis (if purging) Hyponatremia (due to manipulation of water intake)
	Blood urea nitrogen/creatinine	Increased blood urea nitrogen
	Glucose	Normal or low
	Calcium/phosphate/magnesium	Normal or low
	Electrocardiogram	Bradycardia, T-wave inversions, ST depression (anorexia) Prolonged QTc interval (bulimia, if hypokalemic)
Patients with anorexia	ESR[a]	Normal or low
	Urinalysis	Decreased specific gravity
	Liver function tests	Elevated
	Cholesterol	Elevated
	Serum protein/albumin	Low
	TSH/T_4[a]	Normal/normal to low
	Bone density scan	Osteopenia (if amenorrhea >6 months)
Patients with bulimia	Serum amylase	Elevated if vomiting

[a]Beneficial for ruling out other conditions in the differential.
ESR, erythrocyte sedimentation rate; TSH, thyroid-stimulating hormone; T_4, thyroxine.

the typical or underweight patient. Many patients with eating disorders have comorbid psychiatric conditions (e.g., depression, obsessive-compulsive disorder) or a family history of such.

Anorexia is the condition of intentionally limiting caloric intake to achieve excessive weight loss (actual weight <85% of expected body weight). Patients with anorexia have a distorted body image and an extreme fear of becoming fat. Females develop *amenorrhea*; in fact, the absence of menses for at least three consecutive cycles is a diagnostic criterion for the condition and may even precede significant weight loss. The typical patient with anorexia is an outwardly successful, compulsive white female with a poor self-image, but males and adolescents of other cultural and ethnic groups are also affected. Patients with prolonged amenorrhea develop osteopenia and are at an increased risk for osteoporosis later in life. Amenorrhea generally occurs when actual weight falls below 85% of ideal body weight for age and height; however, amenorrhea may precede significant weight loss in many patients and can be a valuable early indicator of anorexia.

Patients with *bulimia* have episodes of binge eating followed by either purging (through vomiting or laxatives) or other behaviors designed to prevent weight gain (excessive exercise). The behavior merits the diagnosis of bulimia if the binging occurs more than twice weekly for at least 3 months. Bulimia is not associated with menstrual irregularities.

The history should address the patient's diet, eating/purging/exercise behaviors, body image, family dynamics, stressors, and mental state. Anorexics may complain of abdominal pains and constipation, symptoms of gallstones, feeling faint, and cold intolerance. Bulimics who vomit can develop chest pain or hematemesis. An examination may reveal tooth decay and/or knuckle abrasions or calluses due to vomiting.

Anorexia and bulimia are clinical diagnoses; however, laboratory tests may be helpful when complications are suspected or hospitalization is being considered. Table 24-12 lists some suggested laboratory tests for adolescents with

TABLE 24-13
ANOREXIA AND BULIMIA: DIFFERENTIAL DIAGNOSES

Anorexia	Bulimia
Malignancy	Achalasia
Inflammatory bowel disease	Increased intracranial pressure
Malabsorption conditions	Pregnancy
Chronic infections	Infectious vomiting
Endocrine disorders (thyroid disease, Addison disease, diabetes)	Metabolic disease
	Endocrine disease

TABLE 24-14
ANOREXIA AND BULIMIA: INDICATIONS FOR HOSPITALIZATION

Both Conditions
Failure to improve with outpatient therapy
Hypokalemia (serum potassium <3.2 mmol/L)
Hypochloremia (serum chloride <88 mmol/L)
Cardiac arrhythmias/prolonged QTc interval/bradycardia
Medical complications requiring inpatient intervention

Anorexia
Unstable vital signs
Severe weight loss (>25% to 30% below ideal body weight)
Need for enteral nutrition (food refusal)
Arrested pubertal development

eating disorders. The differential diagnoses for anorexia and bulimia are found in Table 24-13. Table 24-14 lists indications for hospitalization.

For anorexia, treatment is aimed at nutritional therapy to provide adequate weight gain for growth and the return of menses. In hospitalized patients who are severely underweight, refeeding that is too rapid may lead to edema and/or hypophosphatemia, with resultant cardiac failure, hemolytic anemia, and/or coma. Psychological therapy, in the form of individual, family, and/or group counseling, is beneficial in both anorexia and bulimia. Selective serotonin reuptake inhibitors (i.e., fluoxetine) are thought to be of some benefit in both disorders, although recent anecdotal evidence linking their use to an increased risk of suicide in adolescents suggests caution.

CHRONIC ILLNESS IN THE ADOLESCENT

Optimal management of chronic illness or a handicapping condition in the adolescent requires a thorough understanding of the psychological and cognitive tasks that should be achieved during this time. Table 24-15 discusses factors related to illness that may interfere with the normal transition from child to adult during this vulnerable developmental stage. Patients with both visible and nonvisible chronic conditions are at increased risk of depression and other emotional problems, especially if complications of the illness occur at unpredictable intervals and are beyond the patient's control. An involved and available primary care physician can play an instrumental role in facilitating the transition to adult behavior.

As with any adolescent, the patient should be treated as a full partner in the formulation of a treatment plan. Compliance improves when an adolescent is fully educated

TABLE 24-15

EFFECTS OF CHRONIC ILLNESS ON PSYCHOSOCIAL DEVELOPMENT OF ADOLESCENTS

Achievement of Independence/Separation from Parents

- Typical demands of managing chronic illness require dependence on family members and physician.
- Demand for more independence may lead to refusal to adhere to medical regimen or rejection of medical advice.
- Time and energy devoted to illness management take precedence over preparing to meet future professional and financial responsibilities.

Achievement of Satisfactory Body Image and Positive Self-Esteem

- Conditions that are visible (acne, deformity) or cause a delay in puberty (diabetes) lead to low self-esteem.

Peer Relationships

- Patient may look or feel different from peers at a time when they are desperately trying to be the same.
- Patient may feel or actually be rejected by peers.
- Peer relationships are limited by increased absences from school and other activities.

about the condition, given a chance to have concerns heard and addressed, and allowed to assist in the creation of an appropriate treatment regimen. Other issues related to adherence are discussed earlier in the Adolescent Health Maintenance Visit section. It is particularly important that adolescents with chronic illness and their families plan for transition to adult health care services in order to avoid delay or interruption of care.

SOURCES

Alexander KA. Diagnosis and management of human papillomavirus infections. *Pediatr Infect Dis J.* 2005;24:1007–1008.

American Academy of Pediatrics, Committee in Adolescence. Identifying and treating eating disorders. *Pediatrics.* 2003;111:204–211.

American Academy of Pediatrics, Committee on Practice and Ambulatory Medicine. Recommendations for pediatric and preventative health care. *Pediatrics.* 1995;96:373.

American Academy of Pediatrics, Committee on Psychosocial Aspects of Child and Family Health. *Guidelines for Health Supervision III.* Elk Grove Village, IL: American Academy of Pediatrics; 1996.

American Psychiatric Association. *Diagnostic and Statistical Manual of Mental Disorders.* 4th ed. Washington, DC: American Psychiatric Association; 1994.

Burgess A, Holstrum L. Rape trauma syndrome. *Am J Psychiatry.* 1974; 131:981.

Centers for Disease Control and Prevention. 2006 guidelines for treatment of sexually transmitted diseases. *Morb Mortal Wkly Rep.* 2006; 55:1–94.

Centers for Disease Control and Prevention. Youth risk behavior surveillance—United States, 1999. *Morb Mortal Wkly Rep.* 2000;49:1–96.

Fisher M. Treatment of eating disorders in children, adolescents, and young adults. *Pediatr Rev.* 2006;27:5–15.

Fortenberry JD, Neinstein LS. Overview of sexually transmitted diseases. In: Neinstein LS, ed. *Adolescent health care: a practical guide.* Philadelphia: Lippincott Williams &Wilkins; 2002:1085–1117.

Gutgesell ME, Payne N. Issues of adolescent psychological development in the 21st century. *Pediatr Rev.* 2004;25:79–85.

Marcell AV, Bell DL. Making the most of the adolescents male health visit. *Contemp Pediatr.* 2006;23:50–63.

Neinstein LS, Farmer M. Teenage pregnancy. In: Neinstein LS, ed. *Adolescent health care: a practical guide.* Philadelphia: Lippincott Williams &Wilkins; 2002:809–833.

Onufer CN, Marks J, Gibson A. New momentum on building a medical home for the child with a chronic health problem. *Contemp Pediatr.* 2006;23:65–73.

Rimsza ME. Counseling the adolescent about contraception. *Pediatr Rev.* 2003;24:162–170.

Rimsza ME. Dysfunctional uterine bleeding. *Pediatr Rev.* 2002;23:227–233.

Rosen DS. Physiologic growth and development during adolescence. *Pediatr Rev.* 2004;25:194–200.

Tanner JM. *Growth at Adolescence.* Oxford, United Kingdom: Blackwell; 1962.

QUESTIONS

1. At a routine health maintenance visit for a 12-year-old girl, you note that the patient has formed breasts with projection of the areola above the contour of the breast. Her mother asks you when you think her daughter might "get her period." You reply that her daughter will likely attain menses:

A) any time
B) 12 months from now
C) 18 months from now
D) 24 months from now
E) Her daughter should have already started menstruating.

2. A 13-year-old boy comes to your office with a complaint of "chest pain." He says that the right side of his chest is sore when he lies down on it. You note a 1.5-cm firm nodule directly behind his right nipple associated with minimal enlargement of the right breast area. The history is negative for constitutional symptoms, and there is no erythema, warmth, streaking, or lymphadenopathy. Which of the following is the most appropriate next step in the management of this patient?

A) Chest radiograph
B) Localized ultrasonography
C) Computed tomography of the area without contrast
D) Computed tomography of the area with contrast
E) Reassure the patient that the condition is normal in adolescent males and should resolve spontaneously.

3. In males, peak height velocity is achieved at what genital sexual maturity rating (SMR) stage?

A) SMR 1
B) SMR 2
C) SMR 3

D) SMR 4
E) SMR 5

4. The percentage of high school seniors who report that they have engaged in sexual intercourse at least once is closest to which of the following?
A) 25%
B) 40%
C) 50%
D) 66%
E) 90%

5. Which of the following is the most opportune time to begin counseling a patient regarding abstinence, other forms of contraception, and safe sex practices?
A) At the earliest adolescent health maintenance visit (approximately age 11 to 12 years)
B) When the patient reports that he or she is considering having sex
C) When the patient reports that he or she is having sex
D) When the patient has a positive screening test for a sexually transmitted disease
E) When the patient is considering marriage

6. Which of the following is a true statement regarding the treatment of primary dysmenorrhea?
A) Primary dysmenorrhea is usually present from the onset of menarche.
B) Combined oral contraceptive pills are a first-line treatment of primary dysmenorrhea.
C) Acetaminophen is a first-line treatment of primary dysmenorrhea.
D) Ibuprofen is an appropriate initial treatment of primary dysmenorrhea.
E) Adhering to a healthy diet and moderate exercise schedule are beneficial in the management of primary dysmenorrhea.

7. You see a 17-year-old young woman in your adolescent clinic with a chief complaint of "painful periods." On history, you gather that the pain begins about 7 days prior to the onset of bleeding and lasts for the duration of flow. The patient tells you that her menses have always been painful but that the pain is increasing over time. The patient is also experiencing pain with intercourse. On bimanual examination, you note tenderness in the cul-de-sac area. A pregnancy test and nucleic acid amplification tests for *Neisseria gonorrhoeae* and *Chlamydia trachomatis* are negative. Which of the following is the most likely diagnosis in this patient?
A) Polycystic ovarian syndrome
B) Primary dysmenorrhea
C) Endometriosis
D) Turner syndrome
E) Incomplete abortion

8. Examination of the external genitalia is recommended in all patients with secondary dysmenorrhea in order to rule out which of the following?
A) Uterine fibroid tumors
B) Imperforate hymen
C) Endometriosis
D) Abuse
E) Genital warts

9. A 16-year-old girl reports that she experienced menarche at age 13 years. Her menstrual cycles are now 22 days in length and very regular. The bleeding lasts for 11 days and is not associated with any pain. She usually uses several heavy pads in the first few days and then switches to panty liners for the duration of the bleeding. What aspect of the girl's menstrual history is particularly concerning?
A) She did not achieve menarche until age 13 years.
B) Her menstrual cycles are only 22 days in length.
C) Her bleeding lasts for 11 days.
D) Her cycle is regular when it should still be primarily anovulatory.
E) There is nothing concerning about the girl's menstrual history.

10. What sexually transmitted disease is most likely to be associated with menometrorrhagia?
A) *N. gonorrhoeae*
B) *C. trachomatis*
C) *Trichomonas vaginalis*
D) Herpes simplex virus
E) Human papillomavirus

11. An 18-year-old patient complains of "irregular periods" at her health maintenance visit. Menarche occurred at age 11.5 years. Her cycles last from 14 to 42 days. The bleeding is painless and usually not particularly heavy. She denies sexual activity. The examination reveals an obese patient with acne, facial hirsutism, and pigmented thickening of the skin of the neck and axillae. The external genitalia are normal. This patient's irregular menstrual cycles are most likely caused by which of the following?
A) Anovulation due to laxative use
B) Anovulation due to Cushing syndrome
C) Anovulation due to polycystic ovarian syndrome
D) Anovulation due to hypothyroidism
E) Anovulation due to hyperthyroidism

12. A 15-year-old girl is hospitalized with a diagnosis of dysfunctional uterine bleeding, a hemoglobin level of 8 g per dL, orthostatic hypotension, and active vaginal bleeding. The white blood cell and platelet counts are normal. A pregnancy test is negative. The bleeding slows but does not stop within 24 hours of starting

intravenous conjugated estrogen. Which of the following is the patient's most likely diagnosis?
A) von Willebrand disease
B) Primary dysfunctional uterine bleeding
C) Threatened abortion
D) Chronic liver disease
E) Thrombocytopenia

13. Which of the following is not part of an appropriate outpatient treatment regimen for dysfunctional uterine bleeding?
A) Iron supplementation
B) Combined oral contraceptive pills
C) Progestin-only contraceptive pills
D) Ketoprofen
E) All of the above are appropriate.

14. Which of the following statements regarding sexually transmitted diseases in adolescents is true?
A) Use of a latex or polyurethane condom is not necessary with anal intercourse.
B) Use of a latex or polyurethane condom is not necessary with the withdrawal method.
C) Most infections with sexually transmitted diseases in the adolescent population are asymptomatic.
D) Urethritis in females is not caused by sexually transmitted pathogens.
E) Sexual partners of patients with trichomoniasis do not require evaluation and treatment.

15. A 16-year-old adolescent comes to the clinic with a chief complaint of "pus from my penis" and pain with urinating. He is able to express mucopurulent fluid from the meatus. Gram stain of the fluid reveals multiple white blood cells and Gram-negative intracellular diplococci. Which of the following is the most appropriate treatment for this patient?
A) Ceftriaxone 125 mg intramuscularly (single dose)
B) Metronidazole 2 g orally (PO) (single dose)
C) Metronidazole 500 mg PO twice a day (bid) for 14 days
D) Probenecid 1 g PO (single dose)
E) Doxycycline 100 mg PO bid for 14 days

16. Which of the following forms of contraception has the lowest ideal failure rate?
A) Male condom
B) Combined oral contraceptive pills
C) Depo-medroxyprogesterone acetate
D) Female condom
E) Withdrawal method

17. A 17-year-old girl comes to the walk-in adolescent clinic with a chief complaint of vaginal discharge. She complains that the discharge is foul smelling and increases after sexual intercourse. A sample of the vaginal discharge has a pH of 4.7. Clue cells are seen on the wet mount, and the whiff test is positive. A pregnancy test is positive. What is the recommended treatment for this patient?
A) Metronidazole 500 mg orally (PO) twice a day (bid) for 7 days
B) Metronidazole 2 g PO (single dose)
C) Intravaginal metronidazole once daily (qd) for 5 days
D) Intravaginal clindamycin qd for 7 days
E) This condition cannot be treated because the patient is pregnant.

18. Which of the following is associated with an increased risk of preterm labor in pregnant women?
A) Vaginitis due to *Trichomonas vaginalis*
B) Vaginitis due to bacterial vaginosis
C) Vulvovaginal candidiasis
D) Leukorrhea
E) None of the above

19. Which of the following is not a finding supportive of the diagnosis of pelvic inflammatory disease?
A) Mucopurulent cervical discharge
B) Large number of white blood cells in vaginal secretions
C) Laboratory evidence of infection with *C. trachomatis* or *N. gonorrhoeae*
D) Elevated C-reactive protein and/or erythrocyte sedimentation rate
E) Budding yeast and pseudohyphae on wet mount of vaginal secretions

20. Which of the following patients with genital herpes is NOT a candidate for viral suppressive therapy?
A) An 18-year-old with a severe primary episode of genital herpes
B) A 17-year-old in a stable relationship with a herpes simplex virus–negative partner
C) A 17-year-old with seven recurrences within the past year
D) An 18-year-old patient who requires daily oral steroid therapy for his asthma
E) An 18-year-old patient with three severe recurrences within the past year

21. Which of the following is the most prevalent sexually transmitted disease in the United States?
A) Genital herpes
B) Human papillomavirus
C) Gonorrhea
D) Chlamydia
E) Trichomoniasis

22. Which of the following is the most common clinical presentation of human papillomavirus in adolescents?
A) Cervical dysplasia
B) Cervical carcinoma

C) Urethritis
D) Anogenital warts
E) Asymptomatic

23. Which of the following is NOT a noncontraceptive benefit of combined oral contraceptive pills?
A) Reduction in migraines
B) More predictable, controlled menstrual cycles
C) Improvement in acne
D) Reduced risk of ovarian cancer
E) Reduced risk of pelvic inflammatory disease

24. Which of the following is NOT an absolute contraindication to combined oral contraceptive pills?
A) A history of thromboembolism in the patient
B) A history of coronary artery disease in the patient
C) An illness that results in hypercoagulability in the patient
D) Smoking behavior in the patient
E) A breastfeeding mother requesting contraceptives 48 hours after delivery

25. The mother of one of your patients brings her 17-year-old son to you because "his behavior is out of control." The parent reports that her son has a history of attention-deficit disorder and that his father is in prison for assault. When interviewed alone, the adolescent tells you that he "hates school" because the kids make fun of him for being "poor" and because he is failing two classes. He admits that his friends occasionally steal from houses when the occupants are not at home, but he denies that he has ever been involved. Which of the following factors in this scenario has the highest association with delinquent behavior?
A) History of attention deficit disorder
B) Family member in prison
C) Lack of commitment to education
D) Living in poverty
E) Association with delinquent peers

26. Which of the following is the leading cause of death in the adolescent population of the United States?
A) Motor vehicle injury
B) Firearm injury
C) Homicide
D) Suicide
E) Drowning

27. Which of the following is the most appropriate form of postcoital contraception for a female rape victim who is not currently using any form of contraception?
A) Copper intrauterine device
B) Three 20-μg progestin tablets taken in a single dose as soon as possible after intercourse
C) Two 0.75-mg levonorgestrel pills taken 12 hours apart within 72 hours of intercourse
D) Depo-medroxyprogesterone as soon as possible after intercourse
E) Vaginal spermicide within 24 hours of intercourse

28. A 14-year-old patient is hospitalized on a pediatric medical ward with the diagnosis of severe anorexia nervosa. Her body weight is 74% of predicated ideal body weight, and she has orthostatic hypotension and is quite weak. An electrocardiogram shows bradycardia but no T-wave inversions or ST depression. A nasogastric feeding tube is placed because the patient refuses to eat the required number of calories per day. On the first day of refeeding, the patient suddenly has a seizure and requires intubation. Which of the following is the most likely cause of her neurologic deterioration?
A) Thrombocytopenia with spontaneous intracranial bleeding
B) Hypoglycemia
C) Prolonged QTc interval and cardiac arrest
D) Hypophosphatemia
E) Hypothyroidism

29. Which of the following is NOT an indication for hospitalizing a patient with anorexia nervosa?
A) Severe weight loss
B) Arrested pubertal development
C) Bradycardia
D) Hypokalemia
E) All of the above are indications for hospitalization.

30. Which of the following is NOT associated with increased compliance in the adolescent patient?
A) Parental involvement
B) A clear plan dictated by the physician
C) Medicine calendar
D) Dosage schedule that coincides with other routine activities
E) Involving the adolescent in decisions about his or her health care

31. Several important assessment parameters change during adolescence, becoming consistent with adult values. Which of the following typically remains constant throughout adolescence?
A) Female hemoglobin level
B) Male hemoglobin level
C) Blood pressure
D) Cholesterol
E) Creatinine

32. The female pelvic examination plays an important role in both health maintenance and the diagnosis of abnormalities in the adolescent patient. A pelvic

examination is recommended for the evaluation of each of the following patients EXCEPT:
A) A sexually active 17-year-old patient with dysmenorrhea
B) A sexually active 16-year-old patient in the office for her yearly health maintenance visit
C) A sexually active 17-year-old patient with pelvic pain and vaginal discharge
D) An 18-year-old abstinent patient in the office for her annual health maintenance visit
E) A 15-year-old abstinent patient with primary dysmenorrhea and a normal external genital examination

33. You are seeing a 12-year-old boy in your office for his routine health maintenance visit. You note on examination that he has lengthening of the penis and enlargement of the testes and scrotum. There is sparse growth of slightly pigmented, mostly straight hair at the base of the penis. You record this patient's sexual maturity rating (SMR) as:
A) Genital SMR 3/pubic hair SMR 3
B) Genital SMR 2/pubic hair SMR 2
C) Genital SMR 2/pubic hair SMR 3
D) Genital SMR 3/pubic hair SMR 2
E) Genital SMR 2/pubic hair SMR 1

34. Which of the following gynecologic conditions is not associated with cyclical pain?
A) Dysmenorrhea
B) Amenorrhea
C) Endometriosis
D) Mittelschmerz
E) All of the above are associated with cyclical pain.

35. Which of the following menstrual abnormalities occurs more frequently in patients with bulimia?
A) Amenorrhea
B) Dysmenorrhea
C) Dysfunctional uterine bleeding
D) Menometrorrhagia
E) None of the above

36. A 13-year-old patient comes to your office with a chief complaint of vaginal discharge. She denies sexual activity. She describes the discharge as thin, white, and odorless. Occasionally, she wears a thin panty liner. There are no other symptoms associated with the discharge. She has not begun menstruating. You are correct in telling the patient that:
A) She is likely to start her menses within 6 months.
B) Her discharge is a normal physiologic process.
C) Her discharge does not require specific treatment.
D) Her discharge will eventually resolve spontaneously.
E) All of the above

37. Which of the following is the most successful type of intervention for patients at risk of perpetuating violence?
A) Boot camps
B) Incarceration
C) Community service
D) Limiting exposure to family and media violence from a young age
E) Alternative schools

38. An asymptomatic sexually active adolescent should be offered which of the following screening tests for sexually transmitted diseases at his routine health maintenance visit?
A) Leukocyte esterase urine screen
B) Nucleic acid amplification tests for *C. trachomatis*
C) Nucleic acid amplification tests for *N. gonorrhoeae*
D) A, B, and C
E) B and C

39. Adolescent vision screening:
A) should be carried out only by an experienced ophthalmologist
B) should occur at the beginning of adolescence
C) should occur at the end of adolescence
D) should occur at both the beginning and end of adolescence
E) should occur every 2 to 3 years during adolescence

40. All of the following are true statements about adolescent development EXCEPT:
A) Psychosocial and cognitive development can be reliably predicted by physical development.
B) Important psychological tasks of adolescence include achievement of independence and formation of a positive self-image.
C) Most adolescents achieve the capacity to use formal operational thought at least intermittently by late adolescence.
D) Masturbation often begins in early adolescence.
E) The health maintenance visit early in adolescence is the most opportune time to discuss contraception and encourage abstinence because most people in this age group are not yet sexually active.

41. A 17-year-old black adolescent who is sexually active presents with intense pubic and perianal itching of 3 weeks in duration. His sexual partner is now complaining of the same symptoms, which are worse at night. Which of the following statements regarding this patient's probable condition is TRUE?
A) *Phthirus pubis* infestation is unlikely in this patient given his ethnic background.
B) There is no possibility of spread to the axilla and scalp areas.
C) Both the patient and his sexual partner should be treated with permethrin 1%.
D) The responsible parasite is only spread through intimate sexual contact.

E) The diagnosis of pubic lice infestation requires low-power microscopic examination of scrapings from the lesions.

42. A 15-year-old sexually active girl presents to the emergency department with a chief complaint of progressive right upper quadrant pain of 3 days in duration. This morning, she developed right shoulder discomfort as well. She is nauseous but nontoxic appearing. Her temperature is 38.5°C; otherwise, vital signs are stable. The physical examination is significant for right upper quadrant tenderness. Abdominal ultrasonography reveals normal liver size and architecture, with no gallbladder or pancreatic abnormalities noted. A pelvic examination is positive for cervical motion tenderness and mucoid cervical discharge. Which of the following pathogens is most likely responsible for this patient's abdominal pain?

A) *N. gonorrhoeae*
B) *C. trachomatis*
C) *Ureaplasma urealyticum*
D) *Gardnerella vaginalis*
E) *Mycoplasma hominis*

ANSWERS

1. A	15. A	29. E
2. E	16. B	30. B
3. D	17. A	31. A
4. D	18. B	32. E
5. A	19. E	33. D
6. D	20. A	34. B
7. C	21. B	35. E
8. B	22. E	36. E
9. C	23. A	37. D
10. A	24. D	38. A
11. C	25. E	39. E
12. A	26. A	40. A
13. C	27. C	41. C
14. C	28. D	42. B

Sports Medicine in the Pediatric Patient

25

EVALUATION FOR SPORTS PARTICIPATION

A thorough history and physical examination are indicated for any individual who is considering instituting an exercise program or participating in organized athletics. Historical data of relevance are provided in Table 25-1. In regard to the physical examination, particular attention should be paid to the following:

- Growth parameters
- Vital signs
- Cardiac examination
- Muscle strength and symmetry
- Range of motion and stability of the major joints (including the neck)

TABLE 25-1
PREPARTICIPATION SCREENING EVALUATION: HISTORY

Symptoms
- Chest pain or tightness (particularly when associated with physical exertion)
- Dyspnea at rest or with mild exertion
- Palpitations or irregular heartbeat
- Lightheadedness or syncope

Past Medical History
- Heart murmur
- Rheumatic fever
- Cardiac surgery

Family History
- Hypertrophic cardiomyopathy
- Long QT syndrome
- Marfan syndrome
- Sudden cardiac death prior to 40 years of age

Social History
- Use of anabolic steroids, cocaine, or other illicit drugs

A preparticipation electrocardiogram is indicated for any patient with one or more of the above risk factors.

Additional Aspects of Patient History of Particular Relevance to Sports Participation
- Prior injuries and rehabilitation
- Head injuries resulting in altered consciousness/concussion
- Diagnosis of asthma or any other chronic disease necessitating ongoing care by a physician

Patients with certain chronic conditions may need to modify treatment or refrain from participation in specific sports. The American Academy of Pediatrics recommends that every *Down syndrome* patient who participates in organized sports be evaluated annually with a history and physical examination. Urgent computed tomography or magnetic resonance imaging is indicated in children with symptoms suggesting cord compression (e.g., neck pain/tilt, abnormal gait, increasing clumsiness, changes in bowel/bladder control). Patients with symptomatic atlantoaxial instability are prohibited from participating in activities in which their necks might be placed in hyperextension (e.g., diving, gymnastics). Although the Special Olympics requires documented *radiographic screening* to rule out atlantoaxial instability in asymptomatic children with Down syndrome prior to participation, *the American Academy of Pediatrics has recently dropped this recom-mendation* given the lack of scientific evidence of a link between radiographic instability and subsequent dislocation with cord compression. Currently, asymptomatic children with Down syndrome and radiographic atlantoaxial instability are prohibited by the Special Olympics Committee from participating in activities that place the neck in hyperextension.

An individual *with type 1 diabetes mellitus* needs an additional 10 to 15 g of carbohydrate for every 30 minutes to 1 hour of strenuous physical exercise. Athletes who participate in daily practices or games may require significant downward adjustment of their total insulin dose. Patients with insulin-dependent disease should monitor blood glucose before and after exercise. The supervising physician should provide specific counsel to the patient and family regarding changes in insulin dosing and carbohydrate needs.

As noted in Chapter 21, activities involving sustained physical exertion are contraindicated in patients with *Marfan syndrome* due to a significant risk of sudden cardiac death. Patients without aortic root dilatation or mitral regurgitation may participate in low- and moderate-intensity static sports and low-intensity dynamic sports. All but low-intensity competitive sports are prohibited in patients with aortic root dilatation; strenuous exercise should be avoided in an effort to prevent progressive dilatation and eventual rupture.

HEAT-RELATED ILLNESS

Heat exhaustion occurs when the body's ability to dissipate heat is stressed to capacity. The primary method of heat dispersion is evaporative (i.e., sweating); radiation through vasodilation plays a smaller role. When an individual exercises on a hot day, heat is produced by physical exertion and absorbed from the environment. Factors that increase the risk of heat-related illness include dehydration, lack of acclimation, poor physical conditioning, obesity, and the use of certain medications (e.g., antihistamines, laxatives). The clinical manifestations of heat exhaustion are related to intravascular volume depletion (sweating, vasodilation), electrolyte imbalances (loss in the sweat), and vasodilation and include the following:

- Normal or slightly elevated temperature
- Facial flushing
- Sweating
- Nausea
- Weakness
- Muscle cramps
- Confusion
- Dizziness
- Hypotension (orthostatic or sustained)
- Tachycardia
- Syncope or near-syncope

Recognition and early intervention (rehydration, cooling measures) are vital in the management of heat exhaustion in order to prevent progression to *heat stroke*. Heat stroke presents with significantly *elevated body temperature* (>40°C or 104°F) and signs of *central nervous system dysfunction* (e.g., disorientation, stupor, loss of consciousness). The skin is hot and often dry, although sweating is more typical early in the course. Heat stroke is a medical emergency that requires immediate intervention to affect a positive outcome. Patients who develop shock are at risk for multiorgan system damage and consumptive coagulopathy, which may lead to irreversible functional impairment or death. Ice packs placed at the neck, groin, and axillae should rapidly reduce central temperature to the recommended 38.8°C (101.8°F). Further cooling may precipitate hypothermia. Ice peritoneal lavage is beneficial in the hospital setting. Heat stroke places great demands on the cardiovascular system; cardiac output must increase substantially in order to counteract vasodilation and diminished peripheral vascular resistance. This high-output state may persist for several hours beyond normalization of body temperature.

Patients with heat stroke usually have laboratory evidence of rhabdomyolysis (i.e., elevated serum creatinine phosphokinase concentration and blood urea nitrogen level). Widespread muscle breakdown in the setting of dehydration places the patient at risk for acute renal failure. Renal function should be assessed initially and monitored throughout treatment. Intravenous rehydration is indicated in patients with evidence of central nervous system involvement. Oral rehydration may be sufficient in patients with intact mental function and mild heat exhaustion.

HEAD INJURIES

The subject of head injuries is covered in detail in Chapter 18. Recommendations regarding return to play in athletes who have suffered concussions are based on both the grade of the injury and any history of recent concussions (Table 25-2). Among pediatric patients, soccer is associated with the highest rate of concussion.

EYE INJURIES

The management of eye injuries is covered in Chapter 22.

MOUTH INJURIES

Mouth guards are effective in preventing dental injuries and facial lacerations. Ideally, the mouth guard should be comfortable, cover all tooth surfaces, and not interfere with breathing. Routine use of mouth guards is recommended for athletes who:

- participate in contact sports, including football, soccer, basketball, lacrosse, hockey, and wrestling
- engage in shot put and discus throw (to prevent injuries due to repetitive clenching of the teeth)
- wear braces on their teeth

STRAINS AND SPRAINS

A *strain*, or "pulled muscle," is a tear in muscle or tendinous tissue, usually occurring at a junction of the two. Affected athletes often report a "ripping" sensation at the time of injury, which is followed by pain, muscle spasm, and decreased strength. In contrast, a *sprain* is an injury in which a portion of a ligament or joint capsule is torn as a result of sudden stretching or twisting forces. In both types of soft tissue injury, preventing further injury and limiting associated bleeding and inflammation are the primary goals over the first 48 hours. RICE measures (rest, ice, elevation, compression) are combined with systemic nonsteroidal anti-inflammatory agents to promote early healing and provide analgesia. Although strains and sprains may not be completely healed for up to 2 months, an athlete may return to training when the injury is no longer painful and full range of motion, strength, and stability of the joint have

TABLE 25-2
CONCUSSION IN THE PEDIATRIC ATHLETE: GRADING AND RETURN TO PLAY

Grading of Severity of Concussion

Grade 1 concussion: altered mental status without amnesia or loss of consciousness

Grade 2 concussion: altered mental status with amnesia but without loss of consciousness

Grade 3 concussion: altered mental status or loss of consciousness at 24 hours after injury

Recommendations for Return to Play

Grade 1 Concussion

- Return to play in 20 minutes if asymptomatic (i.e., no headache, dizziness, disorientation, or loss of memory)
- If concussion is accompanied by any of the above symptoms, no return to play until athlete has remained asymptomatic for 1 week.
- If this is the second grade 1 concussion of the season, the athlete may return to play in 2 weeks if asymptomatic for the last week.
- If this is the third grade 1 concussion of the season, the athlete may not return to play for the remainder of the season but may return to competition the following season if asymptomatic.

Grade 2 Concussion

- Consider immediate referral for medical evaluation
- Return to play following asymptomatic period of 1 week
- If the athlete remains symptomatic 1 week following injury, obtain computed tomography of the head.
- If this is the second grade 2 concussion of the season, the athlete may return to play after a period of at least 1 month if asymptomatic for the last week.
- If this is the third grade 2 concussion of the season, the athlete may not return to play for the remainder of the season and should not resume play in any contact sport until asymptomatic for at least 3 to 4 months.

Grade 3 Concussion

- Refer to emergency department and consider computed tomography of the head
- Return to play following a 2-week asymptomatic period
- If this is the second grade 3 concussion of the season, the athlete is prohibited from contact sports for the remainder of the sports season as well as the next season.
- Following a third grade 3 concussion, the patient should be advised to limit participation in organized athletics to noncontact sports only.

been achieved through physical therapy and rehabilitation. The appropriate time to return to activity should be determined by the physician/trainer/therapist rather than the athlete; premature return risks reinjury, which may be more severe than the initial event.

UPPER EXTREMITY INJURIES

Shoulder Injuries

The presentations of *clavicular fracture, shoulder separation,* and *shoulder dislocation* are provided in Chapter 19.

Pitchers, tennis players, and swimmers are subject to the development of *rotator cuff tendonitis,* an overuse injury presenting with shoulder pain that is exacerbated by overhead movements. Weakness of the rotator cuff muscles of the involved shoulder is obvious upon comparison with the nonaffected side. When rest and physical therapy have returned the joint to full-strength, pain-free motion (usually 2 to 6 weeks), the patient is ready for gradual return to overhead arm movements. Patients with associated instability of the glenohumeral joint require more specialized management.

Physiolysis of the proximal humerus, or *Little League shoulder,* is most common in pitchers 11 to 16 years of age. Repetitive throwing motions lead to progressive degeneration of the proximal humeral growth plate. Pain is insidious in onset and exacerbated by throwing. Tenderness to deep palpation is present over the affected area. Plain radiographs reveal widening of the growth plate with associated sclerosis. Premature return to regular throwing places the patient at risk for limb length discrepancy.

Elbow Injuries

Supracondylar fracture of the elbow is covered in Chapter 19.

Medial epicondylitis and Panner disease are two overuse injuries of the elbow diagnosed almost exclusively in young pitchers. Patients with medial epicondylitis (*Little League elbow*) present with the slow progression of medial elbow pain that is not associated with decreased range of motion or "locking" at the joint. *Panner disease* consists of avascular necrosis and subsequent collapse of the capitellum. Pain is located over the lateral aspect of the joint; examination of the elbow is consistent with joint effusion, and range of motion (extension) may be limited. Both respond to rest and appropriate physical therapy.

Wrist Injuries

Gymnasts who present with wrist pain that is insidious in onset and progressive over weeks to months should be evaluated for *physiolysis of the distal radius,* a degenerative stress injury. There is typically no history of antecedent trauma. Range of motion at the wrist joint remains intact, and there is no associated swelling over the distal arm or wrist. Palpation of the distal radius reveals tenderness. Widening of the physis is often noted on plain films of the forearm. Weight bearing at the wrist is prohibited for at least 6 to 8 weeks, although aerobic training is still permitted. Premature return to tumbling and other activities that stress the wrist places the patient at risk for arrested growth at the radial physis and eventual ulnar-radial length discrepancies.

Carpal bone fractures are rare in children, occurring more frequently in adolescents due to completion of ossification. The *scaphoid* is the most commonly fractured carpal bone in the pediatric population, usually resulting from a fall onto the outstretched hand. Swelling on the radial side of the wrist is accompanied by tenderness to palpation of the anatomic snuffbox, where the scaphoid bone articulates with the radius. Fracture of the scaphoid is associated with a high rate of complications compared with other bones of the hand and wrist. Patients with scaphoid bone fractures are at risk for nonunion and resultant avascular necrosis of the bone if the injury remains undiagnosed and the wrist is not properly immobilized in a plaster cast. Abnormal healing requires surgical intervention to repair the damage and prevent significant functional impairment.

LOWER EXTREMITY INJURIES

Deep Thigh Contusions and Hematomas

Any direct blow to the thigh can result in a deep thigh *contusion,* or bleeding in and around the quadriceps/hamstring muscles, which may be mild, moderate, or severe. Mild and moderate injuries respond to RICE measures. If the trauma is significant, it is possible for enough blood to be lost into the potential space for the patient to become symptomatic (e.g., weak, dizzy, tachycardic, hypotensive). Blood loss into a deep thigh hematoma should be suspected in the patient with a history of trauma to the thigh and the delayed (~30 minutes) onset of symptoms of hypovolemia. Fluid resuscitation is indicated for affected patients, along with ice, compression, and referral to an orthopaedic specialist for further evaluation and management. Patients with significant deep thigh contusions are at risk for the development of *myositis ossificans,* bony calcifications within the body of the muscle that cause significant pain and impairment.

Knee Injuries

Pertinent features of the history and physical examination in the major ligamentous and meniscal injuries of the knee are summarized in Table 25-3.

TABLE 25-3
LIGAMENTOUS AND MENISCAL INJURIES OF THE KNEE[a]

Injury	Mechanism	Symptoms	Signs	Management
Anterior cruciate ligament sprain	Twisting or hyperextension at the knee with the foot planted and the knee in full extension	"Pop" in the knee at the time of the injury; knee pain; sensation of instability with lateral movement	Tenderness over the posterior-lateral region of the knee; joint effusion; positive Lachman test	Rest/ice/compression Stabilization in a knee brace Referral for surgical repair
Medial collateral ligament sprain	Lateral valgus stress to a knee in full extension	Tearing sensation in the knee at the time of injury; knee pain and stiffness; sensation of instability with lateral movement	Tenderness over the ligament; swelling; pain and instability on valgus stress test	Rest/ice/compression Stabilization in a knee brace Physical therapy
Meniscal tears	Twisting at the knee with the joint in some degree of flexion	"Pop" in the knee at the time of the injury; knee pain and stiffness; "locking" sensation	Tenderness along the joint line; decreased range of motion; positive McMurray sign	Rest/ice/compression Referral for arthroscopy

[a]These injuries may occur in isolation or in combination.

Prepatellar bursitis can result from an acute injury, such as a direct blow to the anterior knee, or from "wear and tear" due to repetitive flexion/extension with friction at the joint. The affected athlete presents with swelling and tenderness over the patella; range of motion at the knee remains fully intact. Prepatellar bursitis generally resolves with rest and nonsteroidal anti-inflammatory medication. Extensive or recurrent swelling warrants referral to an orthopaedic specialist.

Ankle Injuries

Inversion ankle injuries are the most commonly reported sports injuries in the pediatric population. In adolescents, closure of the growth plates results in injury patterns similar to those in adults. However, the younger athlete with open physes is more likely to sustain a fracture than an isolated sprain (the physis being weaker than associated bones and ligaments). Avulsion fractures often accompany ligamentous injury in this population. Tenderness involving an open growth plate in a skeletally immature patient should be managed as if a fracture is present; these injuries are not always visible on initial plain films. If radiographs demonstrate complete closure of the physis, the management is identical to that for an adult. *Radiographic evaluation* with plain films is indicated for patients when symptoms and findings are primarily medial rather than lateral; when there is point tenderness or deformity over a growth plate, the posterior tip of either malleoli, or the fifth metatarsal; or when the patient is unable to take four steps.

Rest, ice, compression, and elevation comprise the mainstay of treatment over the first 48 hours. Weight bearing is initially limited with crutches but may be advanced with the ankle splinted in an air stirrup as the pain recedes. Early physical therapy and strengthening promote healing and increase stability of the joint. Orthopaedic consultation is reserved for severe sprains, eversion sprains, and sprains with associated fractures.

WEIGHT CUTTING IN SPORTS

Weight cutting is the practice of losing weight rapidly in order to qualify for competition in a lower weight class. The behavior is most common in competitive wrestlers. Various strategies include exercise, dieting, fluid restriction, provoked sweating (e.g., saunas), diuretics, laxatives, and induced vomiting. Weight cutting is an unhealthy activity that can adversely affect performance, energy, and judgment. The American College of Sports Medicine has recommended that weight loss not exceed 2 to 3 lb or 1.5% of body weight per week and that minimum wrestling weight should be calculated based on preseason body composition (percent body fat) rather than ideal body weight.

PERFORMANCE-ENHANCING SUBSTANCES

Current estimates regarding the prevalence of performance-enhancing substance use in adolescents range from 5% to 10%. Most of these individuals are athletes looking to gain an edge over their competitors; a minority comprises nonathletes trying to improve their physical appearances. The history and physical examination are the most effective screening methods for identification of performance-enhancing substance use/abuse in adolescents; specific laboratory tests are expensive, unavailable, or nonexistent. Asking adolescents about their use of supplements and other performance-enhancing substances is important because:

- It permits identification of use/abuse of performance-enhancing substances in many patients.
- It communicates a willingness to discuss the topic.
- It identifies the physician as a source of reliable information regarding performance-enhancing substances.
- It provides an entry to preventive counseling or education regarding risks, adverse effects, and the veracity of claims of benefit.
- Adolescent patients who use anabolic steroids are more likely than their peers to use and abuse other substances, including intravenous drugs.

Dietary supplements (e.g., *creatine*) are the category of performance-enhancing drugs used most commonly by adolescents due to availability. Virtually any substance can be sold as a "supplement" as long as it is not labeled as a "drug" that can treat or cure disease. Anabolic steroids require a prescription, although adolescents can obtain them without documentation through illegal suppliers.

Table 25-4 provides an overview of clinical manifestations associated with the use of several performance-enhancing substances available to adolescent athletes.

THE FEMALE ATHLETE TRIAD

The female athlete triad consists of *disordered eating, exercise-induced amenorrhea,* and *osteoporosis*. It is most common in girls who participate in gymnastics, cheerleading, and long-distance running. "Disordered eating" may include restricting food, fad diets, binging and purging, and taking diuretic or laxative agents. Female athletes can become fixated on weight and develop distortion of body image. Anovulatory cycles and amenorrhea are thought to result from changes in hypothalamic secretion of gonadotrophin-releasing hormone and diminished luteinizing hormone surges. Inadequacy of nutritional intake and alteration in body composition (minimal percent body fat) probably contribute to reported menstrual irregularities. Finally,

TABLE 25-4
OVERVIEW OF PERFORMANCE-ENHANCING SUBSTANCES

Substance	Effects on Performance	Physical Findings	Laboratory Results	Adverse Effects
Anabolic steroids	Documented gains in muscle mass and strength	■ Elevated body mass index ■ Hypertension ■ Acne ■ *Female:* deepening of the voice, hirsutism or hair loss (virilization) ■ *Male:* high-pitched voice, gynecomastia, decrease in testicular size	■ Elevated liver enzyme concentrations ■ Decreased high-density lipoprotein cholesterol level ■ Increased low-density lipoprotein cholesterol level ■ Specific metabolites detectable in urine definitively identify particular substances	■ Behavior changes (e.g., aggression) ■ Emotional lability ■ Mania ■ Psychosis ■ Depression (during withdrawal) ■ Premature closure of the epiphyseal growth plates (in prepubertal users) ■ Dysplasia of collagen predisposing to tendon rupture ■ Diminished sexual desire and decreased sexual function ■ Testicular failure ■ Liver tumors
Androstenedione (dietary supplement; precursor to testosterone)	Purported to produce gains in muscle mass and strength	■ Theoretically the same as for anabolic steroids; no proven efficacy	■ Substance detectable in the urine	■ Theoretically the same as for anabolic steroids
Creatine (dietary supplement)	Enhances the ability of muscles to maintain power in short maximal exertional efforts; not effective unless combined with strength training (e.g., weight lifting); safety profile in adolescents not established	■ Elevated body mass index	■ No specific assay to identify creatine use	■ Muscle cramping ■ Gastrointestinal upset (vomiting, diarrhea) ■ Rash ■ Dyspnea ■ Anxiety ■ Fatigue ■ Myopathy ■ Seizure ■ Arrhythmia ■ Kidney dysfunction (increased serum creatinine, decreased glomerular filtration rate) that is reversible upon discontinuation of the supplement

more than half of a woman's skeletal mass is amassed during adolescence. Low estrogen levels in the amenorrheic adolescent athlete translate to impaired bone formation and active resorption during a time of critical growth. Inadequate mineralization of the bone during adolescence may be irreversible.

Management of a patient with the female athlete triad consists of:

- nutritional counseling, with optimization of intake to meet energy and growth needs
- calcium supplementation, if indicated based on dietary history
- modification of training routines
- psychotherapy to normalize body image and expectations
- hormonal therapy (combination oral estrogen-progesterone pills) in the skeletally mature athlete

SOURCES

Anderson SJ. Lower extremity injuries in youth sports. *Pediatr Clin North Am.* 2002;49:627–641.

Braganza SF, Adam HM. Atlantoaxial dislocation. *Pediatr Rev.* 2003;24:106–107.

Congeni J, Miller S. Supplements and drugs used to enhance athletic performance. *Pediatr Clin North Am.* 2002;49:435–461.

Gomez JE. Upper extremity injuries in youth sports. *Pediatr Clin North Am.* 2002;49:593–626.

Hergenroeder AC, Neinsein LS. Guidelines in sports medicine. In: Neinstein LS, ed. *Adolescent health care: a practical guide.* 4th ed. Philadelphia: Lippincott Williams & Wilkins; 2002:380–438.

Kelly JP, Nichols JS, Filley CM, et al. Concussion in sports: guidelines for the prevention of catastrophic outcome. *JAMA.* 1991;266:2867.

Kirkwood MW, Yeates KO, Wilson PE. Pediatric sport-related concussion: a review of the clinical management of an oft-neglected population. *Pediatrics.* 2006;117:1359–1371.

Koch JL. Performance-enhancing substances and their use among adolescent athletes. *Pediatr Rev.* 2002;23:310–317.

Lerand SJ, Williams JF. The female athlete triad. *Pediatr Rev.* 2006;27:e12–e13.

QUESTIONS

1. An 8-year-old girl with Down syndrome who has been participating in gymnastics classes for 2 years wants to participate in the Special Olympics for the first time. Preparticipation radiographic screening reveals widening of the space between the posterior aspect of the anterior arch of the atlas and the odontoid process. The child has no history of abnormal gait, neck pain, limited neck mobility, head tilt, increasing clumsiness, or changes in bowel or bladder control. No signs of cord compression are noted on physical examination. Which of the following statements regarding this child's participation in the Special Olympics is TRUE?

A) This child will be prohibited from competing in the gymnastics portion of the Special Olympics due to her radiographic findings.
B) This child will be prohibited from competing in any portion of the Special Olympics due to her radiographic findings.
C) This child will be prohibited from competing in any portion of the Special Olympics based on her underlying diagnosis of Down syndrome.
D) This child will be allowed to participate in the gymnastics portion of the Special Olympics.
E) This child will be allowed to participate in the gymnastics portion of the Special Olympics only if computed tomography of the cervical spine rules out atlantoaxial instability.

2. A 10-year-old obese male with Down syndrome comes to your office for his preparticipation sports physical prior to beginning a medical weight loss program that incorporates daily swimming. His mother denies any history of abnormal gait, clumsiness, or change in bowel or bladder control. The patient has a subtle head tilt to the left and mild left-sided tenderness on palpation of the posterior neck; the remainder of the neurologic examination is normal. Which of the following is the most appropriate next step in the management of this patient?

A) Allow the patient to participate in the swimming program as long as he does not dive or engage in the butterfly stroke.
B) Refer the patient for cervical neck films and schedule computed tomography or magnetic resonance imaging of the region as soon as possible.
C) Educate the parent regarding the clinical manifestations of cervical cord compression.
D) Prohibit the patient from participating in the swimming program.
E) Encourage the patient to find ways to exercise that do not involve hyperextension of the neck.

3. A 13-year-old boy with well-controlled type 1 diabetes mellitus has been selected to play on the middle school basketball team. He will be expected to participate in daily 90-minute practices except on the weekends and on game days. Which of the following statements regarding the management of this patient's condition is FALSE?

A) The patient will probably require additional carbohydrate to meet his increased energy needs.
B) The patient will probably require downward adjustment of his insulin dose to account for increased energy expenditures.
C) The patient should limit strenuous exercise to no more than 1 hour a day.
D) The patient should monitor his blood glucose level before and after each practice.
E) The patient's condition does not preclude his participation in organized sports.

4. A 17-year-old high school senior who plays on the football team is in your office for his preparticipation sports physical. His body mass index has increased significantly since last year. Other findings on physical examination include acne (face, shoulders, and back), gynecomastia, and decreased testicular size. This patient's clinical manifestations are most consistent with use of which of the following?

A) Gamma-hydroxy butyrate
B) Androstenedione
C) Creatine
D) Anabolic steroids
E) Ephedra

5. Adolescents who use anabolic steroids as performance-enhancing substances are more likely than their peers to:

A) develop symptomatic hypotensive episodes
B) lose weight
C) develop seizures
D) suffer kidney damage
E) use intravenous drugs

6. The mother of a 14-year-old boy is concerned that her son may be using dietary supplements in an inappropriate manner in order to "bulk up." She is specifically concerned about creatine. Which of the following is most effective for detecting creatine use in adolescent males?

A) Questioning the adolescent about the use of dietary supplements and performance-enhancing substances
B) Measuring the adolescent's serum creatinine concentration
C) Measuring metabolite levels in the adolescent's urine
D) Measuring metabolite levels in the adolescent's serum
E) Comparing the adolescent's weight and height to previous measurements

7. A 7-year-old girl will be participating in basketball camp this year at her local recreation center. A preparticipation physical examination is required prior to registration. Past medical history is noncontributory, and

the review of systems is negative. A maternal uncle has been diagnosed with dilatation of the aortic root due to Marfan syndrome. The physical examination, including assessment of the cardiovascular and pulmonary systems, is normal. Which of the following is the most appropriate next step in the management of this patient?
A) Clear the child for full participation in camp activities.
B) Obtain an electrocardiogram.
C) Clear the child for participation in noncontact activities.
D) Clear the child for participation in low- to moderate-intensity activities only.
E) Prohibit the child from participating in basketball camp.

8. A 15-year-old boy who engages in competitive shot put is in your office for his preparticipation sports assessment. His body mass index is above the 97th percentile for age and height. He reluctantly tells you that he occasionally experiences chest tightness and shortness of breath about 15 minutes into his training sessions. He denies lightheadedness, syncope, or palpitations. A paternal uncle recently died at the age of 52 years following a heart attack. The patient suffered a grade 1 concussion during football season 3 months ago but is no longer symptomatic. Physical examination reveals an obese adolescent male; no other significant findings are identified. You order an electrocardiogram (ECG), which you explain must be obtained prior to approval of his participation in shot put. Which of the following is the most compelling reason for obtaining the ECG in this patient?
A) History of a grade 1 concussion
B) Participation in a sport that places high preload stress on the heart
C) History of chest tightness with activity
D) History of death from myocardial infarction in the paternal uncle
E) High body mass index

9. A 12-year-old boy dressed out in full pads for late-summer football practice appears to faint while standing next to the water cooler. When the trainer reaches him, he is conscious but confused. He is sweating profusely, and his face is flushed. This patient's syncope is most likely to have resulted from which of the following?
A) Benign paroxysmal vertigo
B) Vasovagal syncope
C) Long QT syndrome
D) Heat exhaustion
E) Hypertrophic cardiomyopathy

10. You are the team physician for a summer conditioning "boot camp" for incoming ninth-grade football players. An obese male is carried into the training station by his coaches. He fainted on the field and is now minimally responsive but breathing on his own with a strong pulse. The patient's skin is flushed, and his axillary temperature is 39.8°C. He is not sweating. You have activated emergency medical services. Which of the following is the most important next step in the management of this patient?
A) Try to rouse the patient so that he can drink water.
B) Try to rouse the patient so that he can drink isotonic fluids.
C) Undress the patient and cool him with electric fans.
D) Undress the patient and cool him with wet cloths.
E) Place ice packs at the patient's axillae, groin, and neck and monitor patient temperature.

11. A 15-year-old girl who is a member of the marching band is practicing one summer day in full uniform when she becomes dizzy and confused. Upon arrival to the emergency department, she is awake but disoriented. Her temperature is 37.6°C. Her skin is flushed, and she is sweating profusely. Her mother arrives and tells you that the girl skipped breakfast this morning because she woke up late. You are concerned about the possibility of rhabdomyolysis due to heat-related illness in this child. Which of the following is the most appropriate form of hydration for this patient?
A) Intravenous normal saline bolus
B) Oral rehydration with free water
C) Oral rehydration with fluid that is isotonic and contains glucose
D) Intravenous normal saline at maintenance drip
E) None until the patient urinates

12. Mouth guards are indicated for the prevention of sports-related dental injuries and lacerations during participation in which of the following activities?
A) Lacrosse
B) Wrestling
C) Shot put
D) A and B
E) A, B, and C

13. A 17-year-old basketball player dives into the stands after a loose ball and hits his head on the bleachers. When the trainer reaches him, he is confused about where he is and cannot recall his name. He is taken back to the training room, where his mental status gradually normalizes over the next 5 to 10 minutes. He remembers coming out of the locker room to begin the game but does not remember anything after that, although he now knows who he is and where he is. He is transported to the emergency department via ambulance; both his neurologic examination and computed tomography of the head are normal. He attends school the next day, shows up for practice, and is asymptomatic. This patient may return to play:
A) for today's practice
B) for the next game
C) following an asymptomatic period of 7 days

D) following an asymptomatic period of 14 days
E) following an asymptomatic period of 30 days

14. A 16-year-old ice hockey player who is checked into the boards from behind suffers his third concussion of the winter season. All three episodes involved altered mental status (confusion, dizziness) but no amnesia and no loss of consciousness. The player has remained asymptomatic between head injuries. This player may return to participation in his sport:
A) if he remains asymptomatic for 7 days
B) if he remains asymptomatic for 30 days
C) never
D) during the spring season if he remains asymptomatic
E) 3 to 4 months from now if he remains asymptomatic

15. A 14-year-old girl is playing in the soccer state championship game when she collides head-first with an opposing player. She immediately sits up on the field but is momentarily confused about where she is. There is no loss of consciousness, and she remembers being hit. This girl may return to play:
A) immediately
B) in 20 minutes if she remains asymptomatic and does not develop headache, dizziness, disorientation, loss of memory, nausea, or vomiting
C) after 24 hours have passed as long as she remains asymptomatic and does not develop headache, dizziness, disorientation, loss of memory, nausea, or vomiting
D) after 7 days have passed as long as she has been asymptomatic for the preceding 24 hours
E) after 14 days have passed as long as she has been asymptomatic for the preceding 7 days

16. A 15-year-old girl who plays competitive tennis during the spring and summer and practices year round presents to your office with pain in her right shoulder that has been getting worse over the past 6 weeks. She is right-handed. The pain is exacerbated when she raises the arm above her head. When both elbows are held at the sides close to the body in 90 degrees of flexion, external rotation of the shoulder against resistance is significantly weaker on the right. This patient's shoulder pain most likely results from which of the following?
A) Little League shoulder
B) Intermittent shoulder separation
C) Rotator cuff tendonitis
D) Frozen shoulder
E) Panner disease

17. A 16-year-old young man is practicing pole vaulting with his high school track team when he falls onto his outstretched hand from a height of about 6 feet. Examination of the wrist and hand reveals swelling along the radial side of the wrist and tenderness to palpation of the anatomic snuffbox. Plain radiographs of the wrist demonstrate a complete fracture of the scaphoid bone. Which of the following statements about the treatment/prognosis of this patient's injury is INCORRECT?
A) Fractures of the scaphoid bone have a relatively high rate of nonunion.
B) Immobilization of the wrist in a cast is insufficient treatment for a nondisplaced fracture of the scaphoid bone.
C) Fracture of the scaphoid bone can separate the arterial blood supply to one of the displaced fragments, resulting in avascular necrosis.
D) Nonunion of the scaphoid bone results in functional impairment.
E) Nonunion of the scaphoid bone requires surgical repair.

18. A 9-year-old competitive gymnast presents to your office for evaluation of wrist pain that has been getting progressively worse over the past 2 months. She does not recall any injury to the joint. Physical examination reveals tenderness over the distal radius; swelling is absent, and range of motion is intact at the wrist joint. There are no significant neurovascular findings distal to the wrist. If abnormal, plain radiographs of the wrist are most likely to show which of the following?
A) Widening of the distal physis of the radius
B) Collapse of the scaphoid bone
C) Occult stress fracture of the distal radius
D) An isolated well-demarcated osteolytic lesion within the distal radius
E) Cartilaginous spurs along the articulating surface of the distal radius

19. A 17-year-old soccer player comes to your office complaining of knee pain. She suffered a direct blow to the right anterior knee during practice yesterday. You note tenderness and swelling over the patella; strength and range of motion at the knee joint are intact. There is no evidence of a fracture on plain films of the knee. Which of the following represents the most appropriate immediate management of this patient's injury?
A) Ambulation with crutches initially, with gradual return to weight bearing as tolerated
B) Immobilization in an elastic bandage
C) Immobilization in a cast
D) Rest and nonsteroidal anti-inflammatory medication
E) Immobilization in a knee brace

20. A 17-year-old soccer player was attempting to dribble past a defender when he felt a "pop" in his left knee, followed immediately by pain. He reports that his foot was planted with his leg fully extended and twisting when the injury occurred (to his best recollection). He is

able to bear weight on the leg but feels very uncomfortable when he is asked to suddenly change direction while walking. You note tenderness to palpation over the lateral posterior region of the knee. A Lachman test is positive on the left. This patient's history and physical examination are most consistent with which of the following?
A) Patella fracture
B) Lateral meniscal tear
C) Medial meniscal tear
D) Medial collateral ligament injury
E) Anterior cruciate ligament injury

21. You are providing a lecture about pediatric sports-related injuries to a group of orthopedic interns. You would be correct in telling them each of the following EXCEPT:
A) Eversion ankle injuries are the most commonly reported sports injuries in the pediatric population.
B) In adolescents, closure of the growth plates results in ankle injury patterns similar to those found in adults.
C) The younger athlete with an open physis is more likely to sustain a fracture than an isolated sprain.
D) Avulsion fractures often accompany ligamentous ankle injuries in the pediatric population.
E) Growth plate injuries are not always visible on initial radiographic studies.

22. Radiographic evaluation of the ankle joint is indicated in all of the following patients with ankle injuries EXCEPT:
A) A 16-year-old young man with an eversion sprain and significant medial pain and swelling
B) A 15-year-old menstruating female with an inversion sprain who is able to ambulate five steps with pain
C) An 8-year-old boy with point tenderness over the distal growth plate
D) A 12-year-old girl with point tenderness over the posterior tip of the lateral malleolus
E) A 17-year-old patient with pain in the area of the fifth metatarsal

23. Which of the following interventions is not part of the routine management of an uncomplicated ankle injury in an adolescent?
A) Elevation
B) Ice
C) Orthopaedic consultation
D) Compression
E) Advance of weight bearing as tolerated

24. You are asked to give a 15-minute talk on weight cutting to a group of high school wrestling coaches. You are correct in telling them that minimum wrestling weight should be based on which of the following?
A) Ideal body weight
B) Ideal body composition
C) Preseason body weight
D) Preseason body composition
E) The preceding year's weight and estimated rate of growth

25. A 15-year-old elite baseball player in your office for a routine health maintenance visit tells you that injectable anabolic steroids have been made available to him. He denies using them because he is afraid of needles. However, he has begun taking androstenedione. In counseling the patient regarding his use of this substance, you are correct in telling him each of the following EXCEPT:
A) Androstenedione is detectable in the urine.
B) Androstenedione is purported to increase muscle mass and strength.
C) Androstenedione is a testosterone precursor.
D) Androstenedione is available without a prescription.
E) The effects of androstenedione on adolescent users have been extensively studied.

26. A 14-year-old competitive female gymnast is in your office for a routine health maintenance visit. Her weight today is 1 kg less than her weight at a similar visit last year. The girl's mother tells you that she is concerned about her daughter's restrictive eating habits and obsession with her weight. When you ask the girl how she feels about this, she begins to cry and tell you that she is becoming "too large" to compete in her sport. She does not remember when she last menstruated, but she knows it has been longer than 6 months ago. This patient's persistent amenorrhea places her at increased risk for which of the following?
A) Osteoporosis
B) Infertility
C) Ovarian cysts
D) Endometriosis
E) Vitamin A deficiency

ANSWERS

1. A	10. E	19. D
2. B	11. A	20. E
3. C	12. E	21. A
4. D	13. C	22. B
5. E	14. D	23. C
6. A	15. B	24. D
7. B	16. C	25. E
8. C	17. B	26. A
9. D	18. A	

Substance Use and Abuse

26

EPIDEMIOLOGY OF SUBSTANCE USE

There has been a gradual decline in the rate of substance use/abuse among adolescents since the year 2000. Reported usage patterns for the year 2005 are provided in Table 26-1. The best predictor of individual substance use is substance use among one's peer group. Risk factors for substance use/abuse among adolescents are listed in Table 26-2. The earlier a child is exposed to alcohol, tobacco, and drug use, the more likely that child is to abuse the substance. Alcohol remains the most widely used psychoactive substance across all adolescent age groups. Tobacco, alcohol, and marijuana are considered "gateway" substances; adolescents are most likely to try one of these substances initially because they are readily available and perceived as less harmful than "hard drugs." The consequences of substance use are not limited to the direct physical effects of the substance on the body. Most substances lower inhibition and impair judgment; individuals under the influence of alcohol or drugs are more likely to suffer accidental or intentional injury, commit violence, attempt suicide, and engage in unprotected sexual intercourse. Substance abuse affects psychosocial and cognitive functioning and is associated with increased rates of academic failure, truancy, and delinquency.

Primary care pediatricians are uniquely poised to play a significant role in the prevention, diagnosis, and treatment of substance abuse in children and adolescents. Community intervention can include lobbying for adequate funds for prevention and treatment programs and acting as a source of reliable information for schools and local organizations. All adolescents should be counseled regarding the dangers of drug use/abuse and strategies to minimize those dangers (e.g., avoidance of drinking and driving). At the individual level, age-appropriate anticipatory guidance, questions regarding personal substance use, and preventive counseling should be a part of every adolescent health maintenance visit. Use or abuse of substances should be suspected in any adolescent who presents with weight loss, behavior changes, mood alteration, declining school performance, changes in peer group, and/or involvement with law enforcement or the justice system.

Effective anticipatory guidance encompasses more than just the adolescent. Parental drug use patterns greatly influence adolescent behavior. Parents should be questioned about their attitudes and perceptions as well as any personal substance use or abuse. They should also be informed that parental involvement and supervision serve as important deterrents to substance use in their children. Finally, parents should be encouraged to engage in age-appropriate conversations with their children regarding tobacco, alcohol, and illicit drug use.

Use of multiple substances, often concurrently, is common in adolescents who abuse substances. In addition, street drugs may contain additional agents that are not

TABLE 26-1
RATES OF USE OF TOBACCO, ALCOHOL, AND ILLICIT DRUGS IN ADOLESCENTS (UNITED STATES, 2005)

	9th Grade		12th Grade	
Substance	**Current Use**	**Lifetime Use**	**Current Use**	**Lifetime Use**
Tobacco use[a]	20%	49%	28%	60%
Alcohol use[a]	36%	67%	51%	82%
Marijuana use[a]	17%	29%	23%	48%
Use of any illicit drug[b]	8% (8th grade)	21% (8th grade)	22%	50%

[a]Youth Risk Behavior Surveillance Survey (www.cdc.gov/healthyyouth/yrbs).
[b]Monitoring the Future (www.monitoringthefuture.org).
Current use is defined as use within the past 30 days. Lifetime use is defined as any use during the individual's lifetime; that is, what percentage of adolescents surveyed has *ever* used the substance.

TABLE 26-2
FACTORS THAT AFFECT THE RISK OF ADOLESCENT SUBSTANCE ABUSE

Risk Factors
Association with peers who use substances
Low self-esteem
Poor coping skills
Impulsivity
Psychiatric disorders
ADHD/conduct disorder
Mood disorders (depression, anxiety)
Behavior disorders
Homosexual orientation
History of physical and/or sexual abuse
Anabolic steroid use
Permissive parental attitudes toward substance use
Drug use by parents and older siblings
Poor parental supervision
Lack of after-school supervision
Ready availability of drugs within the community
Poverty
Protective Factors
Social connectedness
Stable relationships within the family
Social success with peers
Involvement in extracurricular activities
Religious beliefs/participation in organized religion
Good self-esteem
Academic success

ADHD, attention-deficit/hyperactivity disorder.

reported to the user. Any adolescent who presents with suspected drug intoxication or overdose should receive urine and drug screening for additional substances that may be contributing to the patient's distress.

INTERVIEWING THE ADOLESCENT REGARDING SUBSTANCE USE

It is unusual for an adolescent to present to the primary health care provider with signs or symptoms of acute intoxication with alcohol or an illicit drug. Therefore, the most effective method of screening adolescents for substance use remains the patient history. Questions regarding substance use should be asked without the parents present. Screening for substance use includes screening for the presence of risk factors associated with drug and alcohol use. In particular, adolescents should be questioned regarding social and family relationships, school performance, sources of conflict or stress, changes in mood or behavior, and engagement in other risky behaviors.

Adolescents are usually more willing to talk about use of alcohol and illicit drugs when approached in a nonjudgmental manner. Questions about substance use in peers can be followed by asking the adolescent about personal use. The physician should be prepared to gather additional information from the adolescent who is engaging in substance use, including specific drugs used, frequency of use, circumstances leading to use, route(s) of administration, and perceived impact on health, relationships, and academic functioning. School attendance, expulsions, and involvement with law enforcement are other areas of interest.

Parental involvement in the management of the adolescent substance user increases compliance. All states allow minors to consent for health care related to diagnosis, assessment, and initial intervention of substance abuse. However, it is unrealistic to expect an adolescent to fund and attend to necessary treatment without parental support. The ideal scenario consists of the adolescent telling the parents about substance use him- or herself, with the physician present to support both parties and enhance communication. Complete honesty with both the adolescent (regarding what information will be shared and what will remain confidential) and the parent (e.g., explaining that some information is regarded as confidential, rather than skirting questions or lying) helps to maintain the doctor-patient relationship. Parents are a source of additional information about the adolescent's behavior, family stressors, and concerns they have for their child. It may be beneficial to contact the school or law enforcement with the expressed consent of the adolescent and parent. A teacher or guidance counselor can provide answers to questions regarding the adolescent's behavior, achievement, and attendance at school, as well as prevailing attitudes and suspected patterns of substance use within the student body.

LABORATORY EVALUATION

Adolescents should not be tested for substances in the urine or blood without their knowledge and consent, even if the parents desire testing. Covert testing is both unethical and detrimental to relationships between the physician and patient *and* the parent(s) and child. Parents who desire testing without the adolescent's knowledge should be questioned about their concerns, educated that the patient history is the most effective method of detecting substance use, and offered an appointment for assessment of their child. The use of screening drug tests during adolescence is limited to:

- assessment of the adolescent with acute alteration in mental status
- assessment of the adolescent who is judged to be a danger to him- or herself or others
- relapse prevention in adolescents who are known drug users and are undergoing treatment
- court-ordered drug testing
- random screening to detect and deter drug use in sports and on the job

Urine drug screens (and less commonly blood screens) are sensitive but lack specificity. Confirmatory tests are highly specific but expensive and not widely available.

That said, *false-negative* results are relatively common in urine drug screening. Intentional adulteration of samples can be achieved by substituting the urine of a nonuser, substituting another substance that resembles urine (e.g., apple juice, tea), diluting the urine by drinking large amounts of water or taking a diuretic, or putting water or other substances into the sample to obscure detection. The patient should be observed by a same-gender monitor during collection of the sample to prohibit tampering. A screen may also be reported as negative if the concentration of the substance in the urine is below the manufacturer's suggested cut-off value. Depending on how heavy and chronic usage is, marijuana can be detected in the urine anywhere from 3 to 30 days after smoking. On the other hand, short-acting barbiturates may persist in the urine for less than a single day. *False-positive* results occur with amphetamines and opiates due to the presence of these substances in medications and foods. A urine screen that is positive for cocaine or alcohol is indicative of use of that substance.

MANAGEMENT OF THE ADOLESCENT SUBSTANCE USER/ABUSER

Decisions regarding intervention are based on substances used, duration and frequency of use, patient willingness to abstain from use, and anticipated withdrawal symptoms (Table 26-3). Early stages of adolescent substance abuse typically consist of occasional recreational use of inhalants,

TABLE 26-3
INTERVENTION FOR THE ADOLESCENT SUBSTANCE USER/ABUSER

Level 1 Intervention (early intervention and outpatient treatment)

Components
Treatment primarily undertaken or managed by the primary care pediatrician, with possible referral to a substance abuse counselor and/or self-help organization (e.g., Alcoholics Anonymous, Narcotics Anonymous)

Appropriate for the patient who:
- is not at risk for withdrawal symptoms
- is willing and cooperative
- has a high likelihood of maintaining abstinence
- has a good social support network

Level 2 Intervention (intensive outpatient treatment)

Components
Hospital- or community-based health clinics with multidisciplinary teams consisting of substance abuse counselors, mental health specialists, and social workers; care coordinated and supervised by the primary care pediatrician

Appropriate for the patient who:
- is not at risk for significant withdrawal symptoms
- has no associated medical issues
- has changes in behavior related to drug use
- is moderately resistant to therapy for substance use
- requires methadone maintenance for opiate withdrawal

Level 3 Intervention (medically monitored intensive inpatient treatment)

Components
Nonhospital inpatient treatment in half-way house, group home, or other type of therapeutic setting

Appropriate for the patient who:
- is at risk for withdrawal symptoms that do not require hospitalization
- needs a change in environment
- has run away
- has had a poor response to intensive outpatient therapy
- is resistant to therapy for substance use
- requires 24-hour structured environment in order to abstain from substance use

Level 4 Intervention (medically managed intensive inpatient treatment)

Components
Dedicated hospital inpatient unit

Appropriate for the patient who:
- is going through withdrawal requiring medical intervention and support
- has one or more severe comorbid psychiatric condition(s) that interfere with the maintenance of abstinence
- is a risk to himself, herself, or others
- has had a poor response to all other therapy options

tobacco, marijuana, or alcohol with friends. No overt behavior changes are detected, and effects on school performance and family relationships are minimal. Patients identified early in the course of social drug use can be managed in the pediatrician's office with education about the physical, psychosocial, and academic consequences of substance use; counseling regarding cessation of use, alternative drug-free activities, and minimizing risk of associated morbidity and mortality (e.g., driving under the influence); negotiation of a contract between the physician and the patient regarding further substance use; frequent office follow-up, with positive reinforcement for maintaining abstinence; and other interventions listed in Table 26-3. Routine drug screening is not indicated during this early stage of drug use.

Referral to a specialized substance abuse program is indicated for any adolescent who:

- begins using a substance regularly
- begins using the substance when alone (i.e., uses the substance solely for the "high" rather than in a social context)
- has noticeable changes in behavior or academic performance related to substance use
- commits illegal acts in order to obtain money for or access to the substance
- is unable or unwilling to remain abstinent following intervention in the primary care physician's office

The physician can be instrumental in discussing treatment programs with the family, tailoring referrals to the patient's specific needs, and reviewing management on a monthly basis to ensure ongoing progression and success.

Unfortunately, substance abuse recovery is a lifelong process, with a significant risk for relapse. Close follow-up will assist in identifying setbacks, which should be anticipated and met with support and additional referral as needed.

USE/ABUSE OF SPECIFIC SUBSTANCES

Alcohol

More teenagers abuse alcohol than any other substance. Although fewer high school seniors admit to regular use of alcohol today compared with 10 years ago, the rate of binge drinking (consumption of more than four drinks in a row within the past 2 weeks) has remained unchanged. Although death from alcohol poisoning is not uncommon, intoxicated adolescents are more likely to require medical evaluation and treatment for intentional or accidental injuries that occur while patients are intoxicated. Examples include motor vehicle accidents related to drinking and driving, drowning, suicide and homicide, and rape.

Ingestion of alcohol results in disinhibition, giddiness, talkativeness, and mild euphoria, all of which make the individual more animated and less anxious in social situations. Ultimately, however, alcohol is a depressant. Continued consumption leads to acute intoxication, characterized by slurred speech, ataxia, agitation or combativeness, aggression, and eventually somnolence. Nausea and vomiting are common. Physical findings associated with intoxication include flushing of the skin, sweating, diminished deep tendon reflexes, sluggish but reactive pupils, and hypoglycemia. Stupor and coma are associated with blood alcohol levels of 300 mg per dL or more. Progressive hypoventilation at higher alcohol concentrations culminates in apnea, cardiorespiratory arrest, and death.

A blood alcohol level, dextrose stick, and urine drug screen are indicated in the patient who presents with alcohol intoxication. As previously stated, adolescents are more likely to use multiple substances than limit themselves to a single agent. Lowered inhibition and impaired judgment resulting from alcohol ingestion may make an adolescent more willing to try an agent that might otherwise be refused. In addition, intoxicated adolescents may unknowingly ingest other substances given to them by peers. Finally, alcohol may potentiate the depressive effects of other substances. Any patient who presents with suspected alcohol intoxication and altered mental status should be screened for the use of other substances with a urine drug test. The patient should not be discharged until mental status has returned to baseline and it has been verified that no other drugs are in the patient's system.

In adults, heavy use of alcohol over a number of years produces cirrhosis, cardiomyopathy, encephalopathy, and peripheral neuropathy. These sequelae are unlikely to manifest in the adolescent age group. Gastritis, characterized by epigastric discomfort, occult blood loss, and occasionally vomiting, is the most frequent complication related to chronic alcohol use in this age group. Pancreatitis also occurs more frequently in adolescents who abuse alcohol. Sudden cessation after chronic abuse results in withdrawal symptoms. Hallucinations, seizures, and delirium tremens are rare in adolescents; however, most report some combination of tremulousness, chills, sweating, agitation, and nausea beginning within 12 hours of abstinence. When withdrawal symptoms are moderate to severe, benzodiazepines are prescribed to prevent seizures and provide some measure of symptomatic relief. Barbiturates may be required for refractory seizures.

Tobacco

Use of tobacco in adolescents, including smoking cigarettes and chewing tobacco, has declined over the past decade. Nicotine, the principle pharmacologically active substance in tobacco, is highly addictive. Most individuals who regularly use tobacco products become physiologically dependent and increasingly tolerant to its effects. It is possible for addiction to occur in some adolescents after smoking only a few cigarettes. Physical changes consistent with cardiac stress occur within minutes of lighting a cigarette, including increases in heart rate, blood pressure, cardiac output, and myocardial oxygen consumption. As a group, adolescents who smoke are more likely than their nonsmoking peers to manifest decreased pulmonary function, increased bronchial reactivity, slower lung growth, pulmonary infections, and chronic respiratory symptoms. Chronic smoking increases lifetime risks for cancer (lung, bladder, stomach, among others), coronary artery and peripheral vascular disease, chronic obstructive pulmonary disease, and osteoporosis. Smokeless tobacco use is associated with gingival recession and increases the lifetime risk of oral cancer.

Nicotine precipitates the release of endogenous opiates. Users report sensations of well-being, increased pain tolerance, decreased cravings for sweets, heightened alertness, and improved concentration. In addition to the physiologic addiction, social customs and interactions associated with smoking may become very difficult to give up. Sudden termination of use precipitates a withdrawal syndrome characterized by anxiety, irritability, headache, insomnia, increased appetite, and an intense craving for cigarettes. These symptoms typically resolve within 4 weeks.

Smoking cessation is one of the most positive decisions that adolescents can make in regard to their health. Smokers should be encouraged to quit and assisted in their efforts. Withdrawal symptoms should be anticipated and discussed. Identifying situations that intensify cravings is beneficial for formulating strategies to meet these challenges. Choosing a target date for quitting is a concrete step in the process. Heavy smokers usually find quitting easier when they can wean their use to 10 to 15 cigarettes a day before attempting abstinence.

Smoking cessation is particularly difficult in patients who smoke more than half a pack per day, smoke within a short time of wakening in the morning, or report intense withdrawal symptoms. Both nicotine replacement therapy and bupropion have proven benefit for adult patients with these characteristics. Nicotine replacement therapy is approved for use in adolescents; its effectiveness in this age group is currently under investigation. A prescription is required for patients under 18 years of age. Adolescents who experience symptoms of nicotine addiction should be offered nicotine replacement therapy to increase their likelihood of success. Nicotine replacement is initiated at a dosage of 1 mg per cigarette per day and adjusted within a few days based on response. Weaning occurs every 2 to 4 weeks. The most common adverse effect of the patch is local irritation. Difficulty sleeping and bad dreams may occur but can be prevented by removing the patch at night and replacing it with another in the morning. Bupropion, an antidepressant, can be safely combined with nicotine replacement therapy and has been proven to boost success rates in adult quitters. Therapy is initiated 7 days prior to the target quitting date and continued for up to 6 months. Bupropion is contraindicated in any patient with a history of seizures.

Any attempt to quit smoking, regardless of whether it proves successful, should be strongly reinforced. Individuals who eventually manage to quit smoking fail an average of seven times before they are able to maintain abstinence.

Marijuana

Marijuana is the most frequently used illicit substance in the adolescent population. Approximately 45% of high school seniors admit to trying marijuana at least once, with approximately 5% reporting daily use. Although it is usually smoked in cigarettes or pipes, marijuana can also be ingested with food or brewed as tea. Smoking the drug produces a euphoric sensation within seconds, which peaks within 30 minutes and lasts up to 3 hours. Acute physiologic effects include tachycardia, peripheral vasodilation, hypertension, and delayed orthostatic responses. The consequences of regular use are similar to those of smoking tobacco. Of note, adolescents who use marijuana may not smoke tobacco cigarettes, and vice versa. Moderate use of marijuana impairs memory and learning; as a group, such students have lower grades and are less likely to graduate from high school than their peers. Heavy use has been associated with psychiatric conditions such as depression, anxiety, and personality disorders. Males may rarely develop gynecomastia. Ten percent of students initiated marijuana use prior to age 13. Males use marijuana more often than females. The use of cigarettes does not necessarily precede the use of marijuana.

Tolerance develops after several days of regular use; chronic abuse results in dependence and addiction. Withdrawal symptoms include irritability, insomnia, agitation, cravings for the drug, and a period of flulike symptoms (e.g., malaise, night sweats, gastrointestinal upset). Symptoms typically resolve within 2 weeks of cessation of use.

Opiates

Although heroin can also be ingested, smoked, and injected, most adolescent heroin users "snort" or "sniff" the drug. Nasal inhalation produces a sensation of euphoria within 30 minutes, accompanied by relaxation, sedation, and increased tolerance to pain. These effects generally last for 3 to 4 hours. Physiologic and behavioral dependence occur within weeks of regular use; however, users never become tolerant of the respiratory effects of the drug. Patients who frequently inhale the drug develop chronic rhinitis and are at risk for ulceration of the nasal septum. Constipation is also common in chronic users. Opiate metabolites are detectable in the urine for 2 to 3 days following last use.

Acute opiate intoxication presents with some combination of the following: dysphoria, nausea, vomiting, pruritus, flushing, bronchospasm, hypoventilation, hypotension, bradycardia, lethargy, and pinpoint pupils. A narcotic overdose produces central nervous system sedation and progressive respiratory depression; hypoxia is the most common cause of death. The management of significant narcotic ingestion is provided in Chapter 4.

Chronic users begin to experience withdrawal symptoms within approximately 4 to 6 hours of their last use:

- Initial, psychological phase (12 to 24 hours)—anxiety, craving for the drug
- Middle, physical phase—yawning, insomnia, sweating, tearing of the eyes, stomach cramps
- Late physical phase—fever, chills, tremors, tachycardia, hypertension, vomiting, diarrhea

Opiate withdrawal is not life threatening.

Intravenous narcotic use has the highest potential for significant adverse outcomes. "Shooting" heroin places the patient at risk for cellulitis, blood-borne infections, bacterial endocarditis, and embolic events. Dependence develops most rapidly with intravenous use, and withdrawal is most intense.

Stimulants

Central nervous system stimulants include prescription and illicit amphetamines and cocaine. Methamphetamine is available in forms that may be ingested, inhaled nasally, administered intravenously, or smoked ("ice"). Smoking the drug provides an immediate euphoric "rush" that is intense but fleeting. Oral use of amphetamines increases energy, improves concentration, and allows the user to stay awake and alert without sleep for long periods. Chronic use leads to insomnia, weight loss, psychotic delusions and hallucinations, and demonstrable cerebrovascular lesions. Stimulant metabolites are detectable in the blood and urine for no more than 2 days following the last use.

Signs of methamphetamine intoxication include euphoria or irritability, agitation, fever, flushing of the skin, sweating, dilated pupils that are slow to react, hyperactive reflexes, tremor, and abdominal cramping/diarrhea. Select patients may become hypervigilant, paranoid, and prone to violence. Toxic ingestion is associated with life-threatening hyperpyrexia, hypertension, ventricular arrhythmias, seizures, loss of consciousness, cerebrovascular stroke, and cardiogenic shock. Treatment is supportive. The conscious patient should be placed in a quiet room with minimal stimulation. Haloperidol or droperidol is administered for significant agitation. A cooling blanket may be needed to reduce a dangerously high fever. Severe hypertension is addressed with antihypertensive medications.

Chronic use of amphetamines does not produce physiologic dependence. Cessation of use is associated with depressive symptoms, anxiety, and impaired concentration. Cravings for the drug peak 48 to 72 hours after last use and typically resolve within a week, although they may recur for months or even years.

Cocaine

Like amphetamines, cocaine is a powerful central nervous system stimulant with peripheral adrenergic effects. Cocaine may be inhaled nasally, injected intravenously, or smoked as crack cocaine. The presentations and physiologic consequences of cocaine use are virtually identical to those described earlier for other stimulants. The most frequent cause of death from cocaine use is cardiac arrhythmia.

Hallucinogens

Most adolescent use of phencyclidine (PCP) occurs when the drug is combined with tobacco or marijuana and smoked. PCP is a dissociative substance that produces sensations of euphoria and relaxation. Users describe vivid visual distortions and hallucinations while under the influence of the drug. Other symptoms associated with PCP use include dry mouth and increased appetite. Vertical or horizontal nystagmus may be present on physical examination. Chronic use of PCP can precipitate disordered thought patterns, paranoia, or a catatonic state. These features are also present in patients with schizophrenia, and substance use is extremely common in the schizophrenic population. Psychotic manifestations that are solely due to hallucinogen use will resolve within a week of discontinuing the drug. Metabolites of PCP are detectable in the urine.

The two most common presentations of PCP intoxication are as follows:

- Severe agitation, paranoia, hallucinations, and possibly seizures
- Catatonic muscular rigidity and a blank stare

Regardless, these patients are typically febrile, tachycardic, and hypertensive.

When present, muscle rigidity carries a significant risk of rhabdomyolysis and subsequent renal compromise. If the serum myoglobin concentration is elevated, aggressive hydration and alkalinization of the urine are indicated to prevent this complication.

Inhalants

Inhalant use is more prevalent in preteens and young adolescents than in high school seniors. These substances (Table 26-4) are inexpensive, readily available, and legal to possess. Inhalant use is usually a group activity. The substance can be inhaled directly from the container, or a rag can be saturated with the substance, which is then held over the nose during several deep inhalations. The rag can also be placed into a bag, which is then secured over the head of the user. Inhalants produce an instantaneous "high." Both the physical effects and the clinical presentation are similar to those of alcohol ingestion. Intoxicated patients develop euphoria, slurred speech, ataxia, delirium, hallucinations, and seizures. The inhalant can usually be

TABLE 26-4
COMMON AGENTS USED AS INHALANTS

Aerosol propellants
Model glue
Rubber cement
Spray paint
Paint thinner
Dry cleaning fluids
Adhesives
Shoe polish
Organic solvents
Gasoline
Propane
Freon

smelled on the breath of the patient during the symptomatic period.

Inhalants are highly lipophilic; chronic use results in demonstrable degeneration of white matter and loss of brain mass. Delinquency and poor school performance are more common in adolescents who use inhalants. Substances used as inhalants may be directly toxic to the liver or kidney. Some inhalants are associated with myocardial irritability, cardiac arrhythmias, and sudden cardiac death, the major cause of death due to inhalant use. Other causes of death include hypoxia due to central nervous system depression and accidental asphyxiation.

SOURCES

Ahrendt DM, Miller MA. Adolescent substance abuse: a simplified approach to drug testing. *Pediatr Ann.* 2005;34:956–963.

American Academy of Pediatrics, Committee on Substance Abuse. Indications for management and referral of patients involved in substance abuse. *Pediatrics.* 2000;106:143–148.

American Academy of Pediatrics, Committee on Substance Abuse. Tobacco, alcohol, and other drugs: the role of the pediatrician in prevention, identification, and management of substance abuse. *Pediatrics.* 2005;115:816–821.

Barangan CJ, Alderman EM. Management of substance abuse. *Pediatr Rev.* 2002;23:123–131.

Brown RT. Risk factors for substance abuse in adolescents. *Pediatr Clin North Am.* 2002;49:247–255.

Casavant MJ. Urine drug screening in adolescents. *Pediatr Clin North Am.* 2002;49:317–327.

Centers for Disease Control and Prevention. Youth risk behavioral surveillance—United States, 2005. *Morbid Mortal Wkly Rep.* 2006; 55:1–108.

Dias PJ. Adolescent substance abuse: assessment in the office. *Pediatr Clin North Am.* 2002;49:269–300.

Forti RJ. Opiate overdose. *Pediatr Rev.* 2007;28:35–36.

Greenhill LL. The science of stimulant abuse. *Pediatr Ann.* 2006;35: 552–557.

Johnston LD, O'Malley PM, Bachman JG, Schulenberg JE. *Monitoring the Future: National Results on Adolescent Drug Use: Overview of Key Findings, 2005.* Bethesda, MD: National Institute on Drug Abuse; 2006.

Kaul P, Coupey SM. Clinical evaluation of substance abuse. *Pediatr Rev.* 2002;23:85–94.

Klein JD, Camenga DR. Tobacco prevention and cessation in pediatric patients. *Pediatr Rev.* 2004;25:17–25.

Legano L. Alcohol. *Pediatr Rev.* 2007;28:153–155.

Levy S, Vaughn BL, Knight JR. Office-based intervention for adolescent substance abuse. *Pediatr Clin North Am.* 2002;49:329–343.

Neuspiel DR. Marijuana. *Pediatr Rev.* 2007;28:156–157.

Schydlower M, ed. *Substance Abuse: A Guide for Health Professionals.* 2nd ed. Elk Grove Village, IL: American Academy of Pediatrics; 2002.

QUESTIONS

1. You screen a 17-year-old boy for substance use and address substance abuse as part of the anticipatory guidance portion of his health maintenance visit. His mother calls you the next day and informs you that she is upset that you have chosen to introduce her son to the topic of "drugs and alcohol" without her knowledge or consent. You would be correct in telling this parent that approximately what percentage of high school seniors admits to trying an illicit drug?

A) 50%
B) 33%
C) 25%
D) 10%
E) <5%

2. A 14-year-old girl is brought to the emergency department by her parents for "acting drunk" when her friends dropped her off after a weekend party. She is somnolent and irritable when roused. She vomits once in the triage area. Vital signs are as follows: temperature, 37.0°C; respiratory rate, 14 breaths per minute; heart rate, 80 beats per minute; and blood pressure, 116/72 mm Hg. You order a dextrose stick, serum glucose, and blood alcohol level. Which of the following additional test results is most important for decisions regarding the acute management of this patient?

A) Serum electrolyte
B) Urine drug screen
C) Urine pregnancy test
D) Serum myoglobin level
E) Electrocardiogram

3. Which of the following is not a risk factor for substance use/abuse in the adolescent?

A) Self-reported homosexual orientation
B) Drug use by older siblings
C) Participation in competitive team or individual sports
D) Use of anabolic steroids (performance-enhancing substances)
E) Permissive parental attitudes toward drug use

4. A 15-year-old who is in your office for his routine health maintenance visit reveals that he has been smoking marijuana daily for almost 6 months. In addition to discussing the effects of his drug use on his social relationships, academic performance, and home life, you are most likely to recommend that the patient do which of the following?

A) Immediately discontinue his marijuana use.
B) Find a group of friends who do not use drugs.
C) Begin daily supplementation with vitamin B_6.
D) Share the fact that he is using marijuana with his parents.
E) Switch to tobacco cigarettes and slowly wean himself away from smoking.

5. The majority of adolescents who admit to substance abuse report that their first experience using drugs involved which of the following?

A) Prescription amphetamines
B) Cocaine
C) Anabolic steroids
D) Inhalants
E) Marijuana

6. Which of the following illicit drugs is most commonly used by adolescents?

A) Marijuana
B) Amphetamines
C) Cocaine
D) Inhalants
E) Gamma-hydroxy butyrate

7. Which of the following is the most commonly abused substance among children and adolescents?

A) Tobacco
B) Alcohol
C) Marijuana
D) Inhalants
E) Amphetamines

8. The parents of a 15-year-old boy are concerned about his declining academic performance and behavior changes. He has been caught skipping school twice in the past month and was recently arrested for vandalizing a county park. The young man is scheduled for a routine health maintenance visit in your office next week, and the parents want his urine tested for drugs without his knowledge. You would be correct in communicating of all of the following to them EXCEPT:

A) Performing a urine drug screen without the patient's knowledge is unethical in this instance.
B) Performing a urine drug screen without the patient's knowledge would undermine your doctor-patient relationship with this adolescent.
C) A urine drug screen that is negative excludes substance use by the patient.
D) You are interested in hearing their concerns about their son.
E) You are willing to discuss substance use and abuse with this young man at the upcoming visit.

9. Obtaining a urine drug screen is appropriate in all of the following patients EXCEPT:

A) A 15-year-old adolescent who has expressed an intention to harm his classmates and admits to thoughts suggesting psychosis in the outpatient clinic
B) A 15-year-old adolescent who is in a treatment program for opiate dependency
C) A 15-year-old adolescent who presents to the emergency department with seizures of unknown origin
D) A 15-year-old adolescent with declining grades whose parents desire that he be tested without his knowledge
E) A 15-year-old adolescent who presents to the emergency department with waxing and waning mental status

10. A 14-year-old girl whose parents are divorced was caught smoking a marijuana joint 5 days ago while in her mother's home. She tells her father that it was the first time she has tried marijuana (and that "I didn't even like it"). She agrees to undergo a urine drug screen in your office. In preparing the girl and her parent for the results, you are correct in telling them which of the following?

A) Obtaining a urine drug screen in this patient is unethical.
B) There is no correlation between regularity of marijuana use and duration of the presence of metabolites in the urine.
C) Marijuana use that occurred <2 days before testing will not be detected in a urine drug screen.
D) Marijuana use that occurred >3 days before testing will not be detected in a urine drug screen.
E) The drug screen may be reported as negative.

11. Which of the following risk factors has the strongest predictive value for drug use in an adolescent?

A) Substance use in his or her peer group
B) Prior physical abuse
C) Having parents who smoke
D) Prenatal exposure to illicit drugs
E) Poverty

12. A 16-year-old girl is caught smoking marijuana with her friends by her parents. She is now in your office for assessment. She admits to smoking marijuana with these same friends on two other occasions over the past 6 months. She has also been to two parties where alcohol was available; she drank fewer than two beers at each event. She denies tobacco use and use of any other illicit drugs. She states that she is sorry that she "broke my parents' trust" and says she is motivated to remain abstinent. Which of the following is the most appropriate management of this patient's drug use?

A) Weekly urine drug screens every Monday morning
B) Office management by her primary care pediatrician with referral to a substance abuse counselor
C) Intensive outpatient treatment at a community health center by a team consisting of a mental health specialist, social worker, and substance abuse counselor
D) Inpatient treatment in a therapeutic community with other adolescent substance users
E) Management on a hospital inpatient unit until withdrawal symptoms have been medically addressed

13. A 17-year-old boy who has been living with his father on the West Coast has moved to Texas (where you practice) to live with his mother. The move was prompted by his dismissal from school for stealing to support his heroin habit. He is ambivalent about committing to a treatment program but admits that his life would be better if he could break his dependence on opiates. His mother is very supportive of him. Which of the following is the most appropriate intervention for the patient at this time?
A) Weekly urine drug screens every Monday morning
B) Office management by his primary care pediatrician with referral to a substance abuse counselor
C) Intensive outpatient treatment with methadone maintenance at a hospital-based clinic center by a team consisting of a mental health specialist, social worker, and substance abuse counselor in communication with his primary care pediatrician
D) Inpatient treatment in a therapeutic community with other adolescent substance users
E) Management on a hospital inpatient unit until withdrawal symptoms have been medically addressed

14. A 15-year-old girl in an intensive outpatient treatment program for abuse of illicit drugs (marijuana, phencyclidine) has failed her fourth urine drug screen in the past 6 weeks. She is currently living with her mother and her mother's boyfriend and tells you that the boyfriend frequently hits her mother but has never hit her. She has a scheduled date in family court for truancy. She denies suicidal or homicidal ideation. Which of the following is the most appropriate treatment option for this patient?
A) Involuntary commitment to a substance abuse facility for adolescents and adults
B) Office management by her primary care pediatrician with referral to a substance abuse counselor
C) Intensive outpatient treatment at a community health center by a team consisting of a mental health specialist, social worker, and substance abuse counselor
D) Inpatient treatment in a therapeutic community with other adolescent substance users
E) Management on a hospital inpatient unit until withdrawal symptoms have been medically addressed

15. A 17-year-old young man is referred to you following his second visit to the emergency department with alcohol poisoning in the past 6 months. He admits that he drinks to excess on the weekends with his friends. He also drinks several beers a day when he is by himself in the afternoons. He is experiencing alteration in his mood that interferes with eating and sleeping. He informs you that he wants to regain control of his life but fails each time he tries to stop drinking. He is "beginning to wonder if life is worth living anymore." Which of the following is the most appropriate intervention for this young man's alcohol abuse?
A) Daily urine drug screens
B) Office management by his primary care pediatrician with referral to a substance abuse counselor and Alcoholics Anonymous
C) Intensive outpatient treatment at a community health center by a team consisting of a mental health specialist, social worker, and substance abuse counselor
D) Inpatient treatment in a therapeutic community with other adolescents who abuse alcohol
E) Management on a hospital inpatient unit until his anticipated withdrawal symptoms have been medically addressed and he has been assessed for a comorbid depressive disorder

16. A 17-year-old patient who has been drinking heavily since he dropped out of school 18 months ago is admitted to the hospital with an infected foot wound. During the night, he becomes agitated and tremulous. About 24 hours after admission, he has a brief seizure. Which of the following medications is indicated for initial management of this patient's alcohol withdrawal?
A) Diazepam
B) Phenytoin
C) Valproate
D) Alprazolam
E) Propranolol

17. A 16-year-old adolescent has spent his evenings and weekends this summer binge drinking with his friends at a lake house. He is most likely to experience which of the following sequelae related to his abuse of alcohol?
A) Cirrhosis
B) Gastritis
C) Peripheral neuropathy
D) Encephalopathy
E) Cardiomyopathy

18. You are invited to your local public school to talk about smoking with a class of eighth-grade students.

You would be correct in telling them all of the following EXCEPT:

A) A person may become dependent on nicotine after smoking only a few cigarettes.
B) Adolescents who smoke suffer from more chronic respiratory symptoms than nonsmokers.
C) A greater percentage of high school students is smoking cigarettes today than 10 years ago.
D) Nicotine increases pain tolerance.
E) Smoking in adolescence results in slower lung growth.

19. A 16-year-old adolescent who is in your office for his routine health maintenance visit is receptive to the idea of quitting cigarette smoking. As part of counseling this patient about smoking cessation, you would be correct in telling him all of the following EXCEPT:

A) Withdrawal symptoms include irritability, difficulty sleeping, increased appetite, and craving for cigarettes.
B) Withdrawal symptoms typically abate within 4 weeks.
C) His attempt to stop smoking may be more successful if he can decrease his daily cigarette count to 10 to 15 per day prior to quitting.
D) Nicotine replacement therapy is available over the counter to assist him in his efforts to remain abstinent.
E) He should set a target date for quitting.

20. Recent surveys suggest that the percentage of high school seniors who have used marijuana at least once is closest to which of the following?

A) <5%
B) 10%
C) 25%
D) 45%
E) 60%

21. A 16-year-old homeless patient is admitted to the hospital with a presumptive diagnosis of septic pulmonary embolism. Within 24 hours of admission, the young man begins complaining of sweating and stomach cramps. He has been unable to sleep since arriving on the unit. When you go to see him, the patient seems very anxious and has difficulty sitting still, but he yawns frequently. His eyes are tearing and he has dilated pupils. This patient is most likely to be suffering withdrawal symptoms related to which of the following?

A) Opiates
B) Amphetamines
C) Alcohol
D) Marijuana
E) Phencyclidine

22. You are giving a lecture to a group of substance abuse chaplains regarding the use of heroin in adolescents. You would be correct in telling them which of the following?

A) Most adolescent opiate users inject the drug.
B) Withdrawal from opiates is not life threatening.
C) Opiate users in withdrawal experience primarily psychological symptoms.
D) Chronic heroin use is associated with diarrhea.
E) The most common cause of death due to heroin use is cardiac arrhythmia.

23. A high school senior honors student is brought to the emergency department by her parents early one morning for "behaving oddly." She reportedly stayed awake all night studying for one of her final examinations. Her mother found her early this morning making spaghetti for herself in the kitchen. Her daughter was extremely anxious and could not sit still or calm herself. At presentation, the girl is very talkative but emotionally labile. Her temperature is 38.3°C, heart rate is 120 beats per minute, respiratory rate is 20 breaths per minute, and blood pressure is 140/90 mm Hg. Her skin is flushed, and her pupils are dilated. Mild hyperreflexia is noted on physical examination. Metabolites of which of the following substances are most likely to be found in this patient's urine?

A) Heroin
B) Phencyclidine
C) Amphetamines
D) Inhalants
E) Barbiturates

24. Recent surveys suggest that the percentage of high school seniors who use marijuana daily is closest to which of the following?

A) 40%
B) 20%
C) 10%
D) <1%
E) 5%

25. An adolescent male is brought to the emergency department for a chief complaint of chest pain. He is difficult to evaluate because he is talking very rapidly, but you gather that he was at a party with some friends when he began to have severe chest pain and called an ambulance. The patient cannot sit still on the gurney to be evaluated. When the nurse attempts to place leads on his chest for an electrocardiogram, he accuses her of trying to kill him and threatens to hurt her. The patient is tachycardic, tachypneic, and hypertensive; his pupils are dilated. Further examination is deferred until security can subdue the patient. You are concerned that the patient may be under the influence of cocaine given his chest pain, behavior, and physical findings. Which of the following medications is most appropriate for addressing the agitation in this patient?

A) Bupropion
B) Chlorpromazine
C) Alprazolam
D) Diphenhydramine
E) Haloperidol

26. Physical tolerance, physical dependence, and physical withdrawal are features of all of the following substances EXCEPT:
A) Amphetamines
B) Alcohol
C) Nicotine
D) Opiates
E) Barbiturates

27. A 13-year-old boy is brought to the emergency department via ambulance with somnolence and slurred speech. He is difficult to rouse. His breath and clothing smell of gasoline. He is intubated and ventilated with 100% oxygen. This patient is most at risk for death due to which of the following?
A) Hypoxia
B) Cardiac arrhythmia
C) Central nervous system depression
D) Liver failure
E) Renal failure

28. Which of the following substances is least likely to be used as an inhalant?
A) Gasoline
B) Propane
C) Bleach
D) Nail polish remover
E) Aerosol propellants

29. You are invited to give a lecture to a group of parents at a neighborhood school regarding inhalant use in adolescents. You would be correct in telling them which of the following?
A) Chronic inhalant use is not associated with changes in brain matter.
B) Chronic inhalant use is not associated with poor academic performance.
C) Chronic inhalant use is not associated with delinquency.
D) Regular inhalant use is more common among preteens and young adolescents than older teens.
E) Chronic inhalant use leads to physical and psychological tolerance and dependence.

ANSWERS

1. A	11. A	21. A
2. B	12. B	22. B
3. C	13. C	23. C
4. D	14. D	24. E
5. E	15. E	25. E
6. A	16. A	26. A
7. B	17. B	27. B
8. C	18. C	28. C
9. D	19. D	29. D
10. E	20. D	

Developmental Pediatrics

27

INTELLIGENCE QUOTIENT AND ACHIEVEMENT TESTING

Intelligence tests assist in the identification and appropriate educational placement of children with mental retardation or academic giftedness. In addition, they provide a measure of a child's potential for learning and academic achievement. The most commonly used *intelligence quotient* (IQ) *tests* in the pediatric population are Wechsler Preschool and Primary Scale of Intelligence–Revised (WPPSI-R; appropriate for children 3 to 7 years of age) and the Wechsler Intelligence Scale–Third Edition (WAIS-III; for children 6 to 16 years of age). Each of these tests generates a *full-scale IQ* score as well as separate scores for *verbal IQ* and *performance IQ*. Mean IQ is set at 100 for all scores, with a standard deviation of 15. "Normal intelligence" is defined by an IQ within two standard deviations of the mean. The older the child is when completing the test, the more closely the IQ score reflects that child's potential for achievement. IQ scores may be less correlative with actual intelligence in children with physical impairments, language barriers, and psychosocial stressors.

Tasks in the verbal performance portions of the tests measure language-based learning and processing. The subject listens to the spoken question and is expected to verbalize the response. In contrast, tasks in the performance part of the tests are activity based and do not require verbal responses. Performance IQ testing evaluates visual-spatial organization, processing, and memory. Many state educational systems consider a difference of more than 15 to 20 points between verbal and performance IQ scores to be indicative of a learning disability.

Achievement testing provides a record of a child's performance in a specific area (e.g., reading, writing, mathematics). Achievement tests permit comparison between a student's performance potential and actual achievement. Students with achievement results that are significantly lower than would be expected based on IQ scores should be evaluated for specific learning disabilities.

MENTAL RETARDATION

An individual is diagnosed with mental retardation (MR) if his or her IQ is ≤70 *and* deficits are noted in adaptive functioning prior to the age of 18 years in at least two of the following areas:

- Communication
- Self-care
- Home living
- Social skills
- Use of community resources
- Self-direction
- Academic skills
- Work
- Leisure
- Health
- Safety

About half of cases result from an identifiable cause (Table 27-1). The classification of MR as mild, moderate, severe, or profound permits long-term planning regarding the patient's predicted potential for academic achievement and independent living (Table 27-2). A specific etiology is more likely to be diagnosed in children with severe and profound MR.

Intelligence tests have a standard error of ±5 points, which partially explains both the overlap in IQ values between classifications and the variability in functioning between patients with the same IQ value. IQ can be estimated in infants and young children by dividing the developmental age by the chronologic age and then multiplying by 100. Adaptive functioning can be quantified through tests such as the Vineland Adaptive Behavior scale or can be assessed indirectly through information gathered from the parents, school, or other knowledgeable sources. Adaptive functioning is likely to improve with appropriate support and instructional assistance, whereas IQ remains relatively fixed.

Diagnostic assessment is indicated for any child with MR. Although the cause remains indeterminate in about half of cases, identification provides information regarding risk of recurrence, anticipated life span, and screening for associated medical conditions. Congenital anomalies and dysmorphisms often guide the direction of further testing. If none are present, initial studies consist of chromosomal analysis and specific testing for fragile X syndrome, the most common heritable cause of MR (Table 27-3). Other studies to consider based on the history and physical examination include plasma and urine amino acid and organic acid levels, serologies for infectious diseases, lead levels, thyroid function tests, and magnetic resonance imaging of

TABLE 27-1
KNOWN CAUSES OF MENTAL RETARDATION

- Genetic disorders
  - Genetic syndromes/chromosomal abnormalities
    - Fragile X syndrome
    - Down syndrome
    - Angelman syndrome
    - Rett syndrome
    - Prader-Willi syndrome (and others)
  - Metabolic disorders
    - Disorders of protein metabolism
    - Disorders of carbohydrate metabolism
    - Disorders of lipid metabolism
  - Neurocutaneous disorders
    - Sturge-Weber syndrome
    - Tuberous sclerosis
- Congenital/perinatal infection
  - Toxoplasmosis
  - Cytomegalovirus
  - Herpes simplex virus
  - Human immunodeficiency virus
  - Rubella
- Perinatal complications
  - Asphyxia
  - Intracranial hemorrhage
  - Kernicterus
  - Protracted hypoglycemia
- Toxin exposure
  - Fetal alcohol syndrome
  - Fetal exposure to opiates; possibly cocaine, tobacco, marijuana
  - Lead
- Hypothyroidism
- Infection
  - Meningitis
  - Encephalitis
- Traumatic brain injury
- Child neglect
- Malnutrition

Sources: American Psychiatric Association's *Diagnostic and Statistical Manual of Mental Disorders DSM-IV-TR*, which classifies mental retardation based on intelligence quotient, and American Association on Intellectual and Developmental Disabilities (www.aaidd.org), which classifies mental retardation based on required level of support (intermittent, limited, extensive, or pervasive).

TABLE 27-2
MILD, MODERATE, SEVERE AND PROFOUND MENTAL RETARDATION

Mild Mental Retardation
- IQ range: 50 to 70 points
- Encompasses approximately 70% of cases of MR
- Patients typically have normal growth and normal physical examinations
- Expected to achieve third- to sixth-grade reading level
- Can often live and work independently as adults
- May marry, have children (unless underlying diagnosis results in infertility)

Moderate Mental Retardation
- IQ range: 35 to 55 points
- Encompasses approximately 10% of cases of MR
- Expected to achieve first- to third-grade reading level
- Usually require supervised living and working arrangements
- Need particular assistance learning life skills (e.g., counting money)
- Unlikely to marry or have children

Severe Mental Retardation
- IQ range: 20 to 40 points
- Encompasses approximately 3% to 4% of cases of MR
- Reading limited to site reading of common words
- Require significant assistance with activities of daily living in a highly structured and supportive environment
- Do not marry or have children

Profound Mental Retardation
- IQ ≤20 to 25 points
- Encompasses approximately 1% to 2% of cases of MR
- Infantile behavior throughout life

the brain. When the etiology remains undiagnosed, the risk of recurrence in future pregnancies is approximately 3%.

COMMUNICATION DISORDERS

Autism

Autism spectrum disorder represents a collection of closely related chronic, nonprogressive developmental conditions involving impairments in social interaction, communication, and behavior (Table 27-4). Autism and Asperger syndrome are both classified as autism spectrum disorders. The incidence of autism in the United States and other industrialized countries seems to be rising over the past decade. Most affected children are diagnosed between 18 months and 3 years of age, but symptoms can be present from infancy (impaired attachment). Autism is thought to be a multifactorial disorder.

Distinguishing an autistic disorder from an isolated speech/language disorder or MR may at times be clinically difficult. In addition, children with autism may have coexisting language and/or cognitive delays. Autism, unlike developmental delay, is characterized by both *delayed development and deviant development.* For example, patients with autism speak and combine words later than their unaffected peers. However, they also are unlikely to respond to their own name despite normal hearing, and they often manifest atypical speech patterns (echolalia, perseverative speech). Children with autism have impairment of social and language skills in excess of what would be expected based on their measured IQ, unlike patients with MR.

Some children with autism benefit from medication designed to target specific symptoms such as anxiety,

TABLE 27-3
FRAGILE X SYNDROME: A REVIEW

Pathogenesis/Heritability
- Fragile X syndrome is the most common inherited cause of mental retardation.
- Genetic defect in the fragile X mental retardation-1 gene (FMR1) on the X chromosome consisting of abnormal repetition of a three nucleotide sequence
- The number of repeats increases with subsequent generations.
- Males with at least 200 repetitions of the sequence have fragile X syndrome.
- Females with at least 200 repetitions of the sequence are carriers of fragile X syndrome and may also be cognitively impaired.
- Patients with the highest number of repeats have the most severe manifestations of the disorder.

Epidemiology
- Experts believe that at least 50% of males who have the full mutation (≥200 repetitions) remain undiagnosed.
- Identification is currently rare prior to late childhood.

Clinical Manifestations
- Mental retardation in 80% of males, 30% of females
- Comorbid attention-deficit/hyperactivity disorder in virtually all males, 50% of females
- High rates of autism, behavior disorders
- Physical characteristics include long, thin face with prominent forehead and nasal bridge; protuberant ears; high, arched palate or cleft; and joint laxity.
- Late-onset macro-orchidism

Diagnosis
- Molecular genetic testing (Southern blot, polymerase chain reaction) for definitive diagnosis
- Assessment for comorbid disorders

Treatment
- None specific
- Treatment for comorbid disorders

hyperactivity, and perseverative behaviors. The most effective management programs combine behavioral interventions, language and social therapies, and parental involvement and support. It is clear is that early recognition and intervention lead to better clinical outcomes. The best prognostic indicator of future success is the extent of language development present during the preschool years.

Language Disorders Not Due to Autism

Up to 15% of preschool-age children meet the diagnostic criteria for speech and/or language delay. Such disorders may involve primarily language, speech, or articulation (Table 27-5). In isolated communication disorders, achievement of language milestones is delayed beyond what would be predicted based on achievement along cognitive and social developmental tracks. Speech and language delay is more common in boys. Of note, language development in boys as a group lags that in girls by an average of only 1 to 2 months. Potential causes of speech and language disorders are noted in Table 27-6.

Children with suspected or confirmed delays in speech and/or language should be referred for full audiologic

TABLE 27-4
SOCIAL, COMMUNICATIVE, AND BEHAVIORAL CHARACTERISTICS OF AUTISM SPECTRUM DISORDER

Social Interaction
- Limited eye contact and facial expression
- Difficulty developing peer relationships
- Indifference to social overtures
- Lack of social reciprocity
- Inflexibility
- No engagement in pretend play

Communication
- Impaired reciprocal communication
- Language development deviant, rather than simply delayed
- Echolalia, perseverative speech

Behaviors
- Restrictive, stereotyped patterns of behavior
- Repetitive, self-stimulatory behaviors (e.g., rocking, spinning)[a]
- Preoccupation or fascination with a single object or subject

[a]Developmentally normal children and patients with mental retardation also engage in these behaviors; their presence should not be considered sensitive or specific for autism.

TABLE 27-5
DIFFERENTIATION OF LANGUAGE, SPEECH, AND ARTICULATION DISORDERS

Language Disorders
- Impairment in acquisition of the native language
- May be expressive and/or receptive
- Individuals are unable to produce or understand the meaning of words
- Vocabulary is limited, and words are misused
- Persistence of grammatical errors
- Difficulty engaging in conversation or following directions
- Higher prevalence of mental health problems in late childhood and beyond

Speech Disorders
- Impairment in the production of speech
- Abnormal voice quality (rhythm, pitch, volume, flow)
- Speech is often unintelligible

Articulation Disorders
- Impairment in ability to articulate and/or sequence speech sounds
- May manifest with substitutions ("wabbit" for "rabbit") that persist beyond the normal age of acquisition
- Children up to 7 years of age with normal speech development may still have difficulty making specific sounds; typically, the final sounds to be acquired are sh, th (think), th (the), s, z, l, r, and zh (treasure).

TABLE 27-6
CAUSES OF DEVELOPMENTAL DELAY IN LANGUAGE

Hearing impairment
- Chronic otitis media with effusion
- Congenital hearing loss
- Acquired hearing loss

Isolated language, speech, or articulation disorder

Motor disability
- Cerebral palsy
- Brain injury
- Muscular dystrophies

Mental retardation

Global developmental delay

Genetic/chromosomal abnormality
- Fragile X syndrome[a]
- Klinefelter syndrome[a]

Autism

Child neglect

Seizure disorder

[a]These patients may present with isolated language delay with or without obvious physical stigmata of their underlying condition.

TABLE 27-7
SPEECH/LANGUAGE DELAY: INDICATIONS FOR REFERRAL

Birth or any age

- No response to sound
- No interest in interacting with other people

4 months

- No drive to communicate

6 to 9 months

- Loss of the ability to coo or babble
- Poor localization of sound

12 months

- Loss of acquired language or social milestones
- No use of "da-da" or "ma-ma"

15 to 18 months

- No use of single words
- Poor comprehension of language

24 months

- Vocabulary <50 words
- No use of two-word phrases
- >50% of speech unintelligible to a stranger

36 months

- Rote memorization of words or phrases
- Frequent echolalia
- Poor voice quality or speech rhythms
- >25% of speech unintelligible to a stranger

48 months

- Inability to participate in conversation
- Dysfluency of initial sounds or parts of words

5 years

- "Developmental dysfluency" that persists beyond the 5th birthday

6 to 7 years

- Immature or inaccurate speech production

[a]In addition, a delay of 25% or greater after 16 to 24 months of age is considered an indication for referral.

assessment. The managements of hearing loss and otitis media with effusion, the most common cause of conductive hearing loss in the preschool-age population, are discussed in Chapter 23. Patients with normal hearing who have coexisting social, cognitive, or motor impairments are referred for comprehensive developmental assessment through public early intervention services or private assessment teams. If the child has normal hearing and otherwise normal development, referral to a speech pathologist is indicated for further assessment, diagnosis, and treatment. Indications for referral are listed in Table 27-7.

Prognosis is related to specific diagnosis and age at identification/intervention. Most communication disorders improve over time with regular therapy. Early speech and language delay has been associated with later impairment in reading skills.

Developmental dysfluency is a normal finding in children between 3 and 4 years of age. Developmental dysfluency is characterized by:

- multiple repetitions of single syllables or words
- no difficulties in communication
- no evidence of tension
- resolution before age 5 years

In contrast, stuttering is disorder of speech fluency that significantly interferes with effective communication. Stuttering is characterized by:

- multiple repetitions of single sounds, rather than whole words ("c-c-c-c-can" rather than "can-can-can-can-can")
- prolongation of initial or terminal sounds in words ("hhhhhhhhigh")
- complete blocking of word sounds
- any of the above accompanied by obvious tension in the muscles of the face and neck
- persistence beyond the age of resolution of developmental dysfluency

Children who stutter should be referred for speech and language evaluation and appropriate therapy. Referral is also appropriate for children younger than 5 years of age with dysfluency characteristics that are more consistent with stuttering. Individualized speech therapy, combined with parental education, improves fluency in the great majority of affected children. Stuttering is a chronic condition that may persist throughout life.

LEARNING DISORDERS

Any condition that results in persistent functional impairment of the immature brain can be considered a *learning disorder*. In contrast, a *learning disability* is present when the individual has significant and persistent difficulty acquiring or using information within a specific domain. The fourth edition of the *Diagnostic and Statistical Manual of Mental Disorders* (DSM-IV Text Revision) recognizes three categories of learning disabilities: developmental speech and language disorders (discussed earlier); academic skills disorders; and learning disabilities not otherwise specified. A child is diagnosed with a learning disorder when his or her functioning in reading, writing, or arithmetic lags behind that of peers by ≥2 years. The diagnosis of learning disability is excluded when the impairment is secondary to MR, global developmental delay, autism, educational deprivation, or physical disabilities. Learning disabilities occur in children of average intelligence as well as those with IQs above and below the mean.

There is wide variability among normally developing children in terms of cognitive ability and academic achievement. A child with delayed acquisition of skills will demonstrate improvement with maturation. In contrast, learning disabilities are present for life. Those that are accompanied by disruptive behavior and poor classroom performance tend to be identified in preschool or elementary school. However, when the presentation is subtle, or the child is able to compensate for the learning disability, the disorder may remain undiagnosed until middle school, high school, or beyond. Newly diagnosed cases of learning disorders peak in the third grade and again in middle school. A single individual may have learning disabilities in more than one area.

The diagnosis of learning disability should be entertained whenever there is a significant discrepancy between a child's academic achievement and the child's perceived ability to learn. For example, a learning disability may be present:

- in a student with a normal IQ score who performs poorly in reading, writing, and/or math
- in a fourth-grade student performing at grade level in math but only at a second-grade level in reading
- in a student with significant differences between performance and verbal IQ scores
- in a student with significant discrepancies between predicted achievement (based on IQ score) and scores on achievement tests in specific subjects

Early psychoeducational testing is indicated for any child suspected of having a learning disability; delay in diagnosis and intervention places the child at risk for school failure, poor self-esteem, and academic disengagement. Students with learning disabilities are at increased risk for psychiatric illness later in life.

Dyslexia, or developmental reading disorder, is the most commonly diagnosed learning disability. Family history of dyslexia and past history of developmental language/articulation disorder are associated with an increased risk of dyslexia. Children with dyslexia have difficulty distinguishing separate sounds in words. Early indicators include difficulties with rhyming words, isolating sounds at the beginning or end of simple words ("What sound does 'CAT' start with?"), learning the sound(s) associated with each letter, and confusing the meanings of words that sound similar. Reading affects every area of academic achievement; thus, dyslexia may be associated with poor school performance in multiple subjects, especially as the curriculum shifts from "learning to read" in the early grades to "reading to learn" in mid-elementary school.

Classroom accommodations that diminish the impact of specific deficits improve the likelihood of successful learning and academic achievement. Examples include oral testing and books on tape for children with dyslexia and use of a keyboard for students with disabilities involving writing. The child is coached in strategies to compensate for the disability, and remedial tutoring is provided in subjects of difficulty.

DISORDERS OF ATTENTION AND IMPULSE CONTROL

Attention-deficit/hyperactivity disorder (ADHD) is the most commonly diagnosed neurodevelopmental health condition in the pediatric population. The three predominant behavioral features of ADHD are *inattentiveness, hyperactivity*, and *impulse control* (Table 27-8). Approximately 5% of school-age children have ADHD; most are diagnosed during the early elementary school years. The disorder is three times more common in males; a positive family history also confers additional risk. *ADHD, predominantly inattentive type* is a variant of ADHD in which inattention is the primary symptom and hyperactivity is minimal or absent; this form is more common in girls. The diagnosis of ADHD requires that symptoms be present in at least two settings (usually school and home). *The absence of characteristic symptoms in the physician's office does not exclude the diagnosis*; the child's behaviors may be suppressed by individualized attention, anxiety, or the novelty of the environment.

ADHD is a clinical diagnosis; laboratory evaluation is noncontributory. ADHD behavioral rating scales

TABLE 27-8
SYMPTOMS OF ATTENTION-DEFICIT/ HYPERACTIVITY DISORDER

Inattentiveness
- Short attention span
- Easily distracted
- Forgetful
- Difficulty following directions
- Difficulty organizing tasks
- Difficulty completing tasks
- Rushing results in careless errors
- Frequently loses things

Hyperactivity
- Fidgets
- Difficulty remaining seated
- Excessively active
- Inappropriate activity level
- Inability to entertain oneself and play quietly
- Talks excessively

Impulsivity
- Difficulty taking turns
- Difficulty waiting
- Often interrupts

(e.g., Conners' Rating Scales) are available in parent and teacher forms. Patients with fragile X syndrome and fetal alcohol syndrome have relatively high rates of ADHD; physical stigmata of these disorders may suggest the underlying condition. Neuroimaging may be indicated in the child with a history of brain injury, seizure disorder, or developmental delay who develops symptoms of ADHD. Disruptive behavior in the classroom is not limited to children with ADHD; students with learning disabilities and others who are unable to satisfactorily complete work that is too difficult for them may also act out at school. Educational assessment is indicated in children with ADHD and academic underachievement in order to evaluate cognitive development and rule out learning disabilities.

A diagnosis of ADHD should be based on criteria outlined in the DSM-IV-Revision manual, not response to stimulants. These medications improve attention in normal children as well as those with ADHD. Similarly, suboptimal response to a stimulant medication does not exclude the diagnosis of ADHD, and it also does not predict the effectiveness of other stimulants or even other formulations of the same medication. Stimulant therapy is beneficial for some patients with MR whose delayed development makes them less attentive and more disruptive than their same-age peers in a mainstream educational setting.

Stimulant medications have demonstrated efficacy in the treatment of ADHD. Three out of four patients with ADHD who begin stimulants experience significant improvement in their core symptoms (i.e., inattentiveness, poor impulse control, hyperactivity). Secondary effects include improved relations with peers, parents, and teachers. A review of available ADHD medications, initial dosages, side effects, and durations of action is provided in Table 27-9. Long-term stimulant use as part of the management of ADHD has not been shown to result in tolerance or dependence. The correct dose of a stimulant is that which provides maximal symptom control with minimal adverse effects. Children should receive their ADHD medications every day and in all settings; "drug holidays" and cessation of therapy over the summer and weekends are no longer recommended. Continuous dosing permits direct parental assessment of treatment effectiveness and familiarizes parents with typical behavior on the drug so that they can more quickly recognize side effects.

Pharmacologic intervention alone is incomplete therapy for ADHD. Additional features may include any of the following: outside tutoring, special education services, classroom accommodations, parental education and anticipatory guidance, cognitive management strategies, counseling, and behavioral therapy. Behavior management involves shaping the behavior of the subject through alteration of the physical or social environment. Stimulant medication is associated with more improvement than behavioral therapy. The addition of behavior management to stimulant therapy does not produce a further decrease in core symptoms but is associated with improved conduct, decreased anxiety, rising academic achievement, and higher parental and teacher satisfaction. Schools should be notified at the initiation of pharmacologic treatment and whenever dosage changes are made. Communicating child-specific behavior management strategies to the teacher assures consistent consequences and rewards for behavior at home and at school.

Comorbid psychiatric disorders are relatively common in patients with ADHD. Oppositional defiant disorder is diagnosed in up to a third of affected patients; other conditions occurring with increased frequency in this population include conduct disorder, anxiety disorder, learning disabilities, and depression. Adolescents with ADHD are more likely than their peers to abuse substances and engage in antisocial behaviors.

Most individuals diagnosed with ADHD as children continue to experience symptoms of the disorder in adulthood. However, since they are generally no longer in a school setting, the behaviors associated with the symptoms are often less obvious. In general, patients with ADHD complete fewer years of formal education and have lower paying jobs than their peers. Patients and their parents should be counseled regarding the chronicity of the disorder and anticipated need for continued educational support and medication throughout one's academic career.

TABLE 27-9
MEDICATION FOR USE IN PATIENTS WITH ADHD

Medication (brand names)	Formulations	Initiation of Treatment	Duration of Action
Stimulant Medications for ADHD			
Dextroamphetamine/levoamphetamine (Adderall) Immediate-release	Tablets	5 mg once or twice a day, advancing every week	4 to 6 hrs
Dextroamphetamine/levoamphetamine (Adderall XR) Extended-release	Capsules	5 mg/day, advancing every week	8 to 12 hrs
Dextroamphetamine (Dexedrine, Dextrostat) Immediate-release	Tablets	5 mg once or twice a day, advancing every week	4 to 6 hrs
Dextroamphetamine (Dexedrine Spansule) Extended-release	Spansule	5 mg/day, advancing every week	6 to 10 hrs
Methylphenidate (Ritalin, Focalin, Methylin) Immediate-release	Tablets; oral suspension (Methylin)	5 mg twice a day, advancing every week (Focalin: 2.5 mg once or twice a day, advancing every week)	Ritalin: 3 to 4 hrs Focalin: 4 to 5 hrs Methylin: 4 to 8 hrs
Methylphenidate [Ritalin-SR, Focalin XR, Methylin SR, Metadate SR, Concerta, Daytrana (patch)] Extended-release	Tablets, capsules, patch	Varies by product; advance every week	6 to 12 hrs, depending on product
Lisdexamfetamine (Vyvanse; a prodrug form of dextroamphetamine metabolized to an active form after ingestion)	Capsule	30 mg once a day, advancing to up to 70 mg	Approx. 12 hrs
Common adverse effects (transient): nausea, headache, tics *Common adverse effects (persistent)*: decreased appetite, weight loss/poor growth, delayed sleep onset *Rare adverse effects*: irritability, syncope, hallucinations, aggressive behavior, seizures; cardiovascular toxicity			
Non-Stimulant Medication for ADHD			
Atomoxetine (norepinephrine reuptake inhibitor) (Strattera)	Capsules	0.5 mg/kg/day (40 mg/day for patients >70 kg); advance every 3 days	18 to 24 hrs
Common adverse effects (transient): nausea, dry mouth, constipation, fatigue *Rare adverse effects*: daytime somnolence, liver damage, suicidal ideation, syncope, aggressive behavior, sexual dysfunction			

The USFDA requires a black box warning on stimulants for sudden cardiovascular events (strokes, sudden death); children with underlying heart disease are particularly at risk.

EDUCATIONAL ASSISTANCE FOR CHILDREN WITH DISABILITIES

Children with disorders that interfere with learning, including MR, learning disabilities, visual or hearing impairment, physical disabilities, and psychiatric or behavioral disturbances, among others, are entitled by federal law to free and appropriate special education services in the least restrictive environment possible. Educational needs and services are determined by the states, and criteria and levels of intervention differ among the states. Examples of services, from the least to the most restrictive, are listed as follows:

- Mainstream classroom; outside assistance through additional tutoring
- Individualized instruction from an educational assistant within a mainstream classroom
- Mainstream classroom; removal to a special educational resource room for specific instruction in problem subjects
- Special educational resource class most of the day; return to mainstream classroom for certain subjects
- Special educational resource classroom at a mainstream education school
- Education at a separate school for children with special needs

The federal government provides financial incentives to the states for early intervention programs for children 0 to 3 years of age who are at risk for learning disorders. Services are designed to assist children with cognitive, physical, communication, social, emotional, or adaptive impairments. Management consists of thorough evaluation of medical, social, and educational needs and provision of needed support in each of those areas.

SCHOOL FAILURE

Many factors influence learning and academic achievement. The list of potential causes of school failure is extensive (Table 27-10); in most cases, academic underachievement results from the interplay of multiple adverse circumstances. The *patient history* is the most important assessment tool for identifying patients with school failure who may benefit from further educational, psychological, or medical assessment. A complete history consists of questions pertaining to a child's home life, potential stressors, emotional health, school performance, previous testing, family history, birth history, early developmental outcomes (particularly language), and social functioning. The physical examination is typically normal. Abnormalities such as micro- or macrocephaly, growth failure, hearing or visual impairment, and dysmorphisms/anomalies may occasionally suggest a previously undiagnosed medical condition. Identification of "soft" neurologic signs (i.e., nonfocal neurologic findings such as clumsiness) is seldom of clinical relevance. In addition to a complete history and physical examination, the child with school learning problems usually warrants thorough educational assessment, including both IQ and achievement testing.

Grade retention is seldom the optimal intervention for school failure. Students who are held back a year are more than twice as likely to eventually drop out as their promoted peers. Risk factors for grade retention include low parental involvement in the child's education, poverty, male gender, racial minority, poor academic performance in early grades, behavior problems, and frequent moves or school transfers. Students who are retained end up being older than their same-grade peers; these children have higher rates of social maladjustment, behavior problems, violence, risky sexual behaviors, and substance use. Grade retention negatively impacts self-esteem and attitude toward school; these trends are difficult to reverse in subsequent grades.

Chronic school failure is associated with increased rates of depression, aggression, juvenile delinquency, substance use, suicide, and teen pregnancy. Long-term consequences of academic failure are not limited to effects on earning potential and vocational opportunities. As a group, adults who did not graduate from high school have shorter life expectancies and are more likely than their educated peers to suffer from chronic health conditions related to lifestyle choices.

TABLE 27-10
FACTORS THAT MAY NEGATIVELY IMPACT SCHOOL PERFORMANCE

Developmental/Behavioral Disorders

Learning disabilities

- Speech and language delay/disorders
- Specific reading, writing, and mathematics learning disabilities

Mental retardation (chromosomal disorders, genetic syndromes, acquired)

Developmental delay

Autism spectrum disorders

Attention-deficit/hyperactivity disorder

Physical Disabilities

Vision impairment

Hearing impairment

Cerebral palsy

Psychiatric Disorders

Depression

Anxiety disorder

Obsessive-compulsive disorder

Conduct disorder

Oppositional defiant disorder

Substance abuse

Medical Conditions

Chronic disease

- Frequent school absences due to disease complications or treatments
- Effects of medication on school performance (particularly antihistamines, anticonvulsants)

Disruptive behaviors resulting from medical conditions

- Tic disorders
- Seizure disorders
- Thyroid dysfunction
- Rheumatologic disorders

Family Environment

Stressors within the family

Parental academic underachievement

Lack of parental or cultural support

Homelessness

Abuse/neglect

Placement in foster care

School Environment

Student-teacher mismatch (temperament, learning style)

Unsafe school environment

Socioeconomic Factors

Poverty

Excessive working outside school

Peer Relationships

Social isolation

Academic underachievement in peer group

Truancy

Participation in Head Start confers an early educational advantage and familiarizes children and parents with behavioral expectations. Reading to children daily during the preschool years promotes early literacy and establishes reading as a family priority. Timely identification of risk factors for school failure and intervention, in the forms of appropriate medical care, developmental or behavioral therapy, parental education, and anticipatory guidance, improves potential for academic, vocational, and social success.

KINDERGARTEN READINESS

Children need to acquire certain skills in order to succeed in kindergarten. They should be able to separate from their parents for several hours at a time, follow directions, play well with other children, communicate their personal needs, and talk about themselves and their experiences. The American Academy of Pediatrics cautions against the use of developmental screening tests as indicators of school readiness or lack thereof. Children who are at risk for delay should be evaluated by qualified practitioners with rigorously standardized developmental examinations before being "held back" or referred for special education services.

SCREENING AND ASSESSMENT

The American Academy of Pediatrics recommends developmental and behavioral screening for all children at every routine health maintenance visit. Validated assessment tools that rely primarily on information gathered from the parents are available and appropriate for use in the primary care setting (Table 27-11). These tests are simple to administer and do not require extensive staff training. The physician may choose separate screening tests for developmental and behavioral assessment; however, some questionnaires screen for deficiencies in both areas.

TABLE 27-11
DEVELOPMENTAL AND BEHAVIORAL SCREENING IN THE PRIMARY CARE SETTING

Developmental Screening Tools

Infant and Child Development Inventories

- Appropriate for use in patients ages 3 months to 6 years
- Parental questionnaires
- Can be completed in <15 minutes
- Good sensitivity, specificity in identification of children with developmental delay

Behavioral Screening Tools

Child Behavior Checklist

- Appropriate for use in patients ages 18 months to 18 years
- Parental questionnaire
- Can be completed in 20 to 30 minutes
- Extensive evaluation of behavior and social competency
- Computerized results with standardized T-scores permit comparison with the norm

Pediatric Symptom Checklist

- Appropriate for use in patients ages 4 to 16 years
- Parental questionnaire
- Can be completed in <10 minutes
- Suggests whether behavioral concerns will be better addressed with psychiatric referral or behavioral interventions

Developmental/Behavioral Screening Tools

Parents' Evaluation of Developmental Status

- Appropriate for children from birth to 8 years of age
- Parental questionnaire
- Can be completed in approximately 2 minutes
- Includes recommendations regarding when to complete additional screens and when to refer for formal testing

SOURCES

American Academy of Pediatrics Committee on Early Childhood, Adoption, and Dependent Care. The inappropriate use of school "readiness" tests. *Pediatrics*. 1995;95:437–438.

American Academy of Pediatrics Committee on Quality Improvement and Subcommittee on Attention-Deficit/Hyperactivity Disorder. Clinical practice guideline: treatment of the school-age child with attention-deficit/hyperactivity disorder. *Pediatrics*. 2001;108:1033–1044.

American Academy of Pediatrics Committee on Quality Improvement and Subcommittee on Attention-Deficit/Hyperactivity Disorder. Diagnosis and evaluation of the child with attention-deficit/hyperactivity disorder. *Pediatrics*. 2000;105:1158–1170.

American Psychiatric Association. *Diagnostic and Statistical Manual of Mental Disorders DSM-IV-TR*. 4th ed. Arlington, VA: American Psychiatric Publishing; 2000.

Byrd RS. School failure: assessment, intervention, and prevention in primary pediatric care. *Pediatr Rev*. 2005;26:227–237.

Feldman HM. Evaluation and management of language and speech disorders in preschool children. *Pediatr Rev*. 2005;26:131–141.

Grizzle KL, Simms MD. Early language development and language learning disabilities. *Pediatr Rev*. 2005;26:274–283.

Moeschler JB, Shevell M. Clinical genetic evaluation of the child with mental retardation or developmental delays. *Pediatrics*. 2006;117:2304–2316.

Phalen JA. Fragile X syndrome. *Pediatr Rev*. 2005;26:181–182.

Rau JD. Is it autism? *Contemp Pediatr*. 2003;20:54–84.

Roberts G, Palfrey JS, Bridgemohan C. A rational approach to the medical evaluation of a child with developmental delay. *Contemp Pediatr*. 2004;21:76–100.

Shaywitz SE, Shaywitz BA. Dyslexia (specific reading disability). *Pediatr Rev*. 2003;24:147–153.

Stein MT, Perrin JM. Diagnosis and treatment of ADHD in school-age children in primary care settings: a synopsis of the AAP practice guidelines. *Pediatr Rev*. 2003;24:92–98.

QUESTIONS

1. Which of the following is the most common heritable cause of mental retardation?
A) Fragile X syndrome
B) Down syndrome
C) Rett syndrome
D) Tuberous sclerosis
E) Hurler syndrome

2. One of your patients, a 6-year-old boy, has been referred for complete developmental assessment due to poor academic performance. The patient's full-scale intelligence quotient is reported to be 64. In order to be diagnosed with mental retardation, the patient must also have which of the following?
A) Evidence of global developmental delay
B) Deficits in adaptive functioning in at least two areas such as social interaction, self-care, safety, and communication
C) At least one congenital anomaly or dysmorphism consistent with a known cause of mental retardation
D) $\geq$200 trinucleotide repeats on the X chromosome OR an demonstrable chromosomal structural or numerical abnormality
E) A maternal Robertsonian translocation

3. At a 4-year health maintenance visit, a mother asks you what kinds of academic activities she should be doing with her daughter to make sure she is ready for kindergarten next year. You reply that her daughter should be able to accomplish all of the following before starting kindergarten EXCEPT:
A) Separate from her parents for several hours at a time
B) Follow directions
C) Know all her letters and letter sounds
D) Play well with other children
E) Communicate her personal needs

4. You are providing a lecture to a group of elementary school teachers about mental retardation. In regard to testing for mental retardation, you would be correct in telling them all of the following EXCEPT:
A) Intelligence tests generally have a standard of error $\pm$5 points.
B) A child's IQ can be estimated by dividing the developmental age by the chronologic age and then multiplying by 100.
C) Adaptive functioning can be quantified through tests such as the Vineland Adaptive Behavior scale.
D) IQ scores are likely to improve dramatically in children with mental retardation who are provided with individualized academic support.
E) All children with suspected mental retardation should receive a thorough diagnostic assessment unless the cause of their condition is known.

5. Which of the following genetic/chromosomal abnormalities is not typically associated with mental retardation?
A) Fragile X syndrome
B) Angelman syndrome
C) Prader-Willi syndrome
D) Down syndrome
E) Turner syndrome

6. A mother brings her 10-year-old son to your office because he is having difficulty in school. He was diagnosed with ADHD about 18 months ago, and his behavior at school has improved on stimulant medication. He was retained in the second grade, and the school has recommended retention again this year. The child has an unusual appearance, with a long, thin face, prominent forehead and nasal bridge, and protuberant ears. His palate is high and arched, and joint laxity is noted on physical examination. Which of the following is most likely to reveal the diagnosis in this patient?
A) Polymerase chain reaction testing of the X chromosome
B) Analysis of the full chromosomal complement
C) Thyroid function tests
D) Questioning the mother about alcohol use during the pregnancy
E) Blood lead level

7. A mother brings her 3-year-old son to your office for evaluation of his stuttering. The child had typical speech and language development at his 3-year routine health maintenance visit and had attained age-appropriate motor, cognitive, and social milestones at that time. The mother reports that he seems to be "thinking faster than he can talk"; he repeats the same word several times before finishing his sentences. The dysfluency is not currently interfering with his ability to communicate, and the child doesn't seem to be bothered by the stuttering. The physical examination is within normal limits. Which of the following is the most appropriate management of this patient?
A) Refer the child for full audiologic assessment.
B) Reassure the mother that developmental dysfluency is a normal occurrence at this age.
C) Refer the child for full developmental assessment.
D) Refer the child to a speech pathologist for isolated fluency assessment.
E) Obtain a tympanogram in the office.

8. The mother of a 4-year-old boy brings her son to your office for evaluation of his stuttering. The child was evaluated 4 months ago by your partner and diagnosed with developmental dysfluency. The mother tells you that the stuttering has become progressively worse and is interfering with his ability to communicate

with both peers and family members. The child has particular difficulty articulating the first syllable of a word, with repetition of the first sound or complete blocking. He is becoming frustrated by his inability to "get his words out." By parental report, the boy has attained age-appropriate motor, language, cognitive, and social developmental milestones. The physical examination is within normal limits. Which of the following is the most appropriate management of this patient?

A) Referral for full audiologic assessment at this time
B) Referral for full speech and language assessment if fluency does not significantly improve by age 5 years
C) Referral for fluency assessment at this time
D) Reassure the parent that the patient has developmental dysfluency.
E) Obtain a tympanogram in the office.

9. A 24-month-old child is in your office for her routine health maintenance visit. Her mother asks you about strategies for dealing with temper tantrums. She reports that her daughter becomes extremely anxious if her daily routine is disrupted, falling to the floor and screaming while covering her ears. The pattern is so disruptive that the mother avoids taking the child away from the home as much as possible. Her daughter's favorite activity consists of methodically pulling books off a lower shelf in the living room, which she will do over and over and which seems to calm her. The child rarely responds to her name and avoids eye contact. In the office, the patient follows neither verbal nor nonverbal instructions. This patient's temper tantrums are most likely due to which of the following?

A) Significant hearing impairment
B) Isolated speech/language disorder
C) Global developmental delay
D) Autism spectrum disorder
E) Hypersensitive temperament

10. A mother brings her 15-month-old child to your office for evaluation of his head banging. She tells you that when the child is in his crib at night, he positions himself on his hands and knees and rocks back and forth banging his head on the headboard of the crib. He seems to find the activity soothing and cannot settle himself to sleep if the behavior is disrupted. The child is otherwise active and happy. By history, the patient has attained normal developmental milestones. There is no evidence of trauma on evaluation of the head; the remainder of the physical examination, including growth parameters, is within normal limits. Which of the following is the most appropriate next step in the management of this patient?

A) Obtain skull radiographs.
B) Obtain computed tomography of the head.
C) Refer the child for specialized evaluation for autistic spectrum disorder.
D) Refer the child for full developmental assessment.
E) Reassure the mother that the child's behavior is normal.

11. Inaccurate production of all of the following speech sounds can be normal up to the age of 7 years EXCEPT:

A) h ("hello")
B) zh ("measure")
C) th ("the")
D) th ("thing")
E) r ("rose")

12. A 5-year-old child is in the office for his routine health maintenance visit prior to starting kindergarten. He has recently been discharged from speech therapy with his mother's approval. The boy was diagnosed with isolated speech/language delay at 24 months of age and attended weekly speech therapy for almost 2 years, with excellent results. This child is at highest risk for which of the following during his academic career?

A) School failure
B) Reading disability
C) Math disability
D) Grade retention
E) Anxiety disorder

13. Which of the following children is most likely to meet the full criteria for the diagnosis of mental retardation?

A) A 4-year-old boy with undiagnosed sensorineural hearing impairment and a full-scale IQ score of 66
B) A 4-year-old boy enrolled in "English as a second language" classes who is tested in English and has a full-scale IQ score of 64
C) A 5-year-old boy with fragile X syndrome and a full-scale IQ score of 63
D) A 3-year-old boy with isolated speech delay and a full-scale IQ score of 72
E) A 7-year-old boy with a 25-point discrepancy between his verbal and performance IQ scores

14. The mother of a 7-year-old boy reports that her son's teacher has suggested that the child be evaluated for ADHD. Educational testing through the public school system demonstrated that the child's IQ was "average," and he is currently passing all his subjects. She is interested in having the child tested. Which of the following is the most appropriate method for determining whether or not her son has ADHD?

A) Conners' Rating Scales for parents, teachers
B) Magnetic resonance imaging of the head
C) Computed tomography of the head
D) Patient history
E) Physical examination

15. The mother of a 5-year-old kindergartener brings you a report completed by the child's primary teacher. The teacher reports that the child is unable to sit still in class and constantly interrupts her. He has difficulty following directions and waiting his turn, and he talks incessantly. His mother reports the same behaviors at home. While the boy is in the office, he sits still on the examining table for the duration of the interview and cooperates with the physical examination, which is unremarkable. You would be correct in telling the mother all of the following regarding the diagnosis of ADHD EXCEPT:
A) Children with ADHD have poor impulse control.
B) Children with ADHD have an increased incidence of learning disabilities.
C) Children with ADHD may have average, below-average, or above-average intelligence.
D) Children with ADHD are most commonly diagnosed in the early elementary school years.
E) The diagnosis of ADHD rests on presence of disruptive behaviors in all settings.

16. Which of the following comorbid psychiatric conditions is most likely to be present in patients with ADHD?
A) Oppositional defiant disorder
B) Autism spectrum disorder
C) Substance abuse and addiction
D) Depression
E) Anxiety disorder

17. An 8-year-old boy has been sent home twice in the past month for disruptive behavior in class. His teacher says that he has difficulty completing his work in a timely fashion. Although his mother tries to help him with his homework, he is disinterested and distracted and usually takes several hours to complete his lessons. Which of the following is the most appropriate initial intervention in this child?
A) A 2-week trial of stimulant medication
B) Complete psychoeducational testing
C) Referral to a child psychiatrist
D) Vision and hearing screening
E) Magnetic resonance imaging of the brain

18. An 11-year-old sixth grader is having trouble with school. She is unable to finish her work on time in the classroom, and her teacher has to send work home with her on the weekends because she is unable to get her homework done during the week. Both the teacher and the girl's mother report that the patient has a short attention span, is forgetful and easily distracted, and has difficulty following directions and completing her work in a timely manner. She often misplaces her workbooks, coat, pencils, and backpack. She fidgets in her seat at school, but otherwise, her behavior is exemplary. Her grades have dropped from all A's and B's in fifth grade to mostly C's and D's in middle school. The girl's physical examination is within normal limits. This patient's clinical history is most characteristic of which of the following?
A) Dyslexia
B) ADHD
C) ADHD, predominantly inattentive type
D) Increased intracranial pressure
E) Global developmental delay

19. Your practice is interested in screening children for behavioral problems at each routine health maintenance visit. You would like a test that will provide standardized T-scores that you can compare with the norm, rather than one that has a single cut-off value for pass/fail. You plan on mailing a parent questionnaire to the parents the week before the visit. Your patient population is generally affluent and educated. Which of the following screening tools is most appropriate for use in your practice, given your stated preferences?
A) Child Behavioral Checklist
B) Child Developmental Inventory (abbreviated screening version)
C) Pediatric Symptom Checklist
D) Parents' Evaluation of Developmental Status
E) Conners' Rating Scales

20. Your clinic is interested in screening children for developmental delay and behavior problems at each visit. You prefer a short parent questionnaire that can be filled out quickly in the waiting room. The clinic serves mostly poor, inner-city families. Many of the parents are uneducated, and some are illiterate, so your staff will need to assist parents who have difficulty understanding and answering the questions. You would rather not have to specially train the staff to administer the test. Which of the following screening tools is most appropriate for your clinic, given your stated preferences?
A) Child Behavioral Checklist
B) Child Developmental Inventory (abbreviated screening version)
C) Pediatric Symptom Checklist
D) Conners' Rating Scales
E) Parents' Evaluation of Developmental Status

21. You have referred a 7-year-old child in your practice for complete neurobehavioral assessment. Results of the Wechsler Intelligence Scale–Third Edition (WAIS-III) include a full-scale IQ score of 85. Which of the following statements regarding this child's IQ score is CORRECT?

A) This child's IQ is one standard deviation above the mean, within the normal range.
B) This child's IQ is one standard deviation below the mean, outside the normal range.
C) This child's IQ is two standard deviations above the mean, outside the normal range.
D) This child's IQ is one standard deviation below the mean, within the normal range.
E) This child's IQ is two standard deviations below the mean, outside the normal range.

22. You have just diagnosed an 8-year-old boy with ADHD. His mother is extremely resistant to placing the boy on stimulant medication for his condition because there is a strong family history of substance abuse, including the boy's natural father. You would be correct in telling this mother all of the following EXCEPT:

A) Behavioral therapy alone is less effective than stimulant therapy alone.
B) The addition of behavioral therapy to stimulant therapy results in a significant decrease in core ADHD symptoms.
C) The chronic use of stimulants for the management of ADHD is not associated with the development of tolerance or dependence.
D) Approximately 75% of patients diagnosed with ADHD will experience significant reduction of core symptoms when placed on stimulant medication.
E) Atomoxetine is a nonstimulant medication approved for use in patients with ADHD.

23. Which of the following adverse effects of stimulant medications used for the treatment of attention deficit-hyperactivity disorder is not transient?

A) Exacerbation of tics
B) Headache
C) Appetite suppression
D) Nausea
E) All of these adverse effects are transient.

24. Adverse effects of grade retention include all of the following EXCEPT:

A) Negative attitudes toward school
B) Increased drop-out rate
C) Interruption of peer relationships
D) Social promotion
E) Low self-esteem

25. Patients who drop out of school are more likely than their peers:

A) to engage in risky sexual behavior and, if female, become pregnant as a teenager
B) to become juvenile delinquents
C) to abuse substances
D) to commit violent acts
E) All of the above

ANSWERS

1. A	10. E	19. A
2. B	11. A	20. E
3. C	12. B	21. D
4. D	13. C	22. B
5. E	14. D	23. C
6. A	15. E	24. D
7. B	16. A	25. E
8. C	17. B	
9. D	18. C	

Psychosocial Issues

28

PSYCHOSOCIAL NEEDS AND DEVELOPMENTAL STAGES

The Prenatal Visit

The American Academy of Pediatrics has set forth five objectives that should be addressed during the prenatal visit:

- Formation of a relationship between the physician and the parents. Parents are introduced to the concept of a medical home for their child. Establishing a rapport with the parents before birth is particularly beneficial when a medical crisis during late pregnancy, birth, or early infancy requires parental counseling and intervention by the pediatrician.
- Collection of basic information from the parents, including ages and occupations, general health, cultural beliefs, parental experiences and expectations, expected impact of the birth on the marriage, reactions of siblings (if any), and child care arrangements.
- Preventive counseling and anticipatory guidance regarding newborn behavior; hospital care of the newborn; risks and benefits of circumcision and control of pain during the procedure; options for infant feeding; benefits of breastfeeding and lactation support services within the office and community; proper and consistent use of infant car seats; and instructions for the timing and scheduling of the first pediatric office visit. The prenatal visit also provides an opportunity to advise the mother about fetal effects of maternal ingestion of alcohol, cigarette smoking, drug use, and poor nutrition.
- Encouragement of positive parenting skills involves helping parents strategize about needs, potential sources of maternal or familial support during the perinatal period and early infancy, division of child care responsibilities, work schedules, and responses to anticipated stressors.
- Identification of risk factors, including but not limited to the following: single mother; adolescent parent(s); history of domestic violence; history of substance abuse; social support (community, extended family); and family medical and personal health histories of the parents. When risk factors are identified, appropriate referrals should be secured.

The Perinatal Period

Maternal-infant bonding is discussed in Chapter 5. Factors which promote effective bonding include early and frequent skin-to-skin contact, placement at the breast in the delivery room, and hospital rooming-in. However, successful maternal-infant bonding can still be achieved when these conditions are not met. A significant minority of women report that they feel bonded to their infant prior to birth. Many parents develop an emotional attachment to their infants during pregnancy. Loss of the child due to fetal demise, early neonatal death, or adoption can provoke significant and sometimes unexpected grief responses. Allowing the parent to see and hold the infant, if desired, may assist in the initial stages and eventual resolution of the mourning process.

Mothers who fail to bond with their infants report feeling indifferent, ambivalent, or hostile toward the child. In rare cases, these emotions may be manifested through neglect or physical abuse of the child. Mothers who suffer from postpartum depression or psychosis and those who experience severe pain during labor are at increased risk for disordered infant attachment.

Postpartum depression is the development of symptoms of a depressive or bipolar disorder within 4 weeks of delivery. Postpartum depression occurs in up to 15% of mothers; postpartum psychosis is much less common. Both conditions disproportionately affect women who suffer from depression before and during their pregnancies. Maternal depression has been shown to impact the cognitive and social development and behavior of infants as young as three months of age (increased fussiness, disordered sleep, feeding difficulties; social withdrawal). The most significant long-term sequelae appear to be associated with insecure attachment. Bonding between the mother and the infant establishes learned attachment patterns that persist throughout life. Pediatricians are in a unique position to assist mothers with postpartum depression by:

- asking all mothers about their attachment to their infants
- identifying mothers who seem to be having difficulty coping with the responsibilities of caring for the infant
- recognizing signs and symptoms associated with depressive disorders
- providing referrals to mental health specialists for evaluation and treatment

- serving as a reliable source of information regarding the effects of maternal psychoactive medication on the breastfeeding infant

The birth of multiples may provoke feelings of guilt when parents become more attached to one infant than the other(s). However, this variable attachment is normal, particularly when one infant requires more intensive medical care than the other. Caring for multiple infants is particularly demanding, both physically and emotionally. Parents of multiples report higher parental stress levels; these families are at increased risk for domestic violence, substance abuse, and divorce. Postpartum depression is also more common in mothers of multiple infants.

Although partners of adolescent mothers may themselves be minors or adults, as a group they are more likely to earn low wages, drop out of school, and have poor parenting skills. The adult fathers are more likely than their adolescent counterparts to remain involved in raising the child and supporting the family financially. Still, more than half of *adolescent fathers* participate in child rearing. Factors associated with increased rates of sustained paternal involvement include attendance at prenatal visits, presence during labor, participation in the delivery room, and performance of caregiving activities in the hospital.

Infancy

Crying is a normal behavior in newborns, yet many new parents are surprised by how much their infants cry. Up to 2 hours of crying a day is normal for neonates; the duration increases by 6 weeks of age to almost 3 hours a day. Colic, which is associated with significant crying between the ages of 6 to 12 weeks, is a syndrome of recurrent irritability that begins acutely and persists for several hours, usually in the late afternoons or evenings. During the attacks, the infant cries inconsolably and may draw the knees to the abdomen. The crying resolves as suddenly and spontaneously as it begins. When the history is consistent with typical infant crying or colic, parents should be reassured that the behavior is normal, counseled in methods of providing comfort to the child, and offered strategies for coping with associated parental stress.

Observation of the interaction between the mother and her infant provides insight into security of attachment and maternal attitudes regarding appropriate care of the child. Feeding not only provides adequate nutrition for growth and development; it also serves as a mutually enjoyable activity and promotes successful bonding. Mothers who engage in inappropriate feeding behaviors, such as using the bottle to quiet the infant who is not hungry and propping the bottle in the infant's mouth without supervision demonstrate poor parenting skills, incomplete understanding of the needs of the child, and/or disordered attachment. Referral for social work evaluation and intervention should be considered in these cases.

Infants and toddlers often engage in rhythmic movements in order to calm themselves. Examples include sucking the thumb and head banging. Head banging may provoke significant parental anxiety. It is more common in boys, usually beginning after the age of 6 months and resolving during the preschool years. Although the behavior is frequently observed in children with developmental disorders, particularly mental retardation and autism spectrum disorder, a significant percentage of typically developing children also engage in head banging. When growth and development are normal, no intervention is warranted beyond counseling the patients to respond by ignoring the behavior or distracting the child. In rare cases, rhythmic behavior may be associated with visual or hearing impairment or may actually represent self-stimulatory behavior in a neglected child.

The Preschool Years

A child is considered toilet trained when he or she has full voluntary control of bowel and bladder function without periodic involuntary soiling. Children become trained at different ages in different cultures. As a group, girls achieve continence a few months earlier than boys. In the United States, about 25% of toddlers are fully toilet trained by age 24 months; this rises to over 95% by 48 months of age. Regardless of cultural norms, children are developmentally ready to begin toilet training when they:

- develop an interest in toilet training
- achieve voluntary control over bladder and bowel function
- can walk to and sit on the toilet without assistance
- can follow two-step commands
- can communicate their need to toilet with words or gestures

Children who are not motivated to learn to use the toilet will often resist parents' efforts. Such resistance should be managed with a break in toilet training until the child expresses an interest. Forcing the child to sit on the toilet for extended periods of time against his or her will precipitates anxiety regarding toileting issues and is rarely successful.

Girls who have not achieved daytime dryness by 4 years of age, and boys by 5 years of age, warrant medical evaluation (see Chapter 16). The management of enuresis is provided in Chapter 16; encopresis, the voluntary withholding of stool with eventual soiling, is discussed in Chapter 12.

Masturbation occurs at all ages but is most prevalent in preschool-age children and adolescents. Young children have an innate curiosity about their own bodies and the bodies of their parents. They may stimulate their genitals with their hands or by rubbing against objects. Masturbation occurs less frequently, and is less overt, in older children prior to the onset of puberty. During adolescence, masturbation becomes more frequent and often results in ejaculation or orgasm. While masturbation is considered a normal behavior, masturbation in public suggests poor awareness of social and cultural norms. Public masturbation in young children is best managed by ignoring or redirecting behavior; punishment should be avoided.

Masturbation which is excessive, compulsive, or injurious must be addressed. Abnormal patterns of masturbation may be associated with irritation of the external genital regions or urethra, vaginal foreign bodies, sexual overstimulation, neglect, or abuse. When masturbation is associated with preexisting genital irritation, treatment of the inflammation may stop the behavior. Masturbation which simulates intercourse in a preschool-age child is strongly suggestive of abuse and warrants referral to local child protective service agencies.

Breath holding spells are paroxysmal episodes that may resemble seizures. The typical presentation involves a child 2 to 3 years of age who begins crying in response to being hurt or frustrated. The child appears to develop trouble breathing, followed by color changes (pallor or cyanosis) and loss of consciousness. The episodes are brief, with return to baseline less than a minute later. Rarely, tonic movements may be noted while the child is limp; their presence has no medical significance, and they are not associated with an increased risk of future epilepsy. Most affected children have no more than a few episodes a month. Parents are taught to modify their reactions in order to discourage the behavior and reward more appropriate expressions of frustration. The condition is typically outgrown by kindergarten.

Sibling rivalry is inevitable. The anticipation of a new baby may result in feelings of insecurity in an existing child; older child may become afraid that something bad will happen to the mother while she is giving birth. Developmental regression is common in younger children. Rarely, a sibling may become physically aggressive toward the infant. Children who are prepared for the arrival of the new baby, allowed to participate in the care of the infant, praised for showing affection toward the infant, and provided adequate time alone with the mother are more likely to accept the new sibling without incident.

Temper tantrums are observed in virtually all children between the ages of 1 to 3 years. Tantrums which occur no more than twice a day in response to an identifiable trigger in a developmentally typical child do not warrant further investigation. Parents should be counseled in behavioral techniques to discourage tantrums and reward more appropriate behavior (Table 28-1). Once learned, these same strategies can be applied to other "problem" behaviors (e.g., hitting, biting). "Time-out" can be used in children as young as 18 to 24 months of age. The child is separated and placed in a chair with no interaction for the duration of the time out (generally 1 minute per year of age). The child is allowed to resume the activity at the end of the time-out as long as he or she has remained in the chair. As with most forms of behavioral intervention, the behavior which prompts the correction will initially increase in frequency prior to extinction.

Pediatricians can be a valuable resource for parents by promoting effective, developmentally-appropriate discipline strategies which increase good behaviors, minimize inappropriate behaviors, and maintain healthy parent-child relationships. Infants benefit from daily structure, which teaches rhythm and predictability. Parents of toddlers should be clear and consistent in communicating expectations and reinforcing good behavior. School-age children can generalize rules to apply to various situations and accept responsibility for their actions. During adolescence, the individual begins to understand the benefits of rules within a society and becomes capable of extrapolating the consequences of personal behavior on oneself and others.

TABLE 28-1
SUCCESSFUL MANAGEMENT OF TEMPER TANTRUMS (AND OTHER PROBLEM BEHAVIORS)

- Prevent temper tantrums by structuring the child's environment to eliminate the most common precipitating conditions (hunger from missed mealtimes; inadequate sleep; expectations beyond developmental age).
- Formulate and communicate consequences of inappropriate behavior.
- Consistently enforce stated consequences, and communicate consequences to all caregivers to ensure uniform responses.
- React calmly.
- Do not reinforce the behavior by giving in to the child's demands.
- Do not punish the child.
- Ignore tantrum behavior, understanding that the tantrums may initially become more frequent.
- Provide positive reinforcement when the child reacts to frustration in an appropriate manner (praise, encouragement, tangible rewards).
- Remove positive reinforcement when the child initiates tantrum behavior.
- Allow the child to experience the natural consequences of his or her behavior (within reason).

Middle Childhood

Fear is a normal and adaptive emotional response to a perceived threat. Typical childhood fears vary according to age; overall, children become less fearful as they grow older. Unrealistic fears which are persistent and debilitating are termed phobias. Phobias can be categorized as specific, social, or agoraphobic (Table 28-2). Phobias are more common in children who have experienced a traumatic event, witnessed fear in their adult caregivers, or been repeatedly subjected to graphic warnings.

Normal childhood fears are managed with reassurance. Discussions with the child may reveal the origin of the fear and the reasoning behind it. Avoidance of the stimulus is appropriate when this does not interfere with activities of daily living (e.g., fear of fireworks). Fears related to physical harm should be thoroughly evaluated and investigated, with involvement of local child protective service agencies if indicated.

Children with specific phobias may respond to graded exposure to the stimulus in a safe environment with the

TABLE 28-2
CATEGORIES OF CHILDHOOD PHOBIAS

Specific Phobias
- Excessive fear of a specific object or situation which impairs functioning and persists for longer than 6 months
- Exposure to the stimulus results in the immediate onset of significant anxiety, characterized by distress, crying, attempted escape, tachycardia, hypertension, and sweating
- Typical onset in childhood

Social Phobia
- Excessive fear associated with anticipated social functions or performance situations which significantly impairs functioning and persists for longer than 6 months
- Thinking about or engaging in the behavior precipitates an anxiety reaction
- May be associated with school refusal
- Typical onset in adolescence
- Attempted self-medication may lead to alcohol or substance use/abuse

Agoraphobia
- Excessive fear of places or situations from which escape might be difficult, embarrassing, or impossible
- Typical onset in early adulthood but may present in adolescence
- Often accompanied by panic disorder

support of a parent. Positive reinforcement is provided for progressive desensitization. Patients with specific phobias which persist despite attempted intervention warrant referral for specialized therapy, which is also indicated for patients with social and agoraphobia. Patients who suffer from phobias often have one or more comorbid psychiatric conditions, including anxiety disorders, obsessive-compulsive disorder, and post-traumatic stress disorder.

Parents of patients in late childhood and early adolescence should be provided with age-appropriate materials for talking with their children about pubertal development and sexual health. Parents who do not allow their children to participate in sexual health educational programs may be under the mistaken impression that these programs encourage early sexual activity. Abstinence-only programs are not effective in delaying the average age of first sexual intercourse. Children in this age range should also be provided with information regarding pregnancy and STD prevention.

Involvement in structured extracurricular activities during the middle school years has a positive impact on self-esteem and social development. Participation in sports provides exercise, fosters motivation, and teaches children to support one another and work together to achieve a goal. Music lessons improve concentration and spatial reasoning. Scouting encourages multiple interests and rewards personal effort and achievement. Children who are provided with opportunities to learn about and experience things outside the classroom secure valuable real-world skills and develop life-long interests. Parents can assist their children in these endeavors by offering diverse participation choices and encouraging children to pursue activities they enjoy. On the other hand, children this age need unstructured time built into their day as well. Overscheduling places the child under stress and may lead to diminished motivation, generalized anxiety, or depression.

An IQ in excess of 130 points qualifies a child as cognitively gifted. Giftedness in other areas (music, artistic ability, athleticism) is less clearly defined but may be just as challenging for the family. Gifted children often have a great deal of energy and curiosity and may manifest behaviors consistent with attention-deficit/hyperactivity disorder when they are not appropriately challenged. The enrichment of gifted children through extracurricular activities and opportunities may place a financial burden on the family and/or consume a great deal of one or both of the parents' time. Treatment which is viewed as preferential by siblings or a spouse fosters resentment and increases interpersonal stress. Some parents begin to allow the child to make decisions for the family, despite an obvious lack of maturity. It is not uncommon for a child who excels in one subject, say math, to have reading abilities closer to those of his peers. Gifted children who skip grades or are advanced in specific subjects may make friends with grade-level but significantly older students; however, a seventh grader who is studying tenth grade math still has the physical, emotional, and social abilities of a seventh grader. Other forms of enrichment include honors classes, acceleration programs, and correspondence and Internet courses.

Adolescence

Few parents are genuinely comfortable discussing issues related to sex, substance use, and risk-taking behaviors with their adolescent children. Given that the onset of adolescence is associated with increased irritability, furtiveness, and heightened sensitivity to embarrassment, adolescents are generally wary of broaching these subjects with their parents as well. Adolescents are more likely to seek information about sexuality from peers, the media, and the internet; adults in authority are rarely consulted voluntarily. However, adolescents do view parents and health care professionals as reliable sources of information regarding sexual health. Age-appropriate discussion of pubertal development and sexual topics should take place at every routine adolescent health maintenance visit. Parents should be encouraged to talk with their adolescent children about their values and expectations; provision of accurate information within the context of these discussions provides adolescents with the tools to make responsible, well-informed choices. Other ways that parents can promote responsible sexual behavior in their adolescent children are provided in Table 28-3.

Sexual experimentation, both same-sex and opposite gender, is a normal adolescent behavior in individuals of all sexual orientations. Most people develop an awareness of their sexual orientation during adolescence, if not before. Homosexual youths often experience a period of confusion regarding sexual identity. Sexual orientation, whether heterosexual or homosexual, is not a choice; it is an inherent and enduring individual property. In contrast, sexual behavior is voluntary.

TABLE 28-3
PREVENTING TEENAGE PREGNANCY: PARENTAL STRATEGIES

Develop close relationships with your children throughout childhood.

Show your children that you value education.

Assist your children in envisioning a personal future which is more attractive than early parenthood.

Provide your children with appropriate supervision.

Monitor your children's activities, including their music, internet use, and television viewing.

Get to know your children's friends and their families.

Discourage early, exclusive dating.

Source: National Campaign to Reduce Teen Pregnancy (www.teenpregnancy.org).

Adolescents who engage in sexual activity with same-gender peers may or may not be homosexual. Homosexual adolescents who refrain from sexual activity with same-gender peers may defer expression of their sexual orientation until adulthood or indefinitely.

Homosexual males are at increased risk for adverse outcomes during adolescence. They are more likely to be physically threatened, drop out of school, use and abuse substances, attempt suicide, and experience homelessness.

Antisocial behavior may be noted in children but usually develops during adolescence. Antisocial behavior (actions which demonstrate a lack of regard for others) is much more common than antisocial personality disorder. Behaviors which are characterized as antisocial include property damage, stealing, engaging in activities which place others in danger, and lying to or conning others for personal enjoyment or benefit. Adolescents who engage in antisocial behavior are more likely than their peers to:

- have low self-esteem
- have difficulty tolerating frustration
- have school failure
- be truant

Antisocial behavior may indicate an underlying psychiatric diagnosis, such as depressive disorders, anxiety disorders, or psychosis. While it may be difficult to distinguish "normal" adolescent rebellion from antisocial behavior, patients who frequently lie and steal, whose behaviors result in physical harm to others, who do not express remorse or a desire to change, and who continue to engage in the behaviors into adulthood are more likely to meet the diagnostic criteria for antisocial personality disorder.

Critical Events in the Life of the Family

Divorce and the Blended Family

Divorce is an emotionally, socially, psychologically, and financially stressful event in the life of the family. The child's reaction to divorce depends on individual characteristics and situational factors (Table 28-4). The adequacy of the child's emotional adjustment to divorce appears to have a persistent effect on subsequent relationships. Children from divorced and blended families are more likely to manifest psychosocial and behavioral difficulties than children of intact families, especially in the first few years after the divorce or remarriage.

TABLE 28-4
FACTORS WHICH AFFECT A CHILD'S RESPONSE TO DIVORCE AND REMARRIAGE

Individual Characteristics

- Children with easy, resilient temperaments and good self-esteem generally experience less difficulty adjusting to divorce and remarriage.
- Children with difficult, resistant temperaments and poor self-esteem generally have more difficulty adjusting to divorce and remarriage.
- The age of the child at the time of divorce is a less significant determinant of adjustment than other individual and situational characteristics.
- Internalizing behaviors such as sad affect, frequent crying, and somatic complaints are more common in adolescents following divorce.
- Externalizing behaviors such as acting out and physical and verbal aggression are more common in adolescents following divorce.
- Children in early adolescence tend to be more resistant to remarriage and participation in a blended family than younger children and older adolescents.

Situation Characteristics

- Parental characteristics which affect a child's reaction to divorce include the adjustment of the parent, the communication style of the parent (withdrawn vs. communicative), and the mental health of the parent.
- The spirit of the divorce impacts the children as well (mutual, one-sided, acrimonious)
- Anticipated changes in the family, including financial losses, necessity of moving, and decreased contact with a parent should also be considered.

Various custodial arrangements may be ordered by the court. The most common are sole custody (a single custodial parent with visitation rights permitted to the second parent) and joint custody. The adjustment of the child appears to be related less to the type of custody than to the presence or absence of consistent involvement with a supportive, well-adjusted, authoritative parent.

The effects of divorce and remarriage on children and adolescents appear to persist into adulthood, being more pronounced in those who have more difficulty adjusting initially. As adults, these individuals report less stable and satisfying intimate relationships and more problems with family and workplace relationships. Divorce rates are higher in children from divorced families.

Death of a Family Member

A child's response to a death in the family varies depending on his or her developmental stage (Table 28-5). Death of an immediate family member results in grieving and

TABLE 28-5
THE CHILD'S RESPONSE TO DEATH

Age: Birth to 2 years

- Experiences death as abandonment
- Disruption of bonds of attachment

Age: 2 to 6 years

- Death considered temporary, reversible
- Child may believe that the death occurred because of something the child did, said, or thought
- Child may express anger toward the person who died

Age: Middle childhood

- Understands that death is final and irreversible
- May begin to fear that other close contacts and family members will die
- May develop psychosomatic complaints

Age: Adolescence

- Understands that death is universal and inevitable
- Grieves for the loss of the comfort of the relationship

stress in the remaining family members. The pediatrician can provide valuable assistance during times of loss by contacting the family, explaining how death of a sibling or parent affects the child, offering support and assistance, and following up with the family at regular intervals.

Psychosomatic Disorders

Young children frequently experience and communicate stress through somatic symptoms, such as "stomachache" or "headache." As they age, complaints such as fatigue, insomnia, pain in the extremities, and neurologic deficits become more common. Somatization is thought to be a learned behavior. Children in families who are uncomfortable discussing negative feelings gain more attention and sympathy from their caregivers for complaining of a stomachache than for expressing their anxiety or disappointment. Chronic pain disorder is a form of somatization characterized by persistent pain rather than physical impairment. In other cases, the child is unconsciously modeling the behavior of an ill family member. Somatization disorders are more common when children experience excessive parental pressure to perform and achieve. High parental anxiety and prior physical or sexual abuse also increase the likelihood of somatization disorders.

Conversion disorder is diagnosed when: motor and/or sensory symptoms suggest a medical condition, but clinical and investigative findings do not conform to any known anatomic or physiologic disorder; the symptoms result in functional impairment; the symptoms are not feigned (as opposed to malingering); and the onset or exacerbation of symptoms follows a readily identifiable psychosocial stressor. In children with existing disease, conversion disorder manifests as physical impairment which is markedly out of proportion to the severity of the illness. In some cases, the functional impairment clearly symbolizes the precipitating stressor. Invariably, the child's behavior is reinforced through both primary (avoidance of the stressor) and secondary (increased parental attention; decreased school attendance) rewards. Children with conversion disorder often demonstrate "la belle indifference," or complete lack of distress related to their functional loss.

Somatization disorders should be differentiated from other psychiatric conditions, including psychosis, malingering, anxiety disorder, Munchausen syndrome by proxy, and undiagnosed organic disease.

Most children with conversion disorder and their families benefit from consultation with a pediatric mental health specialist. Successful management begins with reassuring the family that there is no underlying physical malady, empathizing with the emotional distress of the family, and formation of a physician-parent management partnership. Laboratory and radiographic testing should be kept to a minimum so as to avoid reinforcing the idea that the child is an invalid. The precipitating stressor should be addressed, and the parents should be counseled in behavioral responses that remove secondary gain. Finally, the child should be offered a method of recovery which maintains personal dignity (i.e., administering a harmless "placebo" treatment, or telling the child that the condition will resolve within a week). Success is measured by the child's return to normal functioning and routine activities, not necessarily by resolution of the symptoms. Patients should be screened for comorbid conditions (mood, anxiety disorders) and treated, if indicated. Pharmacologic intervention is reserved for somatization disorders which result in significant impairment and persist for longer than 3 months.

Separation Anxiety Disorder and School Refusal

Separation anxiety is a normal developmental finding from the age of 9 months throughout the preschool years. Children beginning kindergarten often experience mild separation anxiety, which resolves over the first several weeks. When anxiety regarding separation from a parent or caregiver becomes excessive, persistent, and begins to interfere with school attendance and activities outside the home, the individual is diagnosed with separation anxiety disorder. New diagnoses peak between ages 7 to 9 years, but the disorder may begin at any age. Some cases are acute in onset and associated with an obvious triggering event; others develop insidiously. Separation anxiety disorder is a chronic, waxing and waning condition in many patients. Symptoms often recur following a break from school.

Although multifactorial in origin, separation anxiety disorder appears to have a strong heritable component. At least one half of children with separation anxiety disorder are eventually diagnosed with a second anxiety condition, most frequently panic disorder. Depressive disorders are also more common in children with separation anxiety disorder. Environmental conditions which may predispose to the disorder include inadvertent or purposeful parental reinforcement of the anxiety and being raised in a "sheltered" manner which does not permit sufficient opportunity to experience safe separation from the parent. The differential diagnosis of school refusal includes separation anxiety disorder as well as social phobia, agoraphobia, depression, school failure, substance abuse, and conduct disorder. School refusal due to truancy can usually be readily differentiated from separation anxiety disorder. Anxiety regarding separation from the caregiver is the predominant feature of separation anxiety disorder; truancy is usually accompanied by other manifestations of oppositional defiant disorder or conduct disorder.

Many patients with separation anxiety disorder recover completely; however, the condition often persists for years and may be refractory to therapy. Evaluation of separation anxiety disorder begins with the history, including family history of psychiatric disorders; social history; recognition of sources of family and child stress; and identification and quantification of maladaptive behaviors associated with the anxiety. In affected children, the anxiety provoked by separation begins to diminish shortly after the separation occurs; therefore, the most effective method of reversing school refusal in these patients involves returning them to school and immediately withdrawing the parent from the scene. A mental health specialist can teach the child to recognize the physical sensations associated with anxiety and to employ cognitive therapy techniques in managing their fears. Selective serotonin reuptake inhibitors (e.g., fluoxetine, fluvoxamine) have proven beneficial in patients with comorbid anxiety disorders.

Psychotic Behavior and Thought Disorders

Schizophrenia is a psychotic disorder characterized by paranoid delusions, hallucinations (usually auditory), incongruous speech, catatonic or illogical behavior, and extreme social dysfunction. Symptoms are initially noted in late adolescence or early adulthood, and the onset may be abrupt or gradually progressive. Parents often explain away early signs as normal adolescent behavior. Schizophrenia has a strong heritable component; it is as much as ten times more common in first-degree relatives of affected patients than in the general population. Research into possible environmental triggers is ongoing.

Suicide

Suicide is the third leading cause of death among adolescents in the United States. More females attempt suicide, but more males die as a result of their attempts. The ratio of suicide attempts to suicide deaths is between 10- and 30-to-1. Risk factors which increase the likelihood that an adolescent will attempt suicide are listed in Table 28-6. Warning signs are provided in Table 28-7. Any form of self-inflicted harm in children and adolescents may be a sign of attempted suicide or a suicidal gesture. Suicidal behavior, even when interpreted as part of a suicidal gesture, must be taken seriously; suicidal gestures may result in unintentional death. Any patient who has attempted suicide requires at least a brief inpatient hospital stay for psychiatric evaluation. Inpatient psychiatric treatment is indicated for patients who:

- have attempted suicide in a highly lethal manner
- have a history of prior suicide attempt(s)
- would be returning to an environment in which their safety could not be assured
- are personally unlikely, and have parents who are unlikely, to carry through on recommended therapies
- do not deny that they wish to hurt themselves
- are uncommunicative
- are psychotic
- have obsessive thoughts that they cannot control

TABLE 28-6
RISK FACTORS FOR SUICIDE ATTEMPT AND SUICIDE COMPLETION IN THE ADOLESCENT

Factors Which Increase the Risk of Suicide Attempt
Suicidal ideation
Prior suicide attempt
Depression
Substance abuse
History of attention-deficit/hyperactivity disorder
History of conduct disorder
Family history of mental illness
Family history of attempted or completed suicide
Family discord
Victim or witness of domestic violence
History of physical or sexual abuse
Homosexual orientation
Presence of a firearm in the home
Presence of a triggering event
Factors Which Increase the Likelihood of Death from Suicide
Prior suicide attempt
Attempting suicide by jumping or shooting oneself
Attempting suicide at a time and in a place in which the likelihood of discovery and resuscitation are minimal
Clear evidence of a mental or substance abuse disorder

Vulnerable Child Syndrome

Vulnerable child syndrome is a disorder in which the parents of a healthy child view him or her as unusually susceptible to physical disease, psychobehavioral disorders, or developmental abnormalities. This distorted belief may begin in the newborn period when the infant is the product of a difficult pregnancy, labor, and/or delivery. Other factors that predispose to the development of vulnerable child syndrome include fertility problems, preterm birth, postpartum depression, presence of a physical or mental impairment,

TABLE 28-7
POTENTIAL WARNING SIGNS OF SUICIDE IN THE ADOLESCENT

Changes in Affect
Sadness
Withdrawal
Loss of interest in activities
Irritability
Agitation

Changes in Behavior
Motor restlessness
Changes in activity level
Changes in eating habits
Changes in social behavior
Use/abuse of substances

Changes in Functioning
Fatigue
Disordered sleep
Loss of appetite

Warning Statements
Statements of hopelessness ("Nothing can change the way I feel.")
Statements of loneliness ("No one understands me.")
Statements of emptiness ("Life doesn't seem worth living.")
Distorted perception ("My family would be better off without me.")
Statements expressing a wish to harm oneself

history of serious illness in the child, history of a life-threatening or "near-miss" injury, and generalized heightened parental anxiety. In vulnerable child syndrome, excessive parental concern is manifested through frequent doctor visits, requests for medical tests and services, parental anxiety with separation, overprotectiveness, and difficulty setting limits on the child's behavior. Timely intervention and anticipatory guidance can ameliorate parental anxiety and prevent the development of vulnerable child syndrome in many cases. Parents who are at risk for the disorder should be educated in the natural history of vulnerable child syndrome. Parental emotions such as anxiety, dread, fear, and helplessness are natural after a medical illness or injury that is perceived as life-threatening. However, viewing the child as "fragile," sheltering the child, and treating the child in a special or preferential manner are ultimately harmful to both the child and the family unit. Parents should be advised to return to normal family life as soon as possible. Families who have difficulty recovering warrant referral to social services or support groups.

Chronic Illness and Handicapping Conditions

The impact of physical/cognitive impairments and chronic illnesses is not limited to the affected child; the emotional and financial cost is shared by the entire family. Parents of a child with a handicapping condition progress through a fairly predictable cycle of grief (anger, denial, depression). They grieve for the suffering of their child, the loss of the "normal" child, and the changes they anticipate in their lives and the lives of their other children. The rate of progression varies among people; it is normal for one parent to be angry when the other is in denial or depressed. Chronic illnesses and physical/cognitive impairments in a child produce significant stress within the family, leading to higher rates of parental divorce and depression. Siblings are affected by the financial burden of the disease and by the diminished time and emotional energy their parents have to offer them. Pediatricians can assist in this time of adjustment by listening empathetically, assessing the psychosocial needs of the parents and the family as a whole, and referring the family to grief counselors, clergy, organized groups of similarly-affected parents, and medical specialists who can provide information to help them understand the disease and plan for the future. They should also recognize typical transitional periods during which the child and family would benefit from additional evaluation and support, such as when progression of the child's illness requires the addition of medical services or when the child enters kindergarten, middle school, and high school.

Parents may become frustrated with the dearth of therapeutic options available for their child in traditional medicine. It is not unusual for parents to turn to alternative or complementary medicine for additional treatment of the child's condition. They may feel the need to try "everything" that could possibly help their child, or they may be impressed by promises of rapid improvement. Pediatricians should ask whether the parents are considering or undergoing alternative therapies for their child. Primary care physicians can serve as a valuable source of reliable information regarding scientific evidence or lack thereof, risk-benefit ratios, and potential for harm. For example, many dietary interventions have been touted as beneficial for reducing symptoms and improving behavior in patients with attention-deficit/hyperactivity disorder, and activities such as visual training, patterning, and sensory integration are often "recommended" for children with developmental impairments. To date, no sound, peer-reviewed scientific studies have proven the efficacy of any of these treatments.

Domestic Violence

Domestic violence refers to violence against an intimate partner. The cycle of battery usually consists of building tension, a precipitant event, physical battery, a honeymoon period, and increasing tension, which begins another cycle. Pregnancy, attempts to leave the home, and initiation of divorce are important precipitants of the violence, but there are many others. Children who live in a home with intimate partner violence have a 30% to 60% chance of being physically abused themselves. Though domestic violence is found in families of all ethnicities and socioeconomic levels, it is more likely in families:

- of a low socioeconomic class
- that are under significant stress
- in which the caregivers use/alcohol or drugs
- in which the mother's partner is not the biological father of the child
- in which the mother has a psychiatric disorder

Domestic violence should be suspected whenever a woman presents with acute injuries, particularly broken teeth, black eyes, ruptured tympanic membranes, and bruising in typically low-trauma areas; injuries which result in fetal trauma or endanger a pregnancy; substance abuse; or depression. In addition to their risk of being intentionally abused, children in homes with domestic violence can be injured while trying to protect a parent or simply because they are standing in the wrong place at the wrong time. Even in children who are not physically injured, the psychosocial impact of witnessing repeated domestic violence is significant. The overwhelming majority of affected children meet the diagnostic criteria for post-traumatic stress disorder, including reliving the experience in their minds or dreams and maintaining a heightened state of vigilance (evidenced by difficulty sleeping and poor concentration). They are also more likely that their peers to suffer from depression, psychosomatic disorders, learning disabilities, and school failure; to abuse substances; to commit violent physical and sexual acts; and to attempt suicide. Pediatricians are often in a position to screen families for domestic violence in the home. Battered partners should be assisted in locating and accessing support services to ensure their safety and that of their children.

Child Neglect and Abuse

Neglect

Adults may harm children through physical abuse, sexual abuse, psychological (emotional) abuse, and neglect. More children are neglected than abused. Children are considered neglected when the following needs are not met:

- Physical (food, clothing, shelter)
- Medical (routine immunizations, evaluation and treatment for illness)
- Emotional (communication, attachment, cognitive stimulation)
- Educational
- Protective (inadequate supervision)

Neglect is more common in the settings of poverty, parental substance abuse, domestic violence, and limited parental intelligence. Child neglect is the most common cause of primarily nonorganic failure to thrive, characterized by inadequate weight gain with relative sparing of height and head circumference. Infants and young children who are neglected develop impaired attachment and demonstrable delays in language and cognition. They may present with blunted affects or with levels of compliance that are markedly inconsistent with their developmental ages (e.g., a toddler who remains still and quiet for the entire examination, including otoscopy). They are more likely to engage in repetitive, stereotypic behaviors such as rocking for self-stimulation. Older children may be socially withdrawn and have learning disorders.

Child Abuse

Injuries intentionally perpetrated by a caretaker that result in morbidity or mortality constitute physical abuse. Child abuse occurs worldwide among all ethnic groups and socioeconomic classes. The abuse is a related caregiver in 90% of cases. Both abusive and neglectful parents may have severely unrealistic standards for their children's behavior due to ignorance of normal infant and childhood development. Abuse rates are highest in children under the age of 3 years; children under 12 months of age suffer the highest mortality rates, usually resulting from severe intracranial injuries. Siblings of abused children are at increased risk of abuse. Other factors which increase the risk of abuse are listed in Table 28-8. A precipitating event, be it a family crisis or an innocent behavior on the part of the child, serves as the trigger for physical abuse in the setting of these risk factors.

TABLE 28-8
RISK FACTORS FOR CHILD ABUSE

Characteristics of the Child
Physical impairment
Developmental disability
Chronic illness
Product of an unwanted pregnancy
Premature birth
Difficult temperament
Hyperactivity
Behavior disorder

Characteristics of the Parent
History of abuse as a child
Adolescent parent(s)
Substance abuse
Mental illness
Limited cognitive abilities
Inadequate coping mechanisms
Emotional immaturity

Characteristics of the Family
Poverty
Isolation/poor social supports
Family stressors (e.g., unemployment)
Domestic violence
Single parenthood
Multiple births
Multiple young children

Characteristics of the Environment
High poverty rate
High unemployment rate
High rates of violence
High rates of substance use/abuse

Abuse should be considered part of the differential diagnosis whenever a child presents with a traumatic injury. Features of the presentation that are associated with an increased likelihood of physical abuse include:

- injury that is inconsistent with the stated mechanism of injury
- injury that is highly unlikely given the child's developmental stage
- history that changes or evolves over time
- delay in seeking medical attention
- inappropriate affect of the caregiver
- injuries of increasing frequency and/or severity over time
- history of prior investigation by local child protective service agencies

Visible physical findings consistent with abuse are found in the overwhelming majority of affected children. Such signs may include bruises and abrasions in typically low-trauma regions (abdomen, buttocks, ears); burns; identifiable object marks (Fig. 28-1); and bite, pinch, or ligature marks. The dating of bruises is inexact; in general, bruises which are yellow, brown, or green are older and therefore unlikely to be due to acute injury.

The physician should be familiar with the presentations of conditions which may appear similar to abuse. Children with von Willebrand disease bruise easily and may have bruises in various stages of healing. Mongolian spots, linear or circular bruises associated with coining or cupping, eczema, and urticaria pigmentosa may all be mistaken for abusive injuries. Lesions caused by bullous impetigo, scalded skin syndrome, and toxic epidermal necrolysis may look like intentional burn injuries (see Chapter 29).

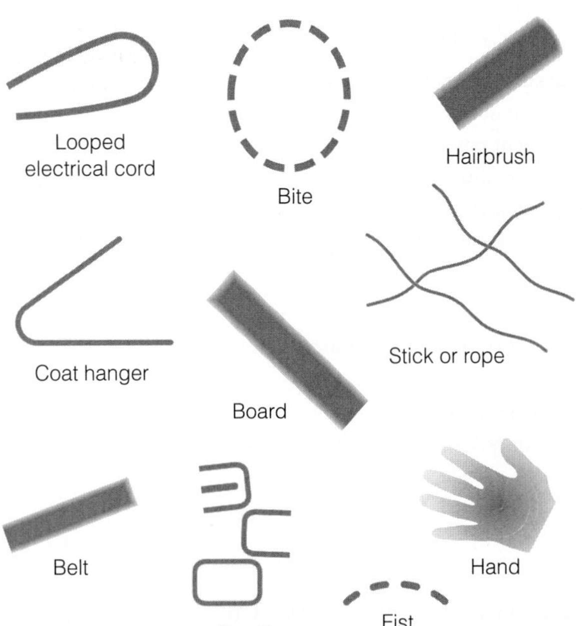

Figure 28-1 Body marks consistent with physical abuse. (From Marino BS, Fine KS. *Blueprints Pediatrics*. 4th ed. Philadelphia: Lippincott Williams & Wilkins; 2006 with permission.)

While most incidences of child abuse do not result in bony fractures, certain fractures do carry a higher specificity for child abuse than others (Table 28-9). Fractures involving the ribs, scapulae, and sternum almost always result from intentional injury in the pediatric patient. A skeletal survey is indicated in any child who is nonverbal or younger than 2 years of age when abuse is suspected. Radionuclide bone scan is more sensitive for subtle signs of acute or healing skeletal trauma; this study should be considered if the skeletal survey provides insufficient images or if plain films are negative and the suspicion for abuse remains high. Another option is to repeat the skeletal survey 2 weeks later to assess for evidence of healing fractures.

Physical abuse does not always leave visible cutaneous findings. Intentional trauma is the most common cause of significant intracranial injury in the first year of life.

Shaken baby syndrome is characterized by intracranial hemorrhaging and retinal hemorrhages in an infant with no external evidence of trauma. Affected infants may present with poor feeding, vomiting, irritability, hypotonia, apnea,

TABLE 28-9

SPECIFICITY OF CERTAIN RADIOGRAPHIC FINDINGS FOR CHILD ABUSE*

High Specificity

Chip fracture of the metaphysis (wrenching or pulling forces)
Buckle handle fractures
Rib fractures (especially posterior rib fractures and rib fractures in nonambulatory children)
Scapular fractures
Fractures of the vertebral spinous processes
Fractures of the sternum

Moderate Specificity

Multiple or bilateral fractures
Fractures in various stages of healing
Epiphyseal separations
Vertebral body fractures
Fractures involving the digits
Complex or multiple skull fractures

Low Specificity (i.e., commonly result from both abuse and accidental injury)

Healing fractures
Clavicular fractures
Long bone shaft fractures
Non-depressed linear skull fractures
Toddler fracture of the tibia
Dislocated elbow

Conditions that may result in radiographic findings suggestive of child abuse: osteogenesis imperfecta; skeletal dysplasia; rickets; osteoid osteoma; hypophosphatemia; congenital syphilis; and infantile cortical hyperostosis.

*Kleinman PK. Skeletal trauma: general considerations. In: Kleinman PK, ed. *Diagnostic imaging of child abuse*. Baltimore, MD: Lippincott Williams & Wilkins; 1987:8–25.

seizures, lethargy, and coma. Repeated episodes of shaking which result in subacute or chronic subdural hematomas may present with a rapidly increasing head circumference and a full, bulging anterior fontanelle. When intracranial hemorrhage is thought to result from abuse, the infant's records should be reviewed for documentation of prophylactic vitamin K administration and possible birth trauma. Fundoscopic examination for hemorrhages is indicated in any infant or young child with suspected head trauma due to shaking (e.g., infants with seizures or coma). Computed tomography is the initial study of choice for documenting intracranial hemorrhaging. Bleeding into the subdural, subarachnoid, and interhemispheric spaces is consistent with shaken baby syndrome; epidural hematomas are more likely to result from accidental injury. Intraparenchymal lesions associated with axonal shearing become evident on magnetic resonance imaging scans days after the episode of abuse.

State laws require the physician to report all cases of suspected abuse to local child protective service agencies (and occasionally law enforcement). HIPAA restrictions do not apply to personal medical records pertinent to investigations of abuse. The reporting physician should discuss the referral with the family and recognize that such action and the subsequent evaluation create enormous stress within the family, even if the report is eventually unsubstantiated. "Unsubstantiated" does not necessarily mean that the abuse did not occur; cases may be reported as unsubstantiated if the child cannot be located or will not confirm the abuse or if the parents refuse to cooperate with the investigating social workers.

When a child abuse case is prosecuted in civil court, conviction requires that the preponderance of evidence (>50%) indicates that the abuse took place. Cases involving serious injury or death are prosecuted in criminal courts, where the standard of proof is significantly higher ("beyond a reasonable doubt," or >99%). In court proceedings, a guardian ad litem is appointed to represent the best interests of the child.

When child abuse is substantiated, the local child protective service agency is responsible for generating and implementing the treatment plan and monitoring the safety of the child. In an effort to keep families together, many neglected and abused children are not removed from their parents and placed in foster care. Physical abuse, sexual abuse, and neglect may continue to occur within the home despite monitoring and intervention. Children who are victims of abuse are more likely to manifest developmental delay, behavior problems, and psychiatric illness. As adults, they may become abusers themselves or suffer from repeated victimization.

Pediatricians can assist in the prevention of child abuse by identifying risk factors for abuse, educating parents about appropriate expectations for their children, referring families to social support services when they are under stress, and counseling parents about acceptable and effective forms of discipline. Regular home visitation programs have been proven to decrease rates of child abuse in families with multiple risk factors.

Munchausen Syndrome by Proxy

Munchausen syndrome by proxy (factitious disorder by proxy) is a rare disorder in which a primary caregiver, almost always the mother, fabricates symptoms or induces signs of organic disease in the child, leading to recurrent, unnecessary medical diagnostic procedures. Munchausen syndrome by proxy is a form of child abuse. As opposed to more typical abuse, the primary motivation seems to be the desire of the parent to assume the "sick role" by proxy in order to obtain ongoing attention from medical personnel. Adults who engage in Munchausen syndrome by proxy:

- often have some degree of medical training or exposure to the practice of medicine
- care for the child exclusively and may be minimally involved with the child's other parent, if at all
- are inordinately concerned for and form unusually close relationships with members of the hospital staff who care for the child
- are almost always cooperative and appreciative
- are more likely than the general population to be diagnosed with a variant of somatoform or fictitious disorder
- are more likely than the general population to have had a previous child die under unclear or suspicious circumstances

The most common presenting features of children who are victims of Munchausen syndrome by proxy are noted in Table 28-10. The nonspecific nature of the complaints often results in significant delay in diagnosis; maintaining a measure of suspicion for this disorder whenever a patient presents with atypical, prolonged, and/or confusing manifestations of disease may substantially decrease the extent of morbidity and mortality. Between 5% to 10% of children affected by Munchausen syndrome by proxy eventually die

TABLE 28-10
MUNCHAUSEN SYNDROME BY PROXY

Presenting Features

Bleeding (intentional trauma or nonaccidental ingestion)

Seizures (fictitious or due to nonaccidental ingestion or salt poisoning)

Lethargy/unconsciousness (nonaccidental ingestion or intentional suffocation)

Apnea (suffocation)

Diarrhea (fictitious or secondary to laxatives)

Vomiting (fictitious or secondary to emetic agents)

Recurrent fever (heating the thermometer or recurrent infection from injection of foreign material into the skin or body)

Rash (abrasive trauma)

Hypoglycemia (nonaccidental ingestion)

Laboratory abnormalities (tampering with the sample, e.g., adding sugar, blood, sand, or pebbles to urine samples; falsifying laboratory results)

from the disorder; those who survive are at high risk for psychiatric disorders (depression, paranoia, inordinate fearfulness regarding their health, chronic invalidism). The risk of death is highest in children who are routinely poisoned or suffocated.

As previously stated, Munchausen by proxy is a form of child abuse, requiring immediate notification of local child protective services. The most effective method of preventing further harm at the hands of the caregiver is removal of the child from the home (foster care placement). Siblings should be interviewed and evaluated for evidence of abuse. Psychiatric assessment and treatment are indicated for both the child and the perpetrator.

Sexual Abuse

Sexual abuse is defined as the involvement of a child in any activity meant to provide sexual gratification to an adult. Girls are two to four times more likely than boys to be sexually victimized as children or adolescents. Sexual abuse may occur in children of any age. Although often highly publicized, molestation by a stranger is relatively uncommon; the vast majority of sexual abuse is committed by a family member or someone else known to the child. Physicians are ethically obligated and required by law to report all cases of suspected child sexual abuse to local law enforcement and child protective service agencies. Care must be taken at each step in the evaluation of the child with suspected sexual abuse; it is up to the court to determine from a review of the medical, forensic, and social work evaluations whether the preponderance of evidence supports the charge of sexual abuse.

Symptoms, behaviors, and physical examination findings which should prompt consideration of sexual abuse are detailed in Table 28-11. Labial adhesions and anal tags are not indicative of sexual abuse. The specificity of vulvar erythema for abuse is so low that this sign is considered of little significance when it occurs in isolation.

When sexual abuse is suspected, great care must be taken during the information-gathering stage. If the possibility of sexual abuse is raised during a visit to the primary care physician, excessive and detailed questioning of the child should be avoided, the child's immediate safety should be ensured, and the child should be referred for evaluation by a sexual abuse team (if one is available). Repetitive interviewing of a child who has allegedly been sexually abused increases the likelihood of leading questions, "learned" responses that appear rote, and recorded inconsistencies. The initial detailed (forensic) interview of the child ideally should be performed by a child-abuse specialist with specific training in proper interview technique. The child should be separated from the caregiver for the duration of the interview. The goal is to obtain valid, reliable information without further traumatizing the child. The interviewer may begin by asking the child to draw pictures, which can be a non-threatening route to opening the discussion. Anatomically-correct dolls can be used instead in very young or nonverbal children; the potential for over-interpretation is a disadvantage to this technique. The information gathered is subsequently used to formulate a treatment plan and identify and prosecute the perpetrator. Verbatim statements by the child obtained during the interview may qualify as admissible evidence in court.

If there is a reported or suspected history of genital contact with an orifice, specimens should be obtained for *Chlamydia trachomatis* and *Neisseria gonorrhoeae* cultures and serum studies for *Treponema palladium*, hepatitis B virus, and HIV. Sexually transmitted disease in a prepubertal child is considered presumptive evidence of sexual abuse. The physician collecting the samples must order "gold standard" forms of testing (e.g., chlamydia and gonorrhea cultures) for each organism; results which are merely "consistent with" or "suggestive of" a sexually-transmitted organism are insufficient evidence of abuse. It must be noted that young children who have perinatal acquisition of *C. trachomatis* or human papillomavirus may have clinical or laboratory evidence of infection with

TABLE 28-11
ELEMENTS OF THE HISTORY AND PHYSICAL EXAMINATION SUSPICIOUS FOR SEXUAL ABUSE

Behaviors
Explicit description of sexual intercourse or other adult sexual behavior
Imitation of sexual intercourse or other adult sexual behavior
Sexualized behavior or sexually acting out
Questions about sexual behavior that are unusually sophisticated for the age of the child
Public masturbation, especially that which is excessive and unresponsive to behavior modification techniques
Self-insertion of foreign bodies into the vagina or anus
Drawings of genitalia or sexual acts
Symptoms
Genital pain*
Genital discharge
Encopresis
Enuresis
Sudden changes in affect, behavior, school performance
Physical Findings#
Anal fissures/tears
Anal dilation
Hymenal tears
Genital or anal abrasions, bruising, or lacerations
Bruising of the inner thighs

*Most cases of genital pain are not due to sexual abuse.
#In the vast majority of cases, sexual abuse does not produce any visible physical findings, such as in cases of oral-genital or hand-genital stimulation, insertion of a small object, or abuse of an older adolescent.

TABLE 28-12
PROPHYLACTIC THERAPY FOR FEMALE PREPUBERTAL AND ADOLESCENT RAPE VICTIMS

Postcoital Emergency Contraception (Plan B):
Two 0.75 mg levonorgestrel pills taken 12 hours apart within 3 days of intercourse (reduces the risk of pregnancy by about 90%)

Prophylactic Antimicrobial Therapy
Neisseria gonorrhoeae and syphilis—Ceftriaxone 125 mg IM (single dose) (all ages)
Chlamydia trachomatis
Children younger than 8 years—Erythromycin 50 mg/kg/day PO divided qid (maximum of 500 mg per dose)
Patients 8 years and older—Azithromycin 1 g PO (single dose) or doxycycline 100 mg PO bid for 7 days (contraindicated during pregnancy)
Trichomoniasis and bacterial vaginosis (adolescents only)—Metronidazole 2 g PO (single dose)
Hepatitis B—vaccinate if not fully vaccinated
HIV—Zidovudine (AZT) 200 mg PO tid or 106 mg per m^2 per dose tid for 4 weeks
PLUS
Lamivudine 150 mg per dose bid or 4 mg per kg per dose bid for 4 weeks
OR (for adolescents)
Combination of 300 mg AZT per 150 mg lamivudine bid for 4 weeks

those organisms. It is rare to find evidence of seminal fluid, which persists for <72 hours, during an evaluation for sexual abuse. Information regarding prophylactic antibiotic treatment and postcoital contraception for female patients who have been raped is provided in Table 28-12.

Parents who are not the perpetrators of sexual abuse understandably have concerns regarding potential effects on the child, including possible transmission of HIV, precocious sexual behavior, loss of virginity, and the "inducement" of homosexuality in boys. The pediatrician can listen to these concerns and offer information and support as needed. Ironically, some families blame the victim of the abuse, either because they believe the child was somehow complicit or because a parent has now been removed from the home and charged with the abuse.

Foster Care Placement

Although placing a child in foster care is meant to protect him or her from continued abuse, removal from the home is typically frightening and traumatic in and of itself. In addition, children who enter the foster care system, as a group, have extremely high rates of physical illnesses/impairments, mental health disorders, developmental disabilities, and school failure. The child may also suffer physical, emotional, or sexual abuse at the hands of foster caregivers. Children in foster care benefit when they continue to be treated by their primary care physician. The pediatrician should remain available for routine health maintenance; bring the child up-to-date on deficient immunizations; review results of developmental and psychosocial testing obtained by child protective service agencies; and monitor response to interventions.

SOURCES

American Academy of Pediatrics Committee on Psychosocial Aspects of Child and Family Health. The prenatal visit. *Pediatrics*. 2001;107: 1456–1458.

American Academy of Pediatrics Committee on Psychosocial Aspects of Child and Family Health and Committee on Adolescence. Sexuality education for children and adolescents. *Pediatrics*. 2001;108: 498–502.

Beers NS. Managing temper tantrums. *Pediatr Rev*. 2003;24:70–71.

Chaudron LH. Postpartum depression: What pediatricians need to know. *Pediatr Rev*. 2003;24:154–161.

Chung EK, Cheng TL. Childhood fears and phobias. *Pediatr Rev*. 2003;24:431–432.

Copelan R. Assessing the potential for violent behavior in children and adolescents. *Pediatr Rev*. 2006:27:e36–e41.

Gushurst CA. Child abuse: Behavioral aspects and other associated problems. *Pediatr Clin North Am*. 2003;50:919–938.

Hanna GL, Fischer DJ, Fluent TE. Separation anxiety disorder and school refusal in children and adolescents. *Pediatr Rev*. 2006;27: 56–63.

Hudson M, Kaplan R. Clinical response to child abuse. *Pediatr Clin North Am*. 2006;53:27–39.

Johnson CF. Sexual abuse in children. *Pediatr Rev*. 2006;27:17–27.

Johnson PL, Flake EM. Maternal depression and child outcomes. *Pediatr Ann*. 2007;36:196–202.

Kleinman PK. Skeletal trauma: General considerations. In: Kleinman PK, ed. *Diagnostic imaging of child abuse*. Baltimore, MD: Lippincott Williams & Wilkins; 1987:8–25.

Lee C. Bonding. *Pediatr Rev*. 2003;24:289–290.

Lieberman AF, Knorr K. The impact of trauma: A developmental framework for infancy and early childhood. *Pediatr Ann*. 2007;36: 209–215.

Lipstein EA. Helping "vulnerable" children—and their parents—lead normal lives. *Contemp Pediatr*. 2006;23:26–37.

Malatack JJ, Consolini D, Mann K, et al. Taking on the parent to save a child: Munchausen syndrome by proxy. *Contemp Pediatr*. 2006;23: 50–63.

McVicar K. Seizure-like states. *Pediatr Rev*. 2006;27:e42–e44.

Meyer TL. Unveiling the secrecy behind masturbation. *Pediatr Rev*. 2002;23:148–149.

Moore JE. Multiple births: The art and science of caring for twins, triplets, and more. *Pediatr Rev*. 2007;28:e9–e15.

National Campaign to Prevent Teen Pregnancy. *Ten tips for parents to help their children avoid teen pregnancy*. Washington, DC: National Campaign to Prevent Teen Pregnancy; 1998.

Serwint JR. The prenatal pediatric visit. *Pediatr Rev*. 2003;24:31–32.

Sharif I. Munchausen syndrome by proxy. *Pediatr Rev*. 2004;25: 215–216.

Sherer S, Radzik M, Neinstein LS. Suicide. In: Neinstein LS, ed. *Adolescent Health Care: A Practical Guide*. 4th ed. Philadelphia, PA: Lippincott Williams & Wilkins. 2002:1443–1453.

Silber TJ, Pao M. Somatization disorders in children and adolescents. *Pediatr Rev*. 2003;24:255–264.

Sieving RE, Oliphant JA, Blum RW. Adolescent sexual behavior and sexual health. *Pediatr Rev*. 2002;23:407–415.

Sirotnak AP, Grigsby T, Krugman RD. Physical abuse of children. *Pediatr Rev*. 2004;25:264–277.

Sparrow JD. Understanding stress in children. *Pediatr Ann*. 2007;36: 187–194.

Tenney-Soeiro R, Wilson C. An update on child abuse and neglect. *Curr Opin Pediatr*. 2004;16:233–237.

Trager JDK, Cohen BA. A private itch and pain: Disease or possible abuse? *Contemp Pediatr*. 2005;22:31–33.

Van Riper M. A change of plans. *Am J Nurs*. 2003;103:71–74.

QUESTIONS

1. A 36-month-old girl is brought to your office for her routine health maintenance visit. She appears well, is following her established growth curves, and has a normal physical examination. A screening urinalysis is positive for glucose but not ketones. When you question the mother, she states that the child ate regular toast for breakfast. She mentions that a paternal grandfather of the child has "bad diabetes," but she doesn't know anymore because the girl's father is no longer involved. The result of a dextrose-stick is 90 mg per dL. You request a first-morning void urine sample the next day; this second specimen is also positive for glucose. An outside laboratory reports a peripheral blood glucose level at 86 mg per dL. Which of the following is the most appropriate next step in the management of this patient?

A) Send a nurse into the bathroom with the child and mother to supervise collection of a clean-catch urine sample in order to prevent tampering.
B) Admit the patient to the hospital for serial urinalysis.
C) Refer the patient for consultation with an endocrinologist.
D) Place the patient on an American Dietetic Association diet for 1 week with repeat urinalysis prior to diet liberalization.
E) Reassure the mother that the condition is benign and will resolve spontaneously.

2. You are providing a lecture about Munchausen syndrome by proxy (factitious disorder of childhood) for a group of family practice interns. You would be correct in telling them all of the following EXCEPT:

A) The caregiver responsible for fabricating or inducing the signs and symptoms of illness is almost always the mother rather than the father of the child.
B) Parents who perpetrate Munchausen syndrome by proxy are unlikely to manifest abnormal illness behavior themselves.
C) Parents who perpetrate Munchausen syndrome by proxy often have some degree of medical training or exposure to the practice of medicine.
D) The child who is a victim of Munchausen syndrome by proxy should be removed from the home at least temporarily.
E) The mortality rate of Munchausen syndrome by proxy is between 5% to 10%.

3. Which of the following actions taken by perpetrators of Munchausen syndrome by proxy (fictitious disorder of childhood) is associated with the highest mortality rate?

A) Injection of foreign material into the skin
B) Fabricating seizure episodes
C) Suffocation
D) Falsification of medical records
E) Inducement of bleeding through cutting

4. Your practice is interested in initiating prenatal visits, and you have been asked to devise a "standardized" form for use at such visits based on American Academy of Pediatrics recommendations. Which of the following is NOT a stated objective of the prenatal visit?

A) Establishment of a relationship between the physician and the parents
B) Collection of basic psychosocial and health information from the parents
C) Provision of information and advice, including anticipatory guidance and preventive counseling
D) Collection of insurance information for preauthorization
E) Identification of and attendance to risk factors

5. A 36-year-old woman with no children who underwent in vitro fertilization with her husband's sperm subsequently delivered twin girls at 32 weeks of gestation. The larger infant had an uncomplicated neonatal course and was discharged to home at a gestational age of 36 weeks. The smaller twin required mechanical ventilation for the first 3 weeks of life but is now breathing on her own and growing. When the mother brings the first twin for a follow-up visit in your office, you ask her how things are going at home. She responds by bursting into tears, explaining that she feels terribly guilty about spending so much time with the twin who is home and "neglecting" her daughter in the hospital. In truth, she much prefers spending time with the infant who is with her today. Which of the following statements regarding this mother's differential reaction to her twins is TRUE?

A) This mother will probably neglect the hospitalized twin when she arrives home.
B) This mother will probably always love the twin who came home first more than her sister.
C) This mother should be referred for grief counseling.
D) This mother should be referred for post-partum depression.
E) It is common for parents of twins to report different levels of bonding with the two infants, particularly when one twin remains hospitalized.

6. The percentage of 5-year-old children with primary nocturnal enuresis is closest to which of the following?

A) <2%
B) 10%
C) 20%
D) 40%
E) 60%

7. Which of the following statements regarding masturbation in the pediatric population is TRUE?

A) Masturbation is rare between the ages of 6 and 11 years.
B) Masturbation is considered a normal part of adolescent development.
C) The toddler or preschool child caught masturbating in public should be punished.
D) Self-induced injury due to masturbation is common in childhood.
E) Typical masturbation in preschool children may include simulation of a sexual act.

8. The parent of an 18-month-old child questions you about when to start toilet training. You answer that readiness to begin toilet training requires that the child achieve all of the following developmental skills EXCEPT:
A) Identification of the parts of the body involved in urination/ defecation
B) The ability to sit on the toilet
C) The ability to concentrate on a task for 10 to 15 minutes without becoming distracted
D) Voluntary control of bowel and bladder reflex functions
E) The ability to follow two-step commands

9. A 30-month-old male is brought to the emergency department by ambulance after his parents report seizure activity. The mother reports that the child was frustrated and crying because the father had put the child in time-out for kicking the family dog. She heard gasping noises and saw the child become pale and limp before collapsing out of the chair. No posturing or shaking movements were noted during the episode, which lasted about 30 seconds. The child is acting well in the emergency department, and the physical examination is normal. The history of this patient's paroxysmal episode is most consistent with which of the following?
A) Generalized seizure
B) Syncope
C) Focal seizure
D) Breath holding spell
E) Temper tantrum

10. The parents of a 2-year-old girl are frustrated by the frequency of the child's temper tantrums. They report that when the child becomes overwhelmed, she responds by throwing herself on the floor and screaming, which may last for up to 5 minutes. The tantrums occur once or twice daily. Physical examination reveals a well-nourished, well-developed child with typical affect. Which of the following is the most appropriate next step in the management of this patient?
A) Referral for behavioral intervention
B) Referral for developmental testing
C) Parental instruction in positive reinforcement
D) Parental instruction in planned ignoring
E) Investigation of parental expectations for the child

11. A father brings his 2-week-old infant to the office for a weight check. The infant is exclusively breastfed and is gaining weight appropriately. When you ask the father how his wife is doing, he tells you that she has an appointment with her obstetrician for later that day to discuss the possibility that she may have postpartum depression. He seems appropriately concerned for both his wife and the infant, and the infant's grandmother is in town for an extended stay to help with the housework and her first grandchild.

After the father leaves the office, a student working with you asks about the effects of maternal depression on the infant. You would be correct in telling her all of the following EXCEPT:
A) Postpartum depression is estimated to occur in <5% of new mothers.
B) Postpartum depression in the mother can affect social development in the infant.
C) Postpartum depression in the mother can affect cognitive development in the infant.
D) Postpartum depression in the mother can affect mother-infant attachment.
E) Infants of mothers with postpartum depression are more likely to manifest disruption of feeding and sleeping.

12. A previously healthy 6-month-old infant was hospitalized with pneumonia due to *Streptococcus pneumoniae.* He required intubation and mechanical ventilation for about 36 hours during his illness. You are seeing the child in your office for follow-up. Which of the following interventions is unlikely to prevent the development of vulnerable child syndrome in this family?
A) Discussing vulnerable child syndrome with the parents
B) Telling the family that they brought the child to the emergency department "just in time"
C) Discussing the natural parental response to serious illness in the child
D) Encouraging the family to return to normal life as soon as possible
E) Scheduling a "routine" follow-up visit for the following week

13. A 17-year-old girl has just given birth to her first child after an uncomplicated pregnancy and delivery. The father of the child, her unmarried partner, is also 17 years of age. Which of the following statements regarding adolescent fathers is INCORRECT?
A) Adolescent fathers are less likely than their peers to graduate from high school.
B) Adolescent fathers tend to have low incomes.
C) Less than half of adolescent fathers participate in the rearing of their child(ren).

D) Adolescent fathers who attend prenatal visits are more likely to remain involved with the child.
E) Adolescent fathers who are present during labor and participate in the delivery room are more likely to remain involved with the child.

14. During the routine health maintenance visit for a 2-month-old boy, his mother reports that she is worried about his "excessive crying." She reports that the child has had crying episodes every evening for the past 2 weeks that last up to 3 hours a night. The infant is inconsolable during the episodes, which begin and end spontaneously. The infant is otherwise well; growth parameters and development are appropriate for age. Which of the following is the most appropriate response to this patient's crying episodes?
A) Schedule the patient for a swallow study.
B) Schedule the patient for an upper gastrointestinal radiographic series.
C) Thicken the infant's feeds.
D) Reassure the mother that the crying is normal.
E) Switch the infant from breast milk or cow milk formula to soy formula.

15. Which of the following behaviors is most closely correlated with a history of sexual abuse?
A) Private masturbation culminating in ejaculation in a 14-year-old boy
B) Masturbation culminating in orgasm in secret in a 16-year-old girl
C) Stimulation of his genitals with his hands in a 4-year-old boy
D) Masturbation against a sliding pole on the playground in a 3-year-old boy
E) Simulation of sexual intercourse while masturbating in a 5-year-old girl

16. You have just diagnosed a 24-month-old child with breath holding spells. His mother is concerned about damage to his brain and desires medical intervention. You would be correct in telling her which of the following?
A) Cardiac pacing is not indicated in this child.
B) The child is unlikely to outgrow the condition.
C) The presence of generalized tonic movements during a breath holding spell is associated with an increased risk of significant central nervous system anoxia.
D) The presence of generalized tonic movements during a breath holding spell is associated with an increased risk of epilepsy.
E) Behavioral therapy has not been found to be beneficial in the management of breath holding spells.

17. A 12-year-old girl who has been fearfully anticipating dissecting a frog in science class for the past week has become fixated on the event. She talks about it daily, even though it is more than 3 weeks away. She has cut science class twice in the past week. She is now resistant to going to school, and becomes agitated and tearful when it is time to leave home. Which of the following features of her history is most consistent with the diagnosis of phobia rather than a normal childhood fear?
A) Duration of the anxiety
B) Functional impairment
C) A specific fear which generalizes over time
D) Avoidance of the fearful stimulus
E) Anxiety associated with the fearful stimulus

18. The parents of a sixth-grade girl inform you that they have asked the girl to be removed from her health education class during discussions regarding pubertal development and sexual health. You would be correct in discussing all of the following with them EXCEPT:
A) The most effective sexual health education programs encourage sexual abstinence messages and provide contraceptive and STD prevention counseling.
B) There are published age-appropriate materials to assist them in discussing pubertal development and sexual health with their child.
C) As a group, adolescents who participate in sexual education programs that limit discussion to abstinence refrain from sexual intercourse for 18 to 24 months longer than adolescents who participate in traditional sexual health programs.
D) The most appropriate time to initiate discussions about pubertal development and sexual health is at the 11-year routine health maintenance visit.
E) Sixty-six percent of high school seniors report that they have engaged in sexual intercourse.

19. The mother of a 17-year-old boy comes to your office to speak with you about her child. The boy has recently told his mother that he believes he may be homosexual. She feels grief regarding her son's sexual orientation but is determined to support him regardless of his "choice." In your counseling of this mother, you would be correct in telling her which of the following?
A) Sexual experimentation with same-gender peers is not a normal behavior during adolescence.
B) Most people do not become aware of their sexual orientation until middle adulthood.
C) Homosexual youths are less likely than their heterosexual peers to experience a period of confusion regarding sexual identity.
D) Sexual orientation, whether heterosexual or homosexual, is not a choice.
E) Adolescents who engage in sexual activity with same-gender peers are homosexual by definition.

20. Which of the following features of antisocial behavior differentiates typical adolescent rebellion from antisocial personality disorder?
A) Persistence of behavior into adulthood
B) Behaviors that result in harm to others

C) Lack of remorse
D) Chronic lying and stealing
E) All of the above

21. At a routine health maintenance visit for a 12-year-old boy, the child's mother tells you privately that she and her husband have filed for divorce, but that they have not yet told their son. She is worried about how the boy will react to the divorce given his age (early adolescent). You would be correct in telling the mother all of the following EXCEPT:
A) The age of the child is a stronger determinant of the child's ability to adjust to divorce than the temperament of the child.
B) Children tend to be more resistance to remarriage of the custodial parent during early adolescence than at other times.
C) Internalizing behaviors are common in adolescents during the period of adjustment to divorce.
D) Externalizing behaviors are common in adolescents during the period of adjustment to divorce.
E) The type of custodial arrangement appears to have less of an effect on the adjustment and subsequent development of the child than the continued involvement of a supportive, communicative, authoritative parent.

22. A 7-year-old boy awakes one morning unable to walk. His mother discovers him sitting up in his bed, in no distress, reading a book. When she attempts to stand him up, he falls to the floor. She believes the boy is malingering, but she allows him to stay home from school. The next day, the boy still cannot walk, so she brings him to your office. There is no history of fever, rash, or sore throat, and there is no family history of inherited neurologic disease. Bowel and bladder control remain completely voluntary. When you question her regarding recent changes in the child's life, she tells you that his father has left them to live with another woman. The child is afebrile with stable vital signs. The physical examination is within normal limits, except that you are not able to assess strength in the lower extremities. Sensation and deep tendon reflexes are intact throughout. This child's neurologic deficit is most likely to result from which of the following?
A) Compression of the spinal cord
B) Conversion disorder
C) Anxiety disorder
D) Schizophrenia
E) Guillain-Barré syndrome

23. A 7-year-old child who presented to your office four days ago with the inability to walk due to the sudden onset of bilateral lower extremity weakness has been diagnosed with conversion disorder. All of the following are appropriate components of the management strategy for conversion disorder EXCEPT:
A) Removal of any secondary gain associated with the child's functional impairment
B) Consultation with a pediatric mental health specialist
C) Hospitalization
D) Reassuring the family that there is no underlying anatomic or neurologic disorder causing the impairment
E) Providing "escape with dignity"

24. You are providing a lecture to a group of school nurses regarding separation anxiety disorder and school refusal. You would be correct in telling them that which of the following is the most effective way to reintroduce a child with separation anxiety disorder and school refusal to school?
A) The child is allowed to complete schoolwork from home for full credit for the duration of the school year.
B) The child is returned to school when drug levels of a selective serotonin reuptake inhibitor are in the therapeutic range.
C) The child is immediately returned to school, with the parent accompanying the child for a diminishing duration of time each day.
D) The child is immediately returned to school, with the parent dropping the child off and exiting the grounds as quickly as possible.
E) The child is immediately returned to school, with an educational specialist accompanying the child for a diminishing duration of time each day.

25. Children with separation anxiety disorder are less likely than their peers:
A) to live in a single-parent home
B) to have a family history of an anxiety disorder
C) to suffer from a comorbid anxiety disorder
D) to suffer from a comorbid depressive disorder
E) to attend school regularly

26. A 13-year-old adolescent patient in your practice is in juvenile court on charges of truancy. He has missed more than 30 school days in the past 3 months. He has no chronic illnesses. When he gets up in the morning, he tells his mother that he does not want to go to school because he is worried that something might happen to her. She allows him to stay home with her many days because he seems depressed. He spends the time playing video games and listening to music but goes out with his friends when they get home from school and on the weekends. The mother has been unsuccessful in convincing the boy to complete his homework assignments. He has been caught vandalizing property twice in the past month. His mother asks you to testify on his behalf because she believes he has separation anxiety disorder. Which of the following features of the boy's history support truancy rather than separation anxiety disorder as the origin of the patient's school refusal?

A) The boy's ability to separate from the parent without difficulty at all other times
B) The boy's avoidance of school attendance
C) The frequency of the boy's absences
D) The boy's refusal to complete his homework
E) The boy's depressed affect

27. A 17-year-old adolescent is brought to your office by his parents for evaluation of his odd behavior. Over the past year, the boy has spent most of the time that he is not in school wandering around the neighborhood talking to himself. A neighbor recently found him sitting at her table eating a sandwich he had made from food in her refrigerator. He has begun pouring over the newspaper every morning in search of messages he believes are directed at him. This patient's behavior is most consistent with which of the following disorders?
A) Major depressive disorder
B) Schizophrenia
C) Generalized anxiety disorder
D) Chronic drug abuse
E) Mental retardation

28. A 15-year-old girl is at a party over the weekend with her boyfriend. The boyfriend breaks up with her at the party. She is very upset and drinks several beers. She goes into the bathroom and cuts her forearm with a razor blade, then calls her parents. She is brought to the emergency department via ambulance. Upon arrival, she is crying and apologizing to her parents, who are understandably upset but appropriately supportive. The physical examination reveals two shallow 5 to 6 cm lacerations on the underside of her left forearm, running parallel to the long axis of the extremity. Which of the following consists of the most appropriate medical response to this girl's self-induced injuries?
A) Discharge home with her parents, with follow-up arranged within seven days
B) Discharge home with her parents, with follow-up arranged within 24 hours
C) Admission to the hospital for psychiatric evaluation
D) Admission to the hospital for psychiatric treatment
E) Admission to the hospital for medical stabilization

29. All of the following increase the risk of suicide completion in the adolescent EXCEPT:
A) Attempting suicide with a gun
B) Attempting suicide by jumping from a great height
C) Attempting suicide at a time during which the individual is unlikely to be discovered prior to death
D) Attempting suicide by cutting oneself
E) Attempting suicide at a location in which the individual is unlikely to be discovered prior to death

30. The presence of a cognitively gifted child within a family can have a negative impact of the functioning of the family unit if:
A) the child is allowed to make decisions for the family
B) the child is treated in a preferential manner
C) a great deal of the family's financial resources support the child's enrichment activities
D) a great deal of one or both parents' time is spent supporting the child's enrichment activities
E) All of the above

31. Which of the following statements regarding the effects of domestic (intimate partner) violence on children in the home is CORRECT?
A) Children who live in a home with intimate partner violence have a 30% to 60% chance of being physically abused themselves.
B) Children who live in a home with intimate partner violence and are not themselves physically abused are not at increased risk for violent injury.
C) Children who live in a home with intimate partner violence are no more likely than their peers to commit acts of physical violence against others.
D) Children who live in a home with intimate partner violence are no more likely than their peers to commit acts of sexual violence against others.
E) The majority of children who witness repetitive intimate partner violence do not meet the diagnostic criteria for post-traumatic stress disorder.

32. Which of the following statements regarding the use of complementary/alternative medicine in children with physical or cognitive impairments is INCORRECT?
A) Parents may be drawn to complementary and alternative medicine because they feel they need to try every possible option.
B) Claims regarding complementary and alternative medicine are governed by the same laws as those regulating traditional medications and treatments.
C) Parents may be drawn to complementary and alternative medicine because they are frustrated by the lack of options offered through traditional medicine.
D) Parents may be drawn to complementary and alternative medicine by promises of rapid improvement.
E) Physicians need to remain knowledgeable about the claims, risks, benefits, and scientific evidence related to complementary and alternative medicine.

33. An infant with Down syndrome is born to the parents of two healthy children. The disorder was unanticipated. The child's mother believes that the diagnosis is in error because a prenatal sonogram demonstrated no abnormalities. The father has not been back to the hospital in the 48 hours since the child's birth because he is too angry at the medical establishment for "missing" the diagnosis. All of the following statements regarding this child's condition are correct EXCEPT:

A) These parents will likely progress though a predictable cycle of grief.
B) The child's condition will increase stress on the family unit.
C) It is not normal for the mother to be in denial while the father is primarily angry.
D) The child's condition will increase stress on the marriage.
E) The child's condition will have an economic impact on the family.

34. A 15-month-old child is in your office for her routine health maintenance visit. She missed her last three appointments and has not received medical care since she was 6 months of age. Her weight percentage has dropped from the 25th percentile nine months ago to the fifth percentile at today's visit. There is a more modest decline in length, and head circumference percentile has not changed. She sits quietly in the chair next to her mother and does not protest when she is moved to the examining table. She remains quiet and still for the duration of the examination. Other than the changes in her growth parameters, the child's physical examination is within normal limits. Which of the following is the most likely cause of this child's growth deceleration?
A) Organic failure to thrive
B) Mental retardation
C) Diabetes
D) Child neglect
E) Renal tubular acidosis

35. You are asked to provide a written summary of the effects of child neglect for use in training potential foster parents. You would be correct in including which of the following statements?
A) Children whose parents abuse alcohol or illicit drugs are no more likely to be neglected than their same-age peers.
B) Inadequate supervision that results in child endangerment is not considered neglect.
C) Parental IQ does not affect a child's risk for neglect.
D) Rates of child neglect are essentially the same across all socioeconomic levels.
E) More children suffer from child neglect than from child abuse.

36. Which of the following people is legally charged with representing the best interests of the child in cases of suspected child abuse by family members?
A) The guardian ad litem
B) The parent(s)
C) The suspected perpetrator
D) The judge
E) A member of the child's extended family

37. Which of the following statements regarding intracranial and retinal forms of injury in child abuse is INCORRECT?
A) Retinal hemorrhages in the setting of significant intracranial injuries are highly specific for physical abuse.
B) Shaken baby syndrome is most common in children 12 to 24 months of age.
C) When all forms of child abuse are considered, shaken baby syndrome has the highest mortality rate.
D) The great majority of serious intracranial injuries in children younger than 12 months of age are due to intentional injury.
E) Cardiopulmonary resuscitation typically results in retinal hemorrhaging.

38. Which of the following radiographic findings is most specific for physical abuse?
A) Oblique spiral fracture of the tibia in a toddler
B) Clavicular fracture
C) Metaphyseal chip fracture
D) Nondisplaced linear skull fracture
E) Fracture of a vertebral body

39. Based on the results of the forensic interview and physical examination, you believe that the sexual abuse of a 7-year-old girl involved genital-to-genital contact, penetration of the vagina, and deposition of seminal fluid. Which of the following statements regarding the further evaluation and treatment of this patient is FALSE?
A) Specimens should be obtained for *Neisseria gonorrhoeae* culture.
B) Specimens should be obtained for *Chlamydia trachomatis* culture.
C) The girl's hepatitis B vaccination status should be reviewed, and the series should be completed if necessary.
D) The girl should receive prophylactic antimicrobial therapy to prevent trichomoniasis.
E) Prophylaxis against HIV should be considered in this child.

40. In providing a lecture to students earning their degrees in social work, you would be correct in informing them of all of the following EXCEPT:
A) The majority of cases of sexual abuse do not involve visible physical findings.
B) Children who are sexually abused usually know their perpetrator.
C) Labial adhesion and anal tags are not signs of sexual abuse.
D) Most complaints of genital pain do not result from sexual abuse.
E) The forensic interview should be conducted in the presence of a supportive caregiver.

ANSWERS

1. A
2. B
3. C
4. D
5. E
6. C
7. B
8. A
9. D
10. E
11. A
12. B
13. C
14. D
15. E
16. A
17. B
18. C
19. D
20. E
21. A
22. B
23. C
24. D
25. E
26. A
27. B
28. C
29. D
30. E
31. A
32. B
33. C
34. D
35. E
36. A
37. B
38. C
39. D
40. E

29 Principles of Critical Care and Emergency Medicine

FEVER

Fever is one of the most common presenting complaints in the pediatric emergency department. Normal human rectal temperature ranges from 97°F to 100.6°F (36.1°C to 38.1°C). Rectal temperature is most indicative of central temperature and is considered the "gold standard." Digital thermometers permit accurate measurement of rectal, oral, and axillary temperature; they are inexpensive and simple to use. Ear-based temperature measurement is a less standardized method. Thermometers containing mercury are no longer recommended for use in children due to the risk of breakage and subsequent heavy metal exposure.

Most fever in children younger than three years of age is viral in origin. Young patients with uncomplicated viral infections typically respond to treatment with an over-the-counter antipyretic with decreased fever and fussiness, increased appetite and activity, and improved comfort level. Recommended dosages are listed in Table 29-1. A sponge bath may also provide a measure of symptomatic relief. Febrile seizures are not uncommon in children under the age of 5 years; such seizures are not prevented by antipyretic therapy but are typically benign (see Chapter 18). Elevation of body temperature increases insensible water loss; however, dehydration is unlikely unless the child also has increased losses through vomiting and/or diarrhea. Since elevation in body temperature increases oxygen consumption and cardiac output, antipyretic medication has an added therapeutic benefit in patients with underlying pulmonary or cardiovascular disease.

TABLE 29-1
RECOMMENDED DOSAGES OF ANTIPYRETICS IN CHILDREN

Acetaminophen
Recommended fever dosing: Maximum of 15 mg/kg/dose every 4 hours, not to exceed 650 mg/dose or 5 doses in 24 hours

Ibuprofen
Recommended fever dosing: Maximum of 10 mg/kg/dose every 6 hours, not to exceed 400 mg/dose or 3 doses in 24 hours

In children between the ages of 3 to 36 months, significant temperature elevation (>39°C/102.2°F) is associated with an increased risk of invasive bacterial disease. In febrile patients in this age range, white blood count $\geq 15.0 \times 10^3$/mcL and absolute neutrophil count $\geq 10.0 \times 10^3$/mcL also have positive predictive value for invasive bacterial infection (e.g., sepsis, meningitis).

Elevation of body temperature beyond 41.0°C (105.8°F) is inconsistent with life. Heat stroke, abnormalities of central thermoregulatory centers (hypothalamus), and malignant hyperthermia may all cause life-threatening elevations in temperature. Malignant hyperthermia is a hypermetabolic state characterized by hyperthermia, metabolic acidosis, cardiac arrhythmias, and muscle rigidity leading to myoglobinuria and elevated serum creatinine kinase levels. Children with underlying neuromuscular disease such as muscular dystrophy are at increased risk for the development of malignant hyperthermia during and immediately following general anesthesia for surgery. Malignant hyperthermia is managed with dantrolene, a muscle relaxant, and supportive care. Depolarizing neuromuscular blocking agents (e.g., succinylcholine) and inhaled anesthetic agents should not be administered to patients with a known history of malignant hyperthermia.

Fever in the neonate younger than 30 days of age is considered a medical emergency. Chapter 5 contains information regarding early-onset neonatal sepsis. Late-onset neonatal sepsis typically presents between 3 to 30 days of life in a former full-term, previously healthy infant who has already been discharged from the newborn nursery. Clinical manifestations include any of the following: fever, irritability, poor feeding, lethargy, hypotonia, bulging fontanelle, and seizures. Any neonate with a rectal temperature ≥38°C should be evaluated with a careful history and physical examination, complete blood count and blood culture, urinalysis and urine culture, and cerebrospinal fluid analysis and culture. The infant is then admitted to the hospital for intravenous antibiotic therapy (ampicillin and cefotaxime) and observation until culture results and susceptibilities are available. Group B streptococci, *Escherichia coli*, and *Listeria monocytogenes* are the most common bacterial pathogens in this age group.

"Fever of unknown origin" (FUO) is defined as documented temperature >38.3°C (101°F) of uncertain etiology on multiple occasions over a 10-day period or more. In children, FUO usually results from a common pediatric infection with an atypically prolonged time course. Diagnostic considerations include the following:

- Infection—urinary tract infection, meningitis, sinusitis, hepatitis, cytomegalovirus (CMV), Epstein-Barr virus (EBV), parasites, cat-scratch disease, Rocky Mountain spotted fever, ehrlichiosis, Lyme disease, brucellosis, leptospirosis, tularemia, endocarditis, septic arthritis, osteomyelitis, intra-abdominal abscess, enteric fever, tuberculosis, HIV, opportunistic infection
- Connective tissue disease—systemic juvenile idiopathic arthritis, systemic lupus erythematosus
- Malignancy—leukemia, lymphoma, neuroblastoma
- Other: inflammatory bowel disease, Kawasaki disease, drug fever, thyrotoxicosis, sarcoidosis, familial dysautonomia (Riley-Day syndrome), factitious fever

The age and gender of the patient narrow the differential diagnosis somewhat. Inflammatory bowel disease and connective tissue disorders are uncommon in younger children. Autoimmune disorders occur more frequently in girls. A thorough history and physical examination suggest the diagnosis in more than half of the children in whom a cause of the fever is found. Sexual history, travel history, current medications, exposure to animals, tick bites, antecedent illness, trauma, associated symptoms, and family history are important areas of inquiry. Different fever patterns (constant, recurrent, cyclical) are more closely associated with particular diagnoses. Conjunctivitis, the absence of tears, rashes, lymphadenopathy, joint tenderness, oral ulcers, thrush, heart murmurs, organomegaly, masses, abdominal tenderness, cutaneous manifestations, joint findings, and mental status changes may suggest a specific cause and guide further evaluation.

Screening laboratory tests include complete blood count and differential, serum electrolytes, blood urea nitrogen (BUN) and creatinine levels, liver function tests, alkaline phosphatase, and urinalysis. Bacterial cultures should be obtained from specimens of blood, urine, stool, and possibly cerebrospinal fluid. Stool may also be sent for viral antigen detection and parasite examination. Additional tests to consider include erythrocyte sedimentation rate (ESR), C-reactive protein, antinuclear antibody, and specific serologic tests for cat-scratch disease, EBV, and other infectious agents. Chest radiographs and skin testing for tuberculosis are typically performed. More expensive and invasive studies may be warranted based on screening results. In about 25% of cases, no etiology is determined and the fever resolves without sequelae.

WOUND CARE

Initial management of traumatic skin wounds is the same regardless of the type of injury (Table 29-2). It is important to obtain a clear and complete history of mechanism of injury if possible, as well as the date of last tetanus inoculation and whether the patient has any underlying systemic or chronic disease.

Certain types of wounds warrant special mention: those associated with a high risk of cosmetic deformity, infection, or other complication based on location or mechanism of injury. Lacerations through the vermillion border of the lip are technically difficult to repair; the perimeter line of the lip must be exactly matched, and the sutures loose enough to accommodate swelling and eventual scar formation. Pain control is achieved through a nerve block rather than local infiltration. Referral to a plastic surgeon should be considered for specialized closure of these wounds.

Puncture wounds carry a high rate of complications. All puncture wounds should be cleansed with normal saline irrigation. Plain films and ultrasonography assist in the location of a foreign body if one is suspected; blind probing is contraindicated. Unless there is a concomitant laceration, the wound should not be closed. Complications of puncture wounds in children include secondary bacterial infection, introduction/retention of a foreign body, abscess formation, and infection of inoculated deep tissues (osteochondritis, osteomyelitis). Factors that impact complication risk include the location of the wound, the depth of the wound, contamination of the wound, and presence of a foreign body. Puncture wounds to the foot through the sole of a shoe may be contaminated with *Pseudomonas* species. The management of puncture wounds with regard to prevention and treatment of secondary infections is discussed in Chapter 20. Wound infections which do not respond to appropriate empiric antibiotic therapy should be cultured and reassessed for retained debris. Surgical consultation is indicated for cases in which: a foreign body is strongly suspected but not confirmed; a puncture wound to the hand or foot places the patient at substantial risk for osteochondritis (suppurative infection of the bone and cartilage); or formation of an abscess requires surgical drainage.

Animal, Pit Viper, and Spider Bites

Animal Bites

The management of animal bites associated with a risk of rabies is detailed in Chapter 10. Post-exposure prophylaxis against rabies is indicated for all patients who have been bitten by an animal that:

- has not been sufficiently vaccinated
- is of unknown or undocumented vaccination status
- is not available for evaluation (euthanasia and examination of the brain) or monitoring

Post-exposure prophylaxis should also be provided to any individual sleeping in a room found to be infested with bats, because humans have been known to acquire infection from bats without history of a known bite. Post-exposure prophylaxis is not indicated for bites from small rodents such as squirrels, hamsters, guinea pigs, gerbils, chipmunks, rats, mice, or lagomorphs (rabbits); these animals succumb to the disease before they become capable of transmitting it. Any wild animal with suspected rabies

TABLE 29-2
INITIAL MANAGEMENT OF OPEN SKIN WOUNDS

Hemostasis (stoppage of blood loss)

- Application of pressure
- Assessment for ongoing arterial bleeding/pulsations
- Estimation of the amount of blood lost

Cleansing and Debridement of the Wound

- Proper cleansing and debridement are the most effective means of preventing secondary wound infection.
- Topical or local analgesic agents or nerve block for pain control prior to cleansing;* conscious sedation may be more appropriate for wounds requiring significant debridement
- Irrigation with *normal saline* under mild pressure from a syringe, with removal of debris; antiseptic agents should not be administered directly into the open wound
- Debridement of devitalized tissue

Closure

- Closure is indicated for wounds which extend into the dermis and wounds which otherwise would not heal by primary intention.
- Wounds which are free of devitalized tissue, inflammation, purulent drainage, and debris (i.e., "clean wounds") can be closed 8 to 12 hours after injury, depending on location. Clean wounds on the face and scalp may be closed even later.
- Puncture wounds, bites, contaminated wounds, and wounds at high risk for secondary infection should be permitted to heal by secondary intention if more than 8 hours have passed since the injury.
- Tissue adhesives are suitable for closure of clean wounds on the face or scalp; inappropriate for use on the oral mucosa, wounds in high-tension/high-impact regions, and wounds on the hands; frequent washing weakens bonding.
- Placement of an adherent dressing; topical antibiotic ointment unnecessary (no difference in infection rates)

Prevention of Tetanus

- Patients who have received ≥3 doses of tetanus toxoid do not require an additional inoculation if the last vaccination was within the past 5 years (or within the past 10 years if the wound is clean and relatively minor).
- Patients between the ages of 4 to 6 years should receive their pre-kindergarten booster vaccination (diphtheria-tetanus-acellular pertussis) at presentation if the booster has not yet been administered.
- Patients with clean, minor wounds who do not have a reliable history of adequate vaccination against tetanus (three doses) should be vaccinated with tetanus-diphtheria toxoid at presentation.
- Both tetanus-diphtheria toxoid and tetanus immune globulin should be administered to certain immunodeficient patients and those with contaminated wounds who do not have a reliable history of adequate vaccination.

Reassessment/Removal of Stitches

- Removal of dressing and reassessment 24 to 48 hours later
- Consider empiric coverage for *Staphylococcus/Streptococcus* species if there is clinical evidence of infection (e.g., purulent discharge); appropriate choices include cephalexin, dicloxacillin (erythromycin in patients who are allergic to penicillin)
- Removal of stitches (facial lacerations within 3 to 5 days; lacerations under tension or in high-impact areas within 10 days; all others within 7 to 8 days)

*Epinephrine-containing preparations should not be used in areas of end circulation, such as the fingers.

must be euthanized for direct fluorescent antibody examination of the brain. Asymptomatic domesticated animals that bite are quarantined for ten days and euthanized if they show signs of the disease. Most local governments require notification of animal control agencies whenever a person is treated for an animal bite.

The management of dog and cat bites, including indications for prophylactic antibiotic administration, is covered in Chapter 20.

Snake Bites

Venomous snakebites in the United States are due almost exclusively to pit vipers (e.g., rattlesnakes, copperheads, water moccasins). Pit vipers can be distinguished from nonvenomous snakes by the presence of the following characteristics: small pits located between the nostril and the eye on either side of the head; elliptical pupils; large, curved fangs; and a triangular-shaped head. Crotalid (pit viper) venom contains neurotoxins, hemorrhagic mediators, digestive enzymes, and metals. Envenomation does not occur with all bites, but when it does, the involved area becomes intensely painful within several minutes, accompanied by perioral numbness and a metallic taste in the mouth. Local and systemic effects develop over 8 to 10 hours:

- Local effects—edema, ecchymosis, hemorrhagic vesicles, muscle fasciculations, regional lymphadenopathy
- Systemic effects—nausea, vomiting, tachycardia, weakness; large envenomations can produce respiratory distress, hypotension, and altered mental status

Placement of a tourniquet and use of a venom extractor are not indicated for patients who have been bitten in the field. Upon arrival to the emergency department, laboratory assessment includes a complete blood count, serum electrolyte levels, blood urea nitrogen, coagulation studies, fibrinogen level, urinalysis, electrolytes, and blood for typing and cross-matching. Crotalid antivenom is reserved for patients with evidence of severe envenomation (e.g., coagulopathies, hypotension).

Spider Bites

The brown recluse is a small spider generally <1.5-cm in length which has a brown violin-shaped mark on the dorsum of the body. The spider is found throughout the Midwest, Southeast, and extreme Southwest. The bite is typically painless, and may remain asymptomatic. Within several hours of the bite, the patient may notice mild pain and itching, followed by the development of erythema around a central pustule. The erythema is most extensive about 3 days after the bite. Local ulceration and necrosis may occur but are not the rule. If the necrotic area is <2-cm in diameter, local wound care is sufficient. Debridement and antibiotic prophylaxis are indicated for cases involving more extensive necrosis. Systemic corticosteroids are of no benefit. Currently, no antivenom exists. Systemic symptoms are extremely rare but may occur early in the course in small children (fever, chills, malaise, joint pain, intravascular hemolysis, and renal failure).

The black widow is a large (up to 1.5 inches in diameter) black spider found throughout the United States. These spiders are easily identifiable due to the dorsal presence of a small red hourglass shape. The bite may initially be painless. Local and systemic effects are seen within 24 hours of the bite, including severe pain, localized muscle tetany, generalized muscle cramping, joint pain, diaphoresis, nausea, tearing, tachycardia, tachypnea, and hypertension. These symptoms are particularly severe in small children; acute renal failure, rhabdomyolysis, shock, and death may occur in these patients. Most cases are appropriately managed with pain control and supportive care. *Latrodectus* antivenom is indicated for any symptomatic patient who is <40 kg in weight or for patients with progressive renal or cardiac failure.

Burns

Burns are the third leading cause of injury in children, behind motor vehicle accidents and drowning, and are the second most frequent cause of accidental death. Boys and children younger than 4 years of age, particularly those with disabilities, are at the greatest risk for burn injury. An estimated 15% to 25% of burns are the result of abuse. The great majority of burns are scald injuries. These may occur in association with spillage of hot food or drinks or be due to bathing injuries. Scald burns that end in straight lines without associated splash marks suggest abuse. Other burn injury patterns consistent with abuse are noted in Figure 29-1. Contact burns result from direct contact with a hot surface (iron, stove). Cigarette contact burns are the most common burn injury in abused children. Flame burns are less frequent but carry a high mortality rate due to associated smoke inhalation injury. Typical scenarios for an electrical burn involve a young child putting conductive material into a wall socket or an infant sucking on the connected end of an extension cord. Chemical burns result from exposure to strong acidic or alkaline material.

Clinical severity is based on affected body surface area and depth. Partial-thickness burns are divided into first-degree and second-degree burns. First-degree burns involve only the epidermis; the skin is red, dry, and tender but does not blister. First-degree burns usually heal within a week with no residual scarring. Second-degree burns may be superficial (less than half the depth of the dermis) or deep (involving most of the dermis but leaving appendages such as sweat glands and hair follicles intact). Superficial partial-thickness burns are often caused by scald injuries. They are painful and exhibit blisters and/or weeping but generally resolve in a few weeks with little scarring. Deep second-degree injuries may or may not be painful. They result in significant scarring and may require skin grafting. Third-degree burns extend into the subcutaneous tissue and are nontender due to sensory nervous tissue loss.

Burned areas should be placed immediately in lukewarm water or covered with wet gauze or cloth. Minor burns (superficial burns involving 10% of the total body surface area

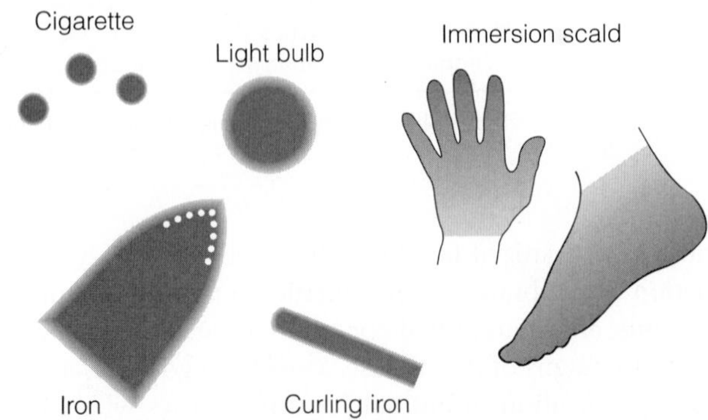

Figure 29-1 Burn injury patterns consistent with abuse. (From Marino BS, Fine KS. *Blueprints Pediatrics*. 4th ed. Philadelphia: Lippincott Williams & Wilkins; 2006 with permission.)

or less) respond to gentle cleansing, silver sulfadiazine (an antimicrobial agent), and daily dressing changes until re-epithelialization occurs. Burns that are severe, circumferential, extensive (more than 10% to 15% of the body), or that involve the face, hands, perineum, or feet require more specialized care. Treatment includes appropriate management of airway, breathing, and circulation issues; effective electrolyte and fluid therapy to account for increased insensible losses; specialized nutritional support; prevention of infection; pain management; excision and skin grafting; optimization of cosmetic recovery; and early mobility and rehabilitation.

The prevention of burns is discussed in Chapter 3.

EVALUATION AND MANAGEMENT OF THE CRITICALLY ILL CHILD

The critically ill or injured child is initially assessed with a primary survey, consisting of rapid evaluation of the following:

- Airway
- Breathing
- Circulation
- Disability
- Exposure

TABLE 29-3
RAPID ASSESSMENT WITH THE PRIMARY SURVEY ("ABCs")

Airway
- Assessment of airway patency
- Immobilization of the cervical spine when indicated (see below)
- Suctioning to remove foreign material
- Positioning with jaw-thrust or chin-lift maneuvers or placement of the head in the "sniffing" position
- Administration of oxygen
- Placement of a stable airway (e.g., endotracheal intubation) if the Glasgow coma score is ≥ 8
- Breslow tape measurement for the type and size of tube; alternatively, use an uncuffed tube in children younger than 8 years of age, with the size of the tube estimated by the following formula: [16+ (age in years)]/4. Use of a cuffed tube in older children, with the size of the tube estimated by the following formula: [9+ (age in years)]/4.

Breathing
- Assessment for adequate spontaneous respirations (chest wall movement, oxygenation)
- Initiation of rescue breathing in the absence of adequate spontaneous respirations

Circulation
- Assessment of adequacy of circulation (central and peripheral pulses, capillary refill, blood pressure)
- *Cardiopulmonary arrest* is defined as the absence of a pulse in the large arteries of an unconscious patient who is not breathing.
- Chest compressions should be initiated in the infant with no detectable brachial pulse or the child/adolescent with no detectable carotid pulse.

The goal of the primary survey is the detection and immediate reversal of life-threatening cardiopulmonary processes. Details are provided in Table 29-3. An algorithm summarizing the initial and secondary assessments of critically ill pediatric patients is provided in Figure 29-2. Current recommendations for health care providers regarding cardiopulmonary resuscitation in infants, children, and adults are reviewed in Figure 29-3. Newborn resuscitation is discussed in Chapter 5.

Management of Shock

Shock ensues when the circulation is no longer adequate to meet the metabolic demands of the body. Changes in the strength of the peripheral and central pulses are a relatively late finding. Heart rate is most closely correlated with intravascular volume status; blood pressure is preserved until the final stages of shock in children. Capillary refill is the most sensitive clinical measure of the adequacy

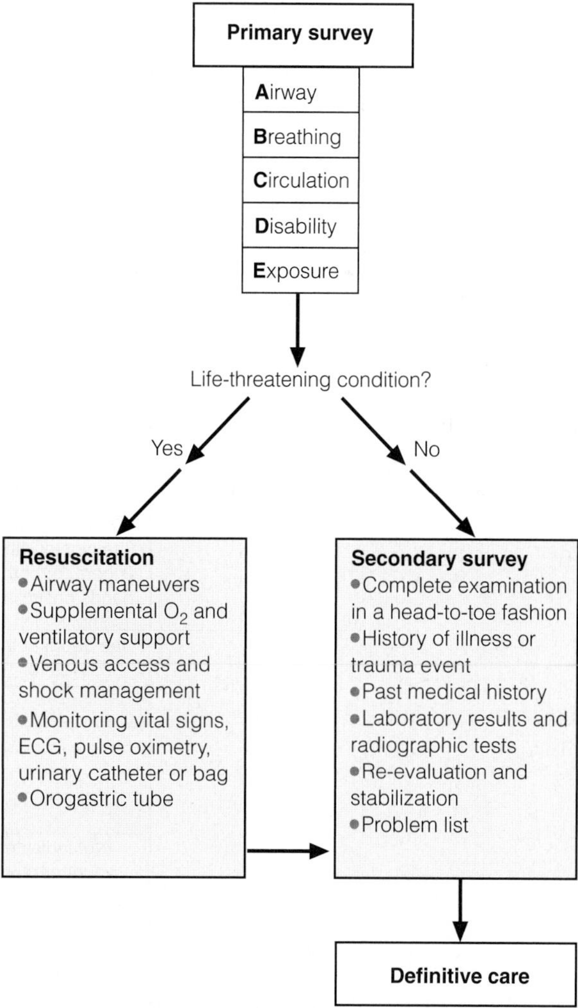

Figure 29-2 Algorithm of the initial assessment of the pediatric patient. (From Marino BS, Fine KS. *Blueprints Pediatrics.* 4th ed. Philadelphia: Lippincott Williams & Wilkins; 2006 with permission.)

Figure 29-3 Review of current recommendations for health care providers regarding cardiopulmonary resuscitation in the infant, child, and adolescent/adult. (*Source:* The American Heart Association 2005 Guidelines for Cardiopulmonary Resuscitation and Emergency Cardiovascular Care. Available at http://www.americanheart.org.)

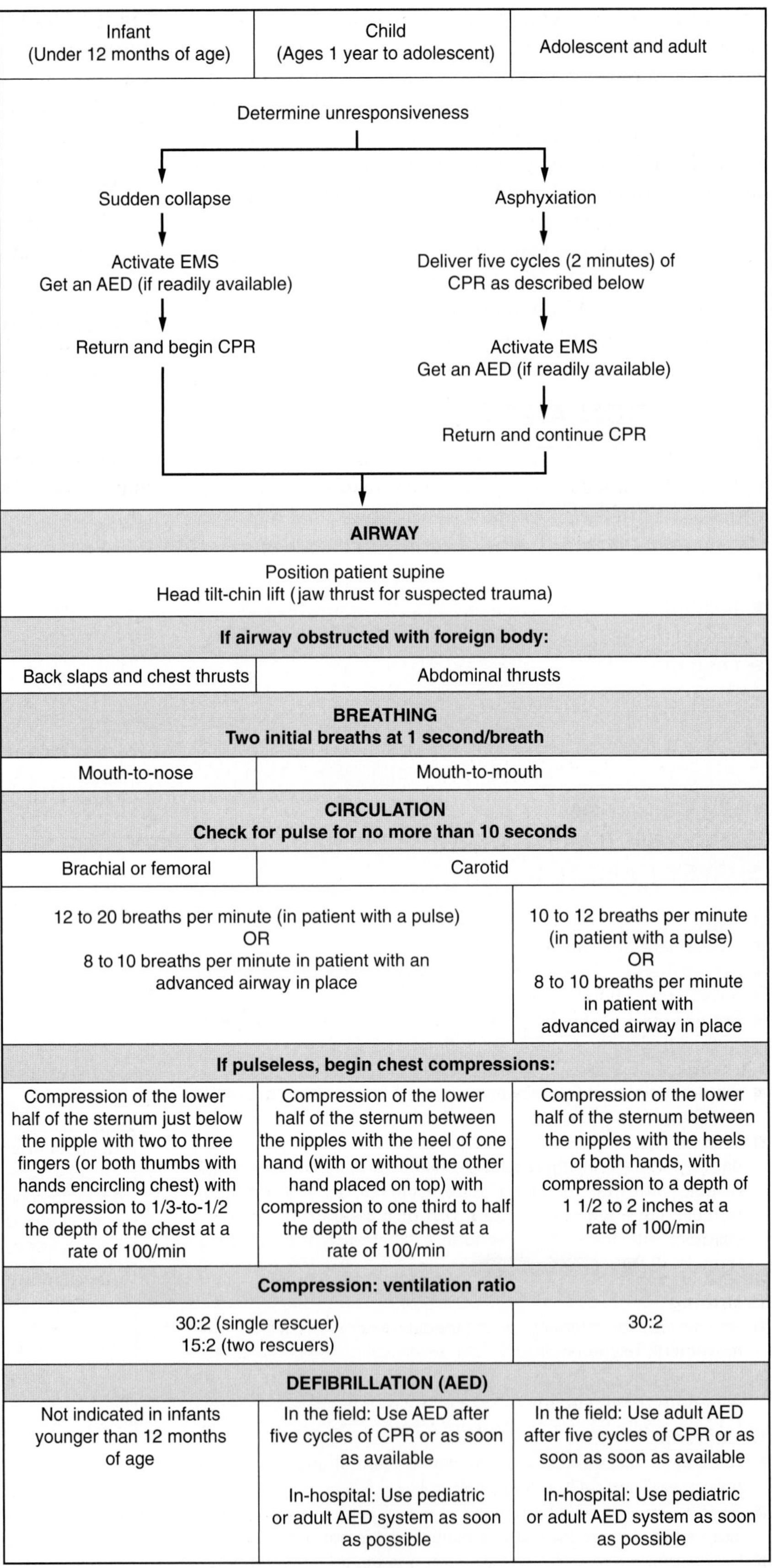

Infant (Under 12 months of age)	Child (Ages 1 year to adolescent)	Adolescent and adult
AIRWAY		
Position patient supine Head tilt-chin lift (jaw thrust for suspected trauma)	Position patient supine Head tilt-chin lift (jaw thrust for suspected trauma)	Position patient supine Head tilt-chin lift (jaw thrust for suspected trauma)
If airway obstructed with foreign body:		
Back slaps and chest thrusts	Abdominal thrusts	Abdominal thrusts
BREATHING **Two initial breaths at 1 second/breath**		
Mouth-to-nose	Mouth-to-mouth	Mouth-to-mouth
CIRCULATION **Check for pulse for no more than 10 seconds**		
Brachial or femoral	Carotid	Carotid
12 to 20 breaths per minute (in patient with a pulse) OR 8 to 10 breaths per minute in patient with an advanced airway in place	12 to 20 breaths per minute (in patient with a pulse) OR 8 to 10 breaths per minute in patient with an advanced airway in place	10 to 12 breaths per minute (in patient with a pulse) OR 8 to 10 breaths per minute in patient with advanced airway in place
If pulseless, begin chest compressions:		
Compression of the lower half of the sternum just below the nipple with two to three fingers (or both thumbs with hands encircling chest) with compression to 1/3-to-1/2 the depth of the chest at a rate of 100/min	Compression of the lower half of the sternum between the nipples with the heel of one hand (with or without the other hand placed on top) with compression to one third to half the depth of the chest at a rate of 100/min	Compression of the lower half of the sternum between the nipples with the heels of both hands, with compression to a depth of 1 1/2 to 2 inches at a rate of 100/min
Compression: ventilation ratio		
30:2 (single rescuer) 15:2 (two rescuers)	30:2 (single rescuer) 15:2 (two rescuers)	30:2
DEFIBRILLATION (AED)		
Not indicated in infants younger than 12 months of age	In the field: Use AED after five cycles of CPR or as soon as available In-hospital: Use pediatric or adult AED system as soon as possible	In the field: Use adult AED after five cycles of CPR or as soon as soon as available In-hospital: Use pediatric or adult AED system as soon as possible

of circulation. Capillary refilling time is a physical manifestation of the effectiveness of peripheral perfusion, which is directly related to cardiac output and peripheral vascular resistance. Normal capillary refill time is <2 seconds. Factors that affect the validity of the test include low ambient temperature (increases capillary refill time), extremity used for the measurement (refill takes longer in the toes than in the fingers), and position of the extremity (should be positioned slightly above the level of the heart to minimize the effects of venous stasis). In children, capillary refill time is also used to assess hydration status, although in this setting its usefulness may be limited primarily to cases of moderate-to-severe hypovolemia.

The different types of shock are outlined in Table 29-4. Shock may result from a single underlying mechanism, a combination of factors, or other conditions (pulmonary embolism, adrenal insufficiency). Frequent re-evaluation of the clinical status of the patient in shock is critical; vital signs and clinical status should be reassessed at a minimum prior to the administration of further boluses or fluids. Careful monitoring of electrolyte levels and indicators of perfusion and hydration status permits optimal resuscitation and prevents morbidity associated with rapid overcorrection.

TABLE 29-4
ETIOLOGIES OF SHOCK

Hypovolemic Shock
- Examples: water/electrolyte losses; hemorrhaging; third spacing of plasma
- Hypovolemic shock is the most common form in children.
- The management of the hypovolemic shock due to fluid loss is discussed in detail in Chapter 7.
- Regardless of the cause of hypovolemic shock, initial fluid resuscitation consists of normal saline or lactated Ringer solution administered as a 20 mg per kg bolus (infants may require more than this to achieve initial stabilization).
- Depending on the cause, additional resuscitative fluids may consist of additional normal isotonic boluses, transfusion of whole blood or packed red cells, or infusion of albumin.

Cardiogenic Shock
- Cardiogenic shock results when the pumping ability of the heart is impaired.
- Examples: ischemic heart disease, congenital heart disease, cardiomyopathy, dysrhythmias, myocarditis, pericardial tamponade
- Possible treatment options, depending on the specific etiology, include surgical repair, balloon angioplasty, and inotropic support.

Septic Shock
- Infection of the bloodstream and release of inflammatory mediators produces decreased vascular resistance, third spacing, hypovolemia, and finally myocardial depression.
- Patients with suspected septic shock should receive immediate infusion of a third-generation cephalosporin (i.e., ceftriaxone) and vancomycin (cefotaxime and ampicillin in infants younger than 3 months of age).

Distributive Shock
- Occurs when an abnormality in vasomotor tone leads to peripheral pooling and effective intravascular hypovolemia.
- Examples: anaphylaxis, head trauma, spinal cord injury, drug toxicity (management of these conditions is discussed in specific previous chapters)

Initial Evaluation of the Trauma Victim

First responders are trained in in-the-field assessment, stabilization, and transport of the trauma victim. This includes evaluation and management of airway patency, breathing, and circulation. In addition, any patient who has sustained significant trauma to the head or neck or who has impaired consciousness following trauma should be immobilized in a cervical collar and secured to a backboard for transport to a tertiary medical facility. Immobilization prevents initial or additional damage to the cervical cord, limiting subsequent impairment. Further assessment for neurologic deficits, vertebral column injury, and cord damage may be deferred until airway, breathing, and circulation have been stabilized.

Any trauma patient with altered mental status or pain/tenderness over the cervical spine warrants thorough work-up for spinal cord injury. Plain films of multiple views of the cervical spine are the initial diagnostic study of choice. Patients with normal mental status and normal spinal films may be removed from the cervical collar. Computed tomography is indicated if films are inadequate for ruling out injury. Patients with a demonstrated fracture involving the spinal column and those with neurologic deficits require magnetic resonance imaging for detailed inspection of the cord. The benefit of routine administration of systemic methylprednisolone to patients with potential spinal cord trauma has been conclusively demonstrated (see Chapter 18).

Determination of Brain Death

Brain death is defined as the irreversible loss of cerebral and brainstem function. Criteria which must be present include a known cause of coma and absent cerebral and brainstem function (as determined by an apnea test and physical findings by two independent physicians) for at least 12 hours in the child ≥12 months of age (longer in neonates and infants). These criteria alone are sufficient for a diagnosis of brain death unless the patient has any of the following conditions: hypothermia, hypotension, cardiovascular shock, a metabolic disorder that may induce coma, presence of toxins or medications known to cause sedation, or extensive injuries that prevent completion of a thorough neurologic evaluation. If any of the above is present, a cerebral radionuclide angiogram should be obtained to assess blood circulation in the brain; the absence of carotid and intracranial arterial blood flow is considered pathognomonic for brain death. Electrocerebral silence on electroencephalography is consistent with but not diagnostic of brain death; however, this study is recommended as an additional measure in children under the age of 12 months. The individual is considered legally dead at the time the criteria are met. The concept of brain death is an important one for both the medical establishment and the family; the diagnosis is beneficial for introducing discussions regarding organ donation but should not be used as a parameter for immediate withdrawal of life support without the family's consent.

SOURCES

Carstairs SD, Tanen DA. Case studies in pediatric toxicology. *Pediatr Ann.* 2005;34:973–980.

Ishimine P. Fever without a source in children 0 to 36 months of age. *Pediatr Clin North Am.* 2006;53:167–194.

Long SS. Distinguishing among prolonged, recurrent, and periodic fever syndromes: Approach of a pediatric infectious diseases subspecialist. *Pediatr Clin North Am.* 2005;52:811–835.

Marino BS. Emergency management: Evaluation of the critically ill or injured child. In: Marino BS, Fine KS. *Pediatric Blueprints.* 4th ed. Philadelphia: Lippincott Wilkins & Williams; 2007:1–9.

Martin BW, Dykes E, Lecky FE. Patterns and risks in spinal trauma. *Arch Dis Child.* 2004;89:860–865.

Murray DL. Fever (the febrile child 3 to 36 months of age). In: Rudolph CD, Rudolph AM, Hostetter MK, et al (eds). *Rudolph's Pediatrics.* 21st ed. New York: McGraw-Hill; 2003:891–892.

Robson MC, Raine T, Smith DJ. Wounds and wound healing. In: Lawrence P, ed. *Essentials of General Surgery.* 4th ed. Philadelphia: Lippincott Wilkins & Williams; 2005:119–125.

Sagerman PJ. Wounds. *Pediatr Rev.* 2005;26:43–49.

QUESTIONS

1. A 12-year-old comatose patient in the critical care unit has been pronounced brain dead. All of the following are required for determination of brain death EXCEPT:

A) An electroencephalogram demonstrating electrocerebral silence
B) Physical findings consistent with absent cerebral function for more than 12 hours
C) Physical findings consistent with absent brainstem function for more than 12 hours
D) A known cause of irreversible coma
E) A positive apnea test

2. When educating new parents about when they should seek medical care for their infant, you would be correct in informing them that the most appropriate method of measuring the child's temperature is with which of the following?

A) Ear-based thermometer
B) Digital thermometer
C) Temporal artery thermometer
D) Forehead strip
E) Mercury thermometer

3. A 12-month-old infant is in your office on the weekend for evaluation of his fever. He has been fussy and has fed poorly for the past 8 hours. He has no upper respiratory symptoms, vomiting, or diarrhea, and there are no known sick contacts. Which of the following is (are) associated with an increased likelihood of invasive bacterial infection?

A) Rectal temperature >39.0° C
B) White blood count $\geq$15.0 × 10^3/mcL
C) Absolute neutrophil count $\geq$10.0 × 10^3/mcL
D) A and B
E) A, B, and C

4. A patient with muscular dystrophy undergoes anesthesia for a dental procedure. In the recovery room, the patient develops a fever of 40.5°C and muscle rigidity. Which of the following medications is most appropriate for the treatment of this patient's fever?

A) Acetaminophen
B) Ibuprofen
C) Ketoprofen
D) Dantrolene
E) Naproxen

5. Which of the following patients is at increased risk for the development of malignant hyperthermia following general anesthesia?

A) The patient with nephrogenic diabetes insipidus who is given sodium thiopental
B) The patient with Hunter syndrome who is given nitrous oxide
C) The patient with Duchenne muscular dystrophy who is given halothane
D) The patient with juvenile idiopathic arthritis who is given succinylcholine
E) The patient with Down syndrome who is given fentanyl

6. A 2-week-old former full-term infant who was previously well is brought to the emergency department with a fever of 38.3°C. Which of the following is the most appropriate evaluation of this patient?

A) Complete blood count and culture; urinalysis and culture; cerebrospinal fluid analysis and culture
B) Complete blood count and culture; urinalysis and culture; cerebrospinal fluid analysis and culture if the peripheral white blood count is $\geq$15 × 10^3/mcL
C) Complete blood count and culture; urinalysis and culture; cerebrospinal fluid analysis and culture if the peripheral absolute neutrophil count is $\geq$10 × 10^3/mcL
D) Complete blood count and culture; urinalysis and culture
E) Complete blood count and culture

7. A 2-week-old former full-term infant who was previously well is brought to the emergency department with a fever of 38.3°C. Following evaluation of the infant, which of the following is the most appropriate management of this patient?

A) Admission to the hospital; intravenous ampicillin and cefotaxime if the peripheral white blood count is $\geq 15 \times 10^3$/mcL
B) Admission to the hospital; intravenous ampicillin and cefotaxime
C) Admission to the hospital; intravenous ampicillin and cefotaxime if the peripheral absolute neutrophil count is $\geq 10 \times 10^3$/mcL
D) Admission to the hospital if the peripheral white blood count is $\geq 15 \times 10^3$/mcL; otherwise discharge to home with follow-up within 24 hours
E) Admission to the hospital if the peripheral absolute neutrophil count is $\geq 10 \times 10^3$/mcL; otherwise discharge to home with follow-up within 24 hours

8. A 3-year-old boy ran into the corner of an end table and split his upper lip at the mid-way point between the philtrum and the right corner of the mouth. The laceration extends through the vermillion border. Which of the following is the most appropriate management of this patient's wound?

A) Allow the wound to heal by secondary intention.
B) Infiltrate the wound with local anesthetic prior to closure in the emergency department.
C) Consult with the plastic surgeon on-call for specialized closure.
D) Repair the wound with a tissue adhesive.
E) Repair the wound with wound closure tape.

9. You are lecturing to a group of students in a physician's assistant program about initial management of open wounds. All of the following are indicated during initial management of an open wound EXCEPT:

A) Adequate control of pain
B) Irrigation with normal saline under mild pressure
C) Hemostasis
D) Infiltration of the wound with an antiseptic agent
E) Debridement of devitalized tissue prior to closure

10. Tetanus immune globulin is indicated for all of the following patients EXCEPT:

A) A 17-year-old unidentified adolescent with a contaminated wound who is in a coma
B) A 17-year-old homeless adolescent with a contaminated wound
C) A 13-year-old boy with a clean wound who is undergoing induction treatment for leukemia
D) A 5-year-old boy with a contaminated wound who is in the foster care system and has no reliable history of completion of his primary tetanus series
E) A 5-year-old boy with a contaminated wound who is up-to-date on his primary immunizations but has not yet received his pre-kindergarten booster vaccinations

11. Post-exposure rabies prophylaxis is indicated for bites from which of the following wild animals?

A) Bat
B) Squirrel
C) Rat
D) Mouse
E) Rabbit

12. Pit vipers can be differentiated from nonvenomous snakes by the presence of all of the following EXCEPT:

A) Small pits located on either side of the head between the eye and nostril
B) An oval-shaped head
C) Large, curved fangs
D) Elliptical pupils
E) It is impossible to differentiate pit vipers from nonvenomous snakes on the basis of appearance.

13. You are providing a lecture to a group of wilderness guides about pit viper bites. You would be correct in telling them which of the following?

A) It is not possible to differentiate pit vipers from nonvenomous snakes based on appearance.
B) Most untreated pit viper bites are fatal.
C) About 25% of pit viper bites do not result in envenomation.
D) Pit viper bites are usually located on the trunk.
E) A tourniquet should be placed prior to transport of the bitten individual to the emergency department.

14. An 18-month-old boy is brought to the emergency department by his father, who tells you that the boy was scalded by hot water in the bathtub. Which of the following burn injury patterns is most consistent with abuse?

A) Involvement limited to the nondominant hand
B) Involvement of both hands with widespread splash marks up the arms
C) Involvement of both distal lower extremities with irregular lines of demarcation
D) Complete involvement of an extremity distal to a circumferential border line without associated splash marks
E) Involvement limited to the distal pads of the index and middle fingers on the dominant hand

15. A 16-year-old boy who was under his house looking for the lawn mower was bitten by a spider. He knocked the spider off his arm and stepped on it immediately. He now presents 18 hours later with severe pain in the muscles surrounding the bite site and muscle cramping in his abdomen and legs. The local reaction to the bite is minimal. Which of the following statements is correct?

A) Antivenom should be administered to this patient immediately.
B) The type of spider that is most likely responsible for this patient's symptoms is not found in the Southeastern United States.
C) This type of spider bite often produces a metallic taste in the mouth.
D) This patient is at significant risk for disseminated intravascular coagulation.
E) Examination of the remains of the spider will most likely reveal a large black spider with a red hourglass shape on the dorsum of the body.

16. An 8-year-old boy who went "camping" with his father in his backyard last night is found to have a bite or sting on his lower left leg. There is significant induration around the site, which consists of two small punctate lesions. Local bruising and hemorrhagic bleb formation are also present. The patient does not recall being bitten or stung. Which of the following is most likely responsible for this patient's localized findings?

A) Brown recluse spider
B) Black widow spider
C) Coral snake
D) Deer tick
E) Hornet

17. Paramedics are called to the home of an 8-month-old boy found unresponsive in the crib by his mother. He has no spontaneous respirations or pulse. Adequate rise of the chest is noted during two initial rescue breaths. Which of the following provides the recommended ratio of chest compressions-to-ventilations in this patient?

A) 15 compressions:1 breath
B) 15 compressions:2 breaths
C) 30 compressions:2 breaths
D) 30 compressions:5 breaths
E) 15 compressions:5 breaths

18. All of the following descriptions of features of infant resuscitation are correct EXCEPT:

A) Back slaps and chest thrusts for dislodgement of a foreign body
B) Chest compression at a rate of 100 per minute
C) Blind finger sweeps by an experienced emergency medical provider
D) Compression of the lower half of the sternum just below the nipple line
E) Compression to a depth of one third to one half the depth of the chest

19. Which of the following interventions should take place prior to any of the others in the unconscious trauma patient?

A) Assessment for neurologic deficits
B) Assessment of circulation
C) Assessment of breathing
D) Immobilization of the cervical spine in a collar and placement of the patient on a backboard
E) Assessment of airway patency

20. Which of the following endotracheal tubes is most appropriate for use during the resuscitation of a 4-year-old boy?

A) Size: 5; cuffed
B) Size: 4; cuffed
C) Size: 3; cuffed
D) Size: 4; uncuffed
E) Size: 5; uncuffed

ANSWERS

1. A	8. C	15. E
2. B	9. D	16. A
3. E	10. E	17. B
4. D	11. A	18. C
5. C	12. B	19. D
6. A	13. C	20. E
7. B	14. D	

30 Pharmacologic Principles in Pediatrics

ADVERSE EFFECTS

Adverse effects of medication may be dose-dependent or idiosyncratic. Dose-dependent adverse reactions are those undesirable consequences that are absent when low doses of the drug are administered but appear at higher dosages. Idiosyncratic reactions are adverse outcomes that occur upon exposure to the drug at any dose. Table 30-1 lists some examples of dose-related and idiosyncratic adverse effects. Some, such as hepatotoxicity, can be either dose-dependent or idiosyncratic, depending on the underlying mechanism.

ALTERNATIVE MEDICINE INTERACTIONS

Supplements and herbal remedies can interact with traditional, prescription medications, resulting in serious adverse effects. For example, St. John's wort, an herbal remedy thought to relieve depression, induces the cytochrome P-450 pathway, resulting in potentially sub-therapeutic serum concentrations of oral contraceptives, digoxin, and oral anticoagulants. Other herbs interfere with platelet function and, when combined with medications with similar properties, can cause coagulopathies. Some documented interactions between commonly used herbal supplements and prescriptive medications are noted as follows:

- Valerian root, which is often taken for insomnia, migraine headaches, or intestinal cramping, has mild sedative effects which may be exacerbated when the herb is taken with alcohol or medications which also cause sedation.
- Ginseng should not be combined with oral anticoagulants, antiplatelet medications, and hypoglycemic agents.
- Echinacea is contraindicated in patients who are also taking immunosuppressant drugs.

TABLE 30-1
EXAMPLES OF DOSE-RELATED AND IDIOSYNCRATIC ADVERSE EFFECTS

Adverse Effects that Are Typically *Dose-Related*

Sedation

Nausea

Bone marrow suppression

Ototoxicity

Hepatotoxicity

- Direct damage to hepatocytes
- Alteration of metabolic pathways
- Examples: acetaminophen, acetylsalicylic acid

Adverse Effects that Are Typically *Idiosyncratic*

Aplastic anemia

Hepatotoxicity

- Hypersensitivity reactions
- Generation of toxic intermediates
- Examples: several anticonvulsants, sulfasalazine, minocycline

ASPIRIN AND OTHER NONSTEROIDAL ANTI-INFLAMMATORY DRUGS

Aspirin is no longer routinely used to treat fever and discomfort in the pediatric population due to its reported association with Reye syndrome. However, this nonsteroidal anti-inflammatory agent is indicated in the management of patients with Kawasaki disease, rheumatic fever, and certain types of inflammatory arthritis. The most common adverse effect of long-term aspirin therapy is gastric ulcer, which presumably results from the drug's inhibition of prostaglandin synthesis. The same mechanism is thought to be responsible for allergic-type symptoms occasionally associated with aspirin use (wheezing, urticaria, angioedema). Long-term aspirin use has been linked to cases of anemia, thrombocytopenia, and impairment of platelet function. Tinnitus and mild hearing loss may also occur; both resolve upon discontinuation of the drug.

Similarly, gastric inflammation and gastric and (less commonly) duodenal ulceration are the most commonly reported adverse effects associated with ibuprofen and other nonsteroidal anti-inflammatory drugs (NSAIDs). Renal complications, including interstitial nephritis and papillary necrosis, are uncommon but serious. Patients managed with long-term courses of ibuprofen and similar NSAIDs should also be monitored for anemia, thrombocytopenia, and elevated liver enzymes. Patients with systemic lupus erythematosus may develop aseptic meningitis when treated with ibuprofen.

CORTICOSTEROIDS AND OTHER IMMUNOSUPPRESSANT DRUGS

Corticosteroids are a class of very potent anti-inflammatory/immunosuppressive drugs. Chronic treatment with a corticosteroid agent suppresses the hypothalamic-pituitary-adrenal axis; sudden discontinuation of the medication results in acute adrenal insufficiency, which may be life-threatening. Adrenal insufficiency is also a concern during periods of physiologic stress, such as infection, trauma, or surgery. In these instances, the steroid dose is increased for a short time to prevent the onset of Addisonian crisis. For surgical procedures, a "stress dose" is administered preoperatively as well.

The immunosuppressive properties of corticosteroids place nonimmune patients at increased risk for complicated varicella when exposed. This risk is magnified in patients with underlying immunodeficiencies; varicella immune globulin (VZIG) is indicated in all such patients within 96 hours of exposure. VZIG should also be considered in otherwise immunocompetent children who have been taking high-dose systemic steroids for more than 14 consecutive days. Patients who are immunosuppressed due to chronic steroid therapy and contract the disease should be treated with acyclovir, and steroid doses should be lowered if possible for the duration of the illness. Other complications of long-term systemic corticosteroid therapy are listed in Table 30-2. Most are dose-related; thus, corticosteroids should be prescribed at the lowest dose for the shortest duration of time that produces improvement in disease.

Three other classes of immunosuppressive drugs are commonly used in children: cytotoxic agents (cyclophosphamide, azathioprine); calcineurin inhibitors (cyclosporine); and antimetabolites (methotrexate). Common adverse effects are listed in Table 30-3.

Pharmacologically-induced chronic immunosuppression carries its own inherent risks. Neutropenia predisposes an individual to infection; moreover, clinical signs of inflammation may be absent or blunted, making diagnosis more difficult. Evaluation of the patient with febrile neutropenia includes a thorough physical examination, complete blood count and blood cultures (at a minimum), and broad-spectrum intravenous antibiotic administration. Empiric therapy is continued until the patient has been afebrile and clinically well for at least 24 to 48 hours and cultures remain negative. Fungal pathogens should be considered in neutropenic patients who remain febrile for several days despite appropriate antibiotic coverage.

TABLE 30-2
ADVERSE EFFECTS OF CHRONIC SYSTEMIC CORTICOSTEROID THERAPY

Growth suppression
Impaired wound healing
Fragile skin/striae
Acne^
Hirsutism
Impaired glucose tolerance
Diabetes
"Cushingoid" appearance
Obesity
Hypertension
Myopathy
Osteopenia
Pathologic fractures
Immunosuppression*
Cataracts
Gastritis/peptic ulcers
Mood changes
Sleep disturbances

^Teenagers undergoing treatment with chronic systemic corticosteroids are prone to development of a characteristic form of acne several weeks after the initiation of therapy. The lesions consist of dome-shaped erythematous papules appearing on the face and trunk; comedones are notably absent. Pre-existing acne may worsen when corticosteroid therapy is initiated.
*A purified protein derivative skin test is indicated prior to the initiation of prolonged high-dose corticosteroid treatment.

CONSCIOUS SEDATION

According to the most recent AAP policy statement regarding sedation in pediatric patients, conscious sedation is defined as "a drug-induced depression of consciousness during

TABLE 30-3
COMMON ADVERSE EFFECTS OF IMMUNOSUPPRESSIVE AGENTS

Cytotoxic Agents (cyclophosphamide, azathioprine)
- Bone marrow suppression
- Immunosuppression/neutropenia
- Increased susceptibility to serious infection

Calcineurin Inhibitors (cyclosporine)
- Gastrointestinal upset
- Gingival hypertrophy
- Hyperkalemia
- Hepatotoxicity
- Renal toxicity
- Dyslipidemia
- Impaired glucose tolerance

Antimetabolites (methotrexate)
- Oral mucous membrane lesions
- Hepatotoxicity
- Gastrointestinal upset
- Increased susceptibility to opportunistic infections
- Bone marrow suppression (uncommon)

TABLE 30-4
SEDATIVES: RECOGNITION AND MANAGEMENT OF OVERDOSE

Benzodiazepines (e.g., midazolam)
- Signs of overdose: respiratory depression, hypotension, hypoxia, central nervous system depression
- Management of overdose: supportive care (including supplemental oxygen); flumazenil

Opiates (e.g., fentanyl)
- Signs of overdose: miosis, respiratory depression, hypoxia, central nervous system depression
- Management of overdose: supportive care; naloxone

Ketamine
- Side effect: hallucinations (if not combined with a benzodiazepine)
- Signs of overdose: prolonged sedation, respiratory depression
- Management of overdose: supportive care

Barbiturates
- Signs of overdose: respiratory depression, hypoxia, bradycardia, hypotension
- Management of overdose: supportive care

Chloral Hydrate
- Signs of overdose: respiratory depression, hypoxia, bradycardia, hypotension, decreased body temperature
- Management of overdose: supportive care

which patients respond purposefully to verbal commands . . . either alone or accompanied by light tactile stimulation." The patient is capable of maintaining a patent airway and breathing spontaneously. Patients who are deeply sedated respond purposely to painful stimuli only and may have airway compromise or impaired respiration. Patients under general anesthesia are unresponsive and require management of airway and breathing.

Conscious sedation is indicated when there is a need to limit anticipated pain associated with a procedure, diminish anxiety, provide amnesia, assure cooperation, limit movement, and return the patient to a conscious state for discharge. Conscious sedation is not appropriate in patients with severe systemic or life-threatening diseases, airway anomalies, tonsillar hypertrophy, or certain emotional or behavioral conditions. Patients who are undergoing conscious sedation for painful procedures require continuous oxygen saturation and heart rate monitoring during the procedure. Intermittent monitoring of respiratory rate and blood pressure is documented during the period of sedation. At least one foot or hand should be left exposed, and the patient's head should be easily accessible for frequent evaluation of airway patency. The facility must have a functioning suction apparatus, as well as the ability to provide oxygen and positive pressure ventilation. Monitoring should continue until the patient has remained alert and asymptomatic for at least 20 minutes.

Table 30-4 lists several of the more commonly prescribed sedatives as well as the clinical manifestations and management of overdose.

PAIN CONTROL

A child's perception of and ability to tolerate pain varies with his or her developmental stage. Newborns experience pain; in fact, infants who undergo repeated painful procedures during the neonatal period develop decreased pain

TABLE 30-5
STRATEGIES FOR DETECTING, QUANTIFYING, AND MANAGING PAIN IN THE PEDIATRIC POPULATION

Pain in Infants—Quantification

Assess physiologic indicators of pain:
- Increased respiratory rate
- Increased heart rate
- Increased blood pressure

Assess behavioral indicators of pain:
- Changes in level of arousal
- Changes in level of activity
- Crying

Determine pain rating based on composite scale of pain in infants (e.g., CRIES, NIPS)

Pain in Infants—Management Strategies

Nonnutritive sucking (pacifier)

Oral sucrose solution prior to the procedure

Skin-to-skin contact with parent

Breastfeeding during procedure

EMLA for circumcision, venipuncture

(continued)

TABLE 30-5
(continued)

Management of pain associated with circumcision:
- Topical analgesic agent
- Dorsal penile nerve block
- Oral sucrose solution prior to the procedure

Pain in Children—Quantification

Assess physiologic indicators of pain:
- Increased respiratory rate
- Increased heart rate
- Increased blood pressure

Assess behavioral indicators of pain:
- Facial expression
- Crying
- Withdrawal or resistance

Elicit self-report of pain through modified self-report scales (≤8 years of age) or adult self-report scales (≥8 years of age)

If self-report is not possible due to developmental or neurologic conditions, determine pain rating based on age-appropriate composite scale of pain in children

Pain in Children—Management

Use of topical and systemic analgesics as appropriate

Parental involvement

Age-appropriate verbal preparation and visual rehearsal

Distraction

Targeted breathing

Physical strategies:
- Transcutaneous electrical nerve stimulation (TENS)
- Application of heat or cold

Relief of pain proceeds in a step-wise manner:

Mild-to-moderate pain
- NSAID
- Addition of an opioid in fixed-dose combination with NSAID for persistent or increasing pain
- Addition of independent (single agent) dosing of opioid

Moderate-to-severe or persistent pain
- Higher doses of opioids or increasingly potent opioid agents
- Round-the-clock basal administration of opioid with bolus doses as needed

tolerance that appears to persist throughout childhood. All patients have the right to adequate control of their pain. Pain management decreases patient and parental anxiety and improves cooperation. Inadequate analgesia seems to create heightened sensitivity to pain in the future. Methods of detecting, quantifying, and managing pain differ depending on the age of the patient (Table 30-5).

Prevention of pain typically requires less medication than control of pain once it has occurred. Pain should be anticipated with procedures such as injections, intravenous line placement, suturing, and setting of bones. Topical analgesic products are available for pretreatment to reduce the pain of needle sticks; conscious sedation is indicated for more lengthy painful procedures.

SOURCES

American Academy of Pediatrics and American Academy of Pediatric Dentistry Joint Statement. Guidelines for the monitoring and management of pediatric patients during and after sedation for diagnostic and therapeutic procedures: An update. *Pediatrics*. 2006;118: 2587–2602.

Cirigliano MD. Herbal treatments in clinical practice. In: Neinstein LS, ed. *Adolescent Health Care: A Practical Guide*. 4th ed. Philadelphia: Lippincott Williams & Wilkins; 2002:1539–1550.

Coddington DA. Corticosteroids. *Pediatr Rev.* 2002;23:146–147.
Collier DN. Nonsteroidal anti-inflammatory drugs and abdominal pain. *Pediatr Rev.* 2007;28:75–77.
Doyle L, Colleti JE. Pediatric procedural sedation and analgesia. *Pediatr Clin North Am.* 2006;53:279–292.
Gedalia A, Shetty AK. Chronic steroid and immunosuppressant therapy in children. *Pediatr Rev.* 2004;25:425–434.
Schechter NL, Berde CB, Yaster M. *Pain in Infants, Children, and Adolescents.* Philadelphia: Lippincott Williams & Wilkins; 2003.
Suchy FJ. Drug- and toxin-induced liver injury. In: Behrman RF, Kliegman RM, Jensen HB, eds. *Nelson Textbook of Pediatrics.* 17th ed. Philadelphia; WB Saunders Co; 2004:1339–1341.
Zempsky WT, Schechter NL. What's new in the management of pain in children. *Pediatr Rev.* 2003;24:337–348.

QUESTIONS

1. Which of the following adverse reactions is most likely to be idiosyncratic rather than dose-related?
A) Aplastic anemia
B) Sedation
C) Nausea
D) Bone marrow suppression
E) Hepatotoxicity

2. A 3-year-old boy with Kawasaki disease and resulting coronary artery aneurysms is being treated with aspirin. Which of the following is the most common complication of long-term aspirin therapy?
A) Esophageal varices
B) Gastric ulcer
C) Reye syndrome
D) Autoimmune hepatitis
E) Aplastic anemia

3. A 14-year-old boy has been taking 800 mg of ibuprofen at least three times a day for the past month for a sore throat associated with "mononucleosis." Urinalysis demonstrates blood in his urine. Which of the following renal complications is most likely to be associated with ibuprofen use?
A) Post-infectious glomerulonephritis
B) Acute tubular necrosis
C) Interstitial nephritis
D) Nephrocalcinosis
E) Hemolytic-uremic syndrome

4. A 9-year-old girl with juvenile dermatomyositis is dependent on chronic systemic corticosteroid therapy for control of her disease. She has been virtually asymptomatic for 3 months when she notices the insidious onset of proximal muscle weakness. She denies pain, and serum muscle enzyme concentrations are within the normal range. Which of the following is the most likely cause of this patient's recent onset of weakness?
A) Misdiagnosed muscular dystrophy
B) Exacerbation of her disease
C) Hysteria
D) Steroid myopathy
E) Fictitious myopathy

5. A 4-year-old girl is receiving multiple immunosuppressive agents as part of induction therapy for acute lymphoblastic leukemia. She is exposed to a visitor who develops chicken pox lesions 48 hours later. The patient has no history of clinical varicella infection or immunization. Which of the following treatment regimens is indicated for this patient? (Note: VZIG—varicella immune globulin)
A) Immediate vaccination against varicella; acyclovir if varicella lesions develop in the patient
B) VZIG, vaccination against varicella, and intravenous acyclovir immediately
C) VZIG and vaccination against varicella immediately
D) VZIG and intravenous acyclovir immediately
E) VZIG immediately; acyclovir if varicella lesions develop in the patient

6. A 6-year-old boy has been dependent on daily systemic corticosteroid therapy (1 mg/kg/day) for control of his rheumatologic disease for the past 3 months. He now requires surgical repair of an inguinal hernia. Which of the following alterations in medical management is indicated in this patient due to scheduled surgery?
A) Preoperative administration of a "stress dose" of steroids, followed by increased dosages in the immediate recovery period
B) Preoperative administration of a "stress dose" of steroids alone
C) Increased dosages of systemic corticosteroids in the immediate recovery period
D) Preoperative administration of a "stress dose" of steroids, followed by increased dosages for the next 4 weeks
E) No change in medication is warranted due to the elective nature of the surgery.

7. Patients undergoing chronic moderate-to-high-dose systemic corticosteroid therapy who are subjected to physiologic stress (trauma, infection, surgery) are most at risk for which of the following complications due to their steroid use?
A) Difficulty with extubation due to restrictive lung changes
B) Adrenal insufficiency
C) Adult respiratory distress syndrome
D) Postoperative pancreatitis
E) Postoperative hepatitis

8. Which of the following patients is under *moderate* sedation (i.e., conscious sedation)?
A) A 12-year-old boy who responds purposefully to painful stimuli only
B) A 12-year-old boy with a normal state of consciousness and minimally impaired coordination
C) A 12-year-old boy with a depressed state of consciousness who responds purposefully to verbal commands and is able to maintain a patent airway
D) A 12-year-old boy with a depressed state of consciousness who is able to maintain a patent airway but requires oxygen therapy
E) A 12-year-old boy who is unresponsive and cannot maintain a patent airway

9. Conscious sedation is most appropriate when:
A) there is a need to limit anticipated pain associated with a procedure
B) there is a need to diminish anxiety associated with a procedure
C) there is a need to limit movement during a procedure
D) there is a need to return the patient to a conscious state for discharge following a procedure
E) All of the above

10. Conscious sedation is contraindicated in all of the following 5-year-old patients undergoing lumbar puncture EXCEPT:
A) The patient who is actively wheezing
B) The patient with extreme tonsillar hypertrophy
C) The patient on chronic midazolam therapy
D) The patient with controlled asthma
E) The patient who is unconscious

11. A 5-year-old boy is undergoing conscious sedation with midazolam, atropine, and ketamine when he becomes hypoxic and hypotensive. Which of the following is the most appropriate next course of action?
A) Supplemental oxygen
B) Supplemental oxygen and naloxone
C) Supplemental oxygen and diphenhydramine
D) Supplemental oxygen and fentanyl
E) Supplemental oxygen and flumazenil

12. When ketamine is not combined with a benzodiazepine during conscious sedation, the patient is at increased risk for the development of which of the following?
A) Hypotension
B) Hallucinations
C) Bradycardia
D) Respiratory depression
E) Coma

13. You are providing a lecture regarding pain management in pediatrics to a group of obstetricians. You are correct in telling them all of the following EXCEPT:
A) A child's ability to tolerate pain varies with his or her developmental stage.
B) Inadequate analgesia seems to result in increased sensitization to pain in the future.
C) Newborns do not experience pain.
D) All patients have the right to adequate control of their pain.
E) Management of pain in the infant decreases parental anxiety.

14. A 36-year-old first-time mother is concerned that her son's circumcision will be very painful for him. You would be correct in telling her which of the following?
A) The perinatal period is a time of decreased sensitivity to pain.
B) Neonates appear to require lower doses of pain medications to produce the same level of analgesia.
C) Pain in the neonatal period is not associated with any change in perception of pain later in childhood.
D) She has a right to expect prevention and control of pain generated during her son's circumcision.
E) Given both the age and size of the infant at circumcision, topical analgesic agents are contraindicated.

ANSWERS

1. A	6. A	11. A
2. B	7. B	12. B
3. C	8. C	13. C
4. D	9. E	14. D
5. E	10. D	

Index

Page numbers followed by *t* indicate tables.
Page numbers followed by *f* indicate figures.

B

C

D

E

H